NURSING PRACTICE AND HEALTH CARE

4TH EDITION

EDITED BY

Sue Hinchliff MSc BA RN RNT

Head of Accreditation, Royal College of Nursing of the United Kingdom, London, UK

Sue Norman RN BEd (Hons) RNT NDNCert Hon DSc

Recent past Chief Executive/Registrar, United Kingdom Central Council for Nursing,
Midwifery and Health Visiting, London, UK

Jane Schober MN RN DipNEd DipN Lond RCNT RNT

Principal Lecturer, School of Nursing and Midwifery, De Montfort University, Leicester, UK

ARNOLD

A member of the Hodder Headline Group
LONDON

First published in Great Britain in 1989 by Arnold
Second edition 1993
Third edition 1998
This fourth edition published in 2003 by Arnold,
a member of the Hodder Headline Group,
338 Euston Road, London NW1 3BH

http://www.arnoldpublishers.com

Distributed in the United States of America by Oxford University Press Inc.,
198 Madison Avenue, New York, NY10016
Oxford is a registered trademark of Oxford University Press

Whilst the advice and information in this book are believed to be true and accurate at the date of going to
press, neither the author[s] nor the publisher can accept any legal responsibility or liability for any errors or
omissions that may be made. In particular (but without limiting the generality of the preceding disclaimer)
every effort has been made to check drug dosages; however it is still possible that errors have been missed.
Furthermore, dosage schedules are constantly being revised and new side-effects recognized. For these
reasons the reader is strongly urged to consult the drug companies' printed instructions before
administering any of the drugs recommended in this book.

British Library Cataloguing in Publication Data
A catalogue record for this book is available from the British Library

Library of Congress Cataloging-in-Publication Data
A catalog record for this book is available from the Library of Congress

ISBN 0 340 808152 (pb)

3 4 5 6 7 8 9 10

Commissioning Editor: Georgina Bentliff
Development Editor: Heather Smith
Project Editor: Anke Ueberberg
Production Controller: Lindsay Smith
Cover Design: Amina Dudhia

Typeset in 10.5/15 Minion by Charon Tec Pvt. Ltd, Chennai, India
Printed and bound in Italy

What do you think about this book? Or any other Arnold title?
Please send your comments to **feedback.arnold@hodder.co.uk**

NURSING PRACTICE
AND HEALTH CARE

CONTENTS

CONTRIBUTORS

Ruth Beretta RN DipN BSc (Hons) MA MSc RNT

Pre-Registration Programme Manager, School of Health and Social Sciences, Coventry University, Coventry, UK

Jane Brown MSc MBA RGN RM

Director of Operations and Clinical Services, Newcastle under Lyme Primary Care Trust, Newcastle under Lyme, UK

Sue Davies PhD MSc (Social Research) BSc RGN RHV

Senior Lecturer in Gerontological Nursing, School of Nursing and Midwifery, University of Sheffield, Sheffield, UK

Marcelle de Sousa RGN RSCN BSc (Hons) Child Health

Adolescent Nurse Specialist, UCL Hospitals NHS Trust, Honorary Lecturer, South Bank University, London, UK

Jacqueline Elton MA BSc (Hons) RN

Senior Nurse, Directorate of Medical and A&E Services, University Hospitals of Leicester NHS Trust, UK

John Fowler MA BA RGN RMN DipN RCNT Cert Ed RNT

Principal Lecturer, School of Nursing and Midwifery, De Montfort University, Leicester, UK

Norma Fryer MA RN RM ADM DipN (A), Cert Ed

Senior Lecturer, Department of Midwifery Studies, University of Central Lancashire, Preston, UK

Paul Gibbons RN DipN DipPhil & Health Care

Chief Nursing Adviser & Director of Corporate Affairs, Argyll & Clyde Health Board, Paisley, Scotland

Faith Gibson PhD MSc (Cancer Nursing) RSCN RGN Onc. Cert Ed RNT

Lecturer in Children's Nursing Research, Centre for Nursing and Allied Health Professionals Research, Great Ormond Street Hospital for Children NHS Trust, London, UK

Nicky Hayes RGN BA (Hons) MSc PG Cert HE

Consultant Nurse, Kings College Hospital, Dulwich, London

Catherine Lawrence MSc RSCN DN(Lon) Dip N Ed(Lon) BSc (Hons)

Principal Lecturer, London South Bank University, London, UK

Alison Loftus-Hills BA BSW MSc

Review Manager, Commission for Health Improvement, Senior Research and Development Fellow, RCN Institute, Radcliffe Infirmary, Oxford, UK

Elizabeth McInnes RN BA (Hons) MPH
Senior Research and Development Fellow, RCN Institute, Radcliffe Infirmary, Oxford, UK

Katrina Neal-Poulson MSc BSc (Hons) RGN FAETC
Director of Nursing and Education, Compton Hospice, Wolverhampton, UK

Michael Nolan PhD B(Ed) MA MSc RN RMN
Professor of Gerontological Nursing, School of Nursing and Midwifery, University of Sheffield, Sheffield, UK

Alison Norman CBE HonDSci RGN RM RHV DMS
Director of Nursing and Operations, Christie Hospital NHS Trust, Manchester, UK

Nigel Northcott PhD MA(Ed) RGN DipN (Lond) PGCEA
Nurse Manager, NHS Professionals (Oxford), and Tutor, RCN Institute, London, UK

Ian Peate RN DipN (Lond) RNT B Ed (Hons) MA (Lond) LLM
Associate Head of Department, Nursing and Midwifery, University of Hertfordshire, Hertfordshire, UK

Yana Richens RGN RM BSc (Hons) MSc
Research and Development Fellow, RCN Institute, Radcliffe Infirmary, Oxford, UK

Jane Salvage BA MSc RGN HonLLD
Visiting Professor, University of Sheffield, Sheffield, UK

Susan Savage MSc BNurs RGN RHV
Professional Officer, Public Involvement, Nursing and Midwifery Council, London, UK

Jane Schober MN RGN DipNEd DipN Lond RCNT RNT
Principal Lecturer, School of Nursing and Midwifery, De Montfort University, Leicester, UK

Sally Taber MA RGN SCM MHSM
Head of Operational Policy, Independent Healthcare Association, UK

Kieron Thayre RN RNT RCNT DipN (Lond) DipNEd (Lond) MSc
Senior Lecturer, Department of Allied Health Professions, University of Hertfordshire, Hertfordshire, UK

Jane Valente BA DipN RN
Senior Nurse, Directorate of Medical and A&E Services, University Hospitals of Leicester NHS Trust, UK

Judy Zur RSCN RGN DN (Lon) BSc (Hons)
Trainer Health Visitor, Hounslow PCT, London, UK (formerly Senior Lecturer LSBU)

FOREWORD

I was delighted to be asked to write the Foreword for the fourth edition of this well respected text, which has helped provide a foundation for nurses in their initial years of study over the past 14 years.

Throughout the period of the preceding three editions nursing has grown ever more complex; it has adopted a surer academic footing; it has acquired more evidence on which to base practice; and it has returned to its roots in competencies for practice. Above all, the profession has refreshed its pledge to the public through a new Code of professional conduct which forms the framework for practice that the public can expect from nurses. There could not be a more appropriate time for a learning resource based on this pledge.

This is a text which goes to the core of nursing and sets out to help nurses care. Caring is not something that can be learned simply from the written word; caring has to be learned in context – and this book will help you to set care in context. It helps to ground you in the rapidly changing environment of health care; it helps you to see how quality care can be assured and why professional practice is regulated; it encourages you to reflect on what practice is and how you can shape it within the multi-professional team; it helps you to think about the issues that impact on care, its delivery and its environment. In short, it helps you on your journey towards being an accountable, licenced practitioner – and maintaining that licence to practise throughout your career. I hope you enjoy your journey.

Jonathan Asbridge
May 2003

PREFACE TO THE FOURTH EDITION

The fourth edition of this extremely popular and successful textbook for pre-registration nurses is a complete revision of the third edition and, as such, reflects the numerous changes which have occurred in nursing in recent years, in particular, the new Code of professional conduct (NMC 2002) and the NMC/UKCC (2000) requirements for educating and training pre-registration nurses. The aim is to provide a core text for nursing students which reflects the range of professional requirements and academic standards necessary to achieve registration and the licence to practise nursing.

As with previous editions, this text is designed to guide, support and inspire readers from all branches of nursing, to consider and learn from a wide range of experts about current professional issues which impact on nursing and health care practice. As well as current professional requirements being addressed and analysed, the needs of patients/clients across the lifespan are also explored. Issues which impact on quality and effective care management and professional decision-making are also included, e.g. ethical dimensions of caring, practitioner–patient relationships, evidence-based practice and risk management. The development of the nurse as a professional is supported by topics which address standards of practice, practitioner support and career development.

Readers should note that the issue of blurring the boundaries in roles between different members of the multi-professional health care team is not addressed here in any detail, since it was felt that there was insufficient literature available to discuss this at length. We hope to address this in the next edition.

The editors recognize that this text is not necessarily read sequentially, rather, the reader is more likely to dip in and out of it. However, in Chapter 1, Jane Salvage provides a thought-provoking analysis of the current changes in nursing and health care policy which underpin many themes within the text and, as such, is the springboard for the whole book.

This edition offers many features within the text, which, we hope, will make it easier to study. These include:

- Boxed introductions at the start of each chapter, to signpost it for the reader
- Boxed summaries at the end of sections to help to recapitulate
- A conclusion at the end of chapters to summarize key issues
- Chapters firmly grounded in practice and professional requirements to facilitate application and analysis
- The inclusion of scenarios and reflective activities to illuminate practice-based issues
- The use of a marginal icon Ⓝ to indicate when the new Code of professional conduct (NMC 2002) is referred to within the text
- Annotated further reading, selected to encourage further study
- The use of colour and shade to highlight many of these key features.

This text is intended to be a valuable resource and guide for your studies. We hope you enjoy using it, whether you are preparing for registration or undertaking a post-registration course of study.

Previous editions have been used widely by those returning to nursing, undertaking an enrolled nurse conversion course or a postgraduate nursing course.

Readers should note that the views expressed are those of individual authors and not necessarily those of the editors.

Sue Hinchliff
Sue Norman
Jane Schober
London 2003

HOW TO USE THIS BOOK

The fourth edition of this popular textbook is designed as an invaluable resource for those studying nursing. As well as the key features listed previously, there are suggestions here to help you use the book effectively.

The editors recognise the importance and value of a textbook which the reader may use sequentially or, as is more likely, a text which you may dip in and out of. If used sequentially, you will find some repetition as different authors discuss and analyse, for example, the NMC Code of professional conduct and NMC competencies for practice in relation to their topic area. This adds to the comprehensiveness and breadth of the text as a range of patient groups and professional themes are featured.

Use this book to aid your studies by:

- Locating your topic or themes in the contents list and index.
- Using the introductions in each chapter to gain an overview of the content.
- Using the reflection points to explore implications for practice and in discussion of key issues with colleagues.
- Referring to summaries and conclusions to focus on outcomes and key arguments.
- Referring to the appendices to substantiate the content of the NMC Code of professional conduct and the NMC competencies.
- Referring to the details within the 'Further Reading', in each chapter, to support the topic.
- Using the address list and web sites to access current data.

REFERENCES TO UKCC AND NMC

You will find many publications and documents referenced under UKCC and NMC in the text. At the time of writing and editing of this book, the regulatory body was re-publishing some of the UKCC documents under the NMC. You may, therefore, find some inconsistencies. However, you should be able to access information about any UKCC or NMC documents references in this book through the NMC website address www.nmc-uk.org.

This is a textbook, which we hope you will use; here we are suggesting ways of doing so more effectively. If you have other thoughts about how it could be improved in terms of content or design, we would be very pleased to hear from you.

CHAPTER 1

NURSING TODAY AND TOMORROW

Jane Salvage

INTRODUCTION

This chapter takes a panoramic view of nursing today. Starting with an overview of the political, social and health status of Europe, it locates nursing in the UK in a wider global context. The World Health Organization's (WHO) Health for All movement and its emphasis on public health are advocated as a helpful policy framework for nursing, although a brief analysis of European health care reform suggests that these approaches are not high on the political agenda. Moving on to assess the role and influence of nursing on health care reform in Europe and the UK, the chapter reaches pessimistic conclusions. However, it points to many interesting developments which demonstrate how nursing is responding to change and being shaped by it. Special attention is paid to changes in the nursing role. Changes at the 'top' and 'bottom' of the profession, also linked to changing patterns of care delivery and a revolution in nursing education, are seen to have potentially far-reaching effects on health care and nursing.

The chapter ends with a plea for a new type of professionalism which looks beyond territorial boundaries and tunes in to the real needs of society and individuals. The weaving together by nurses and patients, in partnership, of the physical, social, emotional and spiritual domains of human life in order to create patterns of care and relationships which are truly holistic and healing is a ripe area for development.

In looking at the future, it is useful to begin by looking at the present – and the past. We need to look at the past both to learn from it and to move on from it. Our attempts to forge a better future are often tragically constrained by the baggage of the past – as current events remind us, whether close to home in Northern Ireland or in countries further afield ravaged by war. In the early 1990s, for example, euphoria over the collapse of the Berlin Wall and the totalitarian systems of Eastern Europe and the former Soviet Union rapidly turned into disillusionment, even despair, and people's intentions to live in peace and harmony evaporated almost overnight. The UK has experienced less dramatic, but nevertheless marked, swings of national mood. After the stagnation of the last years of Conservative government, the election of a new Labour government in 1997 generated a spirit of optimism and willingness to tackle our most intractable problems (such as the troubles in Northern Ireland). Although Labour was re-elected in 2001, by then this optimism was already tinged with disappointment that progress had been slower than expected on many key issues, not least the state of the NHS.

Many nurses, when they look into the future, find their own mood swinging confusingly between optimism and disillusionment. Speculation is rife on the future of the nursing professions and even of the health care system itself. The pace of change is so rapid and the current situation so full of variety and apparently contradictory trends that it is possible to produce evidence to sustain many conflicting prophecies. This chapter develops its own speculations by looking first at the present, at some of the most striking features of the current nursing and health care scenario. It is offered not as an authoritative statement, but as a personal reflection that might encourage you to consider the social and political context of the contribution nursing makes to health; its ideas are drawn from experience, reading and discussion rather than a systematic literature review. The key point of concern is not the nursing profession itself, but the health needs of society and the people it serves – alongside a belief that a healthy profession is an important vehicle for achieving better health for all, and that the need for good nursing is universal and timeless, whatever the current configuration of lay and professional care.

MAP OF THIS CHAPTER

This chapter is written primarily for a UK readership, but any consideration of the future of British nursing cannot ignore the wider European context. Controversy continues to rage about what our relationship with continental Europe should be, and even about the definition of Europe itself. The term is often used as a synonym for the European Union (EU), currently comprising 15 member states, including the UK, but set to expand further in the next few years; 13 countries, mostly in Central and Eastern Europe, have applied for membership and several are likely to join in 2004. The EU's directives and regulations, as agreed by all member states, have a direct and indirect influence on nursing in many ways; for example, the directives on qualifications aim to maintain standards while enabling workforce mobility between countries, thus impacting on nursing education in all 15 member countries. A wider definition of Europe is adopted by other bodies such as WHO, whose European Region comprises 51 member states, including the 15 successor republics of the former Soviet Union, and thus extends territorially from Greenland in the west (a dependency of Denmark) to Vladivostok in Russia's far east, and to the Central Asian republics in the south.

However defined, there is no doubt that Europe will continue to be a major influence, with implications for nursing. This chapter therefore begins with an overview of the current state of Europe and its key health issues. Health care reform and the role of nursing are considered from the perspective of WHO's goal of Health for All and its emphasis on public health as the means to achieve it. Current trends in UK health care and nursing are considered, paying special attention to the question of changing roles. Finally, some ideas are offered for debate about the future of nursing: what strengths can the profession build on to ensure that it equips itself to meet future needs, and what areas of neglect should be addressed?

A EUROPEAN OVERVIEW

When the Cold War ended, Europe once again became whole. After the Second World War the map of Europe had been redrawn and its borders and systems remained fairly stable for 40 years, until the unprecedented changes began in the countries of Central and Eastern Europe and the former Soviet Union in the late 1980s. As the Iron Curtain lifted, countries about which those in the West knew very little took their place on the international stage once more, and we realized that our conception of 'Europe' as essentially the EU was inadequate. Nevertheless, the EU has expanded despite considerable opposition within many member states, and now plays an ever greater part in national affairs. It continues to struggle with the issue of extending membership to Eastern European countries while trying to comprehend and respond to the changes in the east which have had such a major and as yet unmeasurable impact on the rest of the continent.

The accession states awaiting admission to the EU are the most prosperous and successful of the former Communist bloc, but there are still wide disparities, not least in the quality of public health measures, health care delivery and professional skills and training – issues that will impact on the wider European community in many ways with the greater mobility that membership will bring. Many more staff and patients will cross borders in search of work or better care; moreover, health and social problems do not respect national frontiers despite attempts to erect walls around the EU's Fortress Europe. The rapid and alarming spread of AIDS in the east of the region is just one topical example of how the opening up of previously closed societies, greater foreign travel and socio-economic problems can combine to create or exacerbate threats to health.

Eastern Europe paid a heavy price for its gains in freedom and democracy – severe political, economic and cultural problems eroded the fabric of society and drove millions of ordinary people into poverty and sickness in the decade following the fall of the Berlin Wall. This poverty is closely linked with many fatal and debilitating health problems, including communicable and non-communicable diseases; greater maternal and infant mortality; the spread of the smoking, alcohol and drugs epidemics; and the risks of living in unhealthy environments. The social cost of the changes continues to be enormous and it is impossible to predict where it will all lead. Many of these countries are still volatile and armed conflict has taken a terrible toll in the former Yugoslavia, the Caucasus, the Russian Federation and elsewhere. Migration of millions of people within and out of Eastern Europe, whether displaced by war and civil conflict or driven by poverty and lack of opportunity, has accelerated throughout the past decade; combined with mass migration to Europe from other regions such as the Middle East, Africa and South-East Asia, it is a major and intractable social issue that is beginning to play a big part in national and local elections throughout Western Europe.

One indicator of the dramatic changes was the sudden appearance of newly independent countries and new nation states. In 1988, WHO had 32 member states in Europe, but by 2002 it had

51 (for historical and political reasons the WHO European Region includes all 15 former USSR republics, Israel and Turkey, as well as Central/Eastern Europe and the EU). When I joined WHO in 1991 it lacked not only contacts and relationships with many of those Eastern European countries, but also knew little about them. Even the countries themselves lacked information, for a variety of reasons; government chief nurses, for example, might not know the true extent of common health problems or the size of their nursing workforce.

WHO's European nursing and midwifery unit spent 4 years in the early 1990s collecting data and feeding it into individual profiles of nursing and midwifery in 46 countries, later summarized as a description and analysis of the current situation in Europe (Salvage and Heijnen 1997). For the first time, nurses and others could take a comprehensive look at the real picture of nursing and midwifery across Europe, make comparisons and map trends, and undertake further analysis and trend-spotting from a reasonably accurate baseline. No comprehensive update has been undertaken, although some new information is being collected by WHO in the form of a questionnaire asking countries what progress they have made in implementing the 2000 Munich Declaration (see below), and the study remains the best current snapshot of European nursing.

The WHO study and country profiles are used in this chapter to encourage understanding of British nursing in a European context. What emerges time and again is the universal nature of the issues affecting nursing, and the common and often timeless nature of the challenges it faces both in improving the quality of care and in winning recognition of its contribution to health. The vast majority of problems which are assumed to be specific to local situations turn out to be common themes elsewhere, suggesting that long-term solutions lie less in tinkering with systems than in more radical social change, e.g. in the position of women.

THE SOCIOPOLITICAL CONTEXT

Data on nursing and midwifery should be interpreted in the light of the overall social, political and health context of the region. Here are some key facts. The population of Europe (defined here as the member states of the WHO European Region) is around 850 million and is expected to rise slowly. Fertility rates have fallen, marriage is becoming less frequent and divorce is increasing. The population continues to age, with a notable increase in people aged 60–79; 18 of the 20 countries with the world's highest percentages of older people (13–18%) are in the European Region, and the economically active population is also ageing. These statistics indicate complex interlocking factors stemming from sweeping social, political and cultural changes throughout the region. Traditional family and community structures are breaking down, migration to escape war and poverty is soaring, isolation and insecurity are much more marked, and stress – manifested in the growing abuse of drugs and alcohol – is high and increasing. All this and more takes its toll on people's mental and physical health (WHO 2001).

Within nearly every country, East and West, there is a widening health gap between rich and poor; the UK is no exception, as the Black report documented long ago (Townsend et al. 1988). While the rich minority in every country are more healthy and live longer, the majority on low incomes are sicker and die younger. There is also a widening health gap between East and West, with people's health generally improving in the West and deteriorating in the East, mainly attributable to growing poverty; the difference in life expectancy at birth has risen to 6 years. In health services, there is a wide quality-of-care gap between West and East, caused partly by the crisis now engulfing the health care systems of Eastern countries, but also partly attributable to their historical neglect of nursing and midwifery.

The reliable, valid data and sophisticated analysis needed to justify such statements, make comparisons and, most importantly, stimulate progress have historically been difficult to produce, but WHO and others have recently paid more attention to producing health 'league tables' of the type that have become increasingly common in the UK health system. The 2000 World Health Report, *Health Systems: Improving Performance*, took the bold and, in some eyes, controversial step of ranking countries according to such indicators as health levels, expenditure and health service performance (WHO 2000a). Interpretation of the data is a matter of furious debate. The WHO estimate of overall health system attainment for 1997, the latest year for which figures are available, placed Japan in first place and the UK in ninth, rather higher than might be expected for a system so often described as in crisis. Nearly all Western European countries were clustered in the top 30 (of 191 countries), Central Europe in the 29–74 range, most of the countries of the former Yugoslavia in the 70s and 80s, and most of the former USSR in the 80–135 range, above some South-East Asian and most sub-Saharan African countries at the bottom.

HEALTH FOR ALL REVISITED

One of the most exciting moments in my WHO career was waking up somewhere in Central Asia, dazed and jet-lagged, and drawing back the curtains of my 16th-floor hotel window to find a breathtaking panorama of the snow-capped Tien Shan (Celestial Mountains) with a huge, modern building directly beneath. I was in the capital of newly independent Kazakhstan, a new WHO European Region member state, looking down on the Palace of Lenin, venue of the 1978 WHO international conference at which the famous Alma-Ata Declaration was agreed. Like many people, I had hardly realized that Alma-Ata was a place although I had studied the declaration, a remarkably radical statement that both captured and stimulated a new approach to health care. It shifted the emphasis firmly to promoting health and preventing ill health through healthy public policy and primary health care, adopting the latter as the strategy for achieving the goal of health for all the world's population by the year 2000.

By 1984 WHO's European parliament, the Regional Committee for Europe, had used the declaration as the basis of a policy framework setting out the expected improvements in health and describing strategies for achieving them through healthier lifestyles, improvements in the environment, and provision of high quality health services. These strategies, it was proposed, could be implemented using a target approach: 38 Health for All targets and related indicators. The targets were intended to support the formulation of health and health care policies and their implementation in member states, and the indicators would enable comparisons between countries and the monitoring of trends.

The endorsement of this framework by all member states was very encouraging and health policy development took a big step forward. In England, it led to a strategy on the nation's health which, while focusing more on an individualistic, 'lifestyles' approach to health gain than on the wider policy measures also required, was nevertheless a step in the right direction. As yet, however, there has been no real global progress towards the primary target of health for all – equity. Closing the health divide by improving the health of particular population groups, at least to the level of the differences that existed at the beginning of the 1970s, is today's major challenge, in the UK and everywhere else. Important new steps are being taken to tackle it in the UK, beginning with a government review and updating of the aforementioned Black report on inequalities in health, and continuing with comprehensive poverty reduction policies.

As the year 2000 drew nearer and it became ever clearer that the Health for All targets could not be met in the timescale originally envisaged, WHO's member states adopted a World Health Declaration in 1998 outlining a new Health for All policy for the 21st century. Later that year, the European Health for All framework was reviewed, updated and endorsed by the 51 WHO member states, who adopted a new policy framework that reduces the number of specific targets to 21. The overall goal of HEALTH21 is to achieve full health potential for all, with two main aims: to promote and protect people's health throughout their lives; and to reduce the incidence of the main diseases and injuries and alleviate the suffering they cause. Three basic values form its ethical foundation: health as a human right; equity and health and solidarity in action; and participation and accountability for continued health development (WHO 1999).

THE NURSING CONTRIBUTION

The complex backdrop of social, political and economic change must influence any consideration of the future of nursing, just as it has shaped WHO policies. The 1993 WHO publication *Nursing in Action* described visions, goals and policy guidelines which had mostly been developed during the 1980s and earlier through consensus processes involving thousands of nurses from many countries (Salvage 1993). Its forward-thinking view of the nurse's role in helping to achieve the goals of Health for All, summarized in Box 1.1, looks familiar to UK nurses but for many countries it is revolutionary. Yet the First WHO European Conference on Nursing, which laid down the framework for the future of nursing, took place in Vienna in 1988 when the epochal changes had barely begun. This provoked some hard questions as the new Europe of the 1990s took shape. Was the Vienna Declaration and subsequent WHO (and other international) guidance relevant only to Western Europe?

Box 1.1 The Health for All nurse [adapted by the author from the 1988 Vienna Declaration on nursing (Salvage 1993)]

Nursing's mission:
To help individual people, families and groups to determine and achieve their physical, mental and social potential, and to do so in the context of the environment in which they live and work.

The nurse's functions:
- Promotion and maintenance of health
- Prevention of ill health
- Care during illness, rehabilitation and dying

Subsequent developments and policy shifts have actually brought awareness of the key contribution of nurses and midwives further to the fore, although that awareness has not yet been matched by sufficient investment in nursing development. While WHO identifies nurses and midwives as key groups of professionals 'at the hub of the network of services' needed to achieve the goals of HEALTH21, the effective delivery of nursing services is impeded in many countries by a variety of factors. These include the following – which may sound familiar:

- the exclusion of nurses from policy- and decision-making at all levels of the health care system
- shortages of appropriately trained nurses relative to needs
- insufficient financial support
- undervaluing of nursing, and concomitant subordination to medicine
- continuing gender discrimination – nursing everywhere is women's work and shares the characteristic of other female-dominated occupations, i.e. low pay, low status, poor working conditions, few prospects for promotion and poor education.

The Munich Declaration, which was signed at the Second WHO Ministerial Conference on Nursing and Midwifery in Europe in 2000, implicitly underlines this analysis while expressing it in more diplomatic terms (WHO 2000b). Likewise, the International Council of Nurses highlights similar concerns, for example, in its recent position statement on the participation of nurses in health services decision-making and policy development (ICN 2000).

The Munich conference, designed as a follow-up to the pioneering Vienna conference, acknowledged that 'some steps have been taken in Europe towards strengthening the status and making full use of the potential of nurses and midwives'. The terms of the declaration demonstrate, however, how far there is still to go, as WHO's European regional director Marc Danzon acknowledged:

'The key missing ingredient has been strong political support. Ministers of Health will address this challenge in Munich and take action to change it.'

(WHO 2000c)

Yet even within Dr Danzon's own regional office that political support is still lacking; nursing leaders had to lobby hard simply to ensure that the European nursing advisor post, which was allowed to lie vacant for many months, was filled and not downgraded.

The 2000 World Health Report points out that differences in income or health spending are not the only, or even always, the major reasons why some countries perform better than others: 'performance can vary markedly, even in countries with very similar levels of health spending'. This echoes the conclusion of the 1995 WHO Global Expert Committee on Nursing Practice, that there is no direct correlation between the socio-economic condition of a country and the scope of nursing practice: the expectation that rich countries have a more powerful and effective nursing profession than poor ones is not always fulfilled (WHO 1995). The effectiveness of nursing and midwifery across Europe has barely been measured, but it varies widely and cannot always be correlated with prosperity.

Starting points and initial conditions differ widely between countries, and so do the ways they tackle the issues, but it is possible to distinguish some emerging trends. On the positive side, there is a growing awareness throughout the European region of the need to examine the role of nursing. Attitudes towards the position of nursing in society and its role in health care are slowly changing, and the perception of nursing as a low-status occupation requiring minimal training, and the associated undervaluation of humanistic, psychosocial care, is beginning to alter, although the process is very slow and uneven. This is especially marked in the former Communist countries, where the Soviet model of health care, with its almost complete neglect of nursing, gradually superseded existing national nursing traditions. In Romania, for example, all nursing schools were closed in 1978 and were only reopened in 1991 following the overthrow of the Ceausescu regime. In the UK, it has taken decades of painstaking effort to secure greater autonomy for nursing, and even today the real nature of modern nursing work is barely understood outside the profession.

Meanwhile nurses, like all other health care providers, are under increasing pressure to prove they are good value for money, which has spurred greater efforts to measure the outcomes of nursing interventions (particularly in the UK and Northern Europe). Both trends have prompted a growing interest in nursing education and research. Key issues include curriculum review and reorientation to primary health care; new programme development, especially in higher education; training of nurse educators and researchers; provision of high quality educational materials; continuing professional development; and closer links between education, services and research departments.

Visions, goals and guidelines must constantly be reviewed to ensure they are still useful. The spirit of the Munich Declaration is consistent with the Health for All nurse's mission as described in Box 1.1. It lays even greater stress on the public health, health promotion and community development dimensions of the nurse's role, and a new focus on developing the knowledge and evidence base of practice. The Munich conference (WHO 2000b) advocated the role of the 'family health nurse', who works in partnership with individuals and families to help them find their own solutions to their own health needs, acting as a resource on lifestyle and behavioural risk factors, and promoting health in the community. It noted that many different models of community nursing provision were in use across Europe, many already containing elements of the family health nurse role, and agreed to designate 16 pilot sites for its development. In the UK, the concept is being enthusiastically developed in Scotland with strong support from the government chief nurse.

WHO recommends specific actions nurses can take to help their health systems move in this direction (WHO 2000d), based on key principles including:

- the importance of nursing and midwifery as a combined force for health
- the necessity of directing intervention to those most in need
- the value of describing and demonstrating nursing effectiveness
- nurses' and midwives' obligation to engage in leadership and advocacy; in policy-making, legislation and regulation in health and education systems; and in enabling, supporting and teaching individuals, families and communities to promote health and provide care and treatment
- the importance of developing effective teamwork skills and engaging in interdisciplinary teams
- the need to draw out and describe nurses' special contribution as needs assessors, care co-ordinators and care managers as well as clinicians
- the overwhelming significance of developing family health nurses as a force for health improvement.

PRIMARY HEALTH CARE

The 1978 Alma-Ata declaration asserted that primary health care, in its fullest sense, was the route to health for all. It urged governments:

'to give high priority to the full utilization of human resources by defining the technical role, supportive skills, and attitudes required for each category of health worker according to the functions that need to be carried out to ensure effective primary health care'.

This implies that nursing should be a key component of primary health care, and therefore an essential vehicle for health for all. The more recent policy statements and goals, while putting greater emphasis on concepts such as equity and outcome measurement, nevertheless retain the focus on public health and primary health care as the main routes to health gain; thus, by implication, the nurse's role remains as crucial as ever.

Today virtually all the countries of Western Europe have adopted policy goals that propose to shift health care delivery towards primary health care and closer to the community, workplace and home, with less dependence on institutional care. The primary health care approach is certainly better understood by health professionals today, but as Robinson and Elkan (1997) point out:

'there is still a need to educate policy-makers and the public at large that nursing's most effective contributions to the overall health of the population are based in the community'.

Despite the rhetoric, progress in reality has been uneven and slow. Most European countries still support the hospital sector at the expense of the community, too often reinforced in poorer countries by the policies of major aid agencies and bilateral government projects. The strings attached to their loans and grants often reinforce market forces at the expense of equity and social justice; privatization at the expense of socialized health care; and medical power at the expense of multi-professional work and patient power.

Many Western countries state that the development or maintenance of community nursing is a priority, in line with the Munich Declaration, with a trend towards establishing home visiting services to support ageing populations. These services are well established in some countries but relatively underdeveloped in others, east and west. There are relatively few nurses working in the community in the countries of Central and Eastern Europe and the former USSR, owing to poor status, pay and working conditions and a lack of relevant basic and continuing education. These countries are now beginning to redevelop primary health care services and to reassess medical and nursing roles, with promising moves to create better policy, improve training, and foster more autonomy and accountability – although sustainable improvements are few as yet.

In the UK, primary health care nursing is making great strides forward. Following repeated statements from government ministers about their commitment to a 'primary care-led NHS', but a virtually imperceptible shift of care from hospital to the community, the Labour government has finally taken the bull by the horns and made momentous changes to the way primary health care is managed and delivered. Structural changes such as the establishment of primary health care trusts, which will eventually manage 75% of the entire NHS budget, are finally enabling a definitive shift of emphasis and helping ambitious nurses to adopt new roles, introduce innovations and take a lead in organizing and managing services.

Only a few years ago it would have been unthinkable that a nurse should employ a general medical practitioner, but such innovations are becoming more and more common in the pilot schemes enabled by the NHS (Primary Care) Act (1997). They challenge traditional professional hierarchies as well as traditional assumptions about what kind of health care and what kind of practitioner is most effective. Nurses are increasingly the first point of contact for the public, whether in NHS walk-in clinics or via the NHS Direct phone and internet helplines, and they are taking the lead in providing services for many patients with chronic mental and physical conditions. These services tend to be more focused on the patient and the community, and more conscious of public health issues, than many of those provided by GPs. To the dismay of some in the medical establishment, politicians from the Prime Minister downwards have backed these initiatives wholeheartedly. While their support is partly based on their realization that more investment in primary health care could relieve pressure on the overloaded hospital services that create such public disquiet, rather than a blinding flash of illumination about the nursing role, the political imperatives are nevertheless creating exciting and unprecedented opportunities for primary health care nurses to prove their worth – and many are responding with enthusiasm. As a King's Fund report concludes, 'in many respects nurses are the future of primary care' (Gillam 2001).

The overall policy context is broadly more supportive of values which are important to all disciplines of community nursing. There is a greater emphasis on public health, with recognition of the importance of the collective approach; recognition of the importance of partnership and user involvement; and renewed interest in multi-professional working. These values have long been at the heart of community nursing, but are now much more overt in policy documents. However, policy-makers are still unclear about the distinction between 'primary health care', which they too often equate with the personal medical services provided by general medical practitioners, and 'public health' with its roots in the broader vision of Alma Ata and Health for All.

At the same time, there are counteracting pressures to concentrate acute services on more centralized sites, boosted by a major new hospital building programme. The great majority of NHS nurses remain hospital based, and their role is expanding significantly both to meet patients' demands for increasingly complex care regimes based on innovative technologies, and to compensate for medical staff shortages. Progressive thinking encourages bridging the hospital/community divide through a much more flexible pattern of 'seamless' services built around the patient's care pathway rather than traditional institutions or budget systems. Nurses may gradually come to define themselves not as either hospital or community, but in relation to the care group or network in which they work, and they are increasingly likely to develop flexible roles that enable them to work with patients wherever they live and work, as out- or in-patients, according to need.

HEALTH CARE REFORM

Primary health care in the UK and in most other countries is often described by policy-makers as a key aspect of health care reform, which is a major issue everywhere. In the countries of Central and Eastern Europe and the former USSR there is much debate about how far the Soviet model of health care, which dominated all these countries to a greater or lesser extent, can or should be adapted to new needs. Formidable problems are emerging from the efforts to impose rapid change – often too quickly and with incomplete understanding of the policy options, not to mention poor resources. Their concerns about how to find the right balance between public and private health care provision are echoed in Western Europe, where most countries, faced with apparently endless needs and resources that cannot keep pace, are experimenting with different approaches to the structuring and financing of health care systems and the rationing of services. However, there is little evidence to show how health care reform affects health and equity, and only three or four studies have evaluated the implementation of new health reform policies (WHO 2001).

The frequent reference to primary health care in this context is encouraging but seems to be rooted more in rhetoric than reality in many countries. Primary health care is difficult to organize and deliver and its successes are not easily measured in league tables and statistical indicators. It remains the poor relation of acute hospitals, which are not going to give up their lion's share of resources and prestige without a fight. In many western countries the locus of power has shifted from hospital consultants to executive managers, while in the East, where the GP role barely exists, hospital doctors are still in the driving seat and regard health care reform as a synonym for privatization, which they see as the route to improving their own income and status. Either way, west or east, nursing remains marginal and nurses are seen not as active partners in reform discussions but as subordinate workers who carry out others' orders, whether managers or doctors.

In the UK, a radical Conservative government drove health care reform forward on free market principles from the early 1990s, imposing many major changes on the health service. Yet, while many of the changes were ideologically driven, others which were regarded as part of the reform package actually arose from other motivations and other sources. Indeed, it is difficult to generalize about 'reform' for that reason. In any case, as one commentator put it, 'you never start from the Year Zero in the NHS'. Achieving lasting change is much more difficult than it might seem because of entrenched attitudes and structures, especially in a huge organization like the NHS, which is over 50 years old, and lasting changes are likely to be incremental and gradual despite government attempts to force the pace. Nevertheless, it is increasingly acknowledged that health care in Europe as a whole is in a state of 'permanent transition'. Even in the UK, where much health care has been largely free at the point of delivery since the NHS was founded in 1948, the unthinkable is not only being thought but argued out in hot political and public debate as the government presses on with controversial plans to encourage more private provision and public–private partnerships in health and education. There will be no return to the supposedly golden days of the early NHS.

A NEW PATCHWORK OF NURSING SERVICES

One trend unlikely to be reversed in the UK is the growth of the independent health sector, which now accounts for £8 billion (17%) of annual health spending, compared to £40 billion spent on the NHS (Keen 2000). Health care in the UK has always been a mixed economy but the range of providers is greater than ever and likely to grow further, with the non-profit sectors providing more services. Nurses are increasingly likely to be employed outside the NHS, whether by nursing homes, social services, charities or independent nursing agencies.

The 1:5 non-NHS:NHS expenditure ratio given above is just about matched in nursing numbers, with the independent sector in England employing around 55,000 nurses (whole-time equivalent) compared to 256,000 in the NHS in England (RCN 2002). Of those 55,000 registered nurses, over 9000 are working in private hospitals while most of the rest are in nursing and residential homes. The number of nurses working in the independent sector has risen by around 20% in the past few years in the UK overall, probably mostly accounted for by the boom in nursing homes owing to the increase in the elderly population, the gradual withdrawal of the NHS from long-term care provision and new arrangements for insurance-based care. The independent sector will continue to provide a further employment option for many disillusioned NHS nurses, and may come to account for a larger and larger share of the nursing workforce. It also offers promising opportunities for innovation, as entrepreneurial nurses may find more freedom to develop nurse-led initiatives and creative new services there than in the more hidebound NHS structures – and to sell their services to individual or corporate purchasers.

FORGOTTEN RECIPES FOR SUCCESS

The major resource of every health care system, NHS and independent, is the people who work in it, yet discussion of health care reform still focuses obsessively on funding and structures. In the long run the achievements of any service will primarily be influenced not by its choice of structure or funding mechanism, important as these are, but by how well it develops, motivates and deploys its staff. The quality of the contribution of each person, from the top manager to the floor cleaner, is central to success or failure. Major reform of nursing and midwifery should therefore be an important aspect of health care transition, but it rarely is. Although it does not grab the headlines like other measures such as the commercialization of medicine or the emergency supply of drugs, such reform could arguably have a greater long-term impact.

Nurses and midwives, as the largest single group of health professionals in Europe, are fundamental to health care and exert great influence – even if indirectly. If the reform agenda fails to inspire them, its long-term success must be doubtful or even impossible. Around 5 million people work in the nursing services of the 51 WHO European member states, promoting health, preventing disease and providing care. These factors link nursing's fortunes much more closely to the reform of health care systems than is usually recognized, and present a major challenge to every country's health services. Plans for health care reform are unlikely to succeed in isolation and in the absence of concurrent plans for the best use of human resources for health. To put the case at its most extreme, no system can work properly if its best staff have left or are demoralized and demotivated. A comprehensive national health care plan must include these issues as part of its strategy, and tackle them at the same time.

Good management is crucial to success here. People with management capabilities must be identified and trained in order to create a core of managers with modern management skills – a combination of leadership and administrative expertise. Few people, whatever their background, can automatically be good managers without extra training and in-service development. They may be doctors, nurses, other health professionals, experienced managers from other sectors or specially recruited general management trainees. The management style of the organization is also critical: evidence suggests that the most successful organizations are those which motivate their staff, reward them for good work and involve them in decision-making. Good management therefore includes paying attention to organization development and to creating incentives for all staff.

One aspect of organization development which is of special relevance when considering health care reform is the management of change. Professional and management training needs to accept change as the norm, and to give people the capacities to respond effectively in terms of the structures in which they work, the patterns of their work, the tools they use and their responses to new evidence. This is at last being recognized by policy-makers in the UK, where newly-established agencies focusing on policy delivery are producing valuable guidance (see, for example, National Co-ordinating Centre for NHS Service Delivery and Organization 2001). Organizations and individuals who are unable to be flexible and sensitive to change, and to handle its impact on people and institutions, will fail to thrive in the Europe of the future.

VALUE FOR MONEY?

The experiments prompted by health care reform and a more mixed economy of health, with not only nursing homes but other providers, such as voluntary agencies, playing a bigger role in health and social care, have already led to some interesting innovations. Yet, as argued above, the reformers' overriding concern with finance, and the associated structural issues, tends to focus on the historically dominant acute hospitals and medical profession, and is detrimental to nursing and midwifery, which are marginalized. Many countries are aware of the need to tackle such issues as staff recruitment and retention, education and quality of care, but have not taken adequate steps until pressurized by public opinion. In the UK, an endless stream of media stories of poor NHS care, and coverage of the staff shortages that contribute to it, has pushed nursing issues much higher up the political agenda and led to some significant policy decisions. Such attention is long overdue, not least because nurses' salary costs lie at the heart of health service economics.

Nurses, doctors and other health workers are in short supply in many areas and many specialties, but this does not make them immune to criticism. Cash-strapped managers must constantly question whether the same work can be done by a less qualified and therefore 'cheaper' employee. Combined with a traditional tendency to undervalue the often invisible work of the registered nurse, this has prompted many managers to challenge nurses on grounds of both productivity and effectiveness – challenges that seem insulting to people who struggle daily in difficult circumstances to provide high quality care for little financial reward. Yet it cannot be denied that a surprisingly large proportion of the work of health care professionals – doctors, nurses, physiotherapists and others – is ineffective and even harmful. This rather shocking statement is supported by evidence from many countries, including the US and the UK, and is probably true of most countries. Even where clear evidence exists, staff continue to use dangerous or outdated interventions which injure patients and waste money. Perhaps it needed the brutal goad of economics to galvanize a critical mass in the professions into evidence-based practice, stimulating them to scrutinize their work to ensure that it is appropriate and effective. However, the pioneering work done by nurses on audit and research-based practice, long before the medical profession took the issues on board, is yet another unsung story of nursing innovation.

Relevant tools used within the new clinical governance framework, and under the banner of evidence-based practice, include quality assurance systems, clinical audit, clinical research, strategies for research implementation and continuing professional development. The principles underlying these interventions are relevant to any health care system and the tools can be adapted according to its stage of development. The importance of peer and patient review of the effectiveness of health care interventions also points to a new type of professionalism which emphasizes working in partnership with patients and populations – and is linked to another key theme: power-sharing.

NEW ROLES AND NEW PROFESSIONALISM IN THE UK

The nursing professions have always inhabited a rather uncomfortable social space somewhere between the 'true' (i.e. male-dominated, powerful, elitist) professions like medicine and law, proletarian occupations like domestic work and health care assistants, and unpaid 'women's work' in the family home. This has often been regarded as a weakness, and nurse reformers have sought greater power by mimicking the institutions and culture of the true professions. Now, however, it can be seen more clearly that nursing's proletarian nature may be a source of strength and equips it much better for the future than traditional upper-middle-class occupations, whose patrician style is increasingly at odds with ordinary people's expectations and desires. A range of influential organizations is calling for a new type of professionalism to fit the changed circumstances in which we find ourselves (Salvage 2002). In some respects nursing is already moving in this direction, emphasizing therapeutic relationships with patients and introducing important changes in care delivery that give patients more power and more choice, and pay more regard to their individual needs and wishes.

Throughout Europe, consumer demands for greater involvement and control in public services such as health care are also reflected at the macro level. Decentralization is a strong theme of health care reform and indeed of societies in general, promising greater decision-making power at local level. In the UK a good example is the devolution of greater independence to Scotland, Wales, Northern Ireland and the regional assemblies, which are already giving rise to significant differences in health policy and spending. If decentralization is to have any beneficial effect it means devolving authority and responsibility down to the 'lowest' possible levels. People must be given the authority to make decisions on the issues which lie within their competence, whether they are clinical, administrative or support staff. In return for giving them this authority and expecting them to be responsible and accountable for what they do, the organization must offer them proper training and support, and respect the integrity of their decisions.

Power-sharing is not simply a matter for health service staff. Power must also be shared with the users of services. Participative care is essential for effectiveness and efficiency, not just a luxury for consumer-oriented societies. It means involving citizens directly in every stage of health care, from service planning to evaluation; offering them genuine choices based on full information; and evolving new styles of professional behaviour based on doing things with patients rather than to them. After all, people should really be considered not as consumers of health services but as producers of their own health. Ultimately the major human resource of any health care system is its citizens.

CHANGING BOUNDARIES

This panoramic sweep of health, health care and nursing issues in Europe has at many points touched on the question of the nurse's role. Professions like to regard their roles as timeless, wrapped round with self-justifying rhetoric about how indispensable they are, or how they are the only ones who can provide a certain service or uphold certain values. Yet the nursing profession is a relatively new social institution, even though nursing care is as old as humanity itself. Recently, much anguished debate in UK nursing circles has focused on trying to distinguish between what aspects, attributes or values of organized nursing are indeed timeless, and what can or must change as society and its needs and demands change. This is a crucially important debate, but the pressure-cooker atmosphere in which it is conducted does not encourage calm, reasoned reflection; managerial and financial pressures have tended to force nursing into a corner, provoking the fear and uncertainty which lead to territorial defensiveness and introversion rather than a balanced consideration of fitness for purpose. In other words, the debate often starts at the wrong end – with nurses and what they do rather than with patients and what they need.

In a more logical world, many questions about role would be solved by adopting that focus on the client. Proper workforce planning would be an essential component of an effective health care strategy – not as a head-counting, number-crunching pseudo-science, but as a cool consideration of how best to ensure that the profile of the health care labour force is designed to meet people's needs for health care, and of the appropriate steps necessary to match the supply of staff to the demand.

This is a complex exercise involving at least the elements shown in Box 1.2. In real life these logical steps are hard to follow, dogged as they are at every turn by tradition, custom and practice, and vested interests, but the costs of ignoring them are huge – a message that is finally being heard by policy-makers in the UK.

Box 1.2 Elements of successful workforce planning

- Identification of health care needs
- Decisions about how the service aims to meet those needs
- Clarification of the role and functions of each group of staff, including doctors, nurses, other therapists, auxiliary staff and other support workers
- Clarification of the contribution to be made by patients, clients, families and lay carers
- Review of educational initiatives to ensure staff, patients and carers are properly prepared for their roles
- Planning the best mix of grades and skills in the health care team, based on the agreed role and function as well as experience of each member
- Determining the number of staff needed in each grade, and regulating labour supply (recruitment and training) accordingly
- Offering incentives (pay, better working conditions, development opportunities, etc.) to attract and retain high quality staff

A consensus is now developing, albeit slowly and controversially, on reform of the health care professions. While acknowledging how much the patterns and practices of traditional professionalism owe to the dominant ideologies of the 19th century, reform needs to find a way to honour their many achievements and cherish their humanitarian values but help them find expression in more contemporary, productive, socially integrated and egalitarian ways. Health professional roles have never been fixed in stone and the division of labour has constantly shifted, but more rapid, dramatic changes could take place in the current decade than in the preceding century. The 19th century 'lone hero model of masculinity' on which the medical profession was built is increasingly unacceptable to patients, who want more equality and openness, and to fellow professionals as well as many doctors. Nurses, physiotherapists and others, becoming more confident and independent, do not want to be subordinate to doctors, and many younger doctors and those working in Cinderella areas support teamwork and other forms of the new professionalism. This focus on collaboration and teamwork, along with profound changes in the age structure, gender and ethnicity of the professions and different expectations and demands from the public, give traditional professionalism no choice but to evolve.

The government, playing a more interventionist role in order to hasten the professional changes it believes will help deliver its promises, is pushing at a partly open door with its moves to break down professional boundaries and encourage a focus on delivering what the patient wants and needs rather than on worrying about who does what (see, for example, Box 1.3, and DoH 2001a). Scandals like Shipman, Bristol and Alder Hey have undermined medicine's reputation and its leaders face a stark choice: to defend its long-held power and privileges, which could be a bloody and unproductive battle for all concerned, or to relinquish some of what it has cherished in favour of a largely unknown but potentially more exciting and creative future.

Box 1.3 How nurses and therapists will 'shift the boundaries'

From *The NHS Plan* (DoH 2002a):

'NHS employers will be required to empower appropriately qualified nurses, midwives and therapists to undertake a wider range of clinical tasks including the right to make and receive referrals, admit and discharge patients, order investigations and diagnostic tests, run clinics and prescribe drugs...'

Chief Nursing Officer's '10 key roles for nurses' (England):

- To order diagnostic investigations, such as pathology tests and X-rays
- To make and receive referrals direct, say, to a therapist or a pain consultant
- To admit and discharge patients for specified conditions and within agreed protocols
- To manage patient caseloads, say for diabetes or rheumatology
- To run clinics, say, for ophthalmology or dermatology
- To prescribe medicines and treatments
- To carry out a wide range of resuscitation procedures including defibrillation
- To perform minor surgery and outpatient procedures
- To triage patients using the latest IT to the most appropriate health professional
- To take a lead in the way local health services are organized and in the way that they are run

Nursing and the other allied health professions must also scrutinize their own attitudes and practices, especially those which, in the understandable drive for recognition and parity with medicine, have mimicked some undesirable features of traditional professionalism. They too may have something to lose, but a lot more to gain. There is a window of opportunity to re-evaluate the potential of these traditionally subordinate occupations, and to encourage a long overdue focus on the neglected contribution and potential of non-registered health workers, as well as integration of lay carers into the health care team.

NURSING AND SKILL MIX

The changing political climate has spawned many pilot projects which attempt to bring staff organizations and managers together in joint initiatives looking at workforce planning and career structures. Yet policy often follows rather than leads innovation in the field; most 'new' practices are actually an extension, amalgam or adaptation of something that has been tried somewhere else. Earlier exemplars can be found in health services of nearly all the developments now hailed as innovative, including some that demonstrate new forms of professionalism. There have been many attempts to change practice and make it more patient-centred, many barely recorded and poorly disseminated. They have often been isolated, and hard to bring into the mainstream. Many innovative projects are undermined from without and within, and have little lasting impact within and beyond their own sphere. The factors ensuring successful innovation are well researched but not known or poorly heeded by policy-makers or even the innovators themselves. Government and health service leaders need to be much clearer about how they can intervene to accelerate innovation into the mainstream, and make legitimate what is already happening. They need to work at closing the policy–practice loop so that policy and practice interact in a mutually reinforcing, iterative process.

Given the complexity of the issues, change is incremental and traditional and new professionalism continue to coexist. Important changes are already being made or planned on many fronts; whether they can together create a synergistic, unstoppable wave of professional reform is hard to predict. Many previous attempts have been sabotaged by medical opposition, but the medical establishment, driven by enlightened self-interest and itself more diverse, may now be more open to innovation. Policy-makers must act with more determination and focus than hitherto in insisting that the profession moves forward rather than blocks change, while simultaneously reviving and building neglected alliances with progressive groups within medicine, other professionals, service users and other stakeholders.

Many nurses feel threatened by the talk of changing skill mix, shifting roles and breaking down boundaries between the professions. Hindsight has sometimes justified their fears, with employers' talk of changing the skill mix in a team often proving to be code for diluting the skill mix by replacing highly qualified staff with less skilled workers, or for making staff take on increasingly complex tasks without the requisite training or reward. However, official figures show that the nursing workforce, far from being edged out, is actually expanding. The number of registered nurses in the NHS has risen by over 4% in the past 5 years, and the number of non-registered nursing staff by over 11% (RCN 2002), with similar rises in the independent sector. It would appear that skill mix exercises have not had the draconian impact many feared.

Why should this be? Ever more patients are being treated and this high throughput requires high numbers of skilled nurses. There are numerous opportunities for motivated nurses to work as consultants and specialists in hospital and the community, to take over aspects of junior doctors' roles in hospitals, to lead innovative services and even to employ GPs in primary care. Over and above that, nurses remain the core of the health service workforce, essential in keeping the daily work of most services going. Maybe the message that good, efficient care needs to be delivered by registered nurses is beginning to get through.

These role changes spring not only from a genuine search for better quality and responsiveness to patients' needs; they are also a pragmatic response to the vexed question of labour supply and demand. In the mid-1990s, NHS and private employers could pick and choose their nurses; now it is a seller's market. Nurse training places were cut by around 25% in the early 1990s and this disastrously wrong-headed policy is now leading to a shortfall of qualified staff at just the time when their services are in high demand. As a result managers are being forced to dilute their skill mix whether they like it or not. The Labour government has reversed the policy and expanded the number of places again, but students are not yet qualifying in sufficient numbers to fill the vacancies. In a vicious spiral, staff shortages and growing workloads create extra pressure, overworked and stressed staff leave the service, and the situation worsens for those who remain.

It may take many years to repair the damage of earlier ill-advised policy decisions. In the meantime government and health care employers are attempting to fill the gaps by recruiting nurses (and doctors) with overseas qualifications – a politically sensitive initiative at a time when there is a global shortage of skilled staff and many countries are anxious to retain their own nursing and medical graduates rather than see them migrate. The impact on UK health teams is likely to be marked, as foreign-trained health staff may have a different range of skills and knowledge, possibly underpinned by different values and cultural assumptions. Analysis of this impact is yet another dimension that will need to be considered if optimum skill mix is to be achieved.

MINI-DOCTOR OR MAXI-NURSE

The question of the nurse's role has always preoccupied the profession, partly as an expression of its insecurity and partly as a reflection of the difficulty of putting into words many of the most important values and attributes of nursing at its best. Besides, roles rarely remain unchanged for long, and the division of labour within health care has always been contentious. Alongside the efforts – real and imagined – at 'giving away' aspects of the nursing role to support workers or others in generic roles, there is a parallel readjustment of boundaries under way at the top of the practitioner scale.

Both hospital and community nursing seem to be travelling simultaneously down two different and almost contradictory paths. One focuses on taking on aspects of the doctor's role, typically including delegated medical tasks – sometimes because the doctor recognizes the nurse's superior expertise, but more often because the task is routine, unpopular or time-consuming, or is easily delegated. Sometimes nurses take on medical tasks in unpopular locations, with unpopular client groups or at unsocial times such as nights and weekends. Others take on tasks which doctors do not do well, or which they see as trivial, such as giving health advice.

Where it gets confusing is that alternatively, and sometimes in the very same posts, nurses are developing genuinely innovative roles, often with underserved groups such as homeless people or sex workers; meeting care needs of people with specific conditions such as diabetes or asthma; or responding to new developments which create new needs, such as genetic counselling. Some of this work is extremely creative and research is beginning to demonstrate its value to patients. It has been formalized and recognized by government in the creation of the nurse consultant role, seen by many (although not all) not as a mini-doctor but as a maxi-nurse, expanding the nurse's true nursing role.

Therefore, it can be argued that there are two major areas of change, at the top and the bottom of nursing. At the 'top', the most advanced and expert end of the practice spectrum, nurses are taking on ever more adventurous, unorthodox and innovative roles. The nurse practitioner in primary health care is a widely-debated example but there are countless others, where the nurse uses and expands nursing expertise as a complement to the work of other professionals. Clinical specialist nurses in medically defined specialties, mental health nurses in advanced therapeutic roles, theatre nurses performing surgery and community nurses co-ordinating packages of care for elderly or chronically ill people all demonstrate a huge variety of skills and knowledge being attuned to patients' needs. Perhaps it does not really matter whether they are mini-doctors or maxi-nurses if patients are getting better care.

KEY INFLUENCES ON ROLE CHANGE

Such developments are made possible not only by the dynamism and intellect of individual practitioners, but by the willingness of professional colleagues to assimilate these changes and the impact they have on their own practice; the willingness of managers to help professionals reconfigure their services; the willingness of governments and professional and regulatory bodies to lead and enable the changes; and the willingness of patients to accept new types of service and professionals stepping beyond their traditional boundaries.

Other less altruistic factors may be equally important in shaping new roles. The long overdue decision to reduce the number of hours worked by junior hospital doctors was implemented not by employing more doctors to make up the shortfall, but by giving nurses some of their responsibilities. Some have done so happily, some reluctantly; some with extra training, some without. Largely unwittingly this has opened doors which would otherwise have remained closed. Some critics see this as further exploitation of nurses and dilution of the nurse's caring role, while others see it as a gift, an unprecedented chance to revolutionize nursing practice and status.

Either way, it may with hindsight prove to have been one of the biggest levers for change. There are exciting options on offer for those nurses who can put their case persuasively. Yet nursing has been tying itself up in knots: ever sensitive to real or imagined slights from doctors, some bridle at the idea of being duped into doing doctors' dirty work, even if the individual nurse finds it interesting and rewarding. In the prevailing professional paradigm, those who enjoy being medical technicians, such as nurses who have trained to perform minor operations or procedures such as endoscopy, have their authenticity challenged, as though by liking this work they are less caring or are betraying the real values of the profession.

As human beings so often do when confronted with uncertainty, some sectors of nursing opinion have reacted by attempting to exert tight control over these developments – for example, by urging the regulatory bodies to open new registers for 'advanced' or 'expert' practitioners, with specific role descriptions and prescribed clinical and educational experience as a prerequisite for taking on these roles. While it is essential that the public is protected from inadequately prepared practitioners over-stepping the limits of their competence, such moves sometimes seem to be more concerned with internal professional demarcations, rewards and jealousies than with the needs of patients.

At the other end of the spectrum, as discussed, fears are widespread that registered nurses will be replaced by cheaper options such as health care assistants or auxiliary workers. There is nothing new in this: much, if not most, direct, hands-on care in institutions has always been given by unqualified staff, and the profession has continually fought to retain control of these workers and to replace them, wherever possible, with registered nurses. The evidence of the effectiveness of an all-registered nursing workforce is not extensive enough to persuade managers to invest the initial greater cost, even if the staff were available.

What is more noteworthy is the growing professionalization of the health care assistant role. Their numbers are not accurately captured in official statistics, they are not regulated and their title and job content varies from one employer to the next, but the phasing out of the enrolled nurse role, combined with the shortage of registered nurses, means demand for a hands-on nursing worker with some basic skills is soaring. As a sign of their growing importance, members of the Royal College of Nursing decided in 2001 to allow the best qualified health care assistants to apply for membership. With professional body membership secured and regulation on the horizon, demands for better pay, higher status and more training will soon follow.

Taken together, these two trends at both ends of the profession illustrate the fluidity and complexity of nursing's professional status. As university-educated, high-flying practitioners move into semi-medical or more autonomous nursing roles, the top of the profession shifts 'upwards' (these practitioners are starting to demand comparable pay and conditions with doctors). Meanwhile, with the cessation of enrolled nurse training, the gap at the 'bottom' is filled by health care assistants with NVQ training, by experiments with generic workers or multi-skilling and, as always, by nursing auxiliaries and other support workers. These are still the people giving much, if not most, hands-on care in formal settings, casting doubt on the extent of the influence of the much-vaunted changes in care delivery methods and philosophies.

All these developments have different, even contradictory implications. In analysing them we should remember the many reasons underlying role change. Historical, class and gender factors influence the division of labour in health care more strongly than ideals: such factors include government policy decisions which have nothing to do with health; the state of the labour market; the demands/desires of the dominant profession; the demands/desires of the subordinate profession; the attitudes of the employer; the attitudes and aptitudes of the individual nurse; legal constraints; trade union pressure, including restrictive practices; and working conditions, especially for women with children/dependants. The needs of the population or the individual user are probably the least influential factor.

For whatever reason the role of the nurse will continue to evolve. They will be more accountable for their actions and more the judge of their own competence, as expressed in the ethical framework of the *Code of professional conduct* (NMC 2002a). The implementation in 2000 of the UK Human Rights Act (1998) sharpened the focus on the human rights framework within which professional codes operate, placing greater emphasis on the nurse's duty of care at all times and accelerating the shift away from a narrow definition of professional ethics towards a wider focus on citizens' rights (British Medical Association 2001).

All these changes are undoubtedly taking some nurses into areas beyond 'traditional' nursing. They may also lead to some practitioners feeling a stronger identity with non-nurses in the same discipline than with nurses in other disciplines, which could have far-reaching implications for the professional identity and unity of nursing. Meanwhile, provider institutions will continue to enjoy considerable independence in how they interpret and implement government guidance, with ever greater fragmentation of the service. A number of apparently contradictory trends could therefore coexist. For instance, skill mix exercises may well reduce the qualified workforce sharply in some areas while having no impact elsewhere; multi-skilling will be pursued by some employers but not others; pay varies from one part of the country to another; and while some organizations may wish to pursue a traditional model of nursing, others will push the concept to its limits. With such diversity, the challenge is to maintain the focus on what matters most – the patient and client.

AN EDUCATION REVOLUTION

A further factor fuelling these changes is the extraordinary flowering of nursing education and continuing professional development, which increase the academic credibility and currency of nursing as well as the educational level of individual nurses. New professorial chairs have been created, growing numbers of nurses are publishing research studies in books and scholarly journals, and nurse academics are leading faculties of health as well as research units and university departments. The last decade of the 20th century saw dramatic reshaping of pre-registration programmes under the banner of Project 2000, which, despite inevitable teething problems, produced a new generation of nurses. Educated to diploma or degree level in higher education settings, these nurses are more confident, articulate, not content to be medical handmaidens, and committed to continuing their professional and personal development.

Offering both stick and carrot, the then United Kingdom Central Council for Nursing, Midwifery and Health Visiting (UKCC) took the bold step of introducing a requirement that each nurse, midwife and health visitor on the register should prove their entitlement to practise by providing evidence of professional updating (UKCC 1994a). The requirements of its post-registration education and practice (PREP) scheme are modest enough but the move itself was revolutionary and far-reaching. It reinforced the growing commitment to lifelong learning in a focused way and obliged employers and educators to consider how they could meet the continuing education needs of qualified staff. The nursing profession will need to update PREP to keep pace with public expectations and health care developments.

Despite this progress, there were increasing concerns that some newly registered nurses were nevertheless lacking in competence to practise. The relationship of academic study to practice, especially in such a rapidly changing environment, is unclear, while research into education outcomes and fitness for purpose is highly complex and underdeveloped, and its findings do not necessarily point clearly to what changes should be made. However, the UKCC grasped the nettle (UKCC Commission for Nursing and Midwifery Education 1999) and recommended measures that would enable fitness for practice based on health care need. The resulting competencies required on qualification as a nurse (UKCC 2001a) were agreed UK-wide and their implementation supported by government. Time will tell what difference the greater emphasis on supporting learning in practice has made, at a time when clinical areas have experienced extreme workload pressures and staff shortages.

The re-thinking of professional roles and relationships discussed above lays down another challenge to mono-professional education such as nursing and medicine. There is an increasing realization that the development of seamless, patient-centred care needs to start with multi-professional pre-registration education. This idea is not new and many initiatives have been established, such as multi-professional skills laboratories and shared lectures, but following the government's stated goal in the NHS Plan (DoH 2000a), the Department of Health in England is now encouraging a more concerted effort to rethink pre-registration education for health professionals, using four pilot sites to develop new model curricula with significant inter-professional learning components throughout. Success will depend on how far the professions are able to shift towards a truly inter-professional approach to the common goal of patient-centred health care.

LOOKING TO THE FUTURE

All these issues provide endless fuel for controversy in professional nursing circles. They seem important, but nurses sometimes lose sight of the real question: what difference does all this make to patients? Does what people want from their nurses remain fundamentally unchanged, and if so, are we focusing on the right things?

Many nurses believe that the work of the nurse, whatever the setting, draws upon a tradition of caring based around both skills and values. For example, when the four UK government chief nurses brought together an expert group to consider the challenges for nursing and midwifery in the 21st century, the so-called Heathrow debate of 1993, it argued the existence of something called 'the nursing constant', a key subset of characteristics which represented the 'fundamental attributes of a nurse' (DoH 1994a). Though some years have passed since that debate, its conclusions still represent the prevailing view. The nurse's work, it said, includes:

- a co-ordinating function
- a teaching function, for carers, patients and professionals
- developing and maintaining programmes of care
- technical expertise, exercised personally or through others
- concern for the ill, but also for those currently well
- a special responsibility for the frail and vulnerable.

It is hard to dispute these functions, which have been extensively explored in recent years. It is instructive, though, to compare them with the 10 key roles recently outlined by the government chief nurse in England (Box 1.3), which appear superficially more empowering and autonomous but also suggest a return to the task-oriented approach that nursing has spent much effort trying to shake off. It is also worth considering the viewpoint of other health professionals. Is there any reason why a doctor could not sign up to such a description? If, as seems very probable, there is still more that unites than divides the health professions, a new inclusive agenda for the future could be drawn up which concerns itself not so much with drawing lines between different professional territories, but with how the professions' combined skills can best meet patients' needs.

REACTING AGAINST MATERIALISM

The 'nursing constant' alluded to above runs deeper than the rather functional values, attributes and roles listed at Heathrow. Every skilled nurse knows that the subtle processes of healing, of living with disability and of dying a good death have strong psychological, emotional and even spiritual dimensions, although they can be hard to put into words. This is an area where nursing can really come into its own in future.

More and more people, reacting against the gross materialism and greed of the early 21st century, are looking for a spiritual dimension in their lives; seeking healing and meaning in making deeper connections with others, in work and personal life. For a minority this may mean involvement in organized religion, but for most it takes more diffuse forms. In nursing, this spiritual revival glows in the explosion of interest in complementary therapies. From aromatherapy to massage, the ancient healing arts are putting nurses back in touch with values and experiences that are in danger of being destroyed by rapid patient throughputs, cash crises and staff shortages. Indeed, in combination with the deceptively simple acts of 'basic' nursing care, they give nurses the chance to practise the interpersonal and technical skills that attracted them to nursing in the first place.

Nursing's achievements, in complementary therapies and in more mainstream domains, epitomize the type of skills, knowledge and attitudes which could be heavily in demand in the near future. In fact they are heavily in demand now, but society and individuals are still too frightened to acknowledge openly the depth of their need. As the pendulum swings back to humanitarian values, nursing will be increasingly appreciated: not patronizingly, but a true appreciation, at last, of the fact that human beings' physical, intellectual, emotional and spiritual faculties are intertwined; and that caring for another person means paying attention to all those dimensions and their interaction.

Nursing can lead itself and others in that humane direction, but only if nurses can get in touch with their own power and believe in their own potential. This requires what has been dubbed the 'remoralization' of nursing – in both its meanings: raising morale but also reinforcing the moral roots of the profession. This will not be a restrictive Victorian morality, but a reaffirmation of the key values shared by many in every health care occupation and by many service users and carers. It could form the basis of alliances across professional, gender, race, class and cultural divides, in projects and ways of working that not only tolerate but celebrate differences while developing shared visions and goals.

BEYOND ORTHODOX POLICIES

In their necessary efforts to make the world sit up and take notice of them, nurses have emphasized their uniqueness. Healthy self-esteem is essential, but this focus on uniqueness has sometimes been a mask for insecurity. It is time to adopt a different strategy, not least because nurses do not have a monopoly on caring, and such statements alienate potential allies among patients, carers, support workers and other professionals. As argued above, we need a revitalized form of professionalism that empowers patients and involves all colleagues in an interdependent decision-making process that sees responsibility as collective as well as individual.

This does not mean nurses can give up more orthodox forms of political activity, where they have made great strides. Strong professional organizations, trade unions and networks are still vital to fight for nurses' rights, influence decision-making and court public opinion. Better pay, working conditions and child care, better staffing levels, improved education, adequate research funds, a functioning clinical career structure and representation of nurses at the highest levels of management and policy-making are all important aims to be fought for relentlessly.

Not much headway will be made, however, unless nursing works on the issues raised by the new professionalism, such as how to develop specific practitioner strengths without retreating into tribalism, and how to share decision-making with clients and communities. In doing so nurses should remember that they may sometimes feel weak but are actually, in many ways, strong. Nursing is the largest health profession (and the oldest), health services would collapse without it, it enjoys enormous public support and most of the time it provides excellent service.

CONCLUSION

This chapter has taken a panoramic view of nursing today. Starting with an overview of the current political, social and health status of Europe, it has attempted to locate nursing in the UK in a wider global context. WHO's Health for All movement and its emphasis on primary health care have been advocated as a helpful policy framework for nursing. However, despite lip-service to it, a brief analysis of European health care reform showed that Health for All and primary health care are not high on the agenda.

Moving on to assess the role and influence of nursing on health care reform in Europe, this chapter reached largely pessimistic conclusions. However, it pointed to many interesting developments which demonstrate how nursing is responding to change – and being shaped by it, willingly or not. In the UK, policy-makers led by the incoming Labour government have since 1997 been introducing many positive changes that raise the status of nursing and provide new opportunities and challenges to improve the scope and quality of nursing practice in both primary health care and hospitals. Special attention was paid to the prevailing preoccupation with changes in the nursing role, which is not a new phenomenon but has special and current interest. Changes at the 'top' and 'bottom' of the profession, also linked with changing patterns of care delivery and a revolution in nursing education, were seen to have potentially far-reaching effects on health care and nursing.

Finally, the chapter ended with a plea for a new type of professionalism which looks beyond territorial boundaries and tunes in to the real needs of society and individuals. One area seen as ripe for development was the weaving together by nurses, patients and other professionals, in partnership, of the physical, social, emotional and spiritual domains of human life in order to create patterns of care and relationships which are truly holistic and healing. I have included this challenge, along with my other goals for European nursing, in Box 1.4.

Box 1.4 Nursing in Europe: challenges for the next decade

- Maintain a rock-solid commitment to equity and social justice, wherever and whenever nursing care is given
- Challenge the attitudes, forces and traditions that impede progress and perpetuate inequalities within the profession and in society at large
- Welcome and encourage diversity and difference in all its forms, among patients and communities, and within the profession
- Focus on interventions that serve the many rather than the privileged few, leading to a sharper focus on public health and primary health care
- Work towards a new professionalism based on reflective practice, empowerment of patients and colleagues, interdependent decision processes, and engagement rather than detachment
- Recognize that health care is in permanent transition, that change is a way of life and that how we do things counts as much as what we do
- Honour ourselves, our patients and their carers as beings whose physical, intellectual, emotional and spiritual faculties are inextricably intertwined, and reshape our nursing care accordingly
- Taking all this into account, have the courage and vision to risk new styles of leadership that will transform nursing, health care and our world in the 21st century

Peering into the crystal ball may not reveal a clear future, but it shows us that nursing will always be needed, and that its dearest values may be about to make a big comeback. Our troubled world badly needs them.

PRINCIPLES OF PROFESSIONAL PRACTICE

Norma Fryer

INTRODUCTION

The first part of this chapter focuses on the key principles of what it means to be a professional. An overview of the key points in the professional evolution of nursing is provided along with some comparisons with the growth of midwifery as a profession. The chapter explores the values and principles that surround the context of nursing as a 'profession' and the nurse as a 'professional'.

 The second part of the chapter brings together the *Code of professional conduct* (NMC 2002a), which describes the values and responsibilities incumbent on a nurse from which all other guidance and advice is derived, and the competencies required to be fit for practice (UKCC 2001a). The two are part and parcel of each other, forming an explicit pledge to the public on what they can expect from a registered, and therefore licensed, professional practitioner. The *Code* represents a template against which all practitioners should establish and evaluate their individual actions. Throughout, the word 'Council' is used to mean the regulator either in its United Kingdom Central Council for Nursing, Midwifery and Health Visiting (UKCC) or Nursing and Midwifery Council (NMC) form.

Whatever the chosen route to registration as a nurse, midwife or health visitor, a key feature of that achievement is that it denotes membership of a recognized profession. This role and the expectations that accompany being a member of a professional group present many challenges throughout the career of any nurse, midwife or health visitor and deserve specific attention from all those seeking to share the responsibility of such a position.

One of the key features of belonging to a profession is that it holds an acknowledged position within the society it serves. There are therefore certain expectations that are required of all who seek to and subsequently achieve a licence to practise. An integral part of the preparation for achieving this licence is to have an understanding of what is expected from a professional nurse and how this may be nurtured during the course of any programme of education.

The recent changes in the programmes of education for initial registration as a nurse or midwife are aimed at preparing students seeking a career in a particular branch of nursing, or in midwifery, for the diverse and sometimes complex situations that contemporary health care demands. The rapid growth in science and technology, coupled with the increased diversity in social and cultural attitudes and behaviour, have resulted in a major shift in the expectations of those who need the services of health care personnel. To accommodate such changes, there is a constant demand for health care professionals to develop their roles, responsibilities and approaches to practice (UKCC 2001a).

As a measure of the professional commitment to serve and protect the interests and well-being of the public, the professional nurse, midwife or health visitor is required to own and reflect, as part of the licence to practise, the values and responsibilities incumbent on a professional.

DEVELOPMENT OF NURSING AS A PROFESSION

The evolution of nursing as a recognized profession has been the subject of much deliberation (McGann 1992). The early effort for recognition of the professional standing for nursing was much thwarted by its roots as an occupation carried out by women and hence of low social status (Simnett 1986; Dingwall *et al.* 1995). Indeed, the Registrar General's classification of social class still identifies the social status of doctors, dentists, opticians and pharmacists as being superior to that of nurses, midwives, health visitors and those from other professions allied to medicine (Davies 1995).

To be a member of a professional group supports a general view that those who belong to the group provide some kind of personal service to clients. The traditional view of a profession, and usually a male-dominated profession such as medicine or law, is its association with certain features: professional self-governance, professional autonomy and registration of practitioners; setting and monitoring standards for practice and education; having a specialized body of knowledge and a monopoly for practice in certain fields, education in a university and a public ideology of service to clients (Freidson 1970; Jackson 1970).

All health care practitioners in contemporary practice are required to have both the knowledge and understanding of the professional framework for practice and must demonstrate this through their practice. As Fletcher and Buker (1999) explain, although the influence of the regulatory body is focused on registered practitioners, those training for the professions must recognize from the outset, the commitment and responsibilities that 'being a professional' demands and the competencies required in practice to demonstrate that accomplishment.

To explore the current position of nursing and the standards that symbolize its place in the world of the professional practitioner, it is important to examine how nursing has adopted some of the key features of a traditional profession.

PROFESSIONAL SELF-REGULATION AND AUTONOMY

Johnston (1972) asserts a commonly accepted view of a profession as an agent of occupational control of its members. The self-governing nature of a true profession is seen as critical to its success. Professions are legitimized by the state and are therefore bound by certain legal impositions on practice. As such, it was a notable point in history when the Midwives Act (1902) and the Nurses Registration Act (1919) gave statutory recognition to a regulatory framework developed through the work of the Central Midwives Board (CMB) and the General Nursing Council (GNC), respectively.

The move toward state registration did not arouse uniform acceptance from either the medical profession or some sections of the nursing and midwifery professions, which were threatened in different ways by the potential implications of self-regulation (White 1976). The medical profession enjoyed the benefits of self-regulation, autonomy and a monopoly for practice through the establishment of the General Medical Council (GMC) in 1858 (Blane 1988). This was not to be the experience for either nursing or midwifery; professional autonomy was a concept not validated by the 1902 and 1919 Acts. Unlike doctors, nurses and midwives were to be the subject of scrutiny and control from the state and the more powerful influences of the medical profession. A number of contributory reasons have been associated with this. For many years the legacy of Florence Nightingale's leadership style, coupled with the institutionalization of nursing and later midwifery, did little to empower practitioners. Girvin (1998) suggests that while Nightingale was herself a powerful woman and an influential figure in policy-making at the time, the dominance of the medical profession had a lasting impact on the development of nursing as a profession in its own right. Any real impact on the autonomy of the profession was yet to come.

Blane (1988) explains that the 'leading' professions, to which he assigns medicine, differ from the 'lesser' professions, to which he assigns nursing by virtue of the position that access to clients 'is only through the instruction of the leading profession' (p216). His examination of the major differences between the professions of nursing and medicine provides a clear reminder of the subservient role of nursing even in the latter part of 20th century. While the capacity to exercise self-governance evolved through the ceaseless efforts of those determined to see changes, the first major reform to the regulatory framework did not take place until the enactment of the Nurses, Midwives and Health Visitors Act (1979).

These regulatory reforms saw the demise of the CMB and GNC within the UK. They were replaced by one body, the UKCC. This caused much dissent from some factions of the midwifery profession concerned that the absence of a separate regulatory body for midwives would be a retrograde step to its independence from nursing. A separate chapter would be needed to do justice to the position taken by those midwives whose mission had been to maintain a separate identity for midwifery (see Garcia *et al.* 1990 in Further Reading).

Nonetheless, the move towards a larger and more resolute regulatory framework was proposed through the UKCC. In order for the then new Council to project its role and assert greater power on the professional standing of nursing and midwifery, its regulatory function and purpose needed to be more accessible to its registrants. The UKCC reviewed and presented national standards for both education and practice and, as part of its regulatory function, began to issue written advice and guidance on the expected behaviour and conduct to all its registrants. The emphasis on self-governance and autonomy of the individual practitioner became an important feature encouraging practitioners to use the regulatory body as a support and guide to good practice rather than one whose main purpose was punitive.

A much clearer foundation was set from which practice could be monitored and judged. The traditional features of a profession were presented through a framework that required attention to the prevailing values and beliefs of the profession, expressed in a Code of professional conduct and through a set of competencies. These applied not only through standards set for entry and initial registration but were to reflect the requirements for sustaining a licence with a much greater focus on how the values of the profession would ensure an appropriate service to the public.

The 1992 amendment to the Nurses, Midwives and Health Visitors Act (1979) resulted in a proliferation of guidance documents from the Council with a more overt quest to establish a distinct image for the professional nurse, midwife and health visitor. Public protection was at its root and was made explicit. Running parallel to the government's reforms of the NHS in the 1990s was a review of professional regulation. The last Conservative government commissioned an independent review of the two sets of legislation underpinning the regulation of professions allied to medicine, and nurses, midwives and health visitors, respectively. The report (JM Consulting 1998), covering the four National Boards and the UKCC, led to the most recent reforms in professional regulation and culminated in the establishment of the Nursing and Midwifery Council (NMC) in April 2002. Changing professional regulation is part of the modernization of the health service and continues through the initiatives of the present government (DoH 1999a).

Although the focus on self-regulation and the exercise of achieving greater autonomy occupy a continued place in the professional development of nursing, exploration of the practice of nursing has followed a more complex path.

SPECIALIST KNOWLEDGE AND MONOPOLY FOR PRACTICE

Perhaps the most contentious aspect of the search for an enhanced professional standing rests with identifying the distinctive nature of nursing and hence its monopoly for practice. This debate had always divided nursing from midwifery and is one that continues to arouse much discord. While midwifery has within its statute some clearly defined boundaries from which practice is identified and governed (UKCC 1998a), the same cannot be said for nursing. As such, the identification of a 'specialist field of knowledge' that reflects the activity of nursing as a measure of its monopoly for practice, continues to present an important challenge.

Those seeking to enhance the professional standing of nursing sought to compete with the GMC's objective that persons requiring medical aid should be enabled to distinguish between qualified and unqualified practitioners (Blane 1988). The statutory requirement that outlined the activities of a midwife demanded a concerted effort to pursue and eliminate non-*bona fide* midwives from the profession (Robinson 1990). For nursing, the task of policing a 'profession' where such boundaries were more diverse, was problematic. Nonetheless, the emergence of the nurse theorist and the proliferation of the literature in both the UK and the US saw a new approach to this challenge; one that focused on the process as much as the activity of nursing.

The development of a theory for nursing could be said to date back to Florence Nightingale's *Notes on Nursing* (King 1981). Attempts to embrace the essence of nursing were to be explored later through an identification of nursing models and systems of care. In short, the concept of a 'model' for nursing was introduced in an attempt to identify the value, belief or ideology that would underpin the practice of nursing care of individual client groups (Aggleton and Chalmers 2000). Some of the earlier work on models was done by Peplau in the 1950s; the dissemination of other models in the 1970s and 80s aimed to explore the essence of nursing in a more explicit way (Peplau 1988; Orem 1995; Pearson 1996; Roper 2000).

Virginia Henderson, one of the most celebrated authors to explore the concept of nursing models as an inherent feature of a new paradigm for nursing practice, attempted to define the nurse's role:

'… to assist the individual sick or well in the performance of those activities contributing to health or its recovery (or to a peaceful death) that he would perform unaided if he had the necessary strength, will or knowledge'.

(Henderson 1969)

Other efforts to explore the process, rather than the tasks or activities of nursing, brought a revolutionary approach to how care was managed and delivered. The 'Nursing Process' saw the introduction of a more systematic inquiry into how patients' needs would be assessed, planned implemented and evaluated. It brought a new and more structured framework from which nursing could be examined (Christensen 1995). The main purpose of this new dimension was to encourage the skills of decision-making and problem-solving in a more holistic way than had been seen in the more task-orientated approaches of the past.

Benner's work in the 1980s brought a further dimension to the discussion and provoked much debate about the differences between theoretical knowledge and its application in practice (Benner 1984). Benner suggested that the development of skills was not always accompanied by an understanding of theory and that it was important for nurses to have the know *how* as well as the know *what* of practice. This encouraged the shift towards nurses undertaking an increasing number of tasks normally carried out by doctors, exacerbated in part by the growing demand for a decrease in doctors' hours (Greenhalgh and Co. 1994). Over time there has been an almost inevitable expansion in the work carried out by health care assistants to 'fill the gap' left by nurses and a significant shift in the boundaries for practice of all those involved in health care provision.

The growth and development of nursing towards an increase in activities normally carried out by doctors has perhaps failed to clarify the distinctive nature of nursing practice. However, it is towards the changes in education that this chapter now turns, to locate their impact on the professionalization of nursing.

EDUCATION

A distinguishing feature of a profession is the nature of the education of its members and the educational reform of nursing and midwifery has had significant influence on the professional standing of both groups. At the end of the 19th century, the Nightingale Training Schools for Nurses and Midwives provided the first formal education (Woodham Smith 1952). However, it was nearly a century before the move to a university education saw any radical changes in the organization, content and status of programmes of education.

The 1970s saw an acknowledgement for change proposed in the Briggs Report (1972), but this was not enacted until the review of pre-registration programmes in the 1980s (UKCC 1986). This represented a major change in nurse education and professional nursing structures in the UK. It was anticipated that the outcomes of such programmes would see the emergence of a new 'knowledge-able doer' (Slevin 1992).

Such reforms included the introduction of curricular based upon research, opening up new horizons for nurses on both pre- and post-registration programmes (Benner and Wrubel 1989). The value of research as a means to underpin practice was fundamental to the growth and recognition of nursing, not merely as a means of enhancing its professional status but also of replacing outdated practices based on custom rather than grounded in evidence.

One major theme that emerged throughout this new approach to education was the emphasis on the essence of care, described by Kirby and Slein (1992) as a 'new curriculum for care'. Other important elements of problem-solving, critical thinking and reflective practice were formalized as an essential component of the competencies for the nurse of the late 20th century. The study of ethics was introduced where issues relating to moral responsibility were presented in a different way from the pronouncements of the past. The emphasis became that of the individual nurse being required to accept and carry the burden of judgement and decision-making (Hunt 1992). For Hunt the new reforms set out in the Project 2000 report were:

'... underpinned by the notion of a morally responsible and ethically accountable nurse, a nurse who has broken with the unthinking subservience of the past'.

(Hunt 1992, p98)

The introduction of ethics paved the way for a more frank acknowledgement of the client's participation in the care process. Hunt explained how the new curriculum was designed to promote the concept that the nurse must learn to respect the values and desires of the individual patient or client and that students should no longer be treated as 'passive unquestioning recipients' of a limited range of practical skills. This was further enhanced by the legal sanction given through Rule 18 of the Nurses, Midwives and Health Visitors (Amendment) Act (1992) which required that practice should be measured through a set of identified nursing competencies.

In the years that followed, the drive to enhance the professional status of nursing was seen through this new approach to education (Buckenham 1992). A new energy was released that supported an extension of the way the nurse as a professional partner in care should be seen. Overall, the move of nurse and midwife preparation into higher education institutions added the kudos of academic achievement to the professional qualification, with a greater emphasis on research-based practice and an acknowledgement of the shifting boundaries of practice.

However, an evaluation of the Project 2000 programmes of education demonstrated that there were concerns about nurses' fitness for practice at the point of registration (Bartlett *et al.* 1998). As a consequence, the UKCC set up the Commission for Nursing and Midwifery Education to reassess and re-evaluate the preparation for the professional role and:

'to prepare a way forward for pre-registration of nursing and midwifery education that enables fitness for practice based on health care need'.

(UKCC Commission for Nursing and Midwifery Education 1999, section 1)

The resulting *Fitness for Practice* report (UKCC Commission for Nursing and Midwifery Education 1999) identified the need for a more balanced focus on the achievement of both practice-based competencies and those that would reflect the core values of the profession. Therefore, a direct link was made between the accomplishment of competencies for registration and the professional development of the nurse, one that was seen as 'fundamental to the autonomy and accountability of the individual practitioner and therefore fundamental to the *Code of professional conduct*' (UKCC 2001a).

For the first time, the focus on the values and beliefs underpinning practice can be seen to be integrated into pre-registration programmes, strengthening the third and most immutable trademark of a profession – one that seeks to identify the standard of expected conduct and behaviour as a true reflection of the ideology of the time.

PUBLIC IDEOLOGY AND STANDARDS FOR CONDUCT AND BEHAVIOUR

The public perspective and expectation of service provided by the health professional presents the foundation from which all standards for practice and behaviour are determined. Moreover, they represent the core from which the values and beliefs of that profession are confirmed and the root from which codes of conduct and practice are derived.

The trait that identifies the public service element of the role and the relationship between the health care practitioner and the client excites a very different ideology in today's practice compared with the tenets of the past. Efforts to unite the relationship between the patient or client and health professional in a way that facilitates a more equitable partnership are relatively new and have evolved as part of the social and political changes of the 20th century.

Blane (1988) affirms that a duty to serve the public demands that the interests of the client are placed before your own. He claims that the professional is required not to exploit a client's ignorance or their dependence on that profession's specialized knowledge. This somewhat altruistic sentiment has its origins in the first codes of practice from both nursing and medical tenets. Whilst the Hippocratic oath (Faulder 1985) presented the first moral code for medical practice, the early foundations for a nurses' code of practice can be associated with the spirited authority of Florence Nightingale, which would set the scene for what was to come.

The expectations expressed by Nightingale were clear. Nurses had a moral record and a technical record that were scrutinized closely. The moral record had punctuality, quietness, trustworthiness, personal neatness, cleanliness, ward management and order, as values to be pursued. 'Flirtation' was punished by dismissal, with discretion an essential quality. Any failing in this direction was seen as a major deterrent towards the hopes of reforming the nursing profession and elevating its status (Woodham Smith 1952).

Evidence of Nightingale's moral demands is well documented and clearly reflects Victorian ideals. Nevertheless, her perception of the virtue of 'obedience' is often misjudged. There is little doubt that Nightingale expected nurses to recognize the need for observance to certain rules. In doing so she did not expect that compliance with such rules should represent subservience to the doctor. As her *Notes on Nursing* suggest:

'no man, not even a doctor ever gives any other definition of what a nurse should be than *devoted and obedient.* This definition would do just as well for a porter; it might even do for a horse. It seems a commonly received idea among men, and even among women themselves, that it requires nothing but a disappointment in love, or incapacity in other things, to turn a woman into a good nurse'.

(Woodham Smith 1952, p271)

The concept of obedience towards good moral conduct rules remained a dominant feature throughout the first half of the 20th century, a legacy, many would argue, from the somewhat military approach of the Nightingale era. 'Moral and spiritual wholeness' exemplified the ideal nurse (Hector 1968). While this did little to encourage the type of critical thinking and decision-making required of today's practitioner, the power and influence of Florence Nightingale on health care policy was a virtue that would be seen as an asset in contemporary practice.

However, what was to become a redeeming feature of the nurse, which Hector described as a 'crowning quality', was integrity, a characteristic that is fundamental to the professional nurse. The latter part of the 20th century saw for the first time an attempt to encapsulate such values in what was to become the first *International Code of Ethics* (1965, revised 1973), produced by the International Council for Nurses (ICN). This presented a framework which forms the basis of the current *Code of professional conduct* (Singleton and McLaren 1995).

A foundation had been laid for the nursing profession to claim an internationally recognized set of values for its practitioners. In the 1980s the new regulatory body (UKCC) ventured towards a more resolute position, identifying its own standard and values through a written framework for practice. The latter part of the 20th century began to witness nurses who were required to be more empowered in their practice yet able to reflect a professional image that would unite the values and expressions of good conduct.

A NEW PROFESSIONALISM

Davies (1996) described the changes as a move towards a 'new professionalism' required to meet the needs of the 21st century, and expressed some caution that an enhanced professional status may carry the risk of being maligned by those who saw it as an opportunity to exercise professional power. For Salvage (1998) a use of power was seen as a basis for increasing the authority of both the profession of nursing and the professional nurse to make decisions, claiming that it would encourage the individual to be responsible and accountable for what they did. For this to be real and effective, Salvage argued that the evolving new styles of professional behaviour should be based on 'doing things with rather than to' the recipients of health care.

As one of the most insightful authors of the 20th century, Salvage made a plea for a new type of professionalism; one that would look 'beyond territorial boundaries', that would 'tune into' the real needs of society and individuals. She expressed this as something that would result in the development of 'truly holistic and healing patterns of care and relationships' (Salvage 1998, p16). Although Hector's 'moral and spiritual wholeness' may not be embraced in quite the same way by today's recruits, the essence of her plea to maintain 'integrity', as with Florence Nightingale's demand for 'discretion', must be recognized as central to the principles that underpin the professional role of the nurse in the 21st century.

As nursing represents the largest of the health care professions, the new millennium poses new challenges for those who choose to enter the profession. Nursing has a leading role in the provision of health care and this demands a new approach to the development of nursing as a profession.

It should embrace a wider understanding that it need not seek to emulate traditional professional characteristics. Nursing is unique in its framework of caring and as such should be seen as a profession valued for its own contribution to the public health and welfare. This does, however, demand a commitment in both the education of nurses and the practice of nursing to honour certain duties that separate the 'professional practitioner' from other occupational groups not required through any statutory reinforcement to monitor or ensure standards of practice from all its members.

To reflect those qualities that will best serve either the client or the profession, how should the nurses of the new millennium be empowered to promote those values that represent the essence of nursing for the future?

PROFESSIONAL PRACTICE: OLD VALUES AND NEW CULTURE FOR CARE

As a reflection of the values and beliefs of the professions of nursing and midwifery, the guidance from the regulatory body is presented in the form of statutory rules, professional codes, competencies for practice on qualification and advisory documents. Individual accountability is the key and must be applied to the patient or client, the profession, the law and, unless self-employed, to the employer.

Such accountability requires practitioners, on an individual basis, to engage in exploring personal values and ethics in order to participate in seeking shared outcomes with patients and clients, and mutually accepted goals with other professionals. An additional dimension for this has been the hitherto unprecedented expectations of society, increasingly aware of the rights and information so often denied in the past and more enlightened to the shortfalls and fallibility of the health service. A new culture for care has arisen where it has become necessary to formalize an ethical framework for practice to complement those of the profession and the law. Greater consideration is given to the duty of care that underpins the nurse's role, now represented within the regulatory framework, employment contract, health care legislation and through the requests and demands of individual patients or clients.

To examine this duty of care further, the remainder of the chapter focuses on how the *Code of professional conduct* acts as a template on which all professional dimensions of practice are grounded.

SUMMARY

Membership of a professional group requires achievement and maintenance of competence and behaviour that justify the trust and confidence of the public in that profession. The development of nursing and midwifery as professions through regulation, the nature of practice, education and public expectations, have been enhanced both nationally and internationally. The result is a distinct set of values and beliefs that provide a robust and unique framework for the health care practice that the public need and expect. However, maintaining the momentum of that development may mean that nursing does not have to continue to emulate all the traditional characteristics of a profession. There is a new professionalism and culture of care emerging that seeks to 'work with' rather than 'do to' patients and clients. The practice of individual accountability within a robust framework of professional values and beliefs is the key.

THE *CODE OF PROFESSIONAL CONDUCT* AS A FRAMEWORK FOR PROFESSIONAL PRACTICE

The *Code of professional conduct* was initially drawn up by the UKCC under the powers of the Nurses, Midwives and Health Visitors Act (1979). One of the first activities of the new NMC was to publish a new *Code of professional conduct* (NMC 2002a) as a reminder that it is 'the single most important document published by the regulatory body' (NMC 2002b). The new *Code* replaced the 1992 version and two other guidance documents – the UKCC (1992) *Scope of Professional Practice* and the UKCC (1996a) *Guidelines for Professional Practice* – and applies to all nurses and midwives. The *Midwives Rules and Code of Professional Practice* (UKCC 1998a) has a unique place in the process of registration for midwives. Although these rules are not shared by the nursing profession, many of the key principles of good practice contained within them have equal application to nursing.

The *Code of professional conduct* presents the professional framework from which practice is judged. The seven guiding principles (see below, Box 2.2) represent the shared values of all eight UK regulators of health care professionals (NMC 2002a). This is an important presentation of unity to patients and clients who should have confidence that all health care professionals work within the same frame of values. The eight health care regulatory bodies are:

- The Nursing and Midwifery Council
- The Health Professions Council
- The General Medical Council
- The General Dental Council
- The General Optical Council
- The General Chiropractic Council
- The General Osteopathic Council
- The Royal Pharmaceutical Society of Great Britain.

The *Code* encompasses key principles that combine professional duties with patient's rights and, to that end, provides an ethical dimension of accepted behaviour that would satisfy the expectations of the community. The emphasis on public protection and the accountability of each registered practitioner to enact this cannot be overstated. This has far reaching implications in terms of the demands it places on each individual's accountability as it involves how people behave not only to clients but also to each other as professionals and to society.

Singleton and McLaren (1995, p135) suggest that professional codes function as a 'framework for decision-making which enshrines contemporary views of professional morality'. They add that the content of a code should be interpreted as a guide to professional conduct and moral obligation within caring relationships which are based upon trust, worth and dignity. For Hunt (1992), a professional code seeks not to resolve moral problems but to present enforceable minimum standards for practice that act as directives to be used as 'reminders' rather than 'resolutions'.

THE *CODE* AND COMPETENCIES FOR PRACTICE

The standards set by the regulatory body are met through the successful achievement of a series of competencies that combine a number of different aspects of practice. These are currently expressed as 'domains' and fall into four categories (UKCC 2001a):

- care delivery
- care management
- personal and professional development
- professional and ethical practice.

Entry to the profession is therefore seen through the development of knowledge and expertise that embrace clinical activity, interpersonal skills and a commitment to the values of the profession. In acknowledgement of this, the Council expects that an 'acceptance and internalisation of the *Code of professional conduct*' be seen as an inherent part of the process leading to registration (UKCC 2001a, section 32).

The regulatory body captured the essence of this as part of the new educational philosophy for the 21st century:

'The UKCC values the rights implicit in the social contract between the profession and society to participate in the health care of the individuals, families and communities. Such rights also carry obligations. These include not only the responsibility to provide safe and effective care but also responsibility for the highest standards of professional conduct and ethical practice'.

(UKCC 2001a, section 31)

The standards set by the regulatory body apply from the moment a commitment is made to enter a programme of study (UKCC 1998b). It is, therefore, incumbent upon all students to grasp the link between the competencies for practice and the guiding principles that underpin the *Code of professional conduct* which apply to all practice interventions. The principles outlined within the *Code* need to be examined with reference to those competencies; ones that reflect the 'being' rather than the 'doing' element of nursing.

REFLECTION POINT

Consider how aware you were when you started your programme of the existence of the *Code of professional conduct* and its connection with the competencies you will require on registration.

THE *CODE* AND PRINCIPLES FOR PRACTICE

The *Code of professional conduct* (NMC 2002a) presents an unequivocal message to reflect the personal accountability and sense of moral responsibility that an individual practitioner must convey to his/her role (Box 2.1).

Box 2.1 Professional accountability (NMC 2002a, section 1.2)

As a registered nurse or midwife you must:
- Protect and support the health of the individual patients and clients
- Protect and support the wider community
- Act in such a way that justifies the trust and confidence the public have in you
- Uphold and enhance the good reputation of the professions

Each of these requirements is expressed within seven guiding principles that reflect the personal accountability each nurse or midwife has in caring for patients and clients (Box 2.2). An expansion of these principles prompts a series of expected behaviours from which practice is judged. Each of these principles will be considered in turn with an opening reference to the competency for practice that relates to the principle.

Box 2.2 Principles for practice (NMC 2002a)

- Respect the patient or client as an individual
- Obtain consent before you give any treatment or care
- Co-operate with others in the team
- Protect confidential information
- Maintain your professional knowledge and competence
- Be trustworthy
- Act to identify and minimize risk

Respect the patient or client as an individual (*Code* section 2)

The related competencies for practice [Professional and ethical practice domain (UKCC 2001a)] are:

- practise in a fair and anti-discriminatory way, acknowledging the differences in beliefs and cultural practices of individuals and groups
- maintain support and acknowledge the rights of individuals or groups in the health care setting
- provide care which demonstrates sensitivity to the diversity of patients.

The recognition of respect for the individual needs and preferences of patients and clients lies at the heart of the therapeutic relationship; it reflects the personal responsibility assigned to each nurse or midwife to consider the importance of the partnership with the patient or client.

Each practitioner needs to recognize the rights of the individual, accept the uniqueness and diversity of people and to exercise respect and dignity towards others regardless of their differences. Without doubt this may present a major challenge at times, either when decisions made by patients and clients are in conflict with those of the professional, or where opposing values may have to be addressed through compromise.

Emphasis is also placed on 'maintaining appropriate professional boundaries' within the professional relationship, and how the interests may be promoted of those patients and clients who may need support in gaining access to health and social care.

REFLECTION POINT

From your clinical placements so far, think back to an occasion when you or your colleagues felt a patient's or client's rights had not been sufficiently addressed. How did you feel about this? What could have been done differently?

Within this section of the *Code*, the Council acknowledges the right of a nurse or midwife to conscientiously object to the participation in certain activities that may transgress his/her own moral framework or religious belief (Box 2.3; see also Chapter 4). For some, this may appear to contradict the *Code* in that it suggests that the right of the practitioner be protected over and above that of the patient or client.

Box 2.3 Reporting concerns (NMC 2002a)

You must report to a relevant person or authority, at the earliest possible time, any conscientious objection that may be relevant to your professional practice. You must continue to provide best care to the best of your ability until alternative arrangements are implemented.

As one of the more contentious elements of the *Code*, it seeks to preserve certain human or moral concerns that a practitioner may wish to express. However, there are limitations to the application of this right based upon the current legal position which identifies only two areas where a practitioner has the right, conscientiously to object to take part in treatment or care. These are through the Abortion Act (1967), which gives a practitioner the right to refuse to take part in an abortion, and the Human Fertilisation and Embryology Act (1992), which provides rights to refuse to take part in technical procedures in assisted conception.

The expression of a patient's right to a choice in health care matters has, by tradition, been driven largely by the health professional. This, as noted above, was primarily the domain of the doctor, although many nurses and midwives were not without fault in their affirmation of an equally dominant position within the patient–client relationship. As Girvin (1998) explains, the institutionalization and socialization required to survive the hierarchical styles of management seen in both public and private sector environments, paved the way for a type of behaviour that was to infiltrate all professional groups.

However, the paternalistic values associated with that approach have, as a result of the growing demands and expectations of a society far more willing to express dissatisfaction with the health service, seen the emergence of a different paradigm of care. Hence, we have seen a shift towards a more equitable relationship between carer and cared for; one that can and should no longer tolerate a lack of respect for the autonomy of the patient or client.

Perhaps the strongest reinforcement for this shift has been through the Human Rights Act (1998), which came into force in the UK in October 2000 and gave further effect to the rights enshrined in the European Court on Human Rights. The Act provides the legal support, within existing case law, for the courts to exercise a more forceful expression of individual rights. Those parts of the Act most likely to affect health care practice are identified through a series of Articles (Box 2.4).

Box 2.4 Legislation underpinning individual rights [taken from the Human Rights Act (1998) (cited in DoH 2001b)]

- Article 2: Protection of right to life
- Article 3: Prohibition of torture, inhumane or degrading treatment or punishment
- Article 5: Right to liberty and security
- Article 8: Respect for private and family life
- Article 9: Freedom of thought, conscience and religion
- Article 14: Prohibition of discrimination in enjoyment of Convention rights

The Council expects that the appropriate emphasis is given to the right, a patient or client has to make choices, reinforcing that the registered practitioner must not practise in a way which assumes that they know what is best for the patient or client. This is the position that underpins the second principle.

Obtain consent before you give any treatment or care (*Code* section 3)

The related competencies for practice [Professional and ethical practice domain (UKCC 2001a)] are:

- act to ensure that the rights of individuals and groups are not compromised
- respect the values, customs and beliefs of individuals and groups.

The principle relating to obtaining consent prior to giving any treatment or care brings with it respect for patient or client autonomy, while recognizing the complex demands that characterize the overriding professional duty of care. On the one hand, it elevates the rights of a patient to accept or refuse care or treatment, while presenting on the other, a duty to ensure that these rights are not violated irrespective of any potential harm that may be envisaged by the professional.

There are 11 requirements within this principle that seek to establish the current professional and legal position relating to the rights of patients and clients to receive information that should be 'accurate, truthful and presented in such a way that makes it easily understood' (NMC 2002a, section 3.1). It reinforces the principle of respect for autonomy for those legally competent to participate in the planning of their own care programme, making it clear that 'no one has the right to give consent on behalf of another competent adult' (NMC 2002a, section 3.9). Although the *Code* does not state explicitly that this right applies equally to individuals who lack competence, guidance is given on how to apply sound ethical practice to those whose capacity to consent is compromised or absent. This includes patients with mental illnesses, children and emergency situations. Emphasis is placed on the validity of the consent and the need for accurate documentation.

As a reminder that working 'with' patients and clients in order to serve their best interests is now much more than rhetoric, nurses must be prepared for many different scenarios. For example, in demonstrating the principle of respect for client autonomy, they may find themselves caring for the 'competent' patient who has both the capacity and ability to express an informed choice. Here, the nurse must demonstrate respect and support for the decisions made by the patient or client. Alternatively, the patient or client has the capacity to consent but may, as Teasdale (1998) suggests, express feelings of vulnerability and powerlessness in their dealings with health professionals and require a nurse to act as an advocate to speak on their behalf. There will also be patients who lack the capacity to be involved in the decision-making process; this may require the nurse to exercise professional and moral judgements for those whose views and wishes about treatment may not be known.

REFLECTION POINT

Pause for a minute to think about situations where you have seen a procedure or intervention well explained to a patient or client and how they responded. How comfortable have you felt sometimes about what a patient or client has agreed to?

The 11 requirements in this section of the *Code* are consistent with recent government legislation resulting from the retention, without informed consent, of body parts, particularly those of children, at a number of hospitals over many years. The government sets out a clear warning about the consequences of disregarding the patient's right to determine what happens to their own, or their dependent's bodies and identifies a framework of the moral and legal requirements and implications regarding a patient's right to autonomy and informed consent (DoH 2001b). The opening remarks set the scene 'A health professional who does not respect this principle may be liable both to legal action by the patient and action by their professional body' (DoH 2001c). This directive currently applies to England only. However, practitioners need to be aware of legislation in each of the four countries of the UK and any local protocol relating to consent.

Co-operation with others in the team (*Code* section 4)

The related competencies for practice are:

- establish and maintain collaborative working relationships with members of the health and social care team [Care management domain (UKCC 2001a)]
- participate in the negotiation and agreement of the care plan with the patient or client and with the carer, family or other friends as appropriate, under the supervision of a registered nurse [Care delivery domain (UKCC 2002)].

The principle makes paramount the involvement of, and respect for, colleagues, patients and their families. The need to communicate and share knowledge for the benefit of the patient or client through effective verbal and written communication processes is not a new phenomenon. However, it is clear that a resounding message was presented to all health care professionals touched by the tragedy that befell patients and their families who were the victims of the events that took place in Bristol in the 1990s (DoH 2001d).

At the heart of this message is the need for co-operation and respect for all those working within a multi-professional team and involved in the organization and delivery of a health care service. Although this is not a new concept and has been seen as fundamental to the activities and role of all nursing and midwifery practitioners for many years, it nevertheless presents a more overt expression of the value placed upon a respect for others working within the health care team as a means of benefiting patients.

This part of the *Code* reminds practitioners of the equally important contribution of the patient and client to the delivery of health care (see Box 2.5). It emphasizes how working with patients, clients and their families is vital to a successful outcome and is now seen as a fundamental component of the current health care agenda. This presents a new paradigm for practice where the patient is the central focus of the health care team's activity, which necessitates practitioners sharing knowledge, skill and expertise while remaining accountable for their individual actions or omissions.

Box 2.5 Co-operation with and respect for the whole team (NMC 2002a)

4.1 The team includes the patient or client, the patient's or client's family, informal carers and health and social professionals from the NHS and voluntary sectors.

4.2 You are expected to work co-operatively within teams and to respect skills and expertise with other members of the team as required for the benefit of patients and clients.

Protection of confidentiality (*Code* section 5)

The related competency for practice [Professional and ethical practice domain (UKCC 2001a)] is:

- practice in accordance with an ethical and legal framework which ensures the primacy of patient and client interest and well-being and respects confidentiality.

Seeking the help and advice of a health care professional almost invariably involves revealing information that people usually regard as private. In addition, it often involves allowing access to the body and, in some cases, property. It places patients and clients in a vulnerable position and one that can be fairly described as unequal in terms of power (see also Chapter 5). This inevitable imbalance places an obligation on all health care practitioners to respect the confidentiality of information that is shared. The tenet of section 5 of the *Code* is a crucial commitment to the public that the trust they place in health care professionals will not be betrayed (Box 2.6).

Box 2.6 Confidentiality of information (NMC 2002a)

5.1 ....you must guard against breaches of confidentiality by protecting information from improper disclosure at all times.

5.3 If you are required to disclose information outside the team that will have personal consequences for the patients or clients you must obtain their consent. If the patient or client withholds consent, or if consent cannot be obtained for whatever reason, disclosure may be made only where:

- it can be justified in the public interest (usually where disclosure is essential to protect the patient or client or someone else from risk or harm)
- they are required by law or order of a court.

REFLECTION POINT

Take a moment to think about the sort of information you give to your own GP, practice nurse or counsellor, and the assumptions you make that they will not share that information with anyone else without your consent.

The protection against disclosure of information other than in the circumstances set out in the *Code* does, nonetheless, pose some difficulties. The ethical value that underpins the need for confidentiality is one of trust; it requires honesty and an openness that respects and recognizes an equal partnership between the patient and practitioner. However, there is an equally compelling obligation to balance this against the professional duty to protect against any harm that may be imposed on a third party. The 'public interest' means the interest of an individual or groups of individuals or of society as a whole. The *Code* gives a specific example in matters relating to child protection where practitioners are reminded that they must act at all times in accordance with national and local policies. In such cases, the practitioner must engage in an exercise of professional and ethical judgement that could involve the need for legal intervention.

Maintaining professional knowledge and competence (*Code* section 6)

The related competencies for practice [Professional and ethical practice domain (UKCC 2001a)] are:

- manage oneself and one's practice, and that of others, in accordance with the Council's *Code of professional conduct*, recognizing one's own abilities and limitations
- consult with a registered nurse when nursing care requires expertise beyond one's current scope of competence
- consult with other health care professionals when individual or group needs fall outside the scope of nursing practice.

The achievement and maintenance of competencies that lead to registration and its continuance is a lifelong process and is essential to the public's confidence in the profession. This section of the *Code* highlights the requirement to keep knowledge and skills up to date with current evidence or research, and to develop any new or enhanced skills through regular learning.

Practitioners may be required to determine the individual interests of each client in sometimes complex situations that may fall outside the scope of a particular practitioner's practice. In such cases, it requires the exercise of professional judgement and skills to make a decision to acknowledge any limits to professional competence and to account for any action or non-action (Box 2.7).

Box 2.7 Maintaining professional knowledge and competence (NMC 2002a)

6.2 To practise competently, you must possess the knowledge, skills and abilities required for lawful, safe and effective practice without direct supervision. You must acknowledge the limitations of your professional competence and only undertake practice and accept responsibility for those activities in which you are competent.

Practitioners are expected to judge the scope of their own practice and are encouraged to exercise self-determination and professional control. Although Schober (1998) suggests that this was something not widely accepted or acknowledged by nurses in the past, when new skills may have been developed in the absence of an adequate post-registration programme of learning, it has now become integral to the demands of exercising personal responsibility. With autonomy comes responsibility, as the following paragraph from the introduction to the *Code* states:

'You are personally accountable for your practice. This means that you are answerable for all your actions or omissions, regardless of advice or directions from another professional'.

(NMC 2002a, section 1.3)

REFLECTION POINT

You may have already been asked to do things that you do not feel sufficiently prepared or supported to undertake, and this will almost certainly continue to happen after you are registered to practise. Ponder for a minute on how you would feel about such a situation and how you might handle it for the patient's and your benefit.

Trust and professional reputation (*Code* section 7)

The related competencies for practice [Professional and ethical practice domain (UKCC 2001a)] are:

● practice in accordance with the NMC *Code of professional conduct*
● demonstrate knowledge of contemporary ethical issues and their impact on nursing and health care
● manage the complexities arising from ethical and legal dilemmas.

The concept of trust when translated into the professional relationship is fundamental to both the individual practitioner's moral standing and that of the reputation of the profession. The *Code* requires practitioners to behave in such a way that will inspire public trust and confidence, where violation of any one of the key principles could do damage to both. The underlying maxim of any code of conduct is the principle of non-maleficence – the duty to prevent harm as a matter of professional integrity (see Chapter 4). This part of the *Code* sets out how this principle should be practised for the protection of the individual and society (Box 2.8).

Box 2.8 Maintaining public trust in the professional (NMC 2002a)

> 7.1 You must behave in such a way that upholds the reputation of the professions. Behaviour that compromises this reputation may call your registration into question even if it is not directly connected to your professional practice.

Avoiding inappropriate use of the registered nurse status in the promotion of products or services or any involvement in financial gain, are examples of where trust of patients and reputation of professionals need to be protected. Equally, the acceptance of gifts, hospitality, favours or loans 'that might be interpreted now or in the future, as an attempt to gain preferential consideration', are inconsistent with the behaviour expected of a professional nurse or midwife. As Blane (1988) points out, any preoccupation with gain transgresses the notion of altruism and is not generally associated or accepted within professional practice. The important element here is, of course, to separate the gratitude that may accompany a patient's or client's discharge from their care in hospital or the community from an offer or proposal that would be dishonourable if accepted.

Abuse of the privileged relationship a professional has with a patient or client can take many forms and covers a wide spectrum. However, evidence from the extreme manifestations of how the professional relationship may be violated has attracted much attention in recent years, leading to criminal charges against both nurses and doctors. The actions of Beverley Allitt (DoH 1994b) and Harold Shipman (Baker 2001) shocked the public and health care professions alike. While extreme, these examples nevertheless demonstrate how individuals, whose practice was way outside the boundaries of accepted moral or legal conduct, managed to enter the profession and maintain their respective licences to practise unimpeded for some time. This begs painful questions about the vigilance and willingness to act in the public interest of all health care professionals.

Without doubt such cases are exceptional, and it is within the context of avoiding harm in all situations involving patients and clients that the notion of trust should be considered. The duty of care and the requirement to prevent harm have both professional and legal standing and require some personal reflection on how an individual's behaviour may be judged. The *Code* does not identify specific examples of conduct that would be seen to be unworthy of a professional nurse or midwife. It does, however, assume an understanding that any evidence to support that the trust or confidence of the public has been damaged, may lead to a judgement by either the profession, the law, the employer or all three.

As part of their statutory function, both the NMC and GMC deal with significant numbers of allegations of professional misconduct each year, where evidence supports the abuse of the therapeutic relationship between patient or client and practitioner. Although the majority do not attract the same media attention as the examples given, any referral to either the NMC or GMC serves as a reminder of the need to preserve the privilege that a licence to practise bestows and the resultant damage and dishonour to both the individual and the profession when standards of practice and behaviour for that profession are disregarded.

REFLECTION POINT

Pause for a minute and think about what you expect of any nurse or midwife caring for a friend or relative or, perhaps yourself. 'Harm' can be done in many different ways of which, sometimes, we are not aware. Think about what tone of voice, facial expression and body posture convey to you. They might seem trivial but they can be the components of persistent abuse in the unequal power relationship between practitioners and patients or clients.

Identifying and minimizing the risk to patients and clients (*Code* section 8)

The related competencies for practice [Professional and ethical practice domain (UKCC 2001a)] are:

- commit to the principle that the primary purpose of the registered nurse is to protect and serve society
- identify unsafe practice and respond appropriately to ensure a safe outcome.

The final section of the *Code* affirms the key ethical principles of non-maleficence (duty to prevent harm) and beneficence (duty to promote good). It goes without saying that the basis of any caring role is the duty to ensure an individual patient or client is free from harm and that a person's best interest are promoted as part of the package of care. Yet, it is in this area that 'doing nothing' or 'not being heard' has led to the tragedies of Bristol, Shipman and many others less well known.

The obligation placed on practitioners to make appropriate professional judgements in aspects of care, driven as much by an ethical framework as by any professional or legal ruling, generates a need for a particular approach to solving problems. It is likely that the challenges that present in practice will exercise the mind of the most diligent practitioner, particularly where these involve the behaviour of colleagues. Dilemmas may arise from the duty that all practitioners have to make their concerns known where there is evidence to suggest that the care to a patient or client may be compromised, whether this relates to the environment of care or the specific care of an individual (Box 2.9). 'Whistleblowing' is never a comfortable thing to do, but using the appropriate channels and evidence plus persevering are all part of 'practising' this principle in the patient's interest.

Box 2.9 Raising concerns about colleagues (NMC 2002a)

> 8.2 You must act quickly to protect patients or clients from risk if you have good reason to believe that you or a colleague, from your own or another profession, may not be fit to practice for reasons of conduct, health or competence. You should be aware of the terms and of legislation that offer protection for people who raise concerns about health and safety issues.

This clearly poses particular demands on the individual practitioner who may be required to challenge the practice of a colleague or expose the shortfalls of a particular health care environment where there may be serious implications for more than one person. At a time when the nursing profession is eager to promote the need for evidence-based knowledge to support practice and a renewed confidence to empower practitioners to challenge poor practice, it is with regret that the recent findings from the Bristol inquiry, the Kennedy Report (DoH 2001d), serve as a reminder of the devastating implications if poor practice goes unchallenged.

The Kennedy Report identified lessons to be learned from the inquiry into the high death rate amongst children undergoing heart surgery in Bristol. It was critical not only of those whose clinical care was substandard, but also exposed numerous damaging aspects of the environment for care and of organizational systems; it serves as a timely warning for all practitioners to revisit the demands of the principles that underlie section 8 of the *Code*. Indeed, section 46 of the Kennedy Report recommends that the relevant codes of practice for nurses, professions allied to medicine and managers should be incorporated into their contracts of employment with hospital trusts or primary care trusts. It also suggests that:

'Trusts should be able to deal as employers with breaches of the relevant code ... independently of any action which the relevant professional body may take'.

(DoH 2001d)

The Bristol inquiry described a 'club culture' within the Bristol Royal Infirmary which could be taken as an indictment of the more traditional professional values no longer accepted in contemporary practice (Anonymous 2001). It is hoped that a collective and professional effort will avoid such events happening again and will repair the damage done to the image of the health professions.

Other elements of this section of the *Code* highlight the importance of reporting concerns to the appropriate person and the value of a written record to support any claims made. It also explains how a nurse's or midwife's duty of care applies at all times, including to care given outside the work place but that such care would only be judged against the particular circumstances arising at the time (Box 2.10).

Box 2.10 Duty of care in an emergency (NMC 2002a)

> 8.5 In an emergency or outside a work setting, you have a professional duty to provide care. The care provided would be judged against what could reasonably be expected from someone with your knowledge, skills and abilities when placed in those particular circumstances.

REFLECTION POINT

You may have already become aware of practice and care environments that cause concern. During your clinical placements you might take the opportunity to discuss how situations like these would be handled. Talking things through with others is important for future practice. It helps to shape your thinking as well as sharing the burden of a dilemma.

This final requirement of the *Code* leaves the registered nurse and midwife in no doubt about the professional demands that accompany a licence to practise. The licence is a privilege as well as a major commitment to the public, that has its own reward. However, many feel the balance of that reward is seriously undervalued in material terms and this view will take much perseverance on the part of the profession and others to change.

CONCLUSION

The choice to enter the profession of nursing brings expectations and anticipations to be explored and owned throughout the journey towards registration. The successful achievement of professional competencies are the result of utilizing opportunities for learning that will lead to academic, clinical and professional success. It will depend upon a number of inter-related experiences throughout the programme of learning that will be given a different priority at different stages of the process.

The traditional values of 'being a professional' are now the subject of much challenge. We have seen that the recognition of the professional element of nursing or midwifery practice is integral to the wider expression of the 'modern' nurse or midwife practitioner. Nevertheless, it is only recently that real emphasis has been placed upon how the professional nurse may use the regulatory framework to enhance both their personal and professional growth in the ever-widening dimensions of health care.

With a licence to practise as a professional nurse or midwife, comes responsibility and the right to act autonomously in the patient's interest. The responsibility and the right are finely balanced. For example, nurses, midwives and health visitors must exercise their autonomy if they believe they have been instructed to carry out any activity that may not be in the best interests of the patient or client. How the individual practitioner demonstrates this right to autonomy is complex and the subject of much discourse. It is through a greater understanding of this right, and the concomitant duty to protect the public by exercising this right, that the principles contained within the *Code of professional conduct* and the competencies for practice should be embraced and applied.

For students of nursing and midwifery working in contemporary practice, it is vital that the professional and ethical perspective on practice is acknowledged as an integral part of the curricular, with equal importance given to those activities relating to care delivery and management. The philosophy behind the approach to learning places great emphasis on the individual student mastering the necessary competencies and recognizing the professional accountability that registration as a nurse or midwife demands. The outcome of learning will be validated by the profession and will confirm (or not) *'fitness for award'* – the assimilation of knowledge and understanding, *'fitness for purpose'* – the acquisition of skills and expertise, and *'fitness for practice'* – the skills and ability to practise safely and effectively without the need for direct supervision. These mark the achievement of competencies relating to the philosophy and values of professional practice, and will confirm the final step towards registration – the licence to practise, and membership of the profession.

CHAPTER 3

MAINTAINING PROFESSIONAL STANDARDS

Susan Savage

INTRODUCTION

This chapter examines how you, when you become a registered nurse, will fulfil your personal responsibility to maintain your professional standards and how your individual practice contributes to the overall standards of the professions. It explores the concept of standards, in particular the professional standards by which you are expected to practise. The chapter provides an introduction to methods which help you to maintain professional standards, such as reflective practice and clinical supervision; it does not, however, intend to give you a step-by-step guide to these and therefore it is recommended that you use the further reading for detailed guidance.

While our role in addressing poor and unacceptable professional standards is considered here, it is important that this does not overshadow the much larger impact of our professional practice in promoting high clinical standards.

It is hoped that at the end of this chapter you will be keen, as well as ready, to enjoy your professional accountability, developing your skills and knowledge to improve nursing practice. It is through you that future professional standards will be developed and maintained.

3

We often hear about standards in professional practice: clinical standards, standards of care, professional standards and so on. Why are we so concerned with standards in health care? Standards are the linchpin of our professional practice. They define the expected behaviour and level of competence required of nurses, midwives and health visitors, and indeed other health professionals. Professional self-regulation provides the framework for these standards. Chapter 2 describes how the Nursing and Midwifery Council (NMC) acts as the regulatory body for nursing, midwifery and health visiting, and how it sets, maintains and improves the standards for our professions. Registration provides the vehicle to fulfil the public expectation of professional standards; it both grants the right for registered nurses and midwives to practise and at the same time places a responsibility on them to maintain professional standards. This is the essence of professional accountability.

This chapter relates to the outcomes and competencies set out in *Requirements for Pre-registration Nursing Programmes* (UKCC 2001a) as follows:

- manage oneself, one's practice and that of others, in accordance with the *Code of professional conduct* (NMC 2002a), recognizing one's own abilities and limitations
- undertake and document a comprehensive, systematic and accurate nursing assessment of the physical, psychological, social and spiritual needs of patients, clients and communities
- based on the best available evidence, apply knowledge and an appropriate repertoire of skills indicative of safe nursing practice.

STANDARDS AND PROFESSIONAL PRACTICE

EXERCISE

Think about when you have used a service, e.g. having a meal in a restaurant, or opening a bank account. Write down what you liked about the service and then what you did not like. For example, you may include aspects of how the experience made you feel, your satisfaction with the cost, whether what you received was as you expected from its description, and whether you were happy with the final product.

Repeat the exercise in relation to when you or someone you know used a health service. Compare your two lists to identify factors that are similar and those that are different.

As you read the next section, think about how the items on your lists relate to the definitions of standards and their components.

WHAT IS A STANDARD?

The *Concise Oxford Dictionary* (1999) definitions of a standard are:

- a level of quality or attainment; a required or agreed level of quality or attainment
- something used as a measure, norm or model in comparative evaluations; (standards) principles of honourable, decent behaviour.

Your standards for a restaurant may have included expectations about the taste and attractiveness of the food when it arrives at the table, i.e. the 'outcome' of the service. You may also have identified expectations about the service, such as how the waiter served you; an aspect of the 'process'. You would also expect the kitchens to be hygienic and meet health and safety standards; this could be considered as relating to the 'structure' of the restaurant. All three components contribute to the overall expectation or objective for the visit to the restaurant, and form Donabedian's framework (1966) of:

- structure
- process
- outcome.

Donabedian based his framework for quality on the systems theory of input, throughput and output, and it has been used widely in the health care setting (e.g. Sale 1996). You will often see the Donabedian framework adapted and expanded to provide a more comprehensive approach to standard setting and monitoring. For example, the Royal College of Nursing (RCN) used it, together with other health care quality approaches such as a problem-solving approach, in a quality assurance cycle to develop its standard setting system for nursing (Morrell *et al.* 1997).

The criteria on which standards should be based, collectively called SMART criteria, have been identified as (Burke and Lugon 1999, p66):

- specific
- measurable
- achievable
- realistic
- time limited.

EXERCISE

People have a right to privacy under the Human Rights Act (1998). When you are caring for patients and clients you have a responsibility to protect their privacy and their dignity. If you were a patient, what would you expect to ensure your privacy was protected and your dignity maintained? During your next clinical placement find out what standards have been set about maintaining privacy and dignity. Can you identify elements of structure, process and outcome? Assess whether the standards meet the SMART criteria. How do the standards compare with your personal expectations?

Burke and Lugon (1999) stated that the SMART criteria are required if a standard is to be meaningful. However, if a standard is based on criteria set by health care professionals, it may be meaningful to the practitioner but meaningless to the patient or client. An extreme, simplistic example would be to set a standard that all patients on a ward will be in bed by 8.00 pm to ensure they have the opportunity for sufficient sleep. It may be specific, measurable, achievable, questionably realistic and assessed over a period of time, and convenient for the staff to implement, but it is certainly not appropriate for all patients and is unlikely to achieve the outcome of sufficient sleep, rendering it meaningless for the patient. The importance of involving people if standards are to be meaningful is looked at below.

VALUES IN STANDARDS AND THE IMPORTANCE OF INVOLVING PEOPLE

Standards are about quality or expectations. On the face of it, it should be straightforward to set a standard and measure against it. Consider your expectations for privacy compared with the standards set in your clinical area. Ideally they should be similar but that may not be the case. What if factors that are most important to the health care user are not appropriately identified? For example, the manager may view a short length of hospital stay as a success criteria but the patient may feel they have had a rushed and premature discharge and this could indicate poor quality to them. This highlights the potential for conflicting expectations of quality. Quality has a subjective dimension and we all bring our own values and beliefs to what it means for us. Similarly, our beliefs and values influence our behaviour in all aspects of life, including our professional behaviour. Jasper (1996) outlines six sources of our personal values:

- religious and moral upbringing
- ethnic origins
- educational opportunities
- social class
- environment in which we grew up
- life experiences.

The next exercise explores how personal values affect our own attitudes and the potential impact on our practice.

Scenario Julie is a registered nurse who lives and works in a small town. As part of her role she runs a smoking cessation clinic and health promotion programmes, currently focusing on alcohol use. After a busy working day Julie regularly goes to the town's local pub with her friends for a drink and a cigarette. It sometimes turns into quite a party – she has been known to get very drunk and start singing around all the tables, unaware of people looking at her. After one such evening another nurse, Laila, confronts Julie saying it is unprofessional behaviour and compromises the reputation of the profession. Julie gets very angry and tells Laila to mind her own business; she's entitled to a private life and can do what she wants.
- Give three words which portray the image of Julie in your mind.
- Give three words which portray the image of Laila in your mind.
- Who do you agree with, Julie or Laila?
- Think about what judgements you have made about each nurse and your own values affecting your choice.
Discuss the scenario with students and registered nurses to compare your response.

It is worth reflecting on your own beliefs about behaviours that affect health: How was your attitude towards smoking and alcohol formed? What values underpin your image of the professional nurse to which you aspire? Have you assumed that others share that image and those values? People's reactions to the scenario will vary from and between the two extremes; that Julie is undermining the reputation of the profession to Julie has every right to behave how she wishes when not on duty. Personal values affect your views of what should be expected in professional standards and in standards of health care.

REFLECTION POINT

Think about Jasper's six sources of personal values to consider how your own values have developed.

It follows that views and values about what is important in health care and its standards are likely to be diverse. Williamson (2000) highlights the relationship of values to standards:

'Standards are descriptions of specific aspects of health care practices to which are attached prescriptive values…the values can be drawn from any field of knowledge or thought, from the highly technical to the everyday, from the scientific research to psychoanalysis, from ethics to evidence, from empirical certainties to professionals' intuitions and beliefs from their experience'.

(Williamson 2000, p190)

It seems vital then, that the values of society, patients and clients and professional groups are recognized in forming a standard.

REFLECTION POINT

Return to your thoughts about maintaining privacy for patients and clients. Think about what values and beliefs of the patient or client might affect their expected standards of privacy. What values underpin the standards you identified during your clinical placement for maintaining patients' and clients' privacy? Are there any conflicts of values between those of the patient or client and those of the health care professional? What issues would this raise in implementing and measuring the standards?

As people's values differ it would follow that their expectations of standards will differ also, but the opposite is often assumed, i.e. it is a matter of course that the health professional and patient will agree. It would seem obvious that all those affected by the standards should be involved in determining those standards, although it is argued that this has not always been the case (Williamson 2000).

EXERCISE

Williamson stated:

'… although patients have a greater stake in standards than health professionals, health care professionals have the power to reject patients' views about what standards should be.'

(Williamson 2000, p190)

- Do you agree or disagree with this statement?
- Why might it affect professionals' views about involving patients and clients in standard setting?
- What benefits arise from involving patients and clients in standards setting?

Think about the balance of power between professionals and patients: you may wish to explore this in more depth when you consider Chapter 5 on Nurse–patient relationships.

The public, from a local through to a national level, rightly expects greater involvement in the decisions of health care and its standards. This is reflected in health care policy across the UK. For example, involvement in all aspects of health care planning, delivery and evaluation is a requirement of all NHS organizations in Wales, as set by the National Assembly for Wales (2001). It has provided organizations with guidelines about public and patient involvement to help them achieve this. Similar moves have emerged in England, where requirements were set for all acute NHS trusts to submit feedback from its inpatient surveys by April 2002 (DoH 2002a). The whole framework for patient and public involvement in the NHS in England is being revised under the Health and Social Care Act (2001) (DoH 2001e). In Scotland the Scottish Executive funded an initiative, *Designed to Involve*, to help health organizations involve people in their work (details can be found at www.designedtoinvolve.org.uk).

Regulatory bodies are also changing to meet public expectation. The NMC is committed and required to have public involvement in all aspects of its work, so that it sets standards that reflect expectations of health service users. It is building on the foundations established by the UKCC in its *Strategy for Public Involvement* (UKCC 2000a). Other statutory bodies, e.g. the Commission for Health Improvement (CHI), also involve people in their work (CHI 2002a).

EXERCISE

- Who was involved in setting the standards for maintaining privacy in your clinical area?
- How were they each involved?
- Are the same people involved in monitoring or reviewing the standards?

List the ways you have seen people being involved in decisions about health care. Seek opinions from health care professionals and from local patient and voluntary organizations about how people are involved in local health services, and see how their views compare. How many ways are used to set, monitor or review standards?

You may find it helpful to learn more about patient and public involvement from the Further Reading list.

OVERVIEW OF STANDARDS IN HEALTH CARE

Within health care other terms are also used that relate to the measurement of behaviours and quality, e.g. 'criteria' and 'benchmarks'. Standards in the health care setting can be broadly classified in terms of professional, clinical and organizational standards.

Professional standards

These define the requirements and expectations of individual practitioners and focus on the individual's conduct, education and competence to practise. It is the legal responsibility of regulatory bodies such as the NMC and the General Medical Council (GMC) to set these standards, e.g. the duties of the NMC are stipulated in the Nursing and Midwifery Order (2001). These are discussed in detail below.

Clinical standards

These relate to specific aspects of care and treatment, which include the health care user's expectations and experience, and measures of outcomes such as the level of improvement of symptoms and conditions. National standards facilitate consistency of practice that is evidence based. In England, the National Institute for Clinical Excellence (NICE) was established to determine standards for treatment and care, e.g. standards for best practice for pressure ulcer risk assessment and prevention were issued in April 2001, to be reviewed in 2005 (NICE 2002). The Clinical Standards Board for Scotland has a similar role.

Earlier in the chapter you considered a standard in clinical practice in relation to maintaining privacy. This is one of eight aspects of nursing care for which benchmarks were set nationally by the Department of Health in England (DoH 2001f). It was felt that benchmark standards in practice were needed to improve the quality of fundamental and essential aspects of care. The standards were developed with patients, professionals and patient representatives and are being used by organizations and health care teams in the NHS in developing standards of care. The aspects of care are listed in Box 3.1. You may find it useful to look at this in more detail in Further Reading, in particular to compare your previous thoughts on standards for privacy with those specified in *The Essence of Care* (DoH 2001f).

Box 3.1 Eight aspects of care for which benchmarks are set (DoH 2001f)

- Principles of self care
- Food and nutrition
- Personal and oral hygiene
- Continence and bladder and bowel care
- Pressure ulcers
- Record keeping
- Safety of clients/patients with mental health needs in acute mental health and general hospital settings
- Privacy and dignity

Organizational standards

These refer to performance measures that indicate how the organization ensures professional and clinical standards are facilitated and upheld. NHS organizations throughout the UK are required to do this through clinical governance, which is defined as:

> 'a framework through which NHS organizations are accountable for continuously improving the quality of their services and safeguarding high standards of care by creating an environment in which excellence in clinical care will flourish'.
>
> *(DoH 1998)*

One of the responsibilities of the CHI is to monitor the implementation of clinical governance in England and Wales. The Clinical Standards Board for Scotland has a similar role. Other organizational standards include those relating to the environment of care, such as health and safety standards, and financial management.

Professional, clinical and organizational standards are inextricably linked in the framework for the quality of health care. Further discussion on clinical and organizational standards in health care can be found in Chapters 8–12, which address the organization of care delivery in different age groups. The concepts of standards and quality in health care are explored in detail in Chapter 4. The remainder of this chapter focuses on professional standards.

SUMMARY

- A standard is a required level of quality or attainment and can also be used to describe principles of expected behaviour.

- A standard should be specific, measurable, achievable, realistic and time limited to be meaningful.
- Our personal values and beliefs influence our expectations of quality and standards.
- Patients, clients and carers should be involved in determining standards in health care and those of health care professionals.

YOUR PROFESSIONAL STANDARDS

Your professional practice is determined by standards, as set out by the regulatory body, the NMC. The statutory framework for professional self-regulation is described in Chapter 2, but it is worth reminding ourselves that the principal function of the NMC, as laid out in the Nursing and Midwifery Order (2002), is to:

'…establish from time to time standards of education, training, conduct and performance for nurses and midwives and to ensure the maintenance of those standards'.

(Part II 3(2))

In doing so, the Council is reminded in its legislation of the primary context in which these standards are set, as it states:

'The main objective of the Council in exercising its functions shall be to safeguard the health and well-being of persons using or needing the services of registrants'.

(Part II 3(4))

You may consider the latter clause to be an obvious statement, but it had only been implied rather than explicitly stated in previous legislation, the Nurses, Midwives and Health Visitors Act (1979). The previous regulatory body for nurses, health visitors and midwives (the UKCC) had adopted the philosophy throughout its work, however. Education, training, conduct and performance are inter-linked, as are the standards relating to them. These standards are described in more detail below.

PROFESSIONAL STANDARDS FOR CONDUCT

Earlier in the chapter we considered the influence of personal values on attitudes to professional standards. The regulatory body sets out standards that indicate expectations of behaviour, including respect, trust, confidentiality and co-operation with others in the health care team. These standards are stated in the *Code of professional conduct* (NMC 2002a; Box 2.2) and are the shared values of all UK health regulatory bodies.

Standards of professional conduct are measured using this *Code*; these in particular relate to the definition of standards regarding expected behaviour or the norm. It tends to be put to the test when it has not been met, e.g. through complaints, rather than exemplifying when such standards have been met. Our challenge as a profession is to demonstrate standards of behaviour in positive terms.

EXERCISE
Refer back to your notes on standards for maintaining privacy. Identify where professional standards for conduct are incorporated in the standards for clinical practice.

In reviewing your standards to maintain privacy you should find that standards of professional conduct are integral to standards in clinical nursing practice. Benchmarking tools such as *The Essence of Care* (DoH 2001f), as discussed earlier in the chapter, help to articulate how the practitioner upholds conduct standards in, for example, maintaining and promoting dignity and respect.

Changing expectations

The *Code* also encapsulates the second meaning of standards, i.e. it reflects principles of honourable and decent behaviour. Setting such standards is challenging since public and professional expectation will change with time. The effect of time on societal values is exemplified by the change in the nature of complaints brought to the regulatory body. Cases cited from the early days of nursing regulation following the introduction of the Nurses Registration Act in 1919 included removal from the register for bearing illegitimate children, adultery and being drunk and disorderly in a public place (Pyne 1998). While unrelated to nursing practice, at that time society viewed such personal behaviour as unacceptable. Today public expectation of standards of behaviour is still reflected in cases that relate to personal behaviour, but only where it is deemed that the behaviour impedes on professional practice.

EXERCISE

The *Code of professional conduct* states:

'1.5 You must adhere to the laws of the country in which you are practising'.

(NMC 2002a, p3)

Possession of cannabis is illegal in the UK.
- What would you think of a registered nurse using cannabis?
- Does this pose any professional issues?
- Do you think the public viewpoint differs from your own?
Repeat the exercise to consider the use of heroin and explore any differences in your response.

To sustain relevance to current practice and to be applicable across the diversity of the professions and the settings in which they practise, standards are generally stated as principles. The current *Code* has, however, been more explicit in directing behaviour than its predecessor set by the UKCC (1992b). For each standard the *Code* gives further detail about how such behaviour is demonstrated. You may find it helpful to become familiar with the full *Code of professional conduct* (NMC 2002a).

Ethical principles in the *Code*

Values and beliefs are intrinsic in ethics and therefore it is not surprising that ethical principles are found throughout the *Code*. You might find it helpful at this point to remind yourself of ethical theories (see the Further Reading list).

The duty of care to patients and clients seems a straightforward principle, but it does not account for the role of the nurse, midwife or health visitor in balancing the needs of the individual with the needs of all those they have responsibility to for providing care. This situation brings two ethical principles head to head; that of respecting an individual's autonomy and as such their rights, versus utilitarianism, where your action would seek to achieve the greatest good for the greatest number of people (or the least harm for the least number). Seedhouse (2000) criticizes codes of conduct for presenting two competing ideologies; in particular reference to the UKCC *Code of professional conduct* (1992b) he states:

'A Code of Practice is not the place to decide between these ideologies. But neither is it the place merely to state them without further comment'.

(Seedhouse 2000, p8)

This being the case we would need to consider how the standards of professional conduct could be depicted. Such dilemmas in practice will continue for as long as the society in which we practise has a multitude of ideologies and the people of that society have many personal and sometimes differing values. The code from the regulatory body cannot be expected to provide more than a framework of principles. Scott (1998) suggests that promoting it as more than this only serves to misguide the practitioner into thinking there are easy, straightforward answers to dilemmas in practice. It cannot be ignored, though, that the *Code of professional conduct* (NMC 2002a) remains the benchmark against which complaints of misconduct are judged.

It is important to have an understanding of the ethical principles affecting practice so as to understand better your choices and those of your patients and clients; this will help you to articulate your rationale for decisions in practice.

Legal aspects affecting standards of conduct

Standards of professional conduct are underpinned by legal requirements in addition to ethical principles. The legal framework reinforces public expectation of professional behaviour. This relates in particular to:

- respecting an individual and their rights: the Human Rights Act (1998)
- consent: understanding of legal competence to give consent or refuse treatment (and variances in legislation regarding age of consent in different countries), e.g. the implications of the Adult with Incapacity (Scotland) Act (2000)
- confidentiality: implications of the Data Protection Act (1998), Access to Health Records Act (1990) and privacy laws under the Human Rights Act (1998).

It is important that you are familiar with the law affecting your practice. The legal implications of professional competence are discussed further later in the chapter.

PROFESSIONAL STANDARDS FOR EDUCATION AND TRAINING

There are standards for education and training that relate to:

- preparation for entry to the register
- requirements to maintain registration
- specific post-registration qualifications.

The focus below is on the first two.

As you prepare to become a qualified nurse you will be developing your competence in practice under supervision. To be eligible for registration you will need to demonstrate that you have achieved the competencies set out by the regulatory body. It is at the point of registration that you become accountable for your competence in practice, i.e. you become personally responsible and must be able to justify your actions in your professional practice. The competencies are set out in the *Requirements for Pre-registration Nursing Programmes* (UKCC 2001a). There are similar competencies specific for the midwifery profession (NMC 2002c). You will be following a structured programme designed to provide you with formal teaching, and support with self-directed learning, and closely linked with practical experience to develop your practical skills and competence in the clinical setting.

Individuals who are registered nurses or midwives in countries outside the UK and the European Union can also apply for registration to practise in the UK. The NMC (2002e) considers whether the preparation and the experience of each applicant meet the standards for registration in the UK.

Lifelong learning

The need for education does not stop when you register. It is only after registration that the application of knowledge is learned and honed, and confidence is gained through experience. It is recognized that we need continually to update ourselves and learn new skills if we are to practise safely in the ever-changing health care setting, a position also adopted by the NMC (2002e). This reflects the NMC's responsibility to safeguard the health and well-being of persons using or needing the services of registrants; to fulfil this legal duty the NMC sets standards for continuing professional development (CPD). Lifelong learning then contributes to the registered practitioner's ability to meet public expectation of standards of practice. This is reflected in the standards for maintaining registration set by the UKCC (Box 3.2). These were also adopted by the NMC in April 2002.

Box 3.2 Standards for maintaining registration (NMC 2002g)

To renew your registration you must:
- Sign a notification of practice (NOP) form
- Sign a declaration that you have met the continuing professional development standard which is to:
  - undertake at least 35 hours of learning activity relevant to your practice during the 3 years prior to your renewal of registration
  - maintain a personal professional profile of your learning activity
  - comply with any request from the NMC to audit how you have met these requirements
- Sign a declaration that you have met the practice standard which is to have:
  - worked in some capacity by virtue of your nursing, midwifery or health visiting qualification during the previous 5 years for a minimum of 750 hours, or
  - successfully undertaken an approved return-to-practice programme.

(Additionally midwives need to give notice of their intention to practise, in accordance with rule 36 of the midwives rules.)

These standards demonstrate the characteristics described earlier; they are specific, measurable and within a time framework. They are also achievable, although some nurses suggest this is quite an onerous task. However, to achieve 35 hours of learning activity in 3 years, you could question how any nurse could avoid undertaking at least 1 hour of learning activity of some form per month in the work setting. Is this standard still realistic when the purpose of such standards is considered? If it is to convey a standard for registration expected by the public, it could be viewed that the expectation is in fact too low. These standards were first introduced in 1995, set before issues of professional competence and regulation of health care professionals were brought under the spotlight. Some examples that raised concern are the criminal cases of Harold Shipman (Anonymous 2002) and Beverley Allitt (DoH 1994b), and public inquiries into health care tragedies, such as the Bristol Royal Infirmary Inquiry (DoH 2001d). It is reasonable to expect, then, that the NMC, in reviewing standards for re-registration, may consider raising these standards in the future.

EXERCISE

Discuss CPD with the registered nurses you have worked with.

- How do they identify their learning needs?
- What types of learning activity have they undertaken?
- Do they feel that the minimum standards for CPD and practice for renewal of registration are sufficient for them to maintain their competence?
- What minimum standards do you think the public would expect?

The importance of lifelong learning for health care professionals is recognized in the NHS. Whilst the Department of Health's framework for lifelong learning applies to the NHS in England only, its principles are applicable across all health care settings (DoH 2001g).

Learning activity

In the last exercise it is likely that a variety of learning activities were described. However, people tend to think learning activity means formal study, such as seminars, conferences and courses, and as a result worry about the cost of learning. But if you think about the different ways in which we learn new things in our life, you will see that it is not all through formal learning. We learn from what we see around us, from what we experience and from our interactions with other people. Therefore, meeting standards for CPD does not need to cost. It can include observing another practitioner as part of learning a new skill, reading and evaluating research articles, reflecting on a particular practice incident. Through your practice you will undoubtedly find more ways to meet your learning requirements.

Your professional profile

Another aspect that has worried people embarking on self-directed learning is how they record it and maintain a professional profile. While various formats have been presented in the professional literature and commercially produced folders are available (Driscoll and Teh 2001), again it does not need to be complicated or cost money. A profile can be built up quite easily in a notebook (or some prefer a computer file) by writing about each learning activity. The questions in Box 3.3 can help structure the notes.

Box 3.3 Questions to help structure your record of self-directed learning (NMC 2002f)

- Where were you working when you did the learning activity? (to show what type of practice you were in)
- What was the learning activity? (to describe what you did, when you did it and how long it took)
- How has it affected your practice? (to show how the learning activity has informed and influenced your work)

Using a variety of ways to learn

You sometimes find that people's learning activity focuses only on tasks, e.g. venepuncture, or learning about conditions affecting clients and patients, e.g. diabetes. But this only provides part of the picture if they are not applied to the essence of nursing practice. Barber (1998) highlighted the range of skills, knowledge and understanding required in practice, stating:

'Nurses need cognitive skills to learn and understand these [interpersonal] processes involved in health; they need empathy and an interest in the human condition; they need insight into their own unique composition, together with an ability to develop personal and interpersonal relationship skills so that they may share these insights with others'.

(Barber 1998, p332)

Therefore, to develop your professional practice, the elements of theoretical knowledge and practical skills need to be incorporated with the understanding of interpersonal relationships, communication and self-awareness within those relationships.

EXERCISE

Barber stated:

'Enriched, self-aware people make good nurses; emotionally impoverished, unaware people do not'.
(Barber 1998, p332)

Do you agree or disagree with this statement? Think about what it means to you and any implications it has for your professional practice.

If lifelong learning is to enhance your ways of knowing, learning activity needs to combine learning new information, evidence or research, and developing skills by applying new knowledge to practice, with reflection on practice. People use preceptorship, mentoring, reflection and clinical supervision to help them achieve this (see also Chapter 17).

Preceptorship and mentorship

The transition from being a student nurse to a registered practitioner who is accountable for their actions has been highlighted earlier in the chapter. It is a time to consolidate learning and accustom yourself to new responsibilities, which, as with all changes, can be stressful. The need for support during this time was recognized by the UKCC, which recommended a period of preceptorship of approximately 4 months. Its purpose is to assist the newly registered practitioner to develop their practice and interpersonal skills within a supportive and constructive learning environment (UKCC 1995). This means the newly qualified nurse is allocated a named nurse, midwife or health visitor (with at least 12 months' experience), working in the same area of practice, who will provide guidance, help, support and advice as required. As such it is a formal arrangement, which also serves to ensure that safety and standards are maintained during the period of transition. Preceptorship was not, however, made mandatory and so was not consistently introduced across the UK at the time of the UKCC's recommendations.

EXERCISE

Find out how preceptorship is organized at the hospital or clinical setting where you are currently or have recently worked. Seek views about the programme from recently qualified nurses.

Sometimes the term mentorship is used interchangeably with preceptorship, which can cause confusion. While mentorship does share the characteristics of support and enabling another individual, it differs in that the mentor plays a wider role in personal, professional and career development. As such the mentor is chosen by the individual rather than allocated and does not necessarily work within the same environment. The relationship tends to be long term, unlike the transitionary period served by preceptorship (Morton-Cooper and Palmer 2000).

Both preceptorship and mentorship are characterized by reflective activity and developing skills in personal learning. Reflection as a tool of learning is described in detail below.

Reflection

Much has been written about reflection. Johns (2000a) stated:

> 'Reflection is a window through which the practitioner can view and focus self within the context of her own lived experience in ways that help her to confront, understand and work towards resolving the contradictions within her practice between what is desirable and actual practice'.
>
> *(Johns 2000a, p34)*

Models for guided or structured reflection (e.g. Gibbs 1988; Johns 2000a; Taylor 2000) assist the process by asking the practitioner key questions about their experience in clinical practice. The choice of model is down to personal preference. Driscoll (2000) provides a straightforward approach to guided reflection in his What? Model which comprises three stages:

- what? – a description of the event
- so what? – an analysis of the event
- now what? – proposed actions following the event.

The practitioner is assisted through these stages with trigger questions (Box 3.4).

Box 3.4 The What? Model of structured reflection and associated trigger questions [reproduced by kind permission of Harcourt Publishers Ltd from Driscoll (2000)]

1 A *description* of the event. WHAT? trigger questions:
   - What is the purpose of returning to this situation?
   - What happened?
   - What did I see/do?
   - What was my reaction to it?
   - What did other people do who were involved in this?

2 An *analysis* of the event. SO WHAT? trigger questions:
- How did I feel at the time of the event?
- Were those feelings I had any different from those of other people who were also involved at the time?
- What are my feelings now, after the event; are they any different from those I experienced at the time?
- Do I still feel troubled, if so, in what way?
- What were the effects of what I did (or did not do)?
- What positive aspects now emerge for me from the event that happened in practice?
- What have I noticed about my behaviour in practice by taking a more measured look at it?
- What observations does any person helping me to reflect on my practice make of the way I acted at the time?

3 Proposed *actions* following the event. NOW WHAT? trigger questions:
- What are the implications for me and others in clinical practice based on what I have described and analysed?
- What difference does it make if I choose to do nothing?
- Where can I get more information to help me face a similar situation again?
- How can I modify my practice if a similar situation were to happen again?
- What help do I need to help me 'action' the reflections?
- Which aspect should be tackled first?
- How will I notice that I am any different in clinical practice?
- What is the main learning that I take from reflecting on my practice in this way?

You may wish to try out a model of reflection to look at an experience in your own practice, and consider which parts you found comfortable and which were more challenging.

Clinical supervision

Clinical supervision is more than reflection: Driscoll (2000) reinforces this, stating:

'For individuals used to reacting to crisis situations, clinical supervision also offers an opportunity to be more proactive about practice – but with others to support the new ideas and thinking, not alone.'

(Driscoll 2000, p195)

But what is clinical supervision? There can be misconceptions about it, ranging from views that it is just chatting with colleagues to believing it is just another term for managerial supervision. This is not the case. Bishop defines clinical supervision as:

'A designated interaction between two or more practitioners, within a safe/supportive environment, which enables a continuum of reflective, critical analysis of care, to ensure quality patient services.'

(Bishop 1998, p8)

It is characterized then by a formal meeting to discuss and explore issues of practice. This may be between two people or a group of practitioners. Clearly, clinical supervision does not 'just happen'; it needs to be prepared for and have devoted time. Increasingly organizations are recognizing the need to help with this and to make time available to undertake clinical supervision. This is because the organization as well as the practitioner can benefit and it links to professional and clinical standards. The goals of clinical supervision have been proposed as (Bishop 1998):

- to safeguard standards of practice
- to develop the individual both professionally and personally
- to promote excellence in health care.

As clinical supervision becomes more established in practice the profession will need to demonstrate its effectiveness in achieving these goals if it is to continue to enjoy support from practitioners and employers alike.

EXERCISE

On one of your clinical placements, find out the views of the team about clinical supervision.
- Do they have clinical supervision? Ask them to describe it and compare this with the definition and characteristics of clinical supervision.
- What do they find helpful or unhelpful about it?
- Who initiates clinical supervision and does the organization support it? Do they have any guidelines available?
- Did they have any preparation before starting clinical supervision?

So far this section has examined the professional standards for education and training and CPD, together with some of the mechanisms available to help you meet them. These alone will not guarantee competence but will contribute to your ability to achieve it. Standards for professional competence are discussed below.

PROFESSIONAL STANDARDS FOR COMPETENCE

Competence has always been part of the standards for professional practice, as indicated in the guidance of the previous regulatory body (UKCC 1992a,b). How lifelong learning supports the development and maintaining individual competence was explored earlier in the chapter. Registered nurses, midwives and health visitors were (and still are) expected to be competent for any aspect of care they give, to acknowledge and, where appropriate, address any limitations of their competence.

However, it is only since the Nursing and Midwifery Order (2002) that the NMC is required to set standards for performance and has powers to deal explicitly with incompetence. Such standards were still in development in 2003, but we can draw on previous work on competence to outline the nature of standards relating to this.

What does competence mean?

The UKCC used the term competence as meaning:

'...the skills and ability to practise safely and effectively without the need for direct supervision'.
(UKCC Commission for Nursing and Midwifery Education 1999, p35)

One example of the competencies set for entry to the register (UKCC 2001a) in relation to care delivery states that the practitioner will be able to:

'Undertake and document a comprehensive, systematic and accurate nursing assessment of the physical, psychological, social and spiritual needs of patients, clients and communities'.

(UKCC 2001a, p13)

EXERCISE
Think about the above competency for nursing assessment. How would you demonstrate your competence? What evidence would you use? You may wish to repeat this for other competencies.

It is likely that you could identify evidence for selecting a valid assessment tool, and demonstrate the assessment by documenting it and the subsequent care plan, which a registered nurse confirmed was accurate and appropriate. Satisfaction expressed by the patient or client in the way in which you did the assessment could provide another indicator. Equally important in achieving competence is how you undertook the assessment, with the appropriate use of interpersonal skills, observation and listening, which may be assessed by another practitioner observing your practice.

In this one example you can see how theoretical knowledge, skills and their application to meet the unique needs of an individual are interwoven to achieve the expected standard of competence.

Levels of competence and the law

Competence is not a static definition; while the standards for entry to the register indicate a certain level of competence, the practitioner continues to develop expertise so their level of competence increases, but also their exposure to new challenges and changes in practice widens. Their professional accountability gives them the freedom to develop their practice to meet the needs of health care users provided it is within their sphere of competence. The question is who defines such competence? In law this has been answered through cases of negligence, specifically the case of Bolam *v* Friern Hospital Management Committee in 1957 is cited (Dimond 1994; Walsh 2000; NMC 2002a). Here the judge defined the expected standard of a skill as:

'the standard of the ordinary skilled man exercising and professing to have that special skill'.

This subsequently provided the benchmark known as the Bolam test. In applying this to nursing practice, the law requires an ordinary standard rather than the highest possible standard of care. This would be founded on evidence, guidelines and protocols for practices of the time, highlighting the importance of keeping your knowledge and skills up to date.

Scope of professional practice

It is exciting that nursing, midwifery and health visiting have the freedom to develop practice to meet the needs of patients and clients. There is very little that the nurse is restricted from doing in practice by law, and the boundaries between the health professional roles are constantly shifting. This is of course with the proviso that the nurse has both the authority and competence to undertake new areas of practice. The standard of care and expertise required by law would be equivalent to the requirements of the professional who would traditionally have provided such care. For example, if a nurse took on the role of first assistant in surgery, they would be required to demonstrate the skills, knowledge and competence that equate to a doctor in that role. The regulatory body set out principles that practitioners are expected to apply if changing the parameters of their practice, originally in the *Scope of Professional Practice* (UKCC 1992a), and subsequently incorporated into the revised *Code of professional conduct* (NMC 2002a):

- it must be in the best interest of patients and clients
- the practitioner must have the skills, knowledge and competence
- they must acknowledge any limitations of personal knowledge and address these
- it must not compromise or fragment existing care
- the practitioner remains personally accountable
- it must not result in inappropriate delegation.

There have been concerns that some practitioners, while having the professional freedom to push the boundaries of their practice, have not had the authority within their employment to do so, which brings conflict between the practitioner's professional accountability and their accountability to their employer. This can leave the practitioner vulnerable and present concerns about patient safety and standards of care. Placing the onus on the practitioner to ensure competence has been criticized (Walsh 2000). However the pitfalls and vulnerability of individuals can be avoided by:

- thorough planning of any proposed shifts of practice boundaries
- involving all those affected by the proposal (which could include colleagues, other professions such as doctors or dieticians, managers, patient representatives)
- not being isolated in making changes
- thorough preparation for new roles through education and training as required by individuals to acquire competence
- use of reflection and clinical supervision to support the practitioner in developing roles and assisting learning
- where appropriate, development of guidelines and protocols for practice to determine expected standards of care
- clear agreement from the employing organization.

In this way, professional accountability can be used to drive, rather than restrict, new ways of working. There have been substantial and rapid changes in practice since the principles for adjusting the scope of practice were introduced in 1992. The UKCC recognized the need for further standards that would denote practice at a level significantly beyond that of initial registration. A generic standard for a higher level of practice was developed around seven aspects of practice:

- providing effective health care
- leading and developing practice
- improving quality and health outcomes
- innovation and changing practice
- evaluation and research
- developing self and others
- working across professional and organizational boundaries.

Each aspect has supporting criteria which a practitioner would be required to meet to achieve the standard (UKCC 2002). While the standard has not been adopted formally within the regulatory framework, it has been used to inform criteria for consultant nurse/health visitor/midwife roles. It will be for the NMC to decide how these standards can be taken forward.

SUMMARY

- The NMC's primary purpose is public protection; to do this it sets professional standards for the education, training, conduct and performance for nurses and midwives.
- Standards of professional behaviour expected of the registered nurse and midwife are set out in The *Code of professional conduct* (NMC 2002a), which is underpinned by ethical principles and legal requirements.
- Lifelong learning is central to maintaining professional standards.
- People learn in different ways; reflecting on your practice is particularly important in developing your knowledge, skills and self-awareness to enhance how you practise in the future.
- Preceptorship, mentorship and clinical supervision are essential mechanisms to support you and help you improve your practice throughout your professional career.
- You will be required to meet the NMC standards for CPD and practice in order to maintain your registration, i.e. to allow you to continue to practise.
- Once registered, you are professionally and legally accountable to practise competently, and you can enjoy professional freedom to develop practice to meet the needs of patients and clients within any parameters determined by your employers.

ISSUES IN PRACTICE

So far this chapter has explored what our clients and we expect in relation to standards of care, and what is needed to fulfil and maintain such standards. In an ideal world we should be able to achieve this. We know, however, that there can be obstacles and challenges to nurses in maintaining standards. This section looks at these issues in practice in more depth.

CHALLENGES TO STANDARDS OF CARE

EXERCISE

While on one of your clinical placements undertake interviews with the following people:
- sister, charge nurse or senior nurse for the clinical area
- another nurse working in the area (maybe a nurse who has been qualified as well as one with less experience)
- another member of the multidisciplinary team, e.g. a physiotherapist or doctor
- a health services manager.

In your questions ask about situations where they feel unable to provide satisfactory care. Explore what factors create or contribute to these situations and how often such occasions arise. Ask each person what their main concerns are and what they do in these situations.

- Have they described similar situations and concerns?
- Do they have different roles and responsibilities in addressing the problems?
- Did they describe any preventative measures for the future?
- If you were in each of their roles, how would you approach the situations they describe?

You may wish to revisit this exercise in different clinical placements and see whether the challenges presented to the health care team vary or are consistent across the clinical settings.

One of the steps to dealing successfully with the realities of practice is feeling prepared and therefore more able to instigate appropriate action. It is worthwhile thinking about how you might deal with some specific issues of practice before you have to deal with them 'for real'. While nurses know they are required to highlight concerns about practice in the interests of patients and clients (NMC 2002a), it is, however, something that can be challenging. Reflective practice and clinical supervision provide a vehicle to explore such challenges.

Concerns about your own limitations of practice

All nurses at some point in their professional practice will face an aspect of practice for which they feel unprepared, either because they have not undertaken a particular skill before or they have not used a skill for sometime and therefore no longer feel competent in it. This needs to be addressed from two aspects. First, you need to seek assistance from a colleague with the appropriate skill to undertake the skill or supervise you in developing your own practice (if assessed as safe to do so).

Sometimes, particularly when everyone is very busy, nurses find this hard to do, as they feel they are putting more pressure on colleagues and fear being viewed as unable to do the job, and so are tempted just to muddle through in the hope it will all be alright. However, if you attempt skills for which you are not prepared, you risk making mistakes, causing injury to the patient or client. Of course, errors do happen in practice, but where a nurse could have prevented one by acknowledging their own limitations rather than hiding them, their accountability is brought into question. Second, having identified a limitation to their practice, the nurse needs to address this by discussing their concern in the first instance with their manager. Sometimes this raises fears that they are not fulfilling their job and will be detrimental to their future, but again the consequences of not doing so would cause the nurse more problems in the long term. Developing insight into your own practice is a skill in itself, and again highlights the importance of using tools such as reflective practice and clinical supervision in maintaining professional standards.

Scenario Jane qualified as a registered mental health nurse 2 months ago. She was working on a ward for people with acute mental health problems; one patient, Geoff, who was experiencing hallucinations, has insulin-dependent diabetes and unstable glucose levels. Jane had learned about caring for people with diabetes but had not administered insulin according to a sliding scale dosage before. There was only one other registered nurse on the ward. Geoff required his insulin in the next 10 minutes, and Jane had to decide what to do.

- What would you do in Jane's situation?
- Are there any steps Jane could have taken to avoid the urgency of the situation and so meet Geoff's health needs more easily?

Concerns about a colleague's professional practice

Understanding your competence and limitations is essential for safe practice; a practitioner who does not have insight into their own practice and the parameters of their competence is particularly unsafe. If you encounter incompetent or unacceptable practice in others, you will need to act. The fear of being seen as telling tales, or being disloyal to colleagues, can be exacerbated by some work cultures which focus on blaming individuals rather than addressing the standards of care in question. It is important to seek support, whether from another trusted colleague or from a representative of a professional organization.

Where out-of-date practice is identified, it could be tackled by introducing evidence for changing practice within the whole team; the team may need to revisit current protocols and clinical guidelines. Alternatively, a training need could be proposed to the clinical leader or manager, from which all the team could benefit. In some circumstances, though, practitioners may not recognize any skill deficit in themselves and therefore need to be made aware of this. Clinical supervision would provide an opportunity to address this. A supportive team would also enable practitioners to raise concerns directly with colleagues. Even with such support, a practitioner may not acknowledge their limitations and be resistant to change; you would then need to raise such concerns with the practitioner's manager. It is expected that the employer would then take appropriate action to address issues of competence, e.g. by requiring retraining, supervision and reassessment of the individual's competence. If, however, on bringing your concern to your manager's attention the issue is not addressed, care risks falling below unacceptable standards, and you would need to take the next steps in reporting your concern. This is reinforced in the expectations set out in the *Code of professional conduct* (NMC 2002a). These steps are described later in the chapter.

ENVIRONMENT OF CARE

Dealing with problems in the environment of care has two elements; dealing with the immediacy of the problem, and then consideration of your contribution to address the problem in the long term to decrease the likelihood of recurrence. In all incidences, though, you can only act and be accountable for those aspects that are within your sphere of responsibility. Again, it is important to seek support so that you do not feel isolated.

The problem requiring immediate action

Scenario Peter is a registered nurse (adult branch) working on an orthopaedic ward. The ward provides care predominantly for older women who have a fractured femur. The ward has three pressure-relieving mattresses that can usually be distributed according to need. However, one woman who had been recovering well after her operation and was expected no longer to need the pressure-relieving mattress suddenly deteriorated, her condition increasing her risk of skin breakdown. The mattress had been reallocated to another patient who had been assessed as having the same level of risk. Peter has to decide what to do: he has insufficient resources to meet the patients' needs.

Think about what your options would be and write down how you would resolve this issue. What factors have you used to make your decisions? Different factors could change the chain of decisions, e.g. if the patient could not be turned, the availability of more staff or limited access to specialist advice (e.g. the specialist nurse for tissue viability was not available for all shifts), or the on-call manager being unable to obtain a further mattress.

There is unlikely to be only one possible course of action but your proposed action would probably show that Peter, true to life, cannot magically find the resources but he can explore his known options within his competence. He can only provide a standard of care within the resources available but he must also make his concerns known so that those with responsibility for resources can make their decisions in full knowledge of current circumstances. The patient or their family may wish to raise their own concerns about resources which, used positively, contribute to addressing future resource issues. Peter has, arguably, exercised his accountability appropriately within his sphere of responsibility at that time.

What happens next?

There may be a sense of relief in having dealt with the immediate problem but you will need to consider if any further action is needed to help prevent the incident recurring. You may have thought of some options, which could include:

● requesting feedback from the manager about their action to address the issue
● gathering evidence about the problem to assess future need
● proposing the development of a protocol, drawing on specialist expertise, to guide decision-making if the issue recurs and to make the risk management explicit.

These options enable Peter to act in a proactive way by anticipating future health needs. However, despite exercising his accountability, the outcome may be out of his control; if the problem deteriorates further below acceptable standards, he may need to reconsider his course of action.

SUMMARY

● Standards of professional practice can be affected both positively and negatively by the environment of care and those working within it.
● At times you will experience limitations to your own practice due to your level of knowledge, skills and competence; as you develop insight into your own practice you will become equipped with ways to deal with this.
● You can play a positive role in preventing poor standards by identifying problems in the environment of care and being proactive in addressing potential problems.

WHEN PRACTICE FALLS BELOW ACCEPTABLE STANDARDS

Sadly, we have seen cases where standards have not been maintained. It is not solely a concern of nursing and midwifery practice, but the entire health professions. Recent public inquiries have presented salutary lessons regarding the consequences for all responsible for providing health care. The Bristol Royal Infirmary Inquiry in 2001, which investigated the deaths of babies and children following heart surgery, uncovered inappropriate and/or unacceptable practice both by individuals and health care organizations (DoH 2001d). This and other inquiries identify:

- the importance of seeing how things can go wrong
- the dire consequences if responsibilities are not fulfilled in identifying problems and raising concerns
- how, following such tragedies, standards must and can be improved.

While it is acknowledged that the report on the Bristol Inquiry (DoH 2001d) is lengthy, it is recommended that you read the events and experiences of parents described within it.

YOUR PROFESSIONAL RESPONSIBILITY IN CIRCUMSTANCES OF UNACCEPTABLE STANDARDS

You have a duty to act to identify and minimize risk to patients and clients (NMC 2002a). Such circumstances could include:

- you recognize that you may be unfit to practise due to reasons of conduct, health or competence
- you witness abusive behaviour or dangerous practice by a colleague, irrespective of the reasons (given by the colleague you suspect) for such actions
- you identify evidence of unacceptable or dangerous practice that has not been addressed
- the environment of care is unsafe.

Initially, you may feel disbelief and doubt your own observations, particularly if those around you give no indication that they think something is wrong. It is not an easy undertaking to raise your concerns but you need to act on your beliefs; better to be wrong yourself than for a patient or client to experience harm if you do not intervene.

Scenario Mary had just started work in a new unit for people with learning disabilities. She was keen to settle in with the team and was looking forward to developing her skills in this sphere of nursing care. On her second day she heard screaming and rushed to see what was happening; she found the manager yelling at a patient, Simon, who would not get up. Mary asked if she could help but the manager sent her away. Other members of the team seemed not to have heard the commotion, but one told her not to worry as the manager occasionally had days like this, but that the residents do not come to any harm. A few days later Mary was attempting to change Simon's bed after he had been incontinent, when she noticed the manager watching her silently. Just as Mary was finishing the manager said, 'You shouldn't bother, the silly fool does it on purpose'. Only Mary and Simon were in earshot. Mary knew standards of care were unacceptable but no-one else seemed to think so. Mary was so worried she left as soon as she had another job.

It appears obvious that Mary should intervene but she felt powerless to do so as other team members colluded with the manager. Where does she go if her manager is the perpetrator and it is her word against the manager?

REPORTING CONCERNS WITHIN AN ORGANIZATION

Organizations are expected to have mechanisms to support an individual who raises concerns, such as specific policies which outline the process and to whom concerns can be made known, including alternatives to their line manager. This is commonly referred to as a whistle-blowing policy. People remain worried, though, about their job security and it is never action that is taken lightly. All workers, whether in the independent sector or the NHS, are afforded protection from victimization and dismissal by the Public Interest Disclosure Act (1998) (England, Scotland and Wales); the Public Interest Disclosure Order (1998) is the equivalent legislation in Northern Ireland. This is providing disclosures are made in line with the requirements of the Act/Order (RCN 2001). It is important then for individuals to become familiar with the requirements in case they need to follow this action.

An Australian research study that asked nurses about reporting concerns indicated that the individual's belief systems affected how they would respond (Ahern and McDonald 2002), which again highlights the importance of your awareness, and reflection on, the impact of personal values on professional behaviour.

REPORTING CONCERNS ABOUT AN INDIVIDUAL PRACTITIONER TO A REGULATORY BODY

Usually, when concerns have been raised about a registered nurse, midwife or health visitor who is thought to be unfit to practise because of ill health, unsatisfactory behaviour or incompetence, the employing organization will report the individual to the NMC. These referrals account for nearly half of the complaints received by the regulatory body (UKCC 2001b).

However, anyone can report their concern about a registered practitioner to the regulatory body of that profession. Each regulatory body will have similar procedures for considering the concern. When the NMC receives an allegation, it investigates the matter to see whether it is an issue for the regulatory body and if, considering the preliminary evidence (including the practitioner's response to the allegations made against them), it believes there is a case to answer. If so, it will proceed to a full public hearing of the case (unless it is a matter of ill health when proceedings remain private). The proceedings are a legal process set out in the Nursing and Midwifery Order (2002), and therefore are similar to a court of law where there is a panel hearing the case, people are sworn in and legal advisors and solicitors are involved.

EXERCISE

Observe a professional conduct hearing. Hearings are held across the four countries of the UK. Contact the NMC (www.nmc-uk.org) to find out when and where cases are to be heard.

If the allegations are proven, the NMC has a range of sanctions in the Nursing and Midwifery Order (2002):

- 'striking off order': the person is removed from the register
- 'suspension order': registration is suspended (for up to 1 year)

- 'conditions of practice order': conditions are imposed with which the person must comply (for up to 3 years)
- 'caution order': the person is cautioned and this is noted on the register (for not less than 1 year and not more than 5 years) [Part V, 29 (5a–d)].

The purpose of such sanctions is to safeguard the public, not to punish the practitioner. However, it is likely that the consequences of the proceedings in removing or restricting registration will feel like a punishment. The sanctions available to the NMC are wider than those to the UKCC, providing greater scope for the practitioner to be assisted in addressing problems in their practice and to then demonstrate that they have achieved the required standards to be eligible to practise once more.

OTHER ASPECTS REGARDING ADDRESSING UNACCEPTABLE STANDARDS OF CARE

So far this chapter has discussed the role of the individual in raising concerns, the importance of an organization listening to and acting on those concerns, and the role of the regulatory bodies in dealing with concerns about individual practitioners. Other parties also play a role in addressing this issue, so the weight of the problem does not rest solely on the practitioner's shoulders. Parties which may uncover a potential problem in standards of care are those who collate information, which may relate to individuals or organizations. These include:

- patient organizations: e.g. health councils (Scotland) and their equivalent in Wales and Northern Ireland; patient advice and liaison services (England); patients' associations and Action for Victims of Medical Accidents (AVMA) may gather a pattern of complaints regarding a particular organization or practitioner
- coroner: aspects of a case or number of cases may trigger alarm
- Health Service Ombudsman: information about complaints or an unresolved complaint may highlight problems in an organization or with an individual practitioner
- National Patient Safety Agency: established in England in 2001 to implement and operate a system of central reporting and analysis for adverse events and errors in practice. Its aim is to improve patient safety by reducing the risk of harm through error (DoH 2001h)
- Commission for Health Improvement (CHI) (England and Wales) and the Clinical Standards Board for Scotland: when gathering information for routine reviews of clinical governance concerns regarding practice may be uncovered.

It is the last of these organizations, the CHI and the Clinical Standards Board for Scotland, which have powers to investigate serious service failures in the NHS when requested by the Secretary of State for Health (England), the National Assembly for Wales, or the Scottish parliament, in their respective countries. The CHI explains such failures to be:

- a breakdown of processes and standards
- a pattern of incidents of widespread public concern
- other issues that remain unresolved through other reviews and investigations (CHI 2002b).

This should ensure issues regarding standards in organizations are addressed, in addition to those regarding individual practitioners being dealt with by the regulatory bodies. What it does not address are concerns about standards in organizations in the private sector. The National Care Standards Commission in England, established in April 2002, was developing this, but it is now proposed that its role in monitoring private health care will be incorporated in an expanding role for the CHI (DoH 2002b).

LEARNING FROM MISTAKES

The lessons to be learned from the Bristol Royal Infirmary Inquiry (DoH 2001d) are highlighted in its nearly 200 recommendations. Learning from errors and changing practice is not solely about individual practitioners but needs action within organizations. This has been given a high priority within the NHS in England, where mechanisms to report errors or adverse incidents, analyse them and implement changes to prevent a recurrence have been introduced. You will find more information in the plans for improving patient safety in England (DoH 2001h).

However, many of the recommendations of the Bristol Royal Infirmary Inquiry refer to aspects of professional standards that have been discussed earlier in the chapter. For example, 37 recommendations relate to aspects of respect and honesty, including consent, information and communication, which were identified earlier as standards for conduct. Issues of competence bring 49 recommendations, incorporating requirements for education and training, such as CPD being a shared activity across the professions. It also advocates widening the notion of competence beyond that of technical competence, highlighting the need for competence in skills such as communication. While the nursing, midwifery and health visiting professions have considered communication to be of high importance for competence in professional practice, we cannot be complacent about our need to improve these standards further and consistently throughout our own and our colleagues' practice. The list of recommendations continues to address aspects of the safety of care and care of an appropriate standard; again aspects which have been the subject of this chapter.

While the recommendations are not, and should not be seen as, performance targets (DoH 2001d), they do provide specific, measurable, achievable, realistic statements. As such they could be used and incorporated as standards by which the quality of professional practice can be measured and expectations defined in the future.

SUMMARY

- You have a duty to identify and minimize risk to patients and clients (NMC 2002a), so you must take action if you identify unacceptable or dangerous practice.
- Patient organizations and other agencies play an important role in identifying problems or risks to standards in professional practice and health care services.
- Organizations should have policies and protocols which enable and encourage people to report their concerns, without fear of reprisal.
- Anyone can report concerns to the regulatory body regarding a registered practitioner considered to be unsafe to practise (the NMC for nurses, health visitors and midwives), although this is often done by the employer.

- While the NMC has authority to address reported concerns about individual practitioners on its register, other statutory bodies have the responsibility to deal with problems in service delivery or organizations.
- Unacceptable standards of care may arise due to a chain of incidents, factors and involvement of a number of different health care professionals; it is important that lessons are learned from incidents of unacceptable standards of care to prevent them from happening again.

CONCLUSION

It would be wrong to leave this chapter without putting the incidence of failure to meet professional standards into perspective. Of the approximately 640,000 nurses and midwives registered with the NMC, only a small minority, considered unsafe to practise, is removed from the register. For example, 104 individuals were removed from the register in 2000–2001 (UKCC 2001b). Conversely, the professions of nursing and midwifery are maintaining and improving professional standards. Individual practitioners who fulfil their individual responsibility contribute to the professions being able to maintain public confidence in professional standards. This demonstrates professional self-regulation in action.

This chapter explored how you can fulfil your individual responsibility in maintaining standards: in understanding what standards are, how they are set and implemented you can appreciate your contribution to professional standards. You will be able to develop your professional practice as an accountable practitioner, effectively using the standards set by the NMC and through lifelong learning. In this way you will be prepared not only for the challenges of professional accountability, but also will be able to enjoy exercising your freedom to practise innovatively in the best interests of your patients and clients.

CHAPTER 4

ETHICAL DIMENSIONS OF PRACTICE

Paul Gibbons

INTRODUCTION

This chapter introduces the ethical dimension of professional nursing practice. A working definition of ethics is established and three major ethical theories are discussed briefly. From this theoretical basis, ethical principles which can guide the practitioner in identifying and addressing difficult situations are outlined and then applied to a range of everyday situations around aspects of day-to-day care, the beginning and end of life and the ethical implications for the population of research, resource allocation and health promotion.

The chapter aims to promote understanding of the competencies for ethical and professional practice required of those completing pre-registration nursing programmes specified by the former regulatory body, the UKCC Commission for Nursing and Midwifery Education (UKCC 1999), and the interpretation of the *Code of professional conduct* issued by the Nursing and Midwifery Council (NMC 2002a).

WHAT ARE ETHICS?

The *New Oxford Dictionary of English* (1998) defines ethics as 'moral principles which govern a person's behaviour or the conduct of an activity'. At a more philosophical level, ethics is defined as 'the branch of knowledge that deals with moral principles'. Therefore, in the context of nursing practice, ethics can be summarized as 'a systematic approach based on moral principles which can underpin practice and assist the practitioner to act in a manner which fulfils the obligation to the public of being a member of a regulated profession'.

Ethics are important in self-regulated professions, including nursing, medicine, allied health professions and the law, in order that both those who practise the professions and, more importantly, those whom they seek to serve, have no doubt about what represents proper practice.

ETHICAL THEORIES

To apply ethics to practice it is necessary to have a basic understanding of three fundamental ethical theories.

- Virtue-based ethics (as typified by Aristotle) which hold that the virtues, including honesty, justice, charity, kindness, compassion and generosity, provide a basis which enables individuals to fulfil their duty to society and contributes to the overall good of society. In return, society rewards its virtuous members. For instance, individuals who act from compassion and charity to relieve third-world hunger or poverty act ethically according to a virtue-based code and in return can expect the approbation of society for their actions.
- Duty-based ethics (as typified in 1781 by Immanuel Kant in his work *Critique of Pure Reason*) are based on the rightness or wrongness of an act and hold that rational human beings have an obligation to act in the correct way and fulfil their duties to society by so doing. Here, the individual who sees it as a duty to give money to relieve third-world hunger or poverty acts ethically according to a duty-based code. Acting from compassion would be less acceptable to a person who believes in duty-based ethics, as it allows for equivocation as to what is duty. For these individuals, their recognition would come from knowing and being seen to have done their duty.
- Consequence-based ethics (as typified by Jeremy Bentham in his 1789 treatise *Introduction to Morals and Legislation* and modified by J.S. Mill in 1863 when he published *Utilitarianism*). This ethical theory, which has continued to be called utilitarianism, holds that the right act in any given circumstance is the one which maximizes the benefit and minimizes the harm to society and individuals within that society. In this instance, the individual who acts ethically is the one who gives money to relieve third-world hunger because humanity as a whole benefits as fewer people die of starvation.

Seldom, if ever, do individuals or societies consciously categorize their ethical decisions in this way. Rather, their actions are aimed at differentiating between right and wrong, or good and bad. Actions and decisions are influenced extrinsically by cultural and religious influences and acquired values. Intrinsic influences include conscience, personal development, education, inherent values and conditioning in society. Ethical principles, distilled from these theoretical frameworks, can provide a useful guide for individual actions.

ETHICAL PRINCIPLES

The first ethical principle for the nurse is *always act in the best interests of your patient.* This principle underpins all the others and is central to the nurse fulfilling their obligation to the patient. In essence, what is being required here is that the practitioner puts the best interests of the patient or client before all others in the course of any interaction with them. This principle is important when considering how abuse of the relationship between a nurse and a patient can be avoided and how the natural prejudices of individual practitioners can get in the way of therapeutic care and jeopardize professional relationships.

Flowing from best interests are two sub-principles; one is the absolute principle of *never harm the patient or client.* The ethical name for this notion is non-maleficence. The second is the principle of *doing good for the patient or client wherever possible.* Ethically, this is known as beneficence.

Alongside best interests and its two sub-principles there are two other ethical principles which inform and guide nursing practice. The first of these is the principle of recognition of the *autonomy* of the individual. Autonomy is the ability of the individual to exercise self-determination; to plan their own actions and act on the plans without interference from others. In recognizing the autonomy of another person, it is also necessary to respect the autonomous decisions which they make. Clearly, autonomy can never be an absolute right. The autonomy of the individual has to be tempered with the best interests of the wider society; especially respect for other people, e.g. no one would support the autonomous actions of a driver who made a decision to ignore a red traffic light at a busy cross roads and who consequently collided with a school bus. This is a simple example of where the law regulates autonomy in the interests of the safety of society. A point which will be considered further when discussing the ethical implications of resources and decision-making, is that respect for the autonomy of individuals does not grant them the right to have their own needs, demands and aspirations met at the expense of other autonomous individuals.

As will be seen later in the chapter, the principle of autonomy, especially with regard to the capacity of individuals to make decisions, is of the utmost importance when dealing with certain types of patient in relation to consent to treatment.

The final principle is justice. Patients and clients have a right to expect that those who nurse them will treat them justly and in accordance with their needs. Justice demands that patients and clients receive the care they require, free from any discrimination. The principle of justice is also important when considering matters of resource allocation.

EXERCISE

Make a list of potential situations where the duty to act in the best interest of the patient can be compromised by failing to respect the principles of autonomy and justice. To make this instinctive do not spend more than 10 minutes completing this activity.

SUMMARY

Three ethical codes have been examined from which stem a number of ethical principles which can underpin nursing practice and guide the nurse in the general approach to providing care.

ETHICS IN PRACTICE

Here the ethical principles are considered further and applied to a number of situations which nurses encounter in their daily practice.

Rights and responsibilities are fundamental to ethical professional practice. The rights of one person or group of people are normally matched by the responsibility of another person, group or agency. The *Code of professional conduct* (NMC 2002a) places a responsibility on registered nurses to act always in the best interests of their patients or clients; therefore, the matched right of the client is the expectation that those giving them professional care will work in this way.

Although the expectation of nursing practice is that the rights of the patient are paramount, nurses, too, have rights. The responsibility for honouring these rights falls on both patients and employers. The most obvious right enjoyed by nurses is the right to respect for their own autonomy and the right to be treated with respect. The responsibility for ensuring personal safety lies both with individuals who have a duty to safeguard themselves and with employers who have a duty to take all reasonable steps to provide an environment in which staff can work safely. Freedom from verbal and physical abuse are not the only rights which nurses can expect to have accorded to them, they also have the right not to be discriminated against or harassed. Most importantly, they have the right not to be asked by patients, clients or colleagues (of any discipline) to act unlawfully or contrary to best professional practice. This is an important area where matters such as being truthful about issues of diagnosis and treatment, euthanasia or assisted suicide are concerned. It is important that all those working directly with patients and their families have access to appropriate professional support to enable them to reflect upon their practice.

EXERCISE

Identify situations where nurses may come under pressure from (a) patients or their relatives, and (b) colleagues, to act in a way which is potentially in conflict with professional rights and responsibilities.

A contentious area of individual rights for some nurses relates to the role of personal conscience. With very limited exceptions, which are written into the law relating to abortion and assisted fertility services, nurses enjoy no more and no less legal protection for their conscience than any other health worker (see Chapter 2). The part played in practice by conscience is recognized in the *Code of professional conduct* which supports individuals in drawing matters of conscience which cause conflict with professional practice to the attention of senior professional colleagues. Common sense dictates that an individual practitioner, finding themselves faced with difficulty caused by a matter of conscience, should be supported and the difficulty resolved wherever possible. The extent to which such a resolution is possible depends on a number of factors. The balancing factor has to be the need of the patient and the needs of the service. Conscience cannot be used as an abdication of professional responsibility to give care to individual patients or groups whose lifestyle, personal habits or diagnosis are offensive to the practitioner. Even in the limited situations where legal recognition of conscience exists, nurses are still expected to provide appropriate treatment and support in emergency situations.

EXERCISE

Think about issues where individual conscience may impact on professional practice and how these can be addressed (a) by the individual nurse and (b) by professional leaders.

The beginning and end of life are unique, in the variety and quantity of ethical problems which can occur. Three issues related to the beginning of life – abortion, management of infertility and sterilization – will be examined. After considering ethical issues relating to the individual and their professional carers during episodes of care, a further three issues related to the end of life – organ transplantation, withdrawing and withholding treatment, and euthanasia – are described from an ethical perspective. Each of these subjects warrants its own chapter and the outline nature of the present coverage must be recognized.

THE BEGINNING OF LIFE

Abortion

The issue of abortion remains a significant ethical dilemma for many health care professionals. When abortion is being spoken about, it generally refers to the termination of pregnancy by medical or surgical means. Abortion is an emotive term which conjures up images of illicit activity in the back streets of towns and cities before the Abortion Act was passed in 1967. However, abortion is also a physiological term for any pregnancy ending spontaneously before the fetus becomes viable.

Legally, medical or surgical abortion is permissible before the 24th week of pregnancy if two doctors form the opinion that continuing with the pregnancy would involve a greater risk to the mental or physical health of the mother than its termination (Abortion Act 1967). As can be seen, the rights of the fetus are not considered in this process and it is this factor which lies at the heart of the ethical dilemma. As the right to life is assumed to be a good thing, questions around the moral consequences of terminating the life of the fetus must arise.

The fundamental issue here is what right to life does a fetus have? Two responses are possible to this question, each of them proving acceptable to those who advocate the individual position supported by that response. The first response, supported by those who would give a woman total control over her body, is that the fetus, being incapable of separate existence from the mother, has no right to life. The second, supported by those of conservative views and certain religious persuasions, is that the fetus has the potential to become a person in their own right and therefore has a complete right to life.

Neither of these extreme positions provides a 'one size fits all' response to this most difficult of issues. The first fails to recognize that from an early point in its development, a fetus has a beating heart, developing nervous system and the presumed ability to feel pain; in short, as the pregnancy progresses towards the 24th week, when viability is assumed, the fetus becomes increasingly sentient and capable of independent existence. Against this background it must be added that in law the fetus has no status until it draws its first breath. The second position fails to acknowledge that in certain circumstances, such as following rape or acts of incest against young people or those vulnerable through learning disability or profound mental health problems, termination of a pregnancy may be justified. A particularly sensitive area in consideration of whether abortion is justified relates to abortion where antenatal testing has revealed that the fetus is suffering physical abnormality. Understandably, those with disabilities and those groups working with them are vehemently opposed to abortion on these grounds, while in a recent court case (Weber 2001) France's highest court recognized that being born with a handicap can justify a successful claim for compensation. In this case, the mother of a child born with a congenital disability argued that if she had been informed of the results of antenatal tests she would have opted for an abortion. As a result of the judgement both she and the child received payment of damages.

EXERCISE

Consider the above case and identify the points it raises in relation to the two positions outlined at the commencement of the consideration of abortion.

In considering the ethics of abortion, it is important that all nurses consider the issues carefully and non-judgementally. As stated earlier, abortion is one of very few areas of activity where nurses have a legal right, except in emergency situations, to voice a conscientious objection to participation. It is important that this right is respected and that nurses who make such a decision are supported. Equally, it is important that those nurses who are willing to participate in abortion services are also supported so that they, in turn, can support women who face what will probably be one of the most difficult decisions of their lives. Recognition must also be given to the fact that the psychological sequelae of a termination may stay with women for many years, even their whole lifetime. It is interesting to note that at the time of writing (June 2002) a woman has launched an action for damages against an NHS trust for failing to advise her of the psychological impact of having a pregnancy terminated (Dyer 2002).

Management of infertility

The management of infertility is another area of gynaecological practice which can be riddled with ethical dilemmas. Research into treatments for infertility is among the fastest growing areas for clinical study. Techniques currently available span the whole range of interventions from artificial insemination of a naturally produced ovum by a woman's husband/partner or an anonymous donor, through *in-vitro* fertilization using naturally occurring or donated ova and sperm, to surrogacy in which a woman carries a child and at birth passes it to another woman to raise as her own child.

The ethical implications of these techniques are manifest, and no more so than the ethical issues surrounding the use and storage of embryos created *in vitro* and then stored by freezing rather than implanted at the point of fertilization. In this situation exactly the same question arises over the status of the embryo as arises over the status of the fetus. Given the conclusion reached relating to approaches to the status of the fetus, it will come as no surprise to discover that identical arguments may apply to the embryo. The same responses to those arguments can also apply. However, in the case of the embryo, the arguments on the potential person from the moment of conception are weakened by the fact that, as science currently stands, without implantation there can be no development beyond a cell mass and therefore no potential person can exist. That said, it would be wrong to assume that the fertilized human embryo can be treated as an item of science. It is widely accepted that the embryo is entitled to special respect on the basis that it represents human tissue.

Genetic manipulation and embryo research

As techniques for developing and modifying embryos evolve, so too do the ethical implications of the technology. For example, can the genetic manipulation of embryos to provide 'spare parts' for their siblings, parents, relatives or even complete strangers ever be acceptable? Can selection of embryos for implantation on grounds of gender ever be justified? The last question raises an interesting topic for ethical debate. The instantaneous response of most people to this question would probably be a firm no; however, if the question is then posed to them in terms of preventing the transmission of diseases such as haemophilia, which are transmitted through the female line but only affect males, a different response may ensue.

Further questions arise about the benefit to society as a whole which may come from research on embryos and yield possible treatments and cures for previously untreatable, distressing and, in some cases, fatal diseases, such as cystic fibrosis. Many people would subscribe to notions of altruism, while others may raise serious and legitimate questions about research on an embryo which cannot benefit directly from the research findings.

A further differentiation needs to be drawn between embryos which are used for research, having been created for implantation and being surplus to the number required, and those specifically created for research purposes. A more pertinent question may be: What should be the fate of stored embryos? For those who subscribe to the cell mass theory, the answer is straightforward, disposal in the same way as any similar collection of cells. For those subscribing to the potential person theory, a real problem exists: human life is sacred and cannot be ended by the action of another individual or body.

It was in an attempt to deal with questions such as these that the Expert Committee under the chairmanship of Dame Mary (later Baroness) Warnock was established. The findings of that Committee gave rise to the Human Fertilization and Embryology Act (1990). In turn, the Act established the Human Fertilization and Embryology Authority, which has to grapple with these issues on a daily basis. With regard to research and embryo retention, the current legal position is that embryos cannot be allowed to develop beyond the 14th day following fertilization and cannot be stored for more than 5 years after fertilization.

Perhaps of all the areas discussed in this chapter, the ethical implications of embryo research and genetic manipulation are going to be both the fastest changing and the most challenging for students of ethics and health care professionals alike.

Control of fertility

Surgical sterilization and chemical and barrier contraception have been accepted elements of clinical practice for many years. In most circumstances, the use of contraception and sterilization give rise to few ethical issues. That said, there are times when nurses may find themselves caring for people in situations where contraception and sterilization are problematic.

Current ethical issues around contraception relate to the prescription and supply of the contraceptive pill in two circumstances: to girls under the age of 16 and as the so-called 'morning after pill'.

In relation to the first issue, the main question is, as it is illegal for a man to have sexual intercourse with a girl under 16 years of age, can a doctor or nurse prescribe or supply the girl with contraceptive pills? This illegality does not prevent some under 16s from engaging in consensual sexual intercourse. Therefore, falling back on the injunctions never to do harm to the patient and to do good wherever possible, discussed earlier, health professionals have to perform a difficult balancing act between denying contraception and running the risk of an unwanted and potentially psychologically devastating pregnancy, or prescribing contraception in the knowledge that sexual intercourse is going to take place and a crime be committed against the girl. Like many of the other issues discussed throughout this chapter, there is no easy answer to this conundrum. In reality, the health professional has to make their own judgement as to the maturity and understanding of the girl, try to offer wise counsel in regard to responsible sexual behaviour and offer advice on the availability and use of contraceptives that have fewer potential side-effects than the contraceptive pill. At the end of the day, knowing that sexual intercourse will take place regardless of whether or not contraception is used, many health professionals would meet the patient's wishes. A separate and equally contentious issue is the debate as to whether or not the girl's parents should be told; this issue will be looked at further below when examining matters of consent.

The issues associated with the 'morning after pill' relate to its mode of action and availability. The 'morning after pill' is effective because it prevents the fertilized embryo implanting into the endometrium and leads to its spontaneous ejection. Those groups and individuals who hold that the embryo has special status, because of its person potential qualities, argue that this mode of action means that the 'morning after pill' leads to an abortion as surely as if medical or surgical termination of the pregnancy had taken place. With regard to availability, those responsible have determined that, subject to training and counselling being available, the 'morning after pill' should be available from pharmacies without prescription for women over 16 years of age. Opponents of contraception and abortion oppose this step on the grounds that pharmacists will have no ready way of establishing with certainty that every woman they supply is over 16 and will act in accordance with the advice given.

EXERCISE

Consider the pros and cons of school nurses being empowered to prescribe the 'morning after' pill to pupils in their care.

When thinking about surgical sterilization, the ethical implications relate to the presumed permanence of the procedure, the consequences of failure and cases where sterilization is proposed (normally for women) in the absence of capacity to consent. Most individuals seeking sterilization do so with the firm intention of preventing future pregnancy. There are a number of lifestyle reasons why this decision may be regretted, e.g. a change in partner, the death of a child or a change of mind about family size. Some sterilizations may be reversible but many are not. For this reason, it is important that the patient receives adequate counselling about the nature of the procedure they are requesting and gives truly informed consent before the operation takes place. The opposite situation is also true; in a very small minority of cases, the effect of the sterilization (especially in men) may not be permanent if the vas deferens become rejoined. Here again, frank discussion of the possibility of rejoining and obtaining fully informed consent before surgery are essential.

The final sterilization matter that has ethical implications relates to individuals who lack the capacity to consent either to sterilization or consensual sexual relationships. This is a matter of profound concern to the parents, other relatives and carers of women of child-bearing age with learning disabilities or mental health problems who are at risk of sexual exploitation and are wholly incapable, through no fault of their own, of managing a pregnancy and caring for a child. Very few such cases ever arise but those that do cause great angst for those who care for and about the person concerned. Ultimately, it may be necessary for the facts to be presented to the courts and a judgement obtained as to the legality and appropriateness of sterilization. The ethical considerations which both health professionals and the courts need to take into account are the same: the need to ensure that the proposed procedure is the only way of protecting the best interests of the woman and that the risks of rendering her incapable of having a child are less than the risks of her being sexually exploited, finding herself pregnant and facing the distress of either having the pregnancy terminated or having a child who may need to be taken into care.

ETHICS IN DAY-TO-DAY CARE

Consent to treatment

In considering the practical ethical implications of day-to-day activities of care, consent to treatment is a useful starting point. Obtaining informed consent before undertaking any activity involving an autonomous individual lies at the heart of ethical practice. Indeed, any member of the care team who treats an autonomous person without their consent not only acts unethically but also potentially breaches both the criminal and civil law.

Beauchamp and Childress (1994) spell out four components, all of which must be fulfilled, to secure informed consent:

- competence
- disclosure
- understanding
- voluntariness.

Before consent can be given or withheld, the person seeking consent must be satisfied that the patient has the intellectual and mental capacity to appreciate what is proposed. The practitioner must give information in an accessible format, which is in line with the patient or client's level of comprehension, about the planned action. This information should include details of the intervention, the potential or actual benefits to the patient or client and any possible alternatives, complications or side-effects. Once this information has been given, it is for the practitioner to satisfy themselves that the patient or client has understood the information and been given the opportunity to ask questions or seek further information, including information from an independent source, if appropriate. The final requirement is for the consent to have been sought free from inducement or pressure. Once these tests have been met, informed consent can be said to have been given or withheld.

For most patients, explicitly giving or withholding consent is something that happens at a fixed point in time before undergoing surgery or other invasive procedure. The patient or client is seen by a health professional, discussion takes place and a document is signed.

For nurses this explicit and documented process is just the tip of the iceberg. By co-operating in their care, e.g. by keeping an appointment for a counselling session or by holding out their arm to allow venepuncture to take place, patients and clients give their implied, but unwritten, consent on a daily basis to both physical and psychological interventions.

REFLECTION POINT

Think about a patient or client you have worked with recently, consider the inter-actions which took place and list ways in which the client gave implied consent.

There will always be areas where the ability of the individual to give consent is less clear. These situations can present those caring for such patients with real dilemmas.

If the patient or client does not have sufficient mental or intellectual competence to understand the information that allows consent to be given or withheld, the practitioner must always act in the best interests of the individual. There should be protocols in place to guide staff involved in determining how best interests can be met when competence is lacking. This guidance should include criteria for the assessment of competence and also highlight the importance of language and method of communication to ensure maximum comprehension.

There may be circumstances when a patient anticipates encroaching incompetence and makes an Advance Directive (also known as a Living Will) specifying the circumstances under which defined treatments would be acceptable or unacceptable. Although such directives have no clear legal status, good practice and acting in the best interests of the patient would normally require clinicians to comply with the patient's wishes where they are satisfied that the patient was competent at the point of making the directive.

All members of the clinical team must bear in mind that in most circumstances no one, including the next of kin, can give consent on behalf of another adult. In certain circumstances, NHS bodies can apply to the courts for permission to carry out treatments on adults who lack the capability to give informed consent in their own right. A legal framework to protect the rights of those who cannot make decisions for themselves already exists in Scotland in the Incapable Adults (Scotland) Act (2000). In the other UK countries, similar legislation is under consideration.

Consent to the administration of medicines is just as important as consent to any other intervention. The nurse must be able to justify administering medication covertly in the same way as any other non-emergency treatment without consent would be justified. Circumstances where patients who are confused, mentally ill or otherwise unco-operative refuse to take oral medication present real challenges to care teams. These situations require skills of persuasion and patience to achieve compliance. Where all such efforts fail, other members of the clinical team, including prescribers and pharmacists, should be involved to ensure that the treatment which is being attempted is the most appropriate drug and preparation. Where, after full consideration, covert administration is agreed as being in the best interests of the patient, the full details of the decision should be entered into the patient record. Such decisions should always be kept under review by senior members of the clinical team and should remain as part of the treatment for as short a period as possible.

EXERCISE

List the possible approaches which can be employed to gain compliance with medicine regimes and avoid the need for covert administration without consent.

Perhaps the most difficult area facing practitioners is the withholding of consent by a competent adult, where the effect is deterioration in health or even death. Providing competence has been established, no intervention is justified apart from exerting influence in a sensitive and professional manner, which avoids any suggestion of coercion, to ensure that the patient is in possession of and understands the facts. To do otherwise is to suborn the right of the competent individual to autonomous self-determination. This important principle of consent was re-affirmed in 2002 by Dame Elizabeth Butler-Sloss, the President of the Family Division of the High Court in England and Wales. The case concerned Miss B whose respiration was maintained by a ventilator following damage to her spinal cord caused by a haemorrhage. Miss B requested the clinical team caring for her to withdraw her ventilation. Her request, which was refused, was made in the knowledge that she would probably die. On appeal to the High Court, the President decided that Miss B had the competence to understand her request and the probable outcome and thus found that her autonomy was infringed by the refusal of the clinical team to comply with her wishes. The appeal was allowed and Miss B was subsequently transferred to another hospital where the clinical team were prepared to comply with her request, her ventilation was withdrawn and she died peacefully. She was also awarded nominal damages against the first NHS trust for their failure to comply with her wishes.

Another complex area of consent relates to children and young people. For children who, because of their age and immaturity, cannot satisfy the four criteria for informed consent, consent can be given by the parents (or those with parental responsibility). In England, Wales and Northern Ireland, a young person is normally deemed competent to give consent on their own behalf at the age of 16. However, since the 'Gillick' case in 1984, if the practitioner seeking consent believes a young person under 16 has the maturity, understanding and competence to understand the details of the proposed intervention, that individual can give consent without parental involvement. In Scotland, 16 year olds have a statutory right to give consent when the practitioner is satisfied they can understand what is planned.

There are certain circumstances where staff are unable to obtain consent, e.g. where a patient is in extremis or where a practitioner witnesses a sudden cardiac arrest. In these and similar emergency circumstances, nurses will normally be deemed to have acted ethically where they provide appropriate treatment within their professional skills, knowledge and experience, and in the patient's best interest.

Nurses must be aware that there will always be a small number of patients in mental health settings who do not have to give consent to treatment if, in the view of psychiatrists and the legally competent authorities, they meet the requirements of the Mental Health Act (1983) operating in England and Wales and the Mental Health (Scotland) Act (1984).

Scenario Mrs Mary Smith is a 78-year-old lady who has fractured the neck of her left femur; she has a degree of heart failure and is mildly deaf. These physical conditions aside, she is well and is completely competent mentally.

You are Mrs Smith's named nurse and accompany the junior doctor who examines her and seeks her consent prior to surgery to fix her hip fracture. Having listened to the doctor, Mrs Smith signs her consent form. Some hours later you discover Mrs Smith is in a distressed state and, on questioning, find that she is unsure what the form was that she signed as, owing to the high level of background noise in the ward, she could not hear the doctor clearly.

Looking at the four components of consent outlined above, what steps must you take to ensure that Mrs Smith is empowered to give her informed consent for the procedure?

Confidentiality

Confidentiality is another area of nursing practice with a significant ethical dimension. Trust and respect lie at the heart of the ethical relationship between the nurse and the patient. Patients must have confidence that nurses will always act in their best interest in all aspects of the professional relationship. This expectation of trust extends beyond the assumption that the practitioner will carry out therapeutic interventions responsibly and using appropriate skills, knowledge and experience. It also embraces the assumption that any information imparted by the patient to the nurse, either formally (as in the clinical history) or informally (social chat over a cup of coffee), will not be used to the client's detriment – that confidentiality will be respected. From the perspective of the nurse, the principle must be that in all but the most extraordinary circumstances, the presumption of clients that their confidentiality will be respected will prevail. The *Code of professional conduct* (NMC 2002a) specifically requires practitioners to 'treat information about patients and clients as confidential' and only to make disclosures outside the team involved in the delivery of care with consent, by order of a court or where the practitioner can justify disclosure in the wider public interest.

Some examples of when a nurse may be justified in breaching confidentiality include:

- a court orders the information to be released
- the practitioner believes that by doing so a serious crime may be avoided or the detection of a serious crime assisted. Here, serious crime would normally mean a serious crime against the person, e.g. murder, manslaughter, rape or child abuse

● there are grounds to believe that the patient or another person may be at risk of death or serious physical or mental injury if information is not disclosed

● there are grounds to believe that there is a significant risk to public health in not disclosing information.

Formally disclosing information about a patient without consent is always a matter of the utmost gravity. Nurses must also bear in mind that informal breaches of confidentiality can take place more easily than formal ones; consider for instance the impact of two colleagues discussing a patient in their care while walking round a supermarket on their way home from duty and being overheard by a relative of the patient. This may seem improbable in a large city but is entirely feasible in a small town. Staff may also come under pressure from other bodies to provide informal information, e.g. by the police investigating crimes where they believe a suspect may have been injured. In this situation, the patient has the same right to respect for their confidentiality as any other hospital patient.

EXERCISE

Consider how inadvertent breaches of confidentiality can take place and how they can be averted.

ETHICAL ISSUES AT THE END OF LIFE

Having considered the importance of consent and confidentiality in day-to-day nursing practice, the chapter's consideration of ethics in practice concludes with ethical issues surrounding death and dying. First, however, it is important to be clear about when life ends. The answer to this question a century ago was straightforward; life ended when the heart ceased to beat, thus ending the supply of oxygenated blood to the brain. All the other main organs of the body stopped operating as a result of the ensuing hypoxia and metabolic disturbance. The advent of intensive care, artificial ventilation, inotropic drugs and mechanical assistance to support the failing heart have changed this view. While these 'artificial aids' remain in place oxygen exchange can continue, the cells can be supplied and one level of life, which we can call physiological life, can continue. Recognition of this in the 1960s and 1970s led to brain stem death being accepted as a defining measure of death in the developed world. In the UK, the process of confirming brain stem death has three phases:

● identifying the cause of the patient's coma and ensuring that it is not reversible, and then ensuring that the coma is not due to any drug overdose or interaction, hypothermia or metabolic disturbance

● performing a standard range of physiological tests to ensure that all centres in the brain stem which control the body's vital functions are destroyed

● ensuring that the patient cannot breathe when artificial supports are withdrawn.

To establish that brain death has occurred, each phase is repeated at least twice over a period of several hours or days.

Organ transplantation

This discussion of when (brain) death occurs is highly relevant when considering the ethical implications of organ transplantation.

In the UK, most transplants are undertaken using freely donated organs from cadavers. In these situations, organs are donated where the person, while alive, carried an organ donor card or expressed a wish to donate, and where no relatives of the person object to the donation and subsequent transplantation. Although the emphasis here is on the wishes of the individual while alive, and the absence of objection by the relatives, the good practice outlined earlier on informed consent can be helpful in assisting those in a bereaved and distressed state to come to terms with the decision they are being asked to make. Where permission is given and the retrieval and transplantation of organs goes ahead, all is well. Significant ethical problems arise where the relatives are unwilling to give permission and health professionals know that there are numerous patients who are likely to die because of a shortage of organs. In this situation it is important that any views expressed by the individual before the final illness are respected by both the relatives and the clinical staff. The nursing staff who have cared for the patient can be advocates for ensuring this respect is granted by both sides. In the absence of any expressed wishes by the patient, the views of the relatives must be paramount and coercive behaviour aimed at securing their agreement must be avoided.

Transplantation using organs from a living donor is potentially far more ethically complex than transplants using cadaver organs. Living donors, usually of kidneys but sometimes of portions of the liver, submit themselves to both short-term (from the significant surgery required to obtain tissue for transplantation) and long-term risks (from the possibility of future harmful effects occasioned as a result of having only one kidney or an incomplete liver). In the UK, living donor transplants are strictly regulated. The purpose of this regulation is to ensure that any decision to make a donation is free from duress and does not involve any payment or other reward. The regulatory system also monitors that the decision to make the donation is made with full information as to the possible consequences for the donor.

A major difficulty facing the UK is the inadequate numbers of organs being made available for transplant. There is little doubt that some patients, who could be saved if an organ were available for transplant, die while they are waiting. To address this, there are those who propose that, rather than carrying a donor card and indicating a willingness for their organs to be used, individuals should have to register their objection to their organs being used, while alive. The ethical implications of such a practice would require detailed consideration to ensure that an individual's autonomy over their body continues to be accorded its proper priority. The establishment of such a register could also represent the start of a slippery slope. A need to register objection to organ usage today could lead to a need to register an objection to other procedures tomorrow, and eventually could bring about a need to register individual objections to life being ended prematurely.

Persistent vegetative state

Another complex area related to the diagnosis of death is the condition known as persistent vegetative state (PVS), where the damage is to the cortex of the brain rather than its stem. This long-term condition leads to respiration and cardiac output being maintained in the absence of consciousness and self-awareness; physiological life continues in the absence of biographical life. Those responsible for the care of patients with this condition and their families face particularly harrowing decisions. As time goes by, it becomes clear that although treatment of any kind is not going to improve the patient's condition, care has to be ongoing, as, in the absence of severe infection or other major organ failure not associated with PVS, the patient's natural lifespan may be unimpaired.

When faced with a patient lying in a hospital bed with eyes open but unseeing, unable to communicate in anyway, unable to undertake any of the activities which were important in health and unable to recognize those close to them, there comes a point where care teams must ask themselves if they are acting in the patient's best interests by working hard to keep them alive. In the UK, the intentional killing of a person is never considered to be in their best interests; however, when curative treatment is not possible, as is the case for PVS, allowing a person to die free from pain and with all possible dignity may be considered to be in their best interests. In the UK, the question was addressed legally in the 1993 case of Airedale NHS Trust *v* Bland. Anthony Bland was one of the spectators who suffered grave injury in the Hillsborough football tragedy in 1989 and remained in PVS until 1992. In that year, the NHS Trust which managed the hospital in which he was receiving care sought the permission of the courts to stop life-sustaining treatment, including artificial feeding and hydration, and to restrict future treatment to those measures which would allow him to die free from pain and with dignity. The courts, including the House of Lords, upheld the argument that withdrawal of treatment could be in the person's best interests.

Once treatment has ended, the patient normally dies from dehydration within a matter of days. Several aspects of the decision to end treatment may be a cause of ethical unease, including the withdrawal of artificial food and nutrition, the inevitability of death and the manner of that death by dehydration. At the end of the day, in addressing these ethical dilemmas, health professionals need to be satisfied that accepting inevitable death is in the best interests of the patient. Only on that basis can the court decide that withdrawal of treatment is lawful and that action can be taken, in accordance with the ethical principles that underpin good nursing practice.

Euthanasia

If the treatment of those with PVS is an area where the ethical and legal considerations are unclear, the position relating to euthanasia, the deliberate, premature, ending of life, is quite clear. In UK law, the intentional ending of a person's life by act or omission is unlawful.

Two forms of euthanasia are often identified, voluntary and involuntary. The latter involves a belief that the person carrying out the process knows what is best for the individual who is bearing the suffering, which the procedure is intended to relieve, and that because of mental or physical frailty their best interests are being met by bringing their life to an end. This is not a position which finds favour even with those who advocate voluntary euthanasia, which involves a person who believes their suffering is intolerable asking those caring for them to take steps to bring their life to an end. The steps sought may be active, e.g. the deliberate administration of a drug or obstruction of the airway, or passive, e.g. failing to do something, such as withholding antibiotic therapy in patients with pneumonia in the knowledge that life will end.

It is noteworthy that opposition to euthanasia is not universal. The Dutch government recognizes that a person who requests, on an ongoing basis, that their life be ended because of very severe mental or physical suffering which cannot be relieved, may be assisted to die. Those who lead resistance to calls for the UK to go down the same road argue that euthanasia is unnecessary where there is sufficient provision of high quality hospice and palliative care.

REFLECTION POINT

If you have experience of caring for patients in the last stage of their lives, think how effective palliative care interventions can help prevent individuals coming to the point where they might seek the assistance of the care team to end their lives.

4

Assisted suicide

Part of the discussion around euthanasia relates to the notion of assisted suicide. Suicide, which, it may be argued, represents perhaps the greatest exercise of personal autonomy available to an individual, has not been unlawful in the UK for the past 40 years. However, to assist a person to take their own life by providing the means or opportunity for them to do so, or by physically participating in the suicidal act, remains both unlawful and unethical. This principle was confirmed in 2002 when Diane Pretty, who suffered from motor neurone disease, sought an undertaking from the Attorney-General for England and Wales that her husband would not be prosecuted under the Suicide Act (1961) for assisting her to take her own life when the suffering from her condition became unbearable. When the Attorney-General declined to give such an undertaking, Mrs Pretty appealed unsuccessfully to the domestic courts and ultimately to the European Court of Human Rights.

An important ethical issue which must be recognized when considering the ethics of the end of life is the doctrine of double effect. This doctrine holds that certain actions, although foreseen, are not intended. Perhaps the best example of this is the administration of powerful opiates to cancer sufferers who have intractable pain. Those prescribing and administering these drugs do so with the intention of relieving the patient's pain, while at the same time recognizing that the respiratory depression which they cause may also hasten death. As long as the intention in giving the drug is to relieve pain and not bring about death, the patient's best interests are served and the care team are not behaving unethically.

SUMMARY

The translation of the ethical codes and principles into the practice of nursing has been considered on a day-to-day basis, as well as at moments of ethical vulnerability – the beginning and end of life.

THE PROFESSIONAL STANDING OF THE NURSE

Above, the focus was on those aspects of the direct care of patients with an ethical dimension. Here, the impact of professional ethics on the nurse is examined.

PROFESSIONAL RELATIONSHIPS

Acting in the best interests of patients requires nurses not only to take matters such as consent, respect and confidentiality seriously, but also to use their practical skills, knowledge and experience appropriately, to recognize the limitations of their ability and to know when to call in other members of the care team. These are all matters which require the nurse to reflect regularly on their practice to ensure that professional relationships contribute to the overall well-being of the patient. Any action or omission on the part of the nurse which abuses the privileged relationship with the patient, be it physical, sexual, emotional or financial abuse or neglect, inducement or coercion by the nurse on the patient, is always against the patient's best interests and therefore unethical and professionally unacceptable.

Disciplinary action by employers and professional regulatory bodies may be taken against a nurse found to have abused the professional relationship with a patient. Where the action or omission is judged to constitute gross misconduct, removal from the professional register may ensue (see Chapter 3). This is the reality of the interface between professional ethics, employment and professional registration.

Relationships which respect ethical boundaries between professions and with other colleagues are as important as relationships between nurse and patient. Health care relies on teamworking and inter-professional co-operation. No single profession working in isolation can meet all the care needs of a patient. Therefore, each member of the team has to recognize and respect the role of the other members. The features of relationships between professions replicate those of the relationship between nurse and patient: trust, honesty and integrity. The best interests of patients are not served by disharmony within the care team with members not trusting each other to play their part, by inter-professional rivalry or by demarcation disputes leading to avoidable gaps in care.

A significant factor in care in recent years has been the extent to which nurses and other professionals have taken over responsibility for roles previously restricted to doctors. Before taking on these roles, nurses must ask themselves whether or not doing so is in the best interests of the patient. Where this is the case, the nurse must ensure that they have the appropriate skills, knowledge, experience and resources to undertake the role safely and effectively. The nurse must also ensure that by taking on new roles, the nursing elements of the patient's care will not suffer. Where these criteria cannot be met, the nurse should not agree to the reallocation of responsibilities and should seek the advice of senior colleagues. The NMC has produced guidance to support the professions in the *Code of professional conduct* (NMC 2002a, Chapter 2).

Just as nurses have taken on roles previously in the remit of doctors, so staff who are not registered nurses have taken on roles previously undertaken by nurses. There is no ethical objection to this but the nurse must be aware that they retain responsibility for acting in the best interests of the patient. This is best done by ensuring that those delivering the care have the skills, knowledge, experience and resources to give the care, by ensuring that delegation is appropriate and adequate supervision is afforded to the direct carer.

PROFESSIONAL COMMUNICATIONS

Clear communication is essential to effective and ethical professional relationships. To maintain professional integrity and act in the best interests of the patient, the nurse must communicate openly and honestly, not only with the patient but also with colleagues within the wider health care team. When communicating with patients, the nurse must ensure that what is being said is actually being understood. Developing a range of communication skills, styles and techniques that best meet the needs of the patient group must be a priority for every registered nurse. This will entail reviewing both verbal and non-verbal communication methods to find the most effective.

An important practical ethical consideration relates to translation and interpretation for patients from ethnic communities whose first language is not English. For convenience and speed, it may seem obvious to use family members (sometimes from extended families) to provide interpretation and translation between the patient and the care team. However, the need to maintain the patient's expectation of confidentiality must be paramount and, wherever possible, except in emergency situations, specialist interpretation and translation services should be used. The use of professional interpreters and translators who are familiar with clinical terminology also diminishes the likelihood of potentially dangerous mistranslation.

Truthfulness in communication with patients is another potentially difficult area for nurses. All practitioners will experience dilemmas over what information should be given to patients and how it should be given. These dilemmas are never more acute than in situations where bad news about a condition or prognosis has to be given. In these situations, the guiding principles must be that the nurse's first duty is always to the patient and the principle of non-maleficence. The general rule must be that the patient must be given truthful answers to direct questions. The skill for the person giving the answer is in assessing how much information the patient can cope with and having the empathy, knowledge and patience to support understanding of the answers. Where direct questions are not asked, patients should still be given sufficient truthful information to meet their needs at that point in time.

> **Scenario** You are the named nurse of James Worth, a 60-year-old man who has just been diagnosed as suffering from a brain tumour. The clinical team believe that Mr Worth must be told of his condition and also told that as no active treatment is possible he can only live for a matter of a few weeks during which time he will require ongoing and increasing care.
>
> Mr Worth's wife and some of his family insist that he be told that he will get better and be back home very shortly. Other members of the family support the view of the clinical team. The differing views lead to increasing tension at visiting times until finally a confrontation takes place just outside the ward but within hearing of Mr Worth who is understandably upset to hear his family confronting each other and asks you and his wife what is happening.
>
> Bearing in mind that the nurse's prime responsibility is to the patient, how would you handle this situation with regard to both Mr Worth and his family?

Communication with colleagues in health care teams is perhaps one of the areas requiring the greatest attention to ensure the best interests of the patient. While each team member has individual roles to fulfil and responsibilities towards the patient, poor communication within and between teams and their members can lead to patient care being adversely affected, with patients being given confusing information and mixed messages. The more complex the patient's care needs and the longer the episode of care, the greater the need for effective and co-ordinated communication. The named nurse or other identified key worker is well placed to be an effective co-ordinator for the whole team; communication is an essential part of the co-ordination process.

Maintaining appropriate records relating to a patient is a key part of the effective communication which serves the patient's best interests. Effective documentation should enable a reader with the requisite professional knowledge to know the patient's history, determine what problems and care needs have been identified, see the plans made for addressing the problems and meeting the identified needs, and find evidence of evaluation and review sufficient to enable care planning to be dynamic in response to changing need. Regardless of whether uni- or multi-professional documentation systems are used, it is the responsibility of the registered nurse to ensure that an adequate and honest record of all aspects of the nursing care given to the patient is maintained in a comprehensive and timely fashion. In compiling records, nurses should be aware that, with very few exceptions, patients have a statutory right to read their records. They should also be aware that patient records are key items of evidence in the handling of complaints, professional conduct proceedings, litigation and inquests or similar enquiries into patient deaths. As nurses may find themselves involved in any of these situations as a witness under oath, the importance of accurate record keeping cannot be over emphasised (NMC 2002a).

REFLECTION POINT

Critically appraise the last patient record you completed before reading the above and the *Code of professional conduct* and list any improvements that could enhance the quality of the documentation.

SUMMARY

The importance of professional relationships for patient care was examined and the need for effective communication and record keeping considered.

ETHICAL ISSUES AFFECTING POPULATIONS

There are a number of situations where the ethical implications of professional practice go beyond the individual patient and affect larger groups within the population. Three such areas are examined: research ethics, the ethical issues relating to resource decision-making and the ethics of health promotion.

DRUG TRIALS

Research is essential in ensuring that the boundaries of health care are advanced for the benefit of the population. Without research many of the interventions and drug treatments now taken for granted would never have come about. For example, if researchers had not examined why an extract of the bark and sap from a particular type of willow tree appeared to be able to relieve pain and reduce fever, salicylic acid would never have been discovered and the humble, yet potentially life-saving, aspirin would never have become available.

Increasingly, nurses will find themselves involved in or conducting research. All research on individuals, who may be patients or healthy volunteers, is regulated by a network of local and regional research ethics committees whose role is to ensure that all research undertaken complies with national and international good practice, including the Declaration of Helsinki (World Medical Association 1999). Important considerations for ethics committees are the design of the study, in terms of ensuring that it will meet its aims and will do so with the lowest number of participants exposed to the lowest risk, the recruitment of participants to ensure that no coercion is used and the quality of documentation relating to patient information and consent. For individual patients the requirements for obtaining informed consent and safeguarding confidentiality are as applicable to research activity as to other interventions.

By its nature, research will always throw up ethical problems. For example, in a drug trial, one group of patients receives the active drug, without them or their doctors knowing it, and shows a marked improvement in their symptoms, while another group in the same trial receives a placebo, again unknown to them or their doctors, and shows no improvement. The dilemma here is at what point does it become unethical to continue the trial, knowing that the active drug is beneficial and would improve the condition of the whole patient group?

ALLOCATION OF RESOURCES

Following on from research ethics, drug trials form a useful case-study bridge to a consideration of the ethical issues around the allocation of scarce resources for heath care. At the point when the drug is licensed and patients who have been in the trial phase need to take the drug on a long-term basis, as part of their therapy, the companies who have developed the drug expect the NHS to take over the funding responsibility which they have previously assumed. Given that newly developed and licensed drugs are frequently much more expensive than existing drugs, service planners and funders are left trying to balance their need to use limited budgets to the best effect for a population with the competing demand of patients and clinicians for access to the latest drug regardless of cost.

Since the foundation of the NHS in 1948 there have always been groups arguing that the NHS is insufficiently funded and now, almost 55 years later, it looks increasingly unlikely that there ever will be a consensus that funding is wholly adequate. Clearly, all additional funding is to be welcomed and will be useful, but the pace of change in technology, combined with the increasing longevity of the population, will probably always outstrip the ability or willingness of the taxpayer to contribute the level of funding required to meet every need or demand.

The question of whether need or demand should be met is a further ethical challenge, with ethical principles being available to support both views. The meeting of need implies that an organization or other body will take a paternalistic view of what the individuals who make up society need and this will become what is available. The meeting of demand recognizes the autonomy of the individual but also disregards the wider good. This dichotomy lies at the heart of debate on the rationing of health care. Regardless of their political persuasion, the government of the day propounds the argument that the UK has a comprehensive health care system which is free at the point of delivery. This is true. What central government never says is whether the system should meet need or demand.

In excess of 95% of the total NHS budget in any year is taken up in the delivery of core services such as emergency ambulances, district nursing, acute medicine and surgery, mental health teams and caring for older people. Each of these areas, together with rare conditions which require very costly treatment to enable individuals to have the best quality of life, competes alongside new drugs and techniques, such as interventional radiology and minimally invasive surgery for a share of the small amount of the NHS cake which is left for development. In this situation, both need (for timely treatment, such as hip replacement, which can make an individual pain-free and promote independence) and demand (for cosmetic surgery or complicated fertility treatment, which would meet a psychological need) remain unmet, giving rise to very real distress for a number of individuals. The fact that individuals lie at the heart of decisions about resource allocation must never be forgotten. Where 60 patients can receive treatment for varicose ulcers for a year for the same cost as one patient can receive the latest drug to treat his schizophrenia for a month, the decision appears easy; easy, that is, for the 60 people who will receive treatment, their families and their carers. But what of the schizophrenic patient, his family and his carers and also the people who have to make the decision? It is not so easy for them.

There is, of course, no simple solution to this problem. What tends to happen is that blunt instruments, such as waiting lists, are used to regulate the service delivered within the resources available and new developments are introduced in a piecemeal fashion as finances allow. The inevitable result of this method of resource allocation is that those with both need and demand accept their lot and carry on, or become dissatisfied and complain, often involving politicians in making representations on their behalf, in the hope that this will bring the desired result. What is needed is an open and inclusive debate aimed at agreeing that the population would be prepared to pay through taxation enough to meet every need and demand – or if this is not the case, reaching agreement on what level of service can be provided within the money taxpayers are willing to pay. On present evidence, none of the main UK political parties seems to have an appetite for such a debate; it looks, therefore, as if the present system will continue. Perhaps the best example of this debate having taken place is in the US state of Oregon where, following wide public and professional debate, the state legislature reached agreement on a list of interventions which are available from publicly-funded providers of health care (Ham 1998).

EXERCISE

Identify treatments to which you would not allocate development funding and explain why. By reference to your peer group identify commonalities or differences.

HEALTH PROMOTION

Society increasingly recognizes the benefit of encouraging people to maximize their own health and well-being by their own efforts, and the NHS devotes increasing resources and the time of health professionals, including nurses, to this end. When considering the promotion of health, it is important to consider the ethical implications of organized activities. Throughout this chapter much emphasis has been laid on a respect for the autonomy of the individual which can only be restrained in exceptional circumstances. Most health promotion initiatives operate by seeking to influence lifestyle and, while this does not directly interfere with individual autonomy (individuals remain free to act in whatever way they see fit, providing it is legal), critics would argue that the line between freedom of action and coercion into taking a course of action which is not the individual's free choice could easily be crossed. A good example of this is the campaign against cigarette smoking. For good reason, much health promotion and educational activity is aimed at reducing the number of people who smoke or getting those who continue to smoke less. As time goes by, the number of places where smoking is permitted reduces and those who cannot cease smoking are increasingly stigmatized. This could be construed as infringement of their autonomy. Conversely, the anti-smoking lobby could lay claim to the moral and ethical high ground by advancing the argument that their efforts to restrict smoking avoids people, who make an autonomous decision not to smoke, receiving passive doses of smoke.

At a macro level, questions must be asked about the ethics of society in relation to health promotion. Sticking with smoking as an example, it is well known that a large proportion of the cost of any tobacco product is government-imposed taxation. This taxation makes an important contribution to the income of the government, part of which is expended on the NHS. The application of the hypothecated 'tobacco tax' funding for public health projects by the NHS in Scotland represents a transparent example of this. Most health promotion professionals would advocate a ban on the advertising of tobacco products. This step has been mooted in the past by governments without coming to fruition. In terms of securing the greatest health benefit for the population, the ethical position would demand that all reasonable steps be taken to minimize the amount of smoking. If such a policy were introduced, the main loser would be the government, both in financial losses from taxation and in political losses, by potentially rendering themselves unelectable in the future. A moot point is the extent to which reduced demand for resources to fund NHS services, by reducing the number of smoking-related illnesses, would offset the reduction in income caused by the loss of taxation. As outlined above, given the increasing needs and demands faced by the NHS, any supportive argument along these lines is probably specious.

A final example of the ethical dilemmas posed by health promotion activities relates to the fluoridation of public water supplies, to prevent tooth decay, especially in young children. The fact that tooth decay can be prevented by adding fluoride to water is well established, as is the fact that in certain parts of the UK fluoride exists naturally. On this basis the health of children and young people could be improved by reducing their likelihood of developing dental caries. In terms of securing the greatest health benefit and minimizing harm to one large cohort of the population, the addition of fluoride is ethically supportable. The other perspective is that where fluoride does not occur naturally, it becomes yet another chemical added to water and forced on the population who have no choice but to drink it and use it for cooking. Where the addition lacks consent, this may be seen as acting against the autonomy of a large proportion of the population, especially those with no natural teeth who cannot derive the intended benefit.

SUMMARY

Moving from the individual to the population, the ethical issues affecting the whole of society, including funding for the NHS, were discussed.

CONCLUSION

This chapter has sought to give a brief overview of a number of important ethical principles and to apply them to the beginning of life, the treatment of adults and children, and issues at the end of life. Also, an overview of the importance of ethics on the population has been given. What has not been given is an answer to every ethical problem which you will face in a career in nursing. It is hoped that pointers have been given which can help you seek solutions (not right or wrong answers) to ethical difficulties, as well as stimulating further exploration.

CHAPTER 5

NURSE–PATIENT RELATIONSHIPS

Katrina Neal

INTRODUCTION

The relationship between nurse and patient can have a major impact on the well-being of both parties. Any satisfaction derived from an inappropriate relationship can quickly turn to dissatisfaction as the relationship inevitably becomes more stressful owing to the secrecy involved. This chapter aims to increase the student nurse's knowledge of the purpose, function and nature of the appropriate relationship between nurse and patient. Potential problems will be highlighted to help prevent the nurse from entering into an inappropriate relationship with a patient.

On completion of this chapter the student nurse should be able to meet the following requirements for pre-registration nursing programmes (UKCC 2001a):

- manage oneself, one's practice, and that of others, in accordance with the *Code of professional conduct* (NMC 2002a), recognizing one's own abilities and limitations
- practise in a fair and anti-discriminatory way, acknowledging the differences in beliefs and cultural practices of individuals or groups
- engage in, develop and disengage from therapeutic relationships through the use of appropriate communication and interpersonal skills.

These competencies are integrated throughout the chapter, with various sections and scenarios being directly applicable to more than one competence. Where sections bear greater relevance to one particular competence, these have been identified.

Similarly, although the scenarios described involve client groups from the four branches of pre-registration training, the principles contained within each scenario are directly transferable to each of the four branches. Therefore, students would benefit from working through all the scenarios regardless of client group.

Nurses relate to patients continuously throughout their working day. The interaction may be formal or casual. In the context of the nurse–patient relationship, regardless of the health or social care setting, it must always be within professional boundaries.

REFLECTION POINT

Think about a good relationship that you are currently involved in. It may be with a friend, relative, colleague or partner.

- What makes it a 'good' relationship?
- What is the balance of power, trust, respect and intimacy in the relationship?
- How does it make you feel?

Now consider a relationship that you have experienced as 'bad'.

- What made it 'bad'?
- What was the balance of power, trust, respect and intimacy in the relationship?
- How did you feel in the relationship?

How could you use these experiences positively to affect your relationships with patients?

PHILOSOPHICAL BASE

Every relationship has a philosophical base shaped by its purpose and needs. The relationship between nurse and patient is based on the patient's need for care, assistance and guidance. It is a relationship that is established solely to meet the patient's needs and, therefore, is therapeutic in nature. It is further shaped by the concepts of power, trust, respect and intimacy.

POWER

The balance of power within the nurse–patient relationship is not equal. The patient requires varying degrees of care, assistance, guidance or support from the nurse and as such is in a vulnerable position. The nurse has access to privileged information, skills and specialist knowledge of value to the patient, which places the nurse in a position of authority. The nurse's privileged and powerful position is recognized in *The Code of professional conduct* which places a professional duty on them to regard the interests and well-being of the patient as paramount. Thus, the nurse has a responsibility to use power to meet the therapeutic goals of the patient.

The appropriate use of professional power, however, is not always easy. Individuals have varying traits and values. Each nurse will exert power in a way that is unique, but must ensure that the process used is adapted to be acceptable to each patient. Patients will also demonstrate their needs in different ways. Most will want to have some involvement in making decisions about their care and treatment. Some will have the confidence and knowledge to be able to articulate this clearly; others will be less certain and some may choose not to be involved. The nurse will need to ascertain the patient's needs in a manner that is sensitive and acceptable to the patient.

The nurse needs consciously to relinquish some power and take on more of a partnership role with the patient in order to give choice and, more importantly, accept the choices the patient makes. Accepting patients' choices about their care and treatment is not usually an issue. However, if the choices made by the patient are in conflict with the professional viewpoint, there is potential for the patient's viewpoint to be discarded in favour of the professional (Kohner 1994). The imbalance of power that favours the professional side of the relationship leads, if not appropriately managed, to the development of paternalism – the 'professional is right' and 'knows best', rather than partnership where the professional sets out the pros and cons and supports the patient's decision.

TRUST

The patient, on entering the health care setting, will place trust in the nurse. This element of trust is critical because, in the nurse–patient relationship, the patient is in a vulnerable position. People become vulnerable whenever their health or usual function is compromised. This vulnerability increases when they enter unfamiliar surroundings, situations or relationships. Some groups of patients – children, older people, those with mental health or learning difficulties, are especially vulnerable.

REFLECTION POINT
Think of a time in your own life when you felt vulnerable or out of your depth? For example, you may have been involved in a court case and had to deal with lawyers or the police; you or a member of your family may have been treated in a health care setting with which you were unfamiliar; you may have experienced a difficult or long labour. Try to recall your feelings and how you perceived those in control of the situation.

The patient's trust in the nurse will be, largely, based on assumption – assumption that they are employed in a health care setting and must, therefore, have unique knowledge and skill, and that they will use their knowledge and skills to provide proper care.

Patients will be aware of the media coverage given to breaches of trust in health care. Many will be familiar with the case of the nurse Beverly Allitt who caused the deaths of children at Grantham and Kesteven General Hospital in 1991 (DoH 1994b), and of Harold Shipman, the GP convicted in 2001 of murdering some of his patients (Baker 2001), and most recently of the retention of children's organs at Alder Hey and other hospitals. Such events raise anxiety and make it more difficult for trusting relationships to develop between health care professionals and patient. This places greater onus on the nurse to demonstrate behaviours and attitudes that justify the patient placing trust in them.

Trust and confidentiality are two sides of the same coin. The patient will assume that the nurse can be trusted to maintain confidences. However, it is impractical to obtain consent every time there is a need to share information with other members of the team, and the nurse will need to ensure, during the early stages of the relationship, that the patient knows that information will be treated as confidential but will be shared, on a need to know basis, with others involved in the delivery of care. Part of the discussion will be to determine the patient's wishes regarding the sharing of information with their family and others.

Special consideration will be required for those patients who are considered incapable of giving permission. Incapability may have a variety of reasons, e.g. lack of consciousness, anaesthesia or mental incapacity, and may be either short or long term. When a patient is considered to be incapable of giving permission, a consensus decision should be sought within the multi-professional team (NMC 2002a).

Building a trusting relationship will greatly improve care and help to reduce stress for the patient. Breaches of confidentiality could have a devastating effect on the patient's ability to place trust in the nurse and thus care should be taken at all times to guard against such breaches by protecting information from improper disclosure. Potential breaches of confidentiality are usually perceived to be associated with information contained in written records; guidance regarding records and record keeping is available from most regulatory bodies including the Nursing and Midwifery Council (NMC). However, verbal communication is a major potential source of disclosure of confidential information, and care should be taken to ensure that it cannot be overheard. Ward handovers, coffee breaks and travelling on public transport are the most likely places for overhearing personal confidential information about patients.

REFLECTION POINT

What is it that your friends/family/others do that encourage you to trust them?

RESPECT

Respect for the patient and their decisions about their health care is fundamental to the relationship. This means identifying the patient's preferences for nursing care and respecting those preferences, as far as is possible, recognizing that there may be restrictions. For example, the patient may prefer a treatment that is unlawful, such as assisted suicide, or for which there is little supportive evidence, such as a new type of alternative therapy, or that you do not have the resources to provide. The nurse obviously must work within the law and thus cannot support or engage in illegal practices. However, the moral rather than legal issues are not as clear cut and require some negotiating. Respect for the patient's decisions and thus for the patient as an autonomous individual may result in uncomfortable compromises for the nurse. Respect for individuals and their autonomy means respecting their ability to make decisions about themselves and ensuring they have choices. This raises issues of mental capacity and informed consent (see Chapter 4).

Part of respect is recognizing the worth of the patient as an individual and maintaining their dignity. Registered nurses are accountable for ensuring that they promote and protect the interests of patients in their care irrespective of gender, age, race, disability, sexuality, culture, economic status, religious or political beliefs. Nurses must be aware of their own beliefs and values, their foundation and their impact on their behaviour.

REFLECTION POINT

- What do you think/feel about caring for a patient with beliefs that are different from your own?
- How do you feel about caring for someone with a different gender orientation or of a different race?
- Do you think people with physical or mental disabilities are equal to you?
- What do you think of people who are alcohol or drug dependent or who have AIDS?

INTIMACY

Intimacy is the ability to join with another human being on an emotional and physical level. It requires a sense of personal identity and confidence in your ability to relate effectively with another human being. Intimacy in the professional nurse–patient relationship relates to activities that the nurse performs with and for the patient. These activities may be physical, psychological, emotional, spiritual or social, or may contain two or more elements. They are not sexual in nature. However, they do require a closeness and understanding between the nurse and patient that requires the patient to be confident in the nurse and their ability and willingness to treat the patient's interests as paramount.

SUMMARY

The philosophical base of relationships has been considered, while highlighting the concepts that shape the relationship between nurse and patient.

PRINCIPLES UNDERPINNING THE NURSE–PATIENT RELATIONSHIP

Nursing is considered to be a profession. A profession has a distinct and substantial body of evidence, with extensive education that has both theory and practice components. Its members (nurses) share a common identity, values, attitudes and behaviours (see Chapter 2).

SELF-REGULATION

The nursing profession regulates itself in order to serve and protect the public. This means that the profession holds its members accountable for their practice and expects them to abide by its *Code of professional conduct*. The *Code* sets out the profession's expectations of its members in terms of standards of conduct. The public expects the profession to set standards for itself, to adhere to them and to call to account any members who breach those standards. Professional self-regulation is underpinned by three principles: promoting good practice, preventing poor practice and intervening in unacceptable practice. This means that evidence of effective practice should be shared with colleagues and actively promoted, while failures in performance must be acknowledged and addressed. The practice of professional self-regulation requires that registered nurses ensure their acts and omissions in practice have, as their core focus, the interests and safety of patients. It is this practice that contributes to patients' experience and perception of the quality of service they receive and is the face of professional self-regulation from the public perspective. For more information see Chapter 2.

COMPETENCE

At the point of registration, nursing students will have demonstrated that they have reached the competencies as outlined in *Requirements for Pre-registration Nursing Programmes* (UKCC 2001a). The *Nursing and Midwifery Order 2002,* section 3(2), requires the NMC to establish from time to time standards of education, training, conduct and performance for nurses and midwives and to ensure maintenance of those standards (see Chapter 3).

A competent nurse possesses the skills and abilities to practise safely without direct supervision. Self-regulation requires registered nurses to practise safely and thus to acknowledge their limitations, while seeking further to develop their knowledge and competence. Acting outside your competence obviously poses a risk to both the patient and the nurse. The primary aim of the nurse is to provide good quality, safe care to patients. As a professional practising self-regulation, the nurse is accountable for everything they do and everything they fail to do but could reasonably have been expected to do. The nurse can reasonably be expected to care for their patients properly. If a decision not to act could cause harm to a patient, then the nurse has a responsibility to act. Failure to do so would be an omission.

The nurse is also accountable for the quality of their delegation, which means they must ensure that the person to whom they delegate a task is competent to undertake that task. Professional accountability is personal to each registered nurse. No one else can accept responsibility on their behalf and thus they must be able to justify their decisions.

TEAMWORK

The nurse is just one component of the multi-professional team (see also Chapter 16). The patient is the primary member and the focus of activity. Other members of the team include medical practitioners, physiotherapists, occupational therapists, social workers, health visitors, other community staff, radiologists, dieticians, social workers, pharmacists, ambulance drivers, porters, domestic staff and many more. The nurse will engage most regularly with those members of the team who are immediately involved in the delivery of health and/or social care to the patient.

For the team to function effectively, role boundaries will need to be negotiated so that roles and responsibilities are clarified. Effective teams result from understanding people and the way they work, and realizing and valuing the fact that people are not all the same, but have different strengths which they can bring to the team as a whole. The multi-disciplinary team needs to value and understand the contribution of all its members. Within the team each practitioner remains accountable for their own practice, even where tasks are delegated.

Communication is an essential part of teamwork and good practice. The principles of effective communication include:

- being greeted warmly
- being listened to
- receiving clear explanations
- being re-assured
- being able to express fear and concern
- being respected
- being given enough time
- being treated as a person, not just a disease.

Each member of the team must communicate effectively and share knowledge, skills and expertise with other members, as required for the benefit of the patient. The patient's perspective must be included.

The patient's health care records are a useful tool of communication within the team, with each member responsible for maintaining their part of the records. The nurse must ensure that the records they keep are an accurate account of treatment, and care planning and delivery. The record should be consecutive and written with the involvement of the patient, where practicable, as soon as possible after the event has occurred. It should provide clear evidence of the care planned, the decisions made, the care delivered and the information shared.

The nurse must treat information about the patient as confidential and use it only for the purpose for which it was given.

REFLECTION POINT

Think about the different types of communication that you have been party to. What forms of communication do you find most helpful? Identify three ways in which they could be used within teams.

CONTINUING PROFESSIONAL DEVELOPMENT

Reaching the point of registration is only the beginning of professional learning. Maintaining competence in an ever-changing and increasingly complex environment requires continuous learning. Patients have come to expect more from nurses as they themselves learn more about health and health care as a result of ever increasing media sources providing information of variable quality. Re-registration standards for nurses require a minimum of 35 hours of learning activity, relevant to area of practice, in each 3-year period. Most nurses will want to do considerably more in order to improve on current areas of competence and develop their practice.

Techniques such as reflective practice provide opportunities for nurses to look closely at the way they work and the care they deliver, and consider changes they could make to improve what they do. Analysing incidents with the help of a senior practitioner who is able to challenge and add another perspective, possibly in a clinical supervision setting, can be equally as beneficial in assisting learning and professional development. Clinical supervision brings nurses and skilled supervisors together to reflect on practice. Its aims are to identify solutions to problems, improve practice and increase understanding of professional issues. Clinical supervision is therefore helpful when considering aspects of the relationship between nurse and patient as it enables gentle probing and challenge in a supportive climate. For more information see Chapters 3 and 17.

SUMMARY

The principles that underpin professional practice, and thus form the foundations of the therapeutic relationship, have been identified.

BOUNDARIES IN THE NURSE–PATIENT RELATIONSHIP

Historically, nurses were helped to avoid emotional involvement with their patients by maintaining a 'distance' from them through a focus on providing physical care only (Arnold and Boggs 1999). Approaches to nursing have, however, become holistic in nature, thus encouraging involvement in all aspects of the person and allowing a 'closeness' to develop. Although this closeness or intimacy is superficial, as it is built on limited personal knowledge about the patient, in practice it may 'feel' much more substantial and robust. This has resulted in professional boundaries becoming less clearly defined and obvious.

Boundaries in all relationships are open to interpretation as they are largely based on the perceptions of the people involved in the relationship. The nurse will have a view of what is appropriate, as will the patient. Hopefully, these views will be similar, but this may not be the case and some negotiation may be required.

Professional boundaries are not solely dependent on the views of the individuals involved in any one specific relationship. They have as their foundation the profession's perception of a 'right' relationship. Professional boundaries are important as they allow nurses and patients to interact safely in a relationship that is developed purely for therapeutic purposes.

PRINCIPLES UNDERPINNING PROFESSIONAL BOUNDARIES

Certain rules or principles must be followed when establishing the boundaries of the relationship:

- the relationship is therapeutic in nature
- the relationship focuses solely on the needs of the patient
- the responsibility for maintaining professional boundaries rests with the nurse
- the professional relationship exists for the duration of the patient's need for care or treatment and may extend for several years post discharge in the case of vulnerable patients.

Within the therapeutic relationship the nurse, as discussed earlier, is the main power bearer and has as their key responsibility the interests and well-being of their patient. The nurse, if they are to enable the patient to make decisions, must chose to relinquish some of their power. This surrendering of power can help to address the imbalance in the relationship and prepare the way for a more collaborative or partnership approach to care to develop. However, the patient must be willing to be an active participant in their care and chose to accept an increase in power and decision-making.

Working in partnerships with patients and directing care toward their needs necessitates good communication. The patient can make an informed choice only if they are given clear information at every stage of the care process. The nurse, in order to determine the most effective and acceptable way to assist and support the patient in decision-making, must actively listen to the patient's concerns. Decisions are based on an individual's values and beliefs. They will encompass knowledge about the hospital or surgery that the patient has received from friends, relatives and the media. Past experiences will have a major impact and will colour the individual's view for good or bad. Horror stories and good news stories will also play a part in the patient's choice of care.

Decision-making is rarely an isolated act. The nurse will contribute to the process by drawing on professional knowledge and skill and ensuring that the patient has sufficient information, in a format that they can understand and find acceptable, to enable them to make informed decisions about their treatment and care. The nurse, with insight of their own values and beliefs, will be aware of potential conflict in the decision-making process. This should be managed to ensure that the patient's decision is not made as a result of coercion or manipulation. The nurse must accept the decision of a competent adult even if they disagree with it. It is good practice to maintain comprehensive records of decisions made and the rationale behind the patient's choices as part of a plan of care negotiated between nurse and patient to meet the patient's needs.

MAINTAINING BOUNDARIES

Breaches of the boundaries of the professional relationship between nurse and patient can occur when there is a lack of understanding of how, why or where these occur.

Boundaries can easily become blurred when the nurse feels the patient has become a friend and bears some responsibility for maintaining them. One way in which the nurse can prevent this happening is to reflect constantly on their practice to ensure it is patient focused. Identifying and openly acknowledging the potential for breaches is an important part of maintaining boundaries.

How, why and where breaches of the therapeutic relationship occur should be considered as part of the nurse's ongoing learning. Examining current therapeutic relationships in one-to-one or small group settings can provide enormous opportunities to identify areas of potential concern. Nurses working in isolation with little opportunity to share their concerns are potentially at a greater risk of breaching the boundaries and should be given additional consideration when local policies and procedures for the management of risk are developed. Practitioners under stress also have a greater incidence of breaching professional boundaries than their less stressed counterparts. Thus, the development of support and learning mechanisms for such practitioners is crucial.

When nurses and patients engage in a close therapeutic relationship, the potential and opportunity for the relationship to develop in an improper manner increases. Vulnerable people can, on occasion, form attachments that they would not normally form, e.g. becoming attached to the nurse whom they found to be particularly helpful, caring or knowledgeable. Emotions aroused in the course of the therapeutic relationship, on the part of either the nurse or the patient, do not necessarily disappear as soon as the patient is discharged from care (Briant and Freshwater 1998). The nurse must very carefully consider whether it is ever appropriate to have anything other than a purely professional relationship with a patient or former patient. Personal relationships with vulnerable patients are never acceptable. To re-emphasise, the responsibility for maintaining the boundaries of the relationship rests solely with the nurse.

DUAL RELATIONSHIPS

Dual relationships – in which the patient already has a relationship with the nurse, e.g. as a business colleague, friend or relative – can raise complex issues for practitioners. Difficulties in maintaining boundaries can occur as the patient's expectations of the nurse will also be the expectations of a friend, relative or business partner. The boundaries to their non-nurse–friend relationship will already be set. The nurse will need to explain the change in boundaries required by their professional caring role as they must ensure that each relationship is kept within its appropriate boundaries.

Dual relationships are common in small and isolated communities where nurses have become expert at managing the boundaries of their roles. Within hospital ward-based settings, managers often arrange for a nurse to work on another ward if that is considered to be necessary for reasons of confidentiality or to spare the patient and nurse embarrassment. However, in isolated communities, or some primary care settings, this may not be possible, placing an even greater responsibility on the nurse to ensure that the principles of the therapeutic relationship are observed.

Scenario Jane is a registered nurse and midwife living and working in a small community in the far north of Scotland. She provides the district nursing and midwifery service for the community. Many of her patients and clients are also personal friends. Jane is loved and respected by the community. She is known not only for her skill and expertise but also for her loyalty and caring friendships. As many of Jane's patients and clients are her personal friends, they are also friends of each other, such is the size of the community.

Maggie, one of Jane's peers and old school friends, is expecting her second baby. Her first pregnancy and delivery had been easy and Maggie expected this one to be no different. Fliss, another school friend of them both, was expecting her first child. The pregnancy was now progressing well following a difficult first trimester. Maggie was attending the clinic for a routine check-up.

Jane:	*'How are you Maggie? Any problems?'*
Maggie:	*'No, bairn's proper lively and I'm feeling okay.'*
Jane:	*'Good, we'd better just check your blood pressure and have a little listen to junior and you'll be done. Have you filled in any evaluation forms for the antenatal classes yet?'*
Maggie:	*'Aye, I have but I thought I'd keep them all together and hand them back at the last! Just in case you don't like my answers, ha! Besides that, have you seen Fliss recently?'*
Jane:	*'Fliss was in this morning. Are you coming to dinner at Morgan's tonight? I think Fliss and Peter will be there.'*
Maggie:	*'No, John and I are visiting his parents tonight, it's his Dad's birthday. I was worried about Fliss yesterday, she looked so peeky. I don't think things between her and Peter are good at the moment, not very understanding in the bedroom department – did she not tell you this very morning at her check up?'*
Jane:	*'That's not for me to say. Confidential information and all that.'*
Maggie:	*'Such a stickler for protocol! How did I know you would say that!'*

Consider:
- What do you think of the discussion between Jane and Maggie?
- Were any boundaries breached in this scenario?
- Would you have done anything different?

Again, the onus for maintaining the boundaries of the therapeutic relationship rests solely with the nurse. Jane has maintained the boundaries while also maintaining her friendships. To have breached confidentiality could have led to a loss of trust from her patients and clients.

LONG-TERM AND REGULAR SERVICE USERS

A sense of 'knowing' the patient as a person will probably increase when patients are present in a health care setting for a long time or are regular users of the service. Obtaining personal information relating to the lifestyle of the patient as an individual is a normal part of human interaction and will increase with each contact. Most probably, the sharing of 'personal' information from nurse to patient will also increase over time. Therefore, when patients remain in the care setting for a considerable length of time or return/receive visits on a regular basis for cyclical treatments, such as cytotoxic therapy, inevitably the depth of the relationship will increase. Some patients may start to view the care setting as 'home' with the nurses occupying the roles of family as contact becomes part of their social norm for the duration of their care. However, it should be remembered that the relationship between nurse and patient remains a professional one that is built on limited knowledge of the real person and their beliefs, values, desires, dislikes, etc.

ACCEPTABLE BEHAVIOURS

The *Code of professional conduct* sets out the principles of professional conduct (NMC 2002a). It provides the nurse and the public with a picture of what is expected of someone who is registered and therefore has a licence to practise nursing on the public. Successful application of these principles requires nurses as individuals to be aware of themselves and their own behaviour/values/beliefs and how these may impact on their patients. For example, a nurse may consider their behaviour to be sound when viewed from their own perspective. However, viewing the same behaviour from the perspective of the patient may provide a different picture. A laugh and joke at the patient's expense may be funny for the nurse but not for the patient!

Over-familiarity, using terms of endearment such as 'luvvie', 'pet' or 'mate', or first names without asking, is disrespectful and may appear cheeky, rude or patronizing to the patient, while the nurse considers she is being 'friendly'. It is not just forms of address that can be misinterpreted in a relationship. Some people are more naturally tactile than others and will think nothing of holding a hand or putting an arm round someone who is upset or distressed. However, such physical contact may not be acceptable to some individuals, while to others supportive physical gestures to demonstrate empathy and give comfort as part of a therapeutic caring relationship are viewed as an integral part of healing. The nurse, as part of their assessment, must use her knowledge and skill to determine the boundaries of therapeutic touch with each patient.

Non-therapeutic touch, swearing, coarse language, religious or racist comments, and comments which belittle the patient are some of the behaviours that can cause distress. The NMC, as the regulatory body for nurses, midwives and health visitors, would view such behaviours as abuse and as such operate a policy of zero tolerance. A nurse demonstrating such behaviours could expect to have their name removed from the professional register for professional misconduct. These types of boundary breaches can occur in organizations where a cultural tolerance of abuse has developed. Within such cultures it is not uncommon to see relationships that have developed beyond the purely therapeutic (Martin 1984).

Scenario Mrs Thread sat quietly by her bed. She was slightly disorientated and bemused after waking up to find herself in hospital. At 78 she was very fit and usually well. The last she could recall she was in her garden pegging out her washing. She listened to the other three patients in the bay chatting but made no attempt to join in. She was thinking about the test she was having later that day. The doctor had explained it, but she couldn't quite remember. It didn't matter, that nice nurse Robert was coming back to go though it again with her.

That afternoon Robert sat next to Mrs Thread and chatted casually with her for a few minutes. She seemed much better orientated than she had that morning and was anxious to know more about the test.

Robert was quite a tactile person. As he chatted and explained the procedure to Mrs Thread, he occasionally patted her knee. She said nothing but on the third occasion she grabbed his hand and gently laid it in his lap. Robert smiled, apologized and continued explaining what would happen. He was just about to place his hand on her knee again when he stopped himself. He swapped the notes he was holding into his other hand so that he could not touch her without stretching awkwardly to do so. She obviously was not a 'touchy' person.

Consider:

● What do you think of Robert's behaviour?

● What, if anything, would you have done differently?

Robert's behaviour was exemplary. He was tactile but quickly discovered that Mrs Thread was not. His smile and apology dealt with any potential awkwardness between them and conveyed that he cared and understood. He knew that he would probably pat her knee again if he did not do something to restrain his hands. He was that type of person.

Scenario Yvette was married with two young children, aged 7 and 5 years. She had been a district nurse for 10 years and enjoyed her job. Because of her children, she worked the twilight shift when her husband was at home to care for them. She had quite a few 'regulars' whom she enjoyed going to visit.

Polly and her husband, Derek, were two such people. Polly suffered from cardiomyopathy and severe rheumatoid arthritis. She was often confined to a wheelchair and regularly suffered pain. Winter was a bad time for her as she always seemed to suffer badly in the cold and damp. Her joints played her up and she became more breathless.

Yvette visited twice a week when Polly was unwell, sometimes resorting to daily visits when things were really bad. Polly would benefit from a spell in hospital but would not consent to go. She preferred to be in her own home with Derek.

Derek and Polly loved to hear about what was going on in the world and would question Yvette about her family. They loved news of the children and their activities, taking an interest in their school photos.

Yvette did not mind sharing this with them, she was proud of her family and was happy to provide some distraction for Derek and Polly.

Derek started saving his one and two pence pieces in a jam jar. When he filled it he gave it to Yvette 'for the children'.

Yvette: 'Oh, thank you, that's very kind but, I'm sorry, I can't accept it.'
Derek: ''f course you can, it's not much – only coppers – and we're so grateful for everything you do for us. The children can spend it on their holiday.'
Yvette: 'Well, only if you're sure.'
Derek: 'That's settled then.'

Over the next 6–7 months Derek gave her lots of 'coppers for the children'. Yvette accepted them graciously. Polly and Derek had a daughter, Mandie, who was about Yvette's age. She was married but had no children. She regularly visited her parents, took them on holidays with her family, and had them to stay for birthdays and Christmas. Mandie arrived to collect her Mum and Dad one Wednesday evening during Yvette's visit. She chatted with Yvette as she helped pack her Mum's bag.

Derek interrupted them: 'Excuse me girls – here you are dear.' He handed Yvette a jam jar. 'The coppers for the children.'
Mandie, opening her purse: 'Oh, are you collecting for charity?'

Consider:
● How would you have managed this situation?
● Would you have accepted the 'coppers for the children'? On what are you basing your answer?

Yvette should have gently refused to accept money explaining that to do so would jeopardize her future as their nurse as it would be a breach of her *Code of professional conduct*. Sharing information about her children was not wrong. Patients should have opportunities to engage in normal conversation. The burden for the professional is knowing where to draw the line between appropriate and inappropriate behaviour. The principles of the nurse–patient relationship state that the therapeutic relationship should focus on the needs of the patient. Neither the conversation nor the acceptance of the 'coppers' were outside this principle as Yvette was not acting in her own or her family's interests. She was probably trying not to offend Derek and Polly. However, by accepting the money she put herself and them in a difficult position. She had opened the gates for them to give her more, and had inadvertently put pressure on them to continue to give more, because from their perspective, what would she think if she suddenly stopped doing it? Would she think they were unhappy with her?

The duty to maintain appropriate boundaries rests with the nurse. Yvette had failed to maintain those boundaries. She should have discussed her difficulty in this situation with her manager and sought help to manage such events in the future.

SUMMARY

The appropriate boundaries to the nurse–patient relationship have been identified and the areas of concern highlighted. Scenarios of right and wrong relationships have been used to raise the student's awareness of the issues to be considered.

5

RECOGNIZING WARNING SIGNS AND INTERVENING IN UNACCEPTABLE PRACTICE

Detecting problems within the professional relationship between the nurse and patient is rarely a simple process. Many incidents remain private and undocumented. However, investigations of alleged abuse have often identified earlier signs of difficulties within the relationship.

REFLECTION POINT
Reflect on the notes that you made at the beginning of this chapter with regard to good and bad relationships, and think about your behaviour in each relationship.

Signs vary depending on the nature of the relationship that is developing. For example, a nurse who is becoming emotionally attached to a patient will display different behaviours from one who dislikes a patient. The patient will also develop different behaviours depending on whether the altered attention is welcomed. The primary aim is to prevent inappropriate relationships from developing by recognizing the warning signs in you and others and taking appropriate action.

DETECTING THE SIGNS

The nurse may exhibit some of the following signs:

- a marked change in behaviour towards a particular patient, such as becoming more friendly, flirtatious, aggressive or controlling
- a marked change in dress – such as wearing more make-up, more revealing clothes (if a uniform is not required), suddenly wearing aftershave
- secrecy and defensiveness, rather than confidentiality, when the nurse discusses the patient's care with colleagues
- spending more time in the work setting close to the patient and appearing reluctant to end the working day
- making unnecessary visits to the patient.

The patient may exhibit the following:

- signs of having inside knowledge of the department, its staff or other patients
- signs of becoming fearful or showing loss of self-esteem
- signs of becoming increasingly withdrawn or of increasing anxiety and loss of concentration
- signs of physical injury, such as unexplained bruises, grazes, swellings and bleeding
- signs of becoming manipulative, unco-operative or aggressive.

Both the nurse and the patient may exhibit:

- subtle changes in body language
- signs of stress.

Obviously emotions will be involved for both parties. The nurse will know how she 'feels' about the patient and will know whether those feelings are appropriate in a professional therapeutic relationship. A good test is to consider, 'Would you like your boss to know what you are thinking/feeling about Ms or Mr X?' Having feelings for a patient is not wrong, it is a part of human nature to develop relationships. However, it becomes wrong the moment the nurse decides to act on their feelings rather than the therapeutic needs of the patient. Therefore, if the answer to this question is 'no', the nurse must ensure that they are able to maintain the relationship within its proper boundaries in order to safeguard the patient.

The nurse can act in a variety of ways, e.g. using chaperones when undertaking intimate procedures, taking care to ensure they are not left alone with the patient in situations where emotions could be disclosed, adhering to local policies and procedures and, if necessary, taking steps to withdraw from the role of carer for that particular patient.

A clinical supervision setting, established within the principles of professional guidance, as outlined in *Supporting Nurses and Midwives through Lifelong Learning* (NMC 2002e) should provide a safe forum in which to explore the relationship and its proper boundaries.

MANAGING INAPPROPRIATE RELATIONSHIPS

Inappropriate relationships are damaging to the nurse as well as the patient. It is important for both parties that the relationship is recognized as such and returned to within the boundaries of a therapeutic relationship. The principles upon which the boundaries to appropriate relationships are developed have as their purpose the protection of the patient and the nurse. Nurses who breach the boundaries of the therapeutic relationship place themselves in a situation that could lead to charges of professional misconduct and result in their names being removed from the professional register (see Chapter 3).

The nurse must consider the affect that breaches of the boundaries could have on the patient. The well-being of the patient is of paramount importance and overrides all other concerns. Breaching the boundaries is to betray the trust that patients place in the nurse to act only in their best interests. The health regulatory bodies report patients losing trust and faith in health care professionals as a result of professional misconduct borne out of inappropriate relationships; there is much anecdotal evidence from the Prevention of Professional Abuse Network (POPAN) to support this. Abused patients suffer anxiety, shock, anger, lack of trust, pain and fear. For some patients their access to future health care is restricted as a result of the damage incurred (Apfel and Simon 1985). Supportive measures such as counselling should be provided as necessary.

The approach toward the nurse should focus on learning from the mistakes in order to prevent a similar occurrence in the future. However, for severe breaches of the boundaries, such as abuse of patients, the nurse involved must be reported to the regulatory body.

RECOGNIZING ABUSE

Abuse within the nurse–patient relationship is the result of the misuse of power or a betrayal of trust, respect or intimacy between the nurse and the patient, which the nurse should know would cause physical or emotional harm to the patient. Abuse takes many forms. Physical, psychological, verbal, sexual, financial/material abuse and neglect have been defined in *Practitioner–Client Relationships and the Prevention of Abuse* (NMC 2002h) (Box 5.1).

Box 5.1 Definitions of abuse and neglect (NMC 2002h)

Physical abuse: any physical contact which harms patients or is likely to cause them unnecessary and avoidable pain and distress. Examples include handling the patient in a rough manner, giving medication inappropriately, poor application of manual handling techniques or unreasonable physical restraint. Physical abuse may cause psychological harm.

Psychological abuse: any verbal or non-verbal behaviour which demonstrates disrespect for the patient and which could be emotionally or psychologically damaging. Examples include mocking, ignoring, coercing, threatening to cause physical harm or denying privacy.

Verbal abuse: any remark made to or about a patient which may reasonably be perceived to be demeaning, disrespectful, humiliating, intimidating, racist, sexist, homophobic, ageist or blasphemous. Examples include making sarcastic remarks, using a condescending tone of voice or using excessive and unwanted familiarity.

Sexual abuse: forcing, inducing or attempting to induce the patient to engage in any form of sexual activity. This encompasses both physical behaviour and remarks of a sexual nature made towards the patient. Examples include touching a patient inappropriately or engaging in sexual discussions which have no relevance to the patient's care.

Financial/material abuse: involves not only illegal acts such as stealing a patient's money or property but also the inappropriate use of a patient's funds, property or resources. Examples include borrowing property or money from a patient or a patient's family member, inappropriate withholding of a patient's money or possessions and the inappropriate handling of, or accounting for, a patient's money or possessions.

Neglect: the refusal or failure on the part of the registered nurse, midwife or health visitor to meet essential care needs of a patient or client. Examples include failure to attend to the personal hygiene of a patient, failure to communicate adequately with the patient and the inappropriate withholding of food, fluids, clothing, medication, medical aids, assistance or equipment.

REPORTING INAPPROPRIATE BEHAVIOURS

Reporting inappropriate behaviours is necessary to protect both parties. Clinical governance arrangements in organizations have as their focus learning from mistakes and 'near misses'. For all incidents, including where misconduct is not proven, the emphasis is on learning and preventing similar mistakes recurring.

Managing the termination of an inappropriate relationship is not within the remit of the student nurse. The role of the student is to report the matter to a person with the authority to manage the situation. This is not always easy, as reporting someone feels very uncomfortable even when this is done to protect a patient from harm. However, the health care organization will have a policy for reporting such concerns. The policy will detail the steps to be taken and the person to whom the concerns should be reported, including alternatives should they be required. The policy will also outline the documentation to be kept which will include the date, time, nature of the incident(s) and the circumstances surrounding the incident(s) (see also Chapter 1).

Once concerns have been raised, the manager will have as their primary aim the safety and well-being of the patient.

Scenario Patrick, 35, is a senior community psychiatric nurse with 5 years' experience in his current role. He has his own caseload and works on his own. He gave up clinical supervision years ago as he had nothing else to learn, he knew the job and types of patients so well. His periods of management supervision with his line manager have also tailed off so that he sees her once every 2 months at most now, as opposed to every 3–4 weeks like he used to. He considers himself to be an expert practitioner in control of his patch.

Martin is 19 years old and very shy. He has been having problems with relationships recently. He says he frightens girls off because he cannot always control his temper. 'It's alright when I'm on a high but when I start coming down, it gets a bit tricky sometimes.'

Martin had been referred to Patrick during his first admission to hospital as he was going to need continued support and monitoring at home. Patrick visited him at home every 2 weeks at first. They got on well and chatted fairly easily. Martin was a bit reserved at first. He appeared to be a bit of a loner and Patrick felt sorry for him. Patrick started taking Martin out to the pub and round to his flat for meals. His life began to revolve around him and he wanted more from the relationship. He started to put pressure on Martin to engage in a physical relationship but Martin refused. Martin became increasingly depressed as Patrick increased the pressure, phoning him several times during the day, sharing his problems, telling him about his work and other clients.

Martin was re-admitted to hospital following a suicide attempt. He would not tell anyone why he wanted to die. He would not talk to the nurses at all. He had been out of hospital for 6 months.

Consider:

- When did the relationship start to go wrong?
- What could have helped prevent this from happening?
- Would the relationship have been within professional boundaries if Patrick had not pressed for a physical relationship?
- Would it have made a difference if it had been a heterosexual relationship?
- Would it have made a difference if the nurse had been female and the patient male?

The relationship started to become inappropriate as soon as Patrick started to take Martin to social events that were not part of a plan of care. The relationship became an attempt to meet Patrick's needs rather than a therapeutic relationship based on Martin's needs. The attempt to develop a physical relationship was sexual abuse. Gender boundaries would not have affected this.

Patrick was obviously working in isolation with neither clinical nor managerial supervision, and thus there was little opportunity for warning signs to be identified. His manager had been remiss by failing to ensure that Patrick was fulfilling his role and responsibilities as outlined in his role profile, and that appropriate safety mechanisms were in place to protect both patient and nurse.

Scenario Julie Pepper is 27 years old. She is single with her own flat in the city. She teaches math at a private girls school. Julie has been referred to the gynaecology clinic with a history of painful periods and occasional heavy bleeding. The senior registrar is completing her history.

Senior registrar:	*'And what about sex?'*
Julie:	*'Sex?'*
Senior registrar:	*'Yes, sex, is it painful?'*
Julie:	*'I don't have sex, I'm a Christian.'*
Senior registrar:	*'What?'*

Julie: *'I don't believe in casual sex – you know – outside of marriage.'*

Senior registrar: *'Oh, right – sorry, I didn't realize. I need to examine you now. Would you remove your lower garments and lay on the couch, I'll be in in a minute.'*

The senior registrar directed Julie into the examination room. Angela Marsh, the nurse, had been standing behind Julie throughout the consultation. She looked Julie up and down, then followed her into the examination room without saying a word. Julie prepared for the examination and waited, a silent Angela in attendance.

On completion of the examination the senior registrar asked Julie to return to the consulting room as soon as she was ready. Angela went with him and left Julie alone. In the consulting room the senior registrar explained his findings to Julie and discussed options for treatment. Julie made her decision and then left to make a follow-up appointment.

Angela never spoke to Julie as she left the consulting room. Five minutes later Julie saw Angela talking to two other nurses. The three of them turned and watched her leave the clinic. They all had 'knowing' smiles on their faces as they looked her up and down. Julie was sure they had been discussing her sexual history. It was obvious they did not respect her Christian beliefs and thought her abnormal. She was hurt and embarrassed and vowed never to go back.

Consider:
- What do you think of Angela's behaviour?
- How should she have interacted with Julie?
- Think about the components shaping the nurse–patient relationship – were they equally balanced?
- Consider the principles underpinning the relationship – were they followed?

Rewrite the scenario as you think it should be.

Angela, as a registered nurse, has a duty to care for Julie, irrespective of her religious beliefs. Instead she has belittled Julie and breached confidentiality by sharing personal information about a patient that was gained in the course of her work, with colleagues not involved in Julie's care. Furthermore, she did not seek consent prior to disclosure.

Angela's silence during the consultation showed a total disregard for Julie and her feelings. She showed no consideration for any anxiety that Julie may have been feeling and made no attempt to comfort her or maintain her dignity during the examination. Her focus of care was not promoting or safeguarding the interests of her patient.

SUMMARY

The inappropriate relationships that may develop between nurse and patient have been discussed and the signs identified that may indicate such a relationship is occurring. Types of abuse and the regulator's perspective have also been highlighted. The action to be taken has also been considered.

ENDING THE NURSE–PATIENT RELATIONSHIP

Planning for the termination of the therapeutic relationship begins on the day of admission to the service. The length of the relationship is determined by the patient's care needs and will start to become clear as initial assessments are undertaken as part of care planning. If comprehensive and accurate, these assessments will provide vital information required to execute an effective discharge. Ensuring that the patient's care needs are met on discharge from the service is a major part of ending the therapeutic relationship and will have been the aim of care and treatment.

The nurse will have given the patient some indication of the length of the relationship, thus reducing any uncertainty. For example, they may indicate that they are providing care for one shift only, for the duration of treatment or until the patient has no further need for nursing care. The nurse will discuss future needs with the patient and start to identify other team members whose services will be required.

Effective discharge planning is a team event with each member having a vital contribution to make if a comprehensive care package is to be provided. Multiple texts exist that detail how to make such arrangements, including comprehensive guidance from the four government health departments in the UK.

RECEIVING GIFTS

Whether or not it is appropriate to accept a gift from a patient is not always clear. The nurse needs to consider why the patient is offering the gift. Is it that the patient is expecting something in return, such as preferential treatment? Is it that the patient's cultural beliefs and values indicate that a gift should be given? Would failure to accept a gift be interpreted as an insult or could it alter the nature of the relationship or cause a further imbalance of power?

The nurse must not solicit gifts from patients. This can happen by accident if due care is not taken. For example, by saying 'Oh what a lovely scarf, it would go beautifully with my new coat. Did you buy it locally?'

The nurse may choose to accept a gift from a client within the following principles:

- the gift giving was initiated by the patient
- the patient is not expecting anything in return
- the patient is mentally competent
- local policy is followed with regard to reporting the acceptance of gifts
- the context in which the gift is offered is considered, including the monetary value and appropriateness of the gift.

Scenario Mrs Jones had attended the local hospice for a year, on and off, before she died. Her family was delighted by the care and support that both she and they received from the nurses. They wanted to give the nurses a gift to say thank you and brought them each a small pottery brooch. The nurses were not sure if they should accept or not. Should they?

The family wish to express their gratitude for the care and attention received, in a way that is acceptable to them. They are not expecting any favours in return. The nurses did not solicit this gift and therefore it is appropriate for them to accept.

GIVING GIFTS

There are occasions when nurses may consider giving gifts to patients, e.g. the patient may be celebrating a birthday or other significant event and may be well known to the nurses, or may not have any family. When such an event occurs the context of the gift-giving should be carefully considered.

REFLECTION POINT

Think about a situation when a patient received a gift from staff. What was the context in which the gift was given? Would you act differently in the future?

A gift may be given when:

- it is part of a therapeutic plan
- it is given from an organization or group of nurses
- it is clear to the patient that the nurses do not expect anything in return
- it does not change the dynamics of the relationship that the nurses have with the patient or make it difficult for other nurses to provide care
- it does not embarrass or cause other negative feelings for the patient.

SUMMARY

The context has been identified in which gifts may be given to or received from patients in order to help you identify the appropriate boundaries in practice.

CONCLUSION

This chapter has raised issues concerning the appropriate relationship between nurse and patient to assist the nurse in maintaining professional boundaries. An attempt has been made to provide a resource in which you can use existing knowledge and skills while enhancing learning. Progression through all aspects of this chapter will have supported your learning around the three key competencies (UKCC 2001a) mentioned at the start and identified ways of managing difficult situations that can occur within the therapeutic relationship. Remember that there is no 'one' answer to the myriad of issues that can and will arise during the span of the relationship between the nurse and patient. However, consideration and application of the principles discussed within this chapter will help guide you in the direction of appropriate relationships in professional practice.

CHAPTER 6

ASSESSMENT: THE FOUNDATIONS OF GOOD PRACTICE

Ruth Beretta

INTRODUCTION

In a health care setting, assessment has been defined as 'the gathering of information and formulation of judgements regarding a person's health, situation, needs and wishes, which should guide further action' (Heath 2000). Carrying out nursing assessments is an essential part of every nurse's day. Whether meeting a patient or client for the first time, or reviewing their care, the question is asked 'What information do I need to be able to nurse this person?', as each person is an individual with unique health care needs.

WHAT IS ASSESSMENT?

Assessment is the first part of the *nursing process* and is about collecting data or information involving the patient or client and their family or carers.

The information or data may be objective or subjective. If it is objective, it is based on measurement, and can be verified by another person, e.g. temperature or body weight. If the information is subjective, it is based on the nurse's ideas, feelings, values and beliefs, e.g. the nurse may have identified that the patient talked rapidly and fiddled with their clothes, and come to the conclusion that the patient is nervous.

The data gathered through assessment identifies the strengths and weaknesses of the patient or client. This assists in the formulation of a plan of care; nursing care can then be provided as per plan and evaluated to review its effectiveness. Evaluation of care results in re-assessment of the patient's or client's needs (see Fig. 6.1). Assessment is therefore an ongoing process and a foundation of good practice.

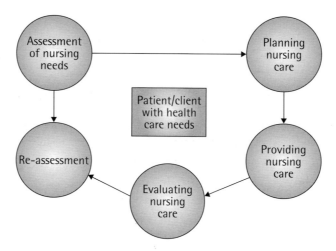

Figure 6.1 Assessment as the first part of the nursing process

THE UKCC REQUIREMENTS AND ASSESSMENT

The *Requirements for Pre-registration Nursing Programmes* (UKCC 2001a) identify the importance of assessment in establishing the foundation of good practice. The specific competencies and their relationship to assessment are identified in Table 6.1.

Table 6.1 UKCC competencies and their relationship to assessment

UKCC domain	UKCC competency	Relationship to assessment
Professional and ethical practice	Practise in accordance with an ethical and legal framework which ensures the primacy of patient and client interest and well-being and respects confidentiality	In the course of assessment, nurses obtain very personal information. The need to respect patient confidentiality and act in a patient's best interest is paramount

(Continued)

Table 6.1 (*Continued*)

UKCC domain	UKCC competency	Relationship to assessment
	Practise in a fair and anti-discriminatory way, acknowledging the differences in beliefs and cultural practices of individuals or groups	On assessment, nurses must make sure they do not allow their personal feelings about a person or their way of life to cloud their judgement about them
Care delivery	Undertake and document a comprehensive, systematic and accurate nursing assessment of physical, psychological, social and spiritual needs of patients, clients and community	Nurses use their ability to interact with others and a range of assessment tools to identify health and social care needs
	Formulate and document a plan of nursing care, where possible in partnership with patients, clients, their carers, family and friends, within a framework of informed consent	Assessment is the first stage of the nursing process. Information collated must reflect the concerns of the patient or client, not just the nurse
Care management	Demonstrate knowledge of effective inter-professional working practices which respect and utilize the contributions of members of the health and social care team	A nursing assessment is unique. However, the information collected completes a package of care with other health care professionals
Personal and professional development	Demonstrate a commitment to the need for continuing personal and professional supervision activities in order to enhance knowledge, skills, values and attitudes needed for safe and effective nursing practice	Assessment should be based on the best available evidence for care

WHEN IS ASSESSMENT CARRIED OUT?

EXERCISE

Jot down the occasions when you think it is important for the nurse to assess patients or clients?

You may have identified the following occasions:

- an assessment is usually carried out when the nurse first meets a patient or client, which may be on admission to hospital, on a visit to a clinic, or in the patient's or client's own home. As identified earlier, the information obtained helps the nurse to establish a plan of care
- assessment may be carried out on a daily basis, to check the relevance of the care plan and to identify whether there is improvement or deterioration in the patient or client. This may mean the care plan has to be updated to accommodate the new information gathered
- assessment is usually carried out before a patient or client is discharged home from hospital, to identify whether there is a need to continue care when the person is at home. This may be a joint assessment involving other members of the multi-professional team, such as the physiotherapist, occupational therapist, social worker and patient's GP

- continuous assessment of patients who are critically ill, e.g. those requiring intensive care. Small children and babies may also need to be continuously assessed. Mentally ill clients who are considered to be at risk of suicide will also require regular assessment.

WHERE DOES THE INFORMATION FOR ASSESSMENT COME FROM?

Within the professional and ethical practice domain of the UKCC requirements (UKCC 2001a), the nurse is advised that patient or client confidentiality is very important and that any information received must be used in the patient's best interest. Nurses must be sure that, if the patient or client is unable to speak for themselves, there is agreement to having a carer or relative speak on their behalf. Nurses must also be sure to have the patient's consent to pass on information to other members of the care team [see sections 5.1, 5.2, 5.3 *Code of professional conduct* (NMC 2002a)].

Patient or client

The patient or client is usually a primary source of data. When questioned, most patients are more than happy to provide information to help plan their care.

Questions put to patients or clients can be 'open' or 'closed'. An open question, e.g. 'tell me how your pain has been over the last few days', gives the person an opportunity to give you their side of the story. A closed question elicits a 'yes' or 'no' type of answer, e.g. 'Are you still in pain?'.

There may be obstacles to using direct questions.

EXERCISE

What situations might make it difficult to use the patient or client as the primary source of information in assessment?

You may have identified some of the following situations. The person being assessed is:

- in severe pain
- emotionally upset
- confused
- too breathless to speak
- unable to communicate in your language
- too deaf to hear your questions
- asleep or unconscious
- a person with a learning disability who uses Makaton or similar sign language to communicate.

This does not mean that the nurse cannot gather information from the patient or client. Means other than verbal questioning can be used to gain information, e.g.:

- visually observing the person:
  - how clean and tidy is the patient? Have they been caring for themselves?
  - what colour is the patient? Pale? Flushed? Cyanosed? Jaundiced?

- what does the patient's facial expression reveal? Pain? Happiness? Anger?
- is the patient bleeding or losing fluid from anywhere?
- what does the patient's position reveal? Are they holding their stomach because they are in pain?
- how mobile is the patient? Can they walk?
- using the sense of smell:
  - does the patient have stale breath, suggesting they have not eaten or drunk for some time?
  - does the patient smell of cigarettes?
  - does the patient smell of urine?
- using the sense of touch:
  - how hot or cold is the patient?
  - does the patient's skin feel clammy or dry?
- using the sense of hearing:
  - does the patient have noisy breathing?
  - does the patient have slurred speech?

Carers, family and friends

If the patient or client is unable to give information to nursing staff for assessment, carers and family members can usually provide useful information relating to the history of the current situation. They will usually also know the person's eating likes and dislikes, hygiene, times of sleep and details of the episode that has brought them to seek health care. The older person, the person with memory disturbance or dementia and the person with an altered perception of themselves or of reality, may need someone to speak on their behalf.

Patient or client records

The patient or client may have a record of previous hospital admissions or episodes of health care. It can be useful to review this record before meeting the patient or client to see whether the information they give you matches up with what you have read about them.

Patient records are also likely to contain results of investigations, such as blood tests and X-rays, a list of current medications the patient may be taking, and reports from other health care professionals, such as physiotherapists or occupational therapists.

HOW IS INFORMATION FOR ASSESSMENT OBTAINED?

Establishing rapport and trust

As considered earlier, the nurse carries out assessments on an almost continuous basis, whether meeting the patient or client for the first time, or in re-assessing or evaluating a package of care, which is ongoing.

Very often, perhaps on admission to hospital, or when being visited by the community nurse at home for the first time, the first nurse the patient sees will be responsible for their assessment and providing information to formulate a plan of care. This means that the relationship between the nurse and the patient must be one where communication can take place easily. Often patients or clients are anxious at the thought of requiring care, and may be nervous and unsure of themselves. The nurse needs to come across as professional and assured, easily developing rapport and trust with the patient. This can be difficult to achieve, especially in an emergency situation.

Scenario José Mendez was very proud of his garden. He spent many hours cultivating his vegetables and regularly won prizes, especially for his garlic and onions. One day, just as he was due to go indoors for tea, he developed severe chest pain. His wife, Maria, frantically rang for the family doctor to visit. However, surgery hours were over and the recorded message advised callers to contact NHS Direct, or dial 999 in an emergency. Uncertain what to do and most concerned at José's continued pain, Maria called for an ambulance.

The ambulance arrived within 10 minutes of the call and the crew told José that he had probably suffered a 'heart attack', best treated in hospital. Maria immediately started to cry, begging to go in the ambulance with her husband. This was agreed and the ambulance made its way to the local hospital, having radioed ahead.

On arrival at hospital, José was still in pain. He looked very ill and was becoming breathless. Maria was crying and waving her arms hysterically as she got out of the ambulance. The ambulance crew quickly got José out of the ambulance and into the lift, and they made their way to the coronary care unit (CCU). The nurse in charge, Andy, greeted them.

Andy welcomed José as Mr Mendez and quickly introduced himself. He told the ambulance crew that a bed had been prepared for José just inside the ward and they wheeled him off. In the meantime, he asked Maria to wait in the waiting room with another nurse, Susie, who would bring her a drink. As she drank her tea and calmed down, Susie asked Maria what had happened to José, and whether he was taking any medications.

Inside the ward, José had been helped into bed, attached to a cardiac monitor and given medication to relieve his pain. An oxygen mask was also put on to help his breathlessness.

Maria joined José after about 15 minutes, by which time he was feeling much better and the pain was subsiding. Both José and Maria were very impressed and felt confident that all would be well.

Can you identify the ways in which the trust of José and Maria was gained and the assessment process was started?

You may have identified the following ways:

- Andy used his interpersonal skills and greeted José by name. This immediately let José and Maria know that the ward was prepared for him and gave them confidence
- although distraught on arrival at hospital, Maria settled down with Susie and was then able to provide information about her husband's condition and his medication, for use in his care plan
- Andy used his visual observation skills quickly to establish that José was in pain and breathless. This meant that José's treatment started almost as soon as he was made comfortable in bed, and was not delayed by his being asked questions which could have been distressing.

The assessment process was under way even before Andy and the CCU nurses had met José and Maria. Andy realized the importance of making a patient feel relaxed and confident, so he made sure that everything was ready when the ambulance crew radioed him. When he first saw José, he realized from the way he was leaning forward on the trolley that he was breathless and grimacing with pain. Andy knew that Maria would be a useful source of information about her husband, but she was too upset to stay at his bedside, so he decided that Susie should keep her company in the visitor's room. Once José's pain was settled, Andy could gain more information by carrying out his own investigation.

Asking questions

It has already been established that, where possible, the patient or client is the primary source for obtaining data for assessment, and that using open or closed questions should provide the necessary information for a care plan to be formulated. But would you know what questions to ask?

EXERCISE

Using a friend or a relative, take about 15 minutes to find out as much as possible about their health. Now compare your questions with those a colleague would have asked.

What questions did you use? Did you find that the questions asked depended on a number of variables, such as the person's age, their experiences of health care, how much they know and understand about health care, and what their expectations are for health?

These variables make asking questions in the process of assessment rather a haphazard affair. However, you may have been guided by the UKCC requirements that:

'…assessment should be comprehensive and systematic, taking into account physical, psychological, social and spiritual needs of patients, clients and community'.

(UKCC 2001a)

SUMMARY

- Assessment is the first part of the nursing process and assists the nurse in identifying patient or client strengths and weaknesses, and in the formulation of a care plan.
- Information obtained at assessment may be subjective or objective.
- Assessment is carried out when the patient or client first meets the nurse, and is then carried out continuously as care is evaluated.
- Information for assessment may come verbally from the patient or client, or it may come from the use of notes, questioning of family and carers, or using the nurse's senses.
- There are links between the process of assessment, the *Requirements for Pre-registration Nursing* (UKCC 2001a) and the *Code of professional conduct* (NMC 2002a), such as the need to respect information gained at assessment as confidential.

NURSING MODELS: A SYSTEMATIC APPROACH TO ASSESSMENT

One way to develop a systematic approach to assessment is through the nursing process, guided by a *nursing model*. Most models originated in the US in the 1960s and aimed to describe what nurses do. One description of a nursing model is 'a mental picture of nursing' (Newton 1991) or a means of guiding, directing and organizing care (Akinsanya *et al.* 1994). To describe what nurses do, most nursing models use a framework, or a series of cue questions, to assess and gain information about the patient or client for formulating a plan of care.

Three nursing models with their frameworks for assessment are considered here – those of Roper *et al.* (1996), Orem (1995) and Peplau (1992).

ROPER, LOGAN AND TIERNEY'S MODEL

This is a British model, developed in the 1970s, which uses as its framework 12 activities of living:

- maintaining a safe environment
- communicating
- breathing
- eating and drinking
- eliminating
- personal cleansing and dressing
- controlling body temperature
- mobilizing
- working and playing
- expressing sexuality
- sleeping
- dying.

Roper *et al.* (1996) consider that assessing how, why, when and where we carry out the activities of living will produce a comprehensive picture of a person's lifestyle and highlight any 'problems' or 'potential problems' which may require nursing care. This is particularly so if the assessment takes into account what the person is like when carrying out the activities of living *usually* and what they are like *now*. Alongside this, Roper *et al.* identify that people move along a continuum from conception to death and, depending on the situation, along a further continuum of complete dependence to complete independence, and possibly back again. They also suggest that the activities will be influenced by physical, psychological, socio-cultural, environmental and politico-economic factors, so the assessment should be unique to the individual and, therefore, *holistic*.

A typical assessment sheet for the Roper, Logan and Tierney model is shown in Table 6.2. Roper *et al.* (1996) suggest it may not be necessary to address every activity of living in every assessment.

Table 6.2 Typical assessment sheet for the Roper, Logan and Tierney model of nursing

Activity of living	Cue issues	Usual routine	Problems: actual/potential
Maintaining a safe environment	External environment: possible dangers or accidents Internal environment: homeostasis		
Communication	Speech, hearing, sight, written, intellectual function, language, pain		

(Continued)

Table 6.2 (*Continued*)

Activity of living	Cue issues	Usual routine	Problems: actual/potential
Breathing	Ability to breathe, cough, phlegm (sputum)		
Eating and drinking	Likes and dislikes, chewing, swallowing, cooking, resources		
Eliminating	Bowel and bladder habits, continence		
Personal cleansing and dressing	Skin condition, cleanliness, type of clothing		
Controlling body temperature	Sensitivity to changes in temperature; elderly, very young		
Mobilizing	Activity and movement		
Working and playing	Exercise, well-being, how time is spent		
Expressing sexuality	Body image, femininity, masculinity		
Sleeping	Patterns of sleeping and waking		
Dying	Awareness of dying or grieving		

OREM'S MODEL

Orem began work on her model in the 1970s, basing it on the concept of 'self-care'. 'Self' is seen as physical, psychological, social and spiritual needs and 'care' as the activities a person carries out to maintain life and develop in a way that is normal for that person (Cavanagh 1991).

To assess a person using this model, the eight *universal self-care requisites* are addressed:

- maintenance of a sufficient intake of air
- maintenance of a sufficient intake of water
- maintenance of a sufficient intake of food
- provision of care associated with elimination processes and excrements
- maintenance of a balance between activity and rest
- maintenance of a balance between solitude and social integration
- prevention of hazards to life, human functioning and human well-being
- promotion of human functioning and development within social groups in accord with human potential, known human limitations and the human desire to be normal (Orem identifies this as 'normacy').

According to Orem, a person is said to be 'healthy' if they have sufficient self-care abilities to meet universal self-care requisites. However, Orem identifies further self-care requisites, depending on the circumstances a person is in. These are the *developmental self-care requisites*, which occur at specific periods of human development, such as infancy, adulthood and old age, and the *health-deviation self-care requisites*, which occur when a person becomes ill, injured or has a disability. It may be that a person is unable to self-care if they have developmental or health deviation self-care requisites to meet. Orem identifies this person as then having a *self-care deficit* and there is then a need for nursing care.

The aim of assessment of a person, using Orem's model of nursing, is the determination of the person's abilities to self-care and the identification of self-care limitations or self-care deficit. A typical assessment sheet for the Orem model is shown in Table 6.3.

Table 6.3 Typical assessment sheet for the Orem model of nursing

Universal self-care requisites	Self-care abilities	Self-care limitations
Maintenance of a sufficient intake of air		
Maintenance of a sufficient intake of water		
Maintenance of a sufficient intake of food		
Provision of care associated with elimination processes and excrement		
Maintenance of a balance between activity and rest		
Maintenance of a balance between solitude and social integration		
Prevention of hazards to life, human functioning and human well-being		
Normacy		

PEPLAU'S MODEL

Peplau originally published writings on interpersonal skills in the early 1950s and it is a development of her thinking that is the basis for her model of nursing. She sees the nurse–patient relationship as the most important issue in nursing and that without it, nursing actions would not be effective. Much of the work published identifying the application of Peplau's model to care is related to patients or clients in a mental health setting, although it can be equally suitable for all client groups (Simpson 1991).

The overwhelming belief within Peplau's model is that the patient or client should be moving towards health, and that the nurse has a number of roles which can educate and empower the person to do this. This will occur within the phases of the nurse–patient relationship.

Phases in the nurse–patient relationship

Peplau sees the nurse and patient or client as passing through four phases of relationship:

- phase of orientation: this identifies the patient or client entering the unknown, with no knowledge of the new environment, the nursing staff or the condition which has brought them to seek health care.

The nurse can expect the patient or client to be anxious and confused, requiring explanations of procedures and routines. Peplau sees the nurse and patient taking the roles of strangers at this time

- phase of identification: this identifies the patient or client finding out more about the reason for health care, the people who can be relied upon for help and advice, and how the patient or client can become more involved in their own care
- phase of exploitation: this identifies the patient or client making full use of the resources around them and moving towards healthy behaviour. Peplau sees this as the patient or client moving from dependence towards independence
- phase of resolution: the patient or client is preparing to live a healthy lifestyle outside of a health care setting. This is the drawing to a close of the nurse–patient relationship which has been so important in providing support and education to move towards health.

Simpson (1991) considers that each phase can be discreet and observed, or they may overlap, and nurses should be aware of this to enable patients or clients to move on.

Roles of nurses

Peplau suggests that as patients or clients move through these phases, the nurse can adopt a number of roles dependent on the situation:

- stranger: Peplau sees this as the opportunity to begin the nurse–patient relationship; it should not be based on presumptions about the person being assessed
- resource: as the person moves through the phases of identification and exploitation, the nurse can be used to gain information, skills or resources to help move towards health
- teacher: the nurse teaches the patient or client how to deal with, for example, a situation, condition or medication
- leader: this may be a flexible role as the patient or client moves towards health, gradually taking more control
- counsellor: Peplau suggests that not all nurses can counsel, but sometimes it is helpful to the patient or client for the nurse just to listen and allow the patient to draw their own conclusions on their progress
- surrogate: this is the nurse acting as a substitute when the person is ill. It is important that, during the phase of resolution, this role is reduced.

Assessment is most likely to occur during the phase of orientation and is about the nurse collecting information. Adopting one or more of the roles may then allow the nurse to make observations of the verbal and non-verbal cues and identify problems for nursing care.

EXERCISE

Using the assessment frameworks of Roper, Logan and Tierney, Orem, and Peplau carry out an assessment of Manjeet and Samantha in the scenarios identified below.

Scenario Manjeet Dhaliwal is admitted to the medical ward with newly diagnosed diabetes. He has recently graduated with a first class honours degree in fine art and is due to start work as a graphic designer. He has been feeling generally unwell and has lost weight, but put this down to the stress of his exams.

Scenario Samantha Temple is 10 years old and had emergency surgery yesterday for appendicitis. She has twin sisters who are 4 years old and her father is currently working abroad. Samantha seems to be very quiet today and says she does not want to get up until her mother arrives to look after her.

For Manjeet, you may have identified the issues outlined in Tables 6.4 using Roper, Logan and Tierney's model, and for Samantha, those in Table 6.5.

Table 6.4 Issues identified in the assessment of Manjeet using Roper, Logan and Tierney's model

Activity of living	Usual routines	Potential/actual problems
Maintaining a safe environment	Fully independent	Blood sugar is unstable. Does not know how to inject insulin
Eating and drinking	Eats 'junk food'. Likes to drink socially about five pints of lager per week	Needs to understand a 'healthy diet' to maintain diabetic control. Fasts each Ramadan
Working and playing	Fully independent. Due to start a new job next week. Played soccer in the university league	Very worried he will not be well enough to start his new job and will not be able to get involved in sport
Expressing sexuality	Independent. Has casual girlfriends at present but 'no one serious'	Worried he will not be able to have a 'normal relationship' with a girl
Dying		Manjeet's uncle died following a major heart attack. He had poorly controlled diabetes

Table 6.5 Issues identified in the assessment of Samantha using Roper, Logan and Tierney's model

Activity of living	Usual routines	Potential/actual problems
Maintaining a safe environment	Fully independent	Samantha has had an operation and may develop a wound infection; she may haemorrhage
Communicating	Usually independent. Likes to read Harry Potter stories	Samantha is quiet and withdrawn. She is shy without her mother present
Eating and drinking	Usually independent. Does not like milk unless really cold. Prefers to eat white bread	Has an intravenous infusion in place until she starts to drink. Has been feeling slightly sick since the operation
Eliminating	Tends to open her bowels three times per week	Bowels not opened since hospital admission
Personal cleansing and dressing	Usually independent. Likes to shower	Has refused to wash without her mother
Controlling body temperature	Independent	Had a raised temperature before going to theatre for surgery; still raised
Working and playing	Fully independent. Enjoys school	Has been very withdrawn and does not interact with other children

For Manjeet, you may have identified the issues outlined in Table 6.6 using Orem's model, and for Samantha those in Table 6.7.

Table 6.6 Issues identified in the assessment of Manjeet using Orem's model

Universal self-care requisites	Self-care abilities	Self-care limitations
Maintenance of a sufficient intake of air	Usually no difficulties Fasts each Ramadam	None
Maintenance of a sufficient intake of water	Usually no difficulties	None
Maintenance of a sufficient intake of food	Eats 'junk food' and drinks five pints of lager per week	Has a knowledge deficit about healthy eating and how to manage during Ramadam
Provision of care associated with elimination processes and excrement	No difficulties	None
Maintenance of a balance between activity and rest	Usually very active; plays soccer	Has been feeling very tired recently
Maintenance of a balance between solitude and social integration	Usually sociable with active life outside university	Worried about socializing with work colleagues
Prevention of hazards to life, human functioning, and human well-being	No difficulties	Does not understand how to inject insulin or check his blood sugar
Normacy	No difficulties	Concerned that he will not be able to have a girlfriend, or that he may suffer an early death, like his uncle who also had diabetes. Now worried his use of alcohol is responsible for his diabetes

Table 6.7 Issues identified in the assessment of Samantha using Orem's model

Universal self-care requisites	Self-care abilities	Self-care limitations
Maintenance of a sufficient intake of air	No difficulties	None
Maintenance of a sufficient intake of water	No difficulties	Has an intravenous infusion. She is not drinking at present
Maintenance of a sufficient intake of food	No difficulties	Has been feeling sick since her operation
Provision of care associated with elimination processes and excrement	No difficulties; opens bowels three times per week	Bowels not opened since admission

(*Continued*)

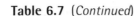

Table 6.7 (*Continued*)

Universal self-care requisites	Self-care abilities	Self-care limitations
Maintenance of a balance between activity and rest	No difficulties, although prefers to be alone than with her twin sisters	Refuses to get up until her mother arrives
Maintenance of a balance between solitude and social integration	Quite shy; misses her father who is away on business	Is withdrawn and has not mixed with the other children
Prevention of hazards to life, human functioning, and human well-being	No difficulties	Has potential for wound infection, haemorrhage and pain
Normacy	No difficulties	Does not like the company of her twin sisters because they like playing with dolls; she prefers to be with her father and go fishing

A possible assessment of Manjeet using Peplau's model is as follows. Phase of orientation – the nurse greeted Manjeet on the ward; he looked very anxious and was leaning forward in his chair as he spoke. The nurse asked if she could sit with him and ask him some questions. He replied that he wanted to get 'this thing sorted out as quickly as possible' and for him to get on with his life. Manjeet said he was to start his first job next week and could not afford for anything to go wrong. He also told the nurse that he had an uncle who had suffered with diabetes and had died at an early age following a heart attack. The nurse made the following notes:

- Manjeet is very anxious about the diagnosis of diabetes. He is not sure what it is, how to manage it or the impact it will have on his life
- Manjeet appears to be highly intelligent and is keen to start his first job. He seems to want to be as independent as possible
- Manjeet has lost weight; his clothes hang loosely on him
- Manjeet had an uncle with diabetes, who died of a heart attack. Manjeet is aware of the need to have his diabetes well controlled, but has no knowledge of what this will entail
- Manjeet says he regrets drinking alcohol because, as strict Muslims, his parents would be disappointed in him.

The nurse then went on to write out Manjeet's care plan, identifying how she could take on the roles of teacher, resource person and counsellor as Manjeet moved through the phases of the relationship.

A possible assessment of Samantha using Peplau's model is as follows. Phase of orientation – Samantha was admitted to the children's surgical ward in the evening, complaining of abdominal pain. This was thought to be due to appendicitis. Samantha's mother came to hospital with her, but was unable to stay because her two other daughters were at home unattended. Samantha's father was working away on business. The staff nurse on the children's ward assessed Samantha and eventually took her to theatre for her operation. He noticed that Samantha was very shy and that her mother answered his questions. He was actually quite pleased when she decided to go home, so he could get to know Samantha a little better. He made the following notes about Samantha and her mother:

- Samantha is hot and in abdominal pain. She probably has appendicitis and will require surgery fairly soon
- Samantha has been vomiting and her mouth is dry
- Samantha is a bright girl but obviously shy. Her mother is used to speaking for her
- the family do not seem to be well supported by an extended family or neighbours, as the younger sisters have been left unattended.

Phase of identification – the staff nurse was not on duty the following morning after Samantha's operation and it was one of the student nurses who tried to strike up a relationship with Samantha. She asked Samantha if she hurt anywhere and if she was ready to get up, have a wash and have something to eat and drink. Samantha seemed surprised that she was allowed up, but she refused to move and said she would not have a wash until her mother arrived. The student nurse went to the nurse in charge to report the following:

- Samantha says she is not in pain but she refuses to move, so she probably does have pain
- Samantha has still had nothing to eat or drink
- Samantha has not passed urine since her operation
- Samantha says she will not move or have a wash until her mother arrives, but her mother rang the ward earlier to say she would not be visiting until after lunchtime.

The nurse in charge used this information to consider the nursing roles that would be needed to move Samantha towards health and through the phases of exploitation and resolution.

REFLECTION POINT
- Which assessment framework did you prefer to use?
- Do you think it is important to have a framework for assessment?
- Which framework makes it easier to be aware of the subjective information available to the nurse at assessment?
- Is there enough specific information identified to be able to formulate a plan of care?

Hopefully, the two scenarios demonstrate some of the issues raised in the UKCC requirements (UKCC 2001a), that nurses:

- 'practise in accordance with an ethical and legal framework which ensures the primacy of patient and client interest and well-being'. The nurse will be made aware that Manjeet is a Muslim, but that he drinks alcohol when he socializes with his friends from university. His parents would be upset if they were aware of this, so the information is important when educating Manjeet how to manage his diabetes, but it is confidential information
- 'practise in a fair and anti-discriminatory way, acknowledging the differences in beliefs and cultural practices of individuals or groups'. The nurse may have been shocked and disappointed that Samantha's mother did not stay with her until she went to the operating theatre, or stay overnight with her. But the nurse must acknowledge that Samantha's sisters also require attention and the nurses must be non-judgemental towards the rest of the family.

However, the scenarios may also serve to highlight a lack of detail in the assessments carried out and that much of the information gathered could *not* be measured or recorded in any systematic manner.

EXERCISE

Identify the ways in which the assessments of José, Manjeet and Samantha lack in detail and accuracy.

Possible omissions you may have identified are listed in Table 6.8.

Table 6.8 Omissions from the assessments

José	Manjeet	Samantha
• How severe was José's chest pain? • How did the nurse in the CCU know it was resolving? • How breathless was José? • Did the oxygen make his breathing better or worse? • How did the nurse know which medication to give?	• How much weight had Manjeet lost? • How different from the 'normal' was Manjeet's blood sugar level to cause him to be diabetic? • How will he know how much insulin he requires?	• How hot was Samantha prior to surgery? Was she the same temperature on return? • How much pain was she in and is that the reason for her not wanting to move? • How dry was her mouth? • How much did she vomit? • How much fluid had she received by the infusion?

It is not possible to provide answers to questions such as those posed in Table 6.8 from the information gleaned using nursing models. However, the UKCC requirements (UKCC 2001a) call for a 'comprehensive, systematic and accurate assessment of the physical, psychological, social and spiritual needs of patient, clients and communities'. Assessment tools, such as recording the temperature, a pain assessment tool, blood sugar testing and a mouth care assessment to name a few, may be required.

SUMMARY

- Nursing models assist in providing a framework to enable a comprehensive assessment of physical, psychological, spiritual and social needs of patients or clients.
- Nursing models may enable you to learn what is the usual behaviour of the patient or client and how this differs from their behaviour when they are ill, or if they can be taught to manage their own health condition.
- It is not sufficient to gather information with nursing models alone; assessment tools are also required to allow the gathering of objective information.

TOOLS FOR ASSESSMENT

Tools for assessment should be able to provide a *valid* and *reliable* measure of the patient's or client's problem or potential problem. Many of the tools used form part of a strategy to minimize the risk a patient or client faces during their period of hospitalization or when in receipt of health care (NMC 2002a).

Two scenarios are used to give examples of how tools can be used.

SCENARIO 1: ALEXANDER ZIOLKOWSKI

Scenario Alexander Ziolkowski had arrived in Britain from Poland during the Second World War. He had settled in the Midlands, where he met and married his wife, Nora. They raised four children, with Alexander working in the coal mining industry for many years. Nora and Alexander's children had now all married and moved away.

Alexander retired at the age of 63, already suffering with chronic lung disease, probably related to his years in the mines. He had bought his house from the colliery, but now is on the council waiting list for a bungalow, as the stairs make him breathless. On his last hospital admission, he had refused to allow the occupational therapist to accompany him home to assess his living circumstances, but now he is wishing he had.

Alexander is admitted to the medical ward with an acute exacerbation of his chronic obstructive pulmonary disease (COPD). He is too breathless to talk on admission and appears *cyanosed* and sweaty. He is wearing an oxygen mask attached to a small cylinder. He refuses to get into the prepared bed, preferring to sit upright in a high-backed chair.

Nora accompanies her husband and tells the nurses on the ward that Alexander has not been downstairs for a week because of his breathlessness. He has been using his oxygen a lot and sometimes gets confused. She says he has not eaten or drunk for several days and she thinks he is losing weight. Nora also says that her husband is a practising Roman Catholic and would like to have last rites performed by Father Joseph if he is going to die.

The nurse allocated to care for Alexander is Mary, who knows him from previous admissions to the ward. She winks at Alexander when he arrives and gives his arm a friendly squeeze, telling him she has a student nurse working with her today and that they would soon 'sort him out'. Mary tells the student they will be using the Roper, Logan and Tierney model of nursing to plan care.

Prioritizing the assessment

You will recall that assessment is not a one-off process, but one occurring continuously. However, with patients as ill as Alexander, it is vital to gain key pieces of information to start the care package, and to make a more detailed assessment later.

EXERCISE

Imagine you are the nurse admitting and assessing Alexander. What information do you need to have straight away?

You may have considered using the 'A, B, C' approach, i.e. A for airway, B for breathing and C for circulation. This is a useful strategy in emergency situations and prompts you to make sure the patient or client is able to survive until a more detailed assessment can be undertaken.

Mary has already noted that Alexander opted to stay in the chair and that he is using oxygen, so she knows his condition is serious. However, she can also see that his breathlessness has not exhausted him completely and that she will have some preliminary information to offer medical staff when they arrive to prescribe medications. The key activity of living for priority assessment is 'breathing' (Jevon and Ewens 2001). Mary asks the following questions:

- Can Alexander breathe?
- Is his airway clear? Is he producing sputum (phlegm) and can he cough it up (expectorate)?
- Is his breathing deep or shallow? Is it noisy?
- How rapid is his breathing? Does he have tachypnoea or bradypnoea?
- Is he having the right amount of oxygen?
- Is he becoming confused because of a lack of oxygen to the brain? (hypoxia)
- Is he in a comfortable position to maintain his breathing or does he need support with more pillows? Does he have dyspnoea or orthopnoea?
- Does he have an acute exacerbation of his condition because of a chest infection?
- Does he have a raised temperature because of infection?
- Does he have a raised pulse because of infection and the extra effort required in breathing? Does he have tachycardia or bradycardia?

To answer these questions, Mary may already have started to use some tools to produce measurements and an accurate assessment.

Assessment of sputum. Mary is aware that patients with COPD regularly produce sputum, especially first thing in the morning. She is particularly interested in the colour and consistency of any sputum produced, as a change in colour to yellow or green, and becoming more sticky and viscid, could indicate infection. Law (2000) identifies that a change of sputum colour may have significance.

Assessment of breathing rate and depth. The normal adult respiratory rate (rate of breathing) is 10–15 breaths per minute (Stocks 1996). Mary is aware of this when recording the number of breaths per minute taken by Alexander, and that rapid breathing (in excess of 20 breaths per minute) is tachypnoea and bradypnoea is a slow rate (less than 12 breaths per minute) (Torrance and Elley 1997). The respiratory rate should always be counted for at least half a minute by observing the rise and fall of the chest. The patient should be unaware that the respirations are being counted as there is an involuntary tendency to change the breathing pattern. In any patient, an increase in the resting respiratory rate of 5 breaths per minute can be a serious indicator of respiratory distress, requiring attention (Place and Graham 2000). The depth of respiration relates to the volume of air moving in and out of the lungs and the position adopted by the patient for breathing. Mary notes that Alexander is having difficulty in breathing (dyspnoea) but also that he is only able to breathe while sitting upright, supported by pillows (orthopnoea).

Assessment of level of oxygen the patient is receiving. Mary checks the oxygen mask that Alexander is wearing and notes that 24% oxygen is being delivered to him. However, he still appears to be cyanosed and confused at times, which could be due to hypoxia. Mary decides to carry out pulse oximetry, which checks the oxygen saturation level of arterial blood (SpO_2) (Place 2000). Pulse oximetry is carried out by attaching a probe to the body (usually the fingertip or ear lobe is used) and a light detector in the probe detects the amount of oxygen absorbed by the haemoglobin, which is usually 95–100%. An SpO_2 of <90% may demonstrate a serious respiratory problem (Sheppard 2000). It is possible to keep a pulse oximetry probe in place for several hours and therefore to monitor the oxygen saturation levels continuously. This is useful for patients like Alexander.

Assessment of body temperature. To assess if Alexander is breathless due to infection or whether the increased activity of breathing rapidly is causing an increase in metabolic rate and raised body temperature (Jevon and Ewens 2001), his temperature is recorded. Mary is aware that the usual body temperature is within a range of 36–37.6°C (Edwards 1997), and that raised temperature is known as pyrexia and lowered body temperature as hypothermia. Body temperature may be recorded at a number of sites, most commonly the mouth, axilla (armpit) and tympanic membrane (eardrum). In Alexander's case, the tympanic route is preferable as he then does not need to be disturbed and a reading can be obtained within approximately 10 seconds.

Assessment of heart rate (pulse). The pulse rate is the number of heart beats in a 60-second period (Marieb 1999). The normal heart rate for an adult is 60–100 beats per minute (Herbert and Alison 1996). A pulse below 60 beats per minute is identified as bradycardia and above 110 beats per minute as tachycardia. Mary expects Alexander's pulse rate to be higher than usual because of his infection, which causes metabolic rate to rise, and because of the extra effort required to breathe.

Already Mary has a significant amount of information, gained from carrying out vital signs and visually observing Alexander, from Nora and from the GP letter, which accompanied him (Table 6.9).

Table 6.9 Assessment of Alexander using the Roper, Logan and Tierney model

Activity of living	Usual routines	Potential/actual problems
Maintaining a safe environment	Has difficulty in negotiating stairs He has been confused over the last week and unable to manage hot drinks safely Has home oxygen and uses it regularly	Confused at times and needs to be observed regularly
Communicating	Usually independent Wears glasses for reading	Too breathless to speak at present He can use a picture board easily
Breathing	Gets out of breath on exertion Does not smoke Uses oxygen at home for at least 6 hours/day	Respiratory rate 24 beats per minute $SpO_2 = 93\%$ Receiving oxygen at 24% Producing green sputum (sample collected)
Eating and drinking	Usually independent but not much of an appetite Has full set of dentures	Mouth is dry – to be assessed later Nutritional assessment later
Eliminating	Has used a bedside commode for last week Usually constipated	Bowels not opened since hospital admission – for further assessment
Personal cleansing and dressing	Daily assisted wash with help of Nora Weekly shower with aid of community helper Cannot put on socks – too breathless	Appears very sweaty on admission Pressure areas not yet assessed
Controlling body temperature	Usually independent	Temp. 37.8°C on admission, pulse 98 beats per minute Fan *in situ*

(Continued)

Table 6.9 (*Continued*)

Activity of living	Usual routines	Potential/actual problems
Mobilizing	Has not been out of the house for a month or downstairs for a week Usually manages stairs	Appears immobile Pressure area risk is high – for assessment later
Working and playing	Retired miner Enjoys watching snooker and football on TV Has no exercise	
Expressing sexuality	Has four children all living away Uses electric shaver. Does not use deodorant spray – makes him cough	Unable to wash and dress with privacy at home
Sleeping	Sleeps with four pillows Has slept in a chair for the last two nights	Rests in a chair Appears drowsy
Dying	A practising Roman Catholic He is aware he is seriously ill	Has asked Father Joseph to be called for last rites if necessary

Alexander's immediate assessment identifies a number of issues related to his ability to breathe, which have to be addressed immediately. However, further issues in relation to other activities of living can be assessed as his condition stabilizes; these are identified under the activities of eating and drinking, personal cleansing and dressing, and mobilizing. The condition of Alexander's dry mouth, his state of nutrition and his pressure areas, with associated risk of developing pressure sores, can be assessed with specific tools.

Oral assessment. Alexander's mouth was said to be dry when he was admitted to the ward. Nora told Mary that her husband had not eaten or drunk for several days. He is receiving oxygen via a face-mask, which also has the effect of drying his mouth and putting him at risk of developing an oral infection (Xavier 2000), further deterring him from eating and drinking. Therefore, assessing Alexander's oral status is important, preferably with an assessment tool that will objectively measure *how* dry or dirty his mouth is.

REFLECTION POINT

Consider the way you start your day: how soon after you get up do you clean your teeth or take a drink to freshen your mouth?

Evans (2001) suggests most of us take a clean, moist and healthy mouth for granted and that when admitting and assessing patients or clients, nurses should be observing for:

- a pink moist tongue, oral mucosa and gums
- teeth/dentures clean and free from debris
- well-fitting dentures
- adequate salivation
- smooth and moist lips
- no difficulties in eating or swallowing.

If some of these features are absent, as well as added complications of treatment, such as medications, and other diseases, such as diabetes or anaemia, the person may be at risk of oral problems. An oral risk assessment tool is identified, where the higher the score of the person assessed, the greater the risk of oral problems and the need for mouth care to be included in the care plan (Table 6.10).

Table 6.10 Oral risk indicator tool (University Hospitals of Leicester 2000)

Mental status		Food/fluid intake		Teeth/dentures/jaw	
Alert	0	Good	0	Clean and free from debris	0
Apathetic	1	Inadequate diet	1	Debris present	1
Sedated	2	Fluids only	2	Denture present top/bottom (delete)	2
Unco-operative	3	No intake	3	Limity jaw mobility	3
Lips		**Tongue**		**Saliva**	
Smooth and moist	0	Pink and moist	0	Present and watery	0
Dry and cracked	1	Coated	1	Thick	1
Bleeding	2	Shiny/red	2	Insufficient/excess	2
Ulcerated	3	Blister/cracked	3	Absent	3
Mucous membranes		**Patient's age**		**Airway**	
Pink and moist	0	16–29	1	Normal	0
Red and coated	1	30–49	2	Humidified oxygen	1
White areas	2	50–69	3	Nebulized therapy	2
Ulcerated	3	70+	4	Open mouth breathing or non-humidified oxygen	3
				Et/oral intubation	4

Additional scores		Risk indicator	
High dose antibiotics	4	Score of 30+	high
Steroids	4	24–29	medium
Radiotherapy	4	Below 23	low
Diabetes	4		
Anaemia	4		
Cytotoxic drugs	4		
Immunocompromised	4		

Nutritional assessment. Alexander has not eaten or drunk for several days due to his breathlessness. Patients who are breathless, and particularly those with chronic lung disease, are known to be at risk of malnutrition (Edwards 1998). When well enough, it would be appropriate to weigh Alexander and compare this weight with what is known to be his usual weight. However, completing a nutritional assessment can be useful, especially if Alexander is to be referred for specialist dietetic support, such as high protein or high calorie drinks because of his difficulty in managing solid food.

Leicestershire Nutrition and Dietetic Services (1998) developed the nutritional screening tool shown in Table 6.11. The risk of poor nutrition is calculated and a care plan devised accordingly.

Table 6.11 Nutritional screening tool (Leicestershire Nutrition and Dietetic Service 1998)

Bodyweight for height		Ability to eat	
Acceptable (BMI 19–25)	0	Able to eat independently	0
Overweight (BMI >25)	2	Ill-fitting dentures/chewing problems	3
Recent significant weight loss	3	Swallowing problems	3
Underweight (BMI <19)	4	Needs to be fed	4
		Complete dysphagia	5
Skin type		**Symptoms**	
Healthy	0	Nausea	2
Dry and flaky	2	Vomiting	2
Oedematous	3	Constipation	2
Poor wound healing	4	Diarrhoea	2
Pressure sore/leg ulcer (all grades)	5		
Appetite and dietary intake		**Psychological state**	
Normal appetite/intake	0	Fully orientated	0
On special diet, e.g. supplements	2	Confused	2
Reduced appetite/intake	3	Depressed/anxious/apathetic	4
No appetite/very poor intake/nil by mouth/clear fluids for 7 days or more	5		
Age		**Total**	
Over 65 years	2		

Patients or clients scoring 10 and above are recommended to be referred for detailed nutritional assessment.
BMI = Body mass index.

Pressure risk assessment. In reviewing the initial assessment of Alexander using the Roper, Logan and Tierney framework (Table 6.9), you will note that under the activities of living of personal cleansing and dressing, and mobility, pressure areas are mentioned. Pressure damage can occur when skin and other tissues are compressed between bone and another surface for a period of time (Pellatt 2001). This causes the blood supply to the tissues to be reduced or cut off, resulting in damage to the skin. The usual result is skin breakdown and the development of a pressure ulcer (bedsore). Alexander has found difficulty in mobilizing because of his breathlessness, and so could be at risk. He has also been sleeping in a chair, putting extra pressure on his sacral area and this again could put him at risk of a pressure ulcer.

Apart from direct pressure, pressure ulcers (sores) can occur by the forces of shearing and friction (Gould 2001). Shearing occurs when tissues are wrenched in opposite directions, e.g. when a patient 'slides down the bed' or the chair. Friction occurs when the skin surface rubs against another surface. Alexander's elbows may be particularly at risk from friction as he uses his elbows to push himself up in the bed or chair to assist his breathing. The sacrum, heels, elbows, hips, knees and ankles pose the greatest risk (Pellatt 2001), but any area under pressure can be damaged. Previous assessments of Alexander's physical condition and his nutritional state also place him at great risk of pressure damage, according to some authors (Waterlow 1985).

Several pressure risk assessment tools have been devised, one of the earliest being the Norton scale (Norton *et al.* 1962), originally for use with older adults (Table 6.12).

Table 6.12 The Norton scale (Norton *et al.* 1962)

Physical condition		Mental state		Activity		Mobility		Incontinence	
Good	4	Alert	4	Ambulant	4	Full	4	Not	4
Fair	3	Apathetic	3	Walks with help	3	Slightly limited	3	Occasionally	3
Poor	2	Confused	2	Chair-bound	2	Very limited	2	Usually urine	2
Very bad	1	Stuporous	1	Bedfast	1	Immobile	1	Double	1

Assessment of risk: under 14 = at risk.

EXERCISE

It has been suggested that the Norton scale is actually subjective and difficult to score. Can you identify any problems with this scale?

You may have identified the lack of specifics within the scale, e.g. what is the difference between a 'fair' and a 'poor' physical condition? How 'occasional' does incontinence need to be before it is used as part of the score? If the patient is catheterized for incontinence of urine, does this give them 'full' continence?

The Waterlow risk assessment (Waterlow 1985) was devised in 1985 and aims to provide much more specific detail about the risk of developing a pressure ulcer (Table 6.13). It gives much more detail and includes factors which the Norton scale does not, e.g. the patient's gender, risk of alterations to the circulation which could be affected by smoking or the effect of anaemia on the skin, and body mass. You will also note that, according to Norton, the patient is at greater risk of pressure damage in bed than sitting in a chair, while the Waterlow scale considers the chair-bound person to be at greater risk and hence has a greater score.

Table 6.13 Waterlow risk assessment (Waterlow 1985)

Build/weight for height		Skin type Visual risk areas		Sex Age		Special risks	
Average	0	Healthy	0	Male	1	Tissue	
Above average	1	Tissue paper	1	Female	2	malnutrition	
Obese	2	Dry	1	14–49	1	Cachexia	8
Below average	3	Oedematous	1	50–64	2	Cardiac failure	5
		Clammy (temp.)	1	65–74	3	PVD	5
		Discoloured	2	75–80	4	Anaemia	2
		Broken/spot	3	81+	5	Smoking	1
Continence		**Mobility**		**Appetite**		**Neurological deficit**	
Complete/ catheterised	0	Full	0	Average	0	Diabetes, MS	4
Occasional incontinence	1	Restless/fidgety	1	Poor	1	CVA	–
Incontinent of faeces	2	Apathetic	2	NG tube/fluids	2	Paraplegia	6
Double incontinence	3	Restricted	3	only		Major surgery/trauma	5
		Inert/traction	4	Nil by mouth/	3	Medication	4
		Chair–bound	5	anorexic			

(PVD = peripheral vascular disease, MS = multiple sclerosis, NG = nasogastric, CVA = cerebrovascular accident).
Score: 10+ at risk; 15+ high risk; 20+ very high risk.

EXERCISE

Using the Norton and Waterlow scales, what scores would you allocate to Alexander? Is he at risk of pressure damage? Do both scales place him at equal risk? Which scale is easier to use?

Identifying a score for the risk of pressure damage is the first part of the assessment process. Appropriate pressure-relieving devices should be used depending on the score obtained. For example, Waterlow advocates the use of a foam mattress for a score of 10+ and an alternating pressure mattress for one of 20+. Pressure-relieving equipment should then also be used in the patient's chair or wheel-chair, bearing in mind the greater risk when sitting.

Pressure risk assessments should be evaluated regularly and documented in the patient's plan of care.

SCENARIO 2: SIMON COOPER

Scenario Simon is a 22-year-old man who lives at home with his mother. He works as a casual labourer at the garden centre. He loves the plants and the aquatic section of the garden centre. As part of his work, he often helps customers carry compost and gravel to their cars. Simon has Down's syndrome.

Simon was admitted to the surgical ward and underwent surgical repair of a right inguinal hernia earlier today. He returns to the ward drowsy but rousable and has received pain relief in theatre.

After completing a full set of post-operative observations on Simon, including pulse, blood pressure, respirations, checking his dressing for leakage, your main concern is to keep him comfortable and free from pain.

Assessing patients for pain

Can you describe what 'pain' is? We all find it difficult, yet most of us have experienced pain at some time of our lives. The International Association for the Study of Pain (1992) suggests pain is:

'an unpleasant sensory and emotional experience associated with actual or potential tissue damage or described in terms of such damage'.

Experiencing pain is a subjective phenomenon and many factors influence the way it is experienced:

- lack of information about what pain is, how it is caused and how it will be relieved, and lack of control over pain, all tend to increase pain
- families and society often 'socialize' people into ways of behaving when in pain, e.g. the British 'stiff upper lip' contrasts with the Mediterranean wailing
- the context in which pain is experienced, e.g. many women expect to have pain in childbirth. Patients recovering from a hip replacement following arthritis of the hip frequently experience no pain because the surgical pain is less than the previous arthritic pain (Hall 2000).

Many patients are now taught to manage their own pain after a surgical operation, using patient-controlled analgesia (PCA), when they deliver a dose of a drug to themselves in response to pain or prior to carrying out movement.

EXERCISE

Make a note of the ways you would assess and identify if Simon is suffering pain.

You may have identified some of the following:

- lack of movement
- groaning
- facial grimaces
- lack of sleep
- rapid pulse.

Simon may exhibit some of these typical pain responses. However, it may be more appropriate to identify pain in a more systematic manner, using a pain assessment scale, e.g. the verbal rating scale (Table 6.14) or visual analogue scale (in which patients are asked to place a mark on a line drawn between the numbers 0 and 10 which represents the intensity of pain; the higher the score, the greater the pain).

Table 6.14 Verbal rating scale

Rating of pain	Score
None	0
Mild	1
Moderate	2
Severe	3

EXERCISE

- From the patient's or client's point of view, what might be the advantages in using a pain assessment tool?
- From the nurse's point of view, what might be the advantages?
- Are there any patients or clients who would have difficulty in using such a scale?

You may have identified the following:

- from the patient's viewpoint, using a rating scale means that every nurse on duty will interpret the pain in the same way, rather than subjectively. It also means that if the pain relief does not take effect within half an hour and the patient is still in pain, there may be the opportunity to review the treatment and find an alternative that will work (evaluation of pain relief)
- from the nurse's viewpoint, this is a means of obtaining an accurate record of what causes pain, how severe the pain is and what helps to relieve it. The score the patient reports may have an impact on the way other activities of living are carried out
- patients such as Simon, who has a learning disability, may have difficulty in using a rating tool like the ones shown. The elderly and very young and those who are confused or partially sighted may also have a problem using such scales.

SUMMARY

- Assessment tools are useful because they allow specific measurements to be made and provide accurate and objective data for assessment.
- Assessment tools can be quite simple, e.g. temperature recording, or sophisticated, e.g. pressure sore risk, nutrition assessment, pain scales and the amount of oxygen carried by the blood.
- Using such tools to measure, assess and evaluate the needs of a patient or client, enables the use of best evidence or research to inform the nursing care the patient or client receives.

CONCLUSION

Assessing patients or clients is a fundamental nursing skill and vital to meeting the needs of patients or clients. Assessment is the first stage of the nursing process and provides the opportunity to reflect the patient's or client's views and concerns about their need for nursing care, not just those of the nurse.

Assessment may be the first time the nurse and patient or client meet and so it is clearly important to develop a trusting and good working relationship from the outset (do not forget, the patient or client will also be assessing you!). This means the nurse needs to have excellent interpersonal and communication skills. Asking the right questions is clearly important, but so is the ability to listen to what is being said and how it is said, particularly when the client may have a communication difficulty. Subjective or objective data may be revealed by assessment. To assist in data gathering, a nursing model with a framework for assessment may be used. This may be used in conjunction with assessment tools, enabling accurate measurement. Using evidence-based tools for assessment means that the same information is available to all members of the multi-professional team and can ensure the care provided is based on the most up-to-date and research-based care.

Following the principles for assessment identifies that it really is the foundation of good practice!

CHAPTER
7

EVIDENCE-BASED PRACTICE

Alison Loftus–Hills, Liz McInnes and Yana Richens

INTRODUCTION

This chapter outlines the core aspects of evidence-based practice and how it relates to your everyday practice as a nurse. It begins with an overview of what evidence-based practice is, and what has driven the 'evidence-based movement' in health care. Evidence-based practice is then placed within the context of other current initiatives aimed at ensuring quality practice care for all patients in the UK.

Next, the chapter aims to give you some of the tools and skills that are essential for evidence-based practice by outlining how you can find and evaluate research evidence on nursing interventions. It takes you through a number of exercises which will help you to develop the skills necessary in doing this, such as searching techniques and critical appraisal skills. An overview of the sources of 'best evidence' is given, including guidelines and systematic reviews, which are both useful tools that place research findings from a number of studies in a synthesized format.

Finally, some of the barriers to evidence-based health care and some of the complexities of implementing evidence in clinical practice are discussed. An overview is given of some approaches to changing practice and possible ways in which you may become involved in improving the quality of practice within the health care setting in which you work.

After reading this chapter and following the various exercises you will understand:

- what evidence-based practice in nursing is
- how evidence-based practice links to other initiatives for ensuring quality of health care across the UK
- how to find and evaluate evidence and the different sources of evidence
- the complexities of implementing evidence in nursing practice and some approaches to enabling this process.

This will allow you to achieve the last of the competencies the UKCC set in 1999 for pre-registration nursing programmes:

'based on the best available evidence, apply knowledge and an appropriate repertoire of skills indicative of safe nursing practice'.

(UKCC Commission for Nursing and Midwifery Education 1999)

OVERVIEW OF EVIDENCE-BASED HEALTH CARE

WHAT IS EVIDENCE-BASED HEALTH CARE?

As a nurse, newly registered or experienced, you will make decisions many times a day about the clinical care that you provide for patients. For example, you may make decisions about what procedure to use, how often to change a dressing or whether a certain course of treatment is working. The decisions you make may be based on a number of different factors or influences which could include: what you were taught in your nurse education, previous clinical experiences or what you are told by the ward manager. Many of your decisions will be made at a subconscious level or on 'automatic pilot' – you do not always question how and why you come to a particular decision.

Evidence-based practice, or evidence-based health care, aims to question the basis of decision-making in health care. Rather than using habit, tradition, intuition or peer opinion, it is about ensuring that decisions about patient care are based on the best available evidence. As Appleby *et al.* (1995) state, evidence-based practice is:

'a shift in the culture of health care provision away from basing decisions on opinion, past practice and precedent towards making more use of science, research and evidence to guide clinical decision-making … [this] requires the evaluation of the effectiveness of medical (and other health care) interventions, dissemination of results and the application of those findings in practice'.

Sackett *et al.* (1997) have defined evidence-based medicine as:

'The conscientious, explicit and judicious use of current best evidence in making decisions about the care of individual patients. The practice of evidence-based medicine means integrating individual clinical expertise with the best available best external clinical evidence from systematic research'.

They go on to highlight that clinical decisions need to be made with the compassionate use of 'individual patients' predicaments, rights and preferences' (Sackett *et al.* 1997). Others have also identified that patient-specific information is another form of evidence to be utilized in the decision-making process (The Clinical Guidelines Education Team 2001).

As such, evidence-based practice is about using *all* available evidence in making clinical decisions in health care practice. There has been much debate and discussion about what constitutes 'evidence' in relation to health care. While evidence from patients and clinical observations is key to good practice, the use of *research-based evidence* in making decisions about patient care is central to evidence-based practice. The challenge for all health care professionals lies in *integrating* different forms of evidence – from research, from their own clinical experience and from the information provided by patients. In doing so, patients' views and preferences are a key consideration. This will be discussed later in this chapter.

EXERCISE

Consider the above definitions of evidence-based health care. What are some of the possible benefits to nurses and patients in using evidence in practice?

The use of high-quality research evidence in conjunction with clinical expertise and patient preferences is seen to have many advantages for improving practice. If evidence is available and appropriately applied it has the potential to:

- improve clinical effectiveness for patients
- make decision-making more transparent, thereby giving greater information to patients as well as health care professionals
- empower clinicians to make informed decisions and question practice
- enable patients to use knowledge to become more informed and involved in decisions about their care
- enable better use of resources by practitioners and purchasers by adopting more effective treatment, at times, leading to better outcomes for patients such as, shorter hospital stays for patients.

ORIGINS OF EVIDENCE-BASED HEALTH CARE

The term 'evidence-based medicine', and subsequently evidence-based health care, seems to have originated from a group of academics and doctors working in Canada who devised different ways of teaching medical students. As Pencheon (1998) points out, they were determined to re-think the process of professional development and use a problem-based, more critical approach to medical education. These developments spread quickly to the UK, with the development of the Centre for Evidence-based Medicine and the UK Cochrane Centre, both based in Oxford.

More generally, however, this work increasingly focused attention on developing evidence-based health care, which has since become central to government policy and health care professionals' education and practice. A number of broader interrelated factors have created an emphasis on outcomes in health care and on ensuring the best possible care for patients. These factors relate more generally to social, economic and political aspects of providing health care.

One of the initial driving factors was the need for *cost containment* in the health care sector. From the early 1970s in the UK and many other western societies, economic recession, inflation and rising unemployment led to a systematic attempt to restructure economies and reduce public expenditure (Flynn 1992). Within health, the need to contain expenditure coincided with:

- rapid increases in demand
- technological advances and
- an increasingly ageing population.

The need to contain costs led to, among other things, a greater focus on measuring and monitoring the effectiveness of different health care interventions in an attempt to eliminate unnecessary expenditure, with the ultimate aim of improving efficiency (Epstein 1990; Flynn 1992). While eliminating unnecessary expenditure is obviously still a key factor driving evidence-based practice, it is also important to highlight that at times the best known treatment is not necessarily the cheapest.

A second origin stems from a response to research which found *substantial and unacceptable differences in the rate of medical procedures* used across geographical regions. This, in turn, led to a generation of further interest and research to investigate the nature of these variations (Epstein 1990). McPherson *et al.* (1981) found significant variations in surgical rates for common procedures, both within the UK and internationally. This study and similar research (Wennberg 1987a) concluded that geographical variation could not account for the differences. Wennberg (1987a) and many others surmised that it was more that the medical profession lacked consensus on the 'best' or most appropriate way to treat patients. These studies highlighted the need, if variation in clinical practice were to be addressed, to centre attention on improving the scientific basis of medicine (Wennberg 1987b). This was not necessarily a new observation and was supported from within the medical profession by some influential and vocal advocates, such as Archie Cochrane. Cochrane (1976) was dominant in demonstrating that clinical practice was often based on poor research findings and that many practices had no research foundation at all.

Alongside these other changes, consumers of health care were demanding to know more about their treatment options, in order to make informed and appropriate decisions, and they had increasing expectations of what the health service should be providing (Ellwood 1988).

The document *Research for Health: A Research and Development Strategy for the NHS* was published in 1991 by the Department of Health (DoH 1991a). It stated that the objective of the strategy was:

> 'to ensure that the content and delivery of care in the NHS is based on high-quality research relevant to improving the health of the nation'.

While the 1980s had seen an increase in the amount of research and effectiveness, and the development of tools such as clinical guidelines, this strategy gave greater impetus (and funding) to research and provided a concrete strategy for its development.

Evidence-based developments within nursing

At the same time, other health professional groups, including nursing, focused increasingly on critically assessing the basis of health care interventions.

In 1993, the *Report of the Taskforce of the Strategy for Research in Nursing, Midwifery and Health Visiting* (DoH 1993a) stated that there was a need to develop research skills across the profession. The taskforce highlighted that, while not all nurses had to be involved directly in research, it was essential for every practitioner to 'develop a capacity for critical thought and basic research literacy'.

These requirements are also reflected in many of the standards set by the United Kingdom Central Council for Nursing, Midwifery and Health Visiting (UKCC) [now the Nursing and Midwifery Council (NMC)]. The guidance provided by the UKCC states that practitioners working at a higher level will (among other things):

- determine therapeutic programmes which are based on evidence, in the interests of patients and clients, and which involve other practitioners where this will improve health outcomes
- make specific interventions based on evidence and which are appropriate to assessed needs, context and culture, in partnership with patients, clients and other professionals
- synthesize, coherently and effectively, knowledge and expertise related to an area of practice
- interpret and evaluate information from diverse sources to make informed judgements about its quality and appropriateness
- actively monitor the effectiveness of current therapeutic programmes and integrate different aspects of practice to improve outcomes for patients and clients (UKCC 1999a,b; UKCC Commission for Nursing and Midwifery Education 1999).

As Cullum *et al.* (1997) stated:

'as the millennium approaches nurses are expected to be able to identify patients' actual and potential health problems; and develop research-based strategies to prevent, ameliorate and comfort. Increasingly, nurses are expected to undertake work historically done by doctors; they are also expected to be empathic communicators who are highly educated, critical thinkers, abreast of all the important research findings'.

EVIDENCE-BASED HEALTH CARE IN THE CONTEXT OF WIDER QUALITY INITIATIVES

It is useful to consider where evidence-based practice sits in relation to other quality initiatives within health care policy.

Clinical governance

Clinical governance is a term you may be familiar with (see also Chapters 3 and 14). It was first developed in 1998 (to be implemented from April 1999). It has been defined as:

'a framework through which NHS organizations are accountable for continuously improving the quality of their services and safeguarding high standards of care by creating an environment in which excellence in clinical care can flourish'.

(NHS Executive 1999a)

Clinical governance is made up of a number of activities, which may not be new but which have now been placed within an overall framework for quality (see Box 7.1 for an overview of some of the main components of clinical governance; examples of clinical governance activities are given in

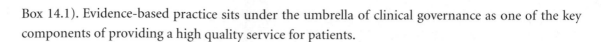

Box 14.1). Evidence-based practice sits under the umbrella of clinical governance as one of the key components of providing a high quality service for patients.

Box 7.1 Some elements of clinical governance

- Clinical audit – local and national programmes
- Use of evidence-based practice
- Clinical supervision
- Clinical risk management policies
- Continuing professional development for professional staff and lifelong learning systems for all staff
- Workforce planning and development, including clinical leadership development
- Systems for remedying poor performance, including responding to complaints (patient/client feedback systems), clinical incident reporting and critical incident analysis, and professional performance procedures

Every staff member working in a health care setting is accountable for the quality of care they provide to patients, including clinicians and non-clinical staff. As a nurse, clinical governance is about becoming involved in quality activities. For example, you may become involved in helping to establish priorities for improvement, by learning from others, voicing any concerns you may have about the quality of patient care in a particular area and working as part of a team to conduct a clinical audit. Actively seeking out training and development opportunities is also a core way of contributing to fulfilling the aims of clinical governance as an individual.

More information on clinical governance can be obtained from two useful guides produced and supplied by the RCN (1998a, 2000a).

Other related quality initiatives

Clinical governance is a key part of an overall larger strategy for quality in the NHS. Box 7.2 summarizes some of the other key components of this broader strategy for quality within the NHS.

Box 7.2 Overview of the strategy for quality in the NHS (adapted from RCN 2000a)

National standards and guidelines:
- National Institute for Clinical Excellence (NICE): not Scotland (provides patients, health care professionals and the public with robust and reliable guidance on current best clinical practice)
- Scottish Inter-Collegiate Guidelines Network (SIGN): provides guidance on best practice for Scotland
- National Service Frameworks (not Scotland): national standards that define service models for a specific service or care group (e.g. cancer care)

Local implementation:
- Clinical governance
- Professional self-regulation
- Lifelong learning

External evaluation and monitoring:
- Commission for Health Improvement (CHI): for England and Wales and by invitation in Northern Ireland (not Scotland). CHI's role is to assess the clinical governance arrangements of every NHS organization, investigate where there is serious failure, check the NHS is following national guidelines and advise the NHS on best practice

- Clinical Standards Board for Scotland
- National Performance Framework (not Scotland)

For more information on policy developments in the NHS, see DoH (1997; 2002b).

PROCESS AND COMPLEXITIES OF PRACTICING EVIDENCE-BASED MEDICINE

As highlighted above, evidence-based practice involves using the best available evidence when making decisions with patients about the care you provide. So, what does this involve and what are some of the issues or problems you may encounter along the way?

Figure 7.1 outlines the key steps of evidence-based practice. In many ways it is similar to the quality improvement cycle of defining practice, measuring practice and changing practice, then re-measuring.

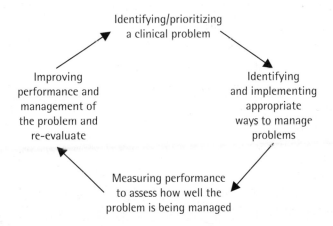

Figure 7.1 Steps of evidence-based practice [adapted from Oxman *et al.* (1994)]

The process of evidence-based practice seems relatively straightforward. It is a matter of asking a clear clinical question, identifying research, appraising it, applying it in practice and then measuring whether it has changed practice and ultimately improved the overall performance of health care. While in some clinical areas you may find this to be the case, in many clinical areas, the process of finding and utilizing evidence is *not* straightforward.

There are still many examples which indicate that despite policy initiatives and educational and practice developments, poor or ritualistic practices still exist within health care settings. Examples within nursing practice include:

- in the nursing management of fever in children, it has been found that practices are not often based on research (Watts *et al.* 2001)
- in one study, 21% of 1200 nurses had not implemented a new research finding in the past 6 months (Bostrom and Suter 1993)
- in leg ulcer management, Luker and Kenrick (1995) found that community nurses' knowledge was often inadequate to be able to treat patients effectively.

There are many reasons for this. In 1981, Hunt published a key article that outlined five main reasons why nurses did not use research in their practice. Nurses:

- did not know about research findings
- did not understand research findings
- did not believe research findings
- did not know how to use research findings
- were not allowed to use research findings.

Many of these reasons for not using research are still relevant today – although possibly with the saturation of education and training, articles, circulars, clinical guidelines and government policies, to a lesser extent.

It is also worth keeping in mind that *generating* nursing research is not always straightforward. For example, in some clinical areas, rigorous research on what is effective may not exist. Given that nursing is a relatively young profession, as compared to medicine, it has a more recent history of research:

'we know much less about the outcomes of nursing, and relatively little evaluative research has been done to distinguish between effective and ineffective nursing practices'.

(Cullum et al. *1997, p32)*

However, Cullum *et al.* (1997) go on to state, 'this is changing' with the development of research programmes and evidence-based initiatives within nursing.

Conversely, in some clinical areas, there may be an overwhelming amount of information to understand and digest, which can make it very confusing to know what is correct, safe and acceptable practice. Watts *et al.* (2001) reviewed 41 internet sites which offered advice about the care of children with fever in the home, and found that only four adhered closely to selected guidelines. As outlined below, finding a good clinical guideline or systematic review of the specific clinical area and appraising it is one way to address this.

You may also find conflicting opinions about the best way to manage a condition reported in the nursing literature or among your colleagues. Again, the management of fever in children provides an example of inconsistent practice (Watts *et al.* 2001), with differing views given about correct management.

SUMMARY

- Evidence-based practice is about questioning the basis of decision-making in health care and ensuring that the best available research evidence is used to inform your practice in conjunction with the appropriate use of clinical expertise and with consideration of patients' views and preferences.
- Evidence-based health care has been driven by political, social and economic factors, including the need for cost containment and a desire to limit unnecessary variation in health care practice. The aim is to apply the right practice to the right patient at the right time (Kitson 1997). Evidence-based practice is a central part of a wider agenda for quality, and is a central component to the delivery of clinical governance.
- Practising in an evidence-based way requires time, a range of skills and an understanding of the limitations of evidence and the complexities of implementing evidence in clinical practice.

HOW CAN I PRACTISE EVIDENCE-BASED HEALTH CARE?

Here the UKCC competencies listed at the beginning of this chapter are addressed:

- determine therapeutic programmes which are based on evidence, in the interests of patients and clients, and which involve other practitioners when this will improve health outcomes
- interpret and evaluate information from diverse sources to make informed judgements about its quality and appropriateness.

Before changing your practice in the light of new research or research cited by colleagues, you should be able to appraise critically the studies and be satisfied that they are of good quality and that the results are applicable to and will benefit your patients. You should also understand the main sources of research evidence, particularly sources of summarized evidence – like systematic reviews and clinical practice guidelines. Understanding these sources of evidence will enable you to give the best possible care to your patients.

Bearing in mind the UKCC competencies now stress an evidence-based approach to clinical decision-making, you may want to access the many guides and courses on critical appraisal that are now widely available, e.g. consult http://cebm.jr2.ox.ac.uk/docs/calendar.html (and other websites listed in Box 7.7).

A brief introduction to critical appraisal is presented and the role of clinical practice guidelines and systematic reviews in providing reliable sources of evidence-based information is emphasized. However, this in no way substitutes for formal training in critical appraisal (courses for health professionals are held all over the UK) or for consulting with a medical librarian who specializes in systematic searching for research studies. As the focus here is on accessing and appraising evidence of effectiveness (i.e. what intervention/therapy works best), the emphasis is on quantitative sources of research evidence, namely systematic reviews and particularly randomized controlled trials (RCTs).

As indicated earlier in this chapter, part of clinical practice involves basing your care on good quality research, to ensure that the care you deliver will result in the best possible outcomes for your patients. It will also enable both you and your patients to make well-informed decisions about the best treatment options for particular conditions.

REFLECTION POINT

Think of an area of clinical practice, whether it is taking a patient's blood pressure, applying a dressing technique or an example from midwifery, such as electronic fetal monitoring. Was there a level of uncertainty about how best to treat patients or were treatment decisions straightforward? Spend some time thinking about the basis of the information/knowledge you were given. How evidence-based do you think the area is?

HOW DO I START?

Above, a common dilemma faced by health care practitioners was introduced – having identified the need for evidence-based information to inform clinical practice, then being unsure of:

- how to access such information and/or
- how to be sure that the sources of evidence are reliable.

If you have concerns that the care you are providing is ineffective or out-of-date, or if you simply do not know what effective care is for a particular clinical condition, a good starting point might be to ask your colleagues if they know of any evidence or research-based interventions that might work for that situation.

Alternatively, you may want to search for research that relates to your clinical dilemma via the web or your hospital library in conjunction with a medical/nursing librarian. There are different sources of evidence. The main three that are relevant and outlined in this chapter are:

- *clinical practice guidelines:* recommendations for the care of individuals by health care professions which are based on the best available evidence (NICE 2001a), e.g. *Clinical Practice Guidelines on the Recognition and Assessment of Acute Pain in Children* (RCN 1999a)
- *systematic reviews:* a rigorous summary of all the research evidence that relates to a specific question (Ciliska *et al.* 2001), e.g. *The Nursing Management of Fever in Children: A Systematic Review* (Watts *et al.* 2001)
- *primary study:* a piece of research investigating a particular question or hypothesis, e.g. a RCT of specialist nurse intervention in heart failure (Blue *et al.* 2001).

There are many databases you can use to search for material relevant to a particular clinical area (Box 7.3).

Box 7.3 Useful databases

PubMed http://www.ncbi.nlm.nih.gov/PubMed: the USA's National Library of Medicine's biomedical bibliographic database is free on the internet. It contains over 11 million references to journal articles, books and other publications. There is an online tutorial for first-time users.

CINAHL (Cumulative Index to Nursing and Allied Health Literature): contains references specifically related to nursing and allied health and relevant articles from the biomedical education, behavioural science and health management literature.

MEDLINE: bibliographic databases which cover medicine, nursing, dentistry and preclinical sciences. Contains over 11 million citations dating back to the mid-1960s.

EMBASE: a comprehensive pharmacological and biomedical database. It contains more than 13 million bibliographic records with abstracts from EMBASE (1974–present) and MEDLINE (1966–present).

Cochrane Library Free access for NHS via National Electronic Library for Health http://www.nelh.nhs.uk.: an excellent up-to-date source of RCTs on many topics. Includes the following databases:

- Cochrane Database of Systematic Reviews (full-text Cochrane systematic reviews of health-care interventions)
- Database of Abstracts and Reviews of Effectiveness (DARE) (abstracts of high quality systematic reviews)
- Cochrane Controlled Trials Register (150,000+ controlled trials)
- NHS Economic Evaluation Database
- Health Technology Assessment Database

Hospital librarians should be able to assist you to use these databases. Alternatively you can contact the RCN Quality Improvement Information Service which can search for guidelines or literature on specific topics (020 7647 3831 or email: qip.hq@rcn.org.uk).

It may be useful to access a relevant guideline, systematic review or research study yourself (or with a team of people) and to critically appraise it for its quality and clinical relevance to decide whether:

- its findings are worth your attention
- if it could be applied to a patient you have cared for.

WHAT IS YOUR CLINICAL QUESTION?

Before you can start searching for evidence, you will need to formulate a clear and focused question. Generally, the clinical question of interest is structured by specifying:

- the patient or problem
- the intervention of interest, and possible comparison interventions
- the outcomes of interest.

For example, you may want to know the current best method for reducing a child's fever:

- is it to administer paracetamol and/or to immerse a child in a tepid bath, or simply to sponge the child?
- is the current ward policy correct in relation to the best available research evidence for managing this clinical problem, or is there one which may be safer, more effective and provide more rapid relief for the patient?
- in short, what is the most clinically effective intervention for managing a child's fever?

This allows you to pinpoint the sort of evidence required to answer your clinical questions and to build a search strategy which can be conducted either by you or a health care librarian (Box 7.4). It also allows you easily to assess if your clinical question is being addressed by the research articles you retrieve.

Box 7.4 Overview of basic searching techniques

For the systematic review on the management of fever in children, Watts *et al.* (2001) entered the following search terms to retrieve relevant papers from the CINAHL database: nurse* or manage* and fever* and child*

The * is a handy way of truncating words or part of a word to find similar word-endings. This form of searching, i.e. *text word* searching, is only one technique to retrieve articles on your topic of interest. There is also thesaurus searching, also called *MeSH* (Medical Subject Headings) in MEDLINE and *De* (descriptors) in CINAHL and other databases, which allows you to search for references under headings taken from a structured list of standardized subject headings. For example, you can guess a heading, such as *decubitus*, enter the term in the thesaurus box, and then explode the term to search on related terms (such as pressure ulcer, bed sore, etc).

The recommendation for optimal searching is to use a combination of both free text and thesaurus searching.

For example, a structured question for determining the effectiveness of different bandaging for the treatment of venous leg ulcers would be broken down into the various components relating to:

- *patients:* patients presenting in outpatient or primary care settings with venous leg ulcers
- *the intervention:* high-compression bandaging for the treatment of venous leg ulcers

- *comparison:* low-compression bandaging
- *outcome:* number of patients healed within 12 weeks.

The question can then be phrased: What is the effectiveness of high-compared to low-compression bandaging as a treatment for venous leg ulcers in patients presenting to primary care or outpatient settings? For the management of a child with fever outlined above, the question would be: Does the available evidence, in terms of outcomes, support the types and timing of the various nursing interventions which are commonly used to reduce fever in non-critically ill children? (Watts *et al.* 2001).

Each of the components (patient, intervention, comparison, outcome) should be reflected in the search strategy. This can be quite complicated and it is best to consult your hospital librarian about the optimal way of doing this or to access websites such as www.shef.ac.uk/~scharr/ir/adept/therapy/searching.htm.

WHAT KINDS OF RESEARCH EVIDENCE ARE THERE?

It is important to be able to identify the best research design to answer the clinical question posed. Different clinical questions require evidence from different research designs. Different designs can variously address questions of prevention, treatment, therapy, interventions, causation, prognosis and harm. Each research design also has a number of potential biases which the reviewer needs to be aware of.

As outlined above, here the focus is on accessing and appraising evidence of *effectiveness*. Thus, the emphasis is on quantitative sources of research evidence, namely systematic reviews and particularly RCTs (Box 7.5). Commonly, study designs are ranked in terms of their value in asking how *effective* a certain health care treatment or intervention is. In order of ranking, this includes:

- systematic reviews and meta-analyses
- RCTs
- quasi-experimental/controlled trials
- cohort
- case-control
- cross-sectional
- case series/reports.

Box 7.5 Quantitative and qualitative research

What is quantitative research?

Quantitative research studies are concerned with how many and how often events occur and what treatment/intervention works best and why, e.g. how many people voted in a certain way? Or what is the best method for preventing the development of pressure ulcers? Statistical techniques are used to summarize and analyse the numerical data collected.

What is qualitative research?

Qualitative research methods aim to understand the ways that people make sense of the world and how they give meaning to it. In health care, qualitative research can explore, among other things, patient and carer experiences of hospitalization and care as well as the views of health care providers. This kind of research gives information which can be valuable understand views and perceptions, for the planning and organization of care and can also generate ideas for further in-depth research.

The important point is that no single design has precedence over another, rather the design chosen must fit the particular research question (Roberts and DiCenso 1999). For a good overview of the different research paradigms and how different forms of knowledge are used see Crookes and Davies (1998).

The above ranking reflects the degree to which the different study designs are susceptible to bias and also their ability to provide evidence on effectiveness of treatments. Systematic reviews are seen as the highest level of evidence because their findings are based on multiple good quality RCTs. Of the study designs, the RCT is graded as being at least risk of bias (see below).

These designs are often translated into 'levels of evidence' with Level Ia being the best or 'highest' level of evidence (Table 7.1). These levels are commonly used in clinical practice guidelines to inform the reader of the strength of evidence underpinning each guideline recommendation.

Table 7.1 Levels of evidence (NICE 2001b)

Level	Type of evidence
Level Ia	Evidence obtained from systematic review or meta-analysis of randomized controlled trials
Level Ib	Evidence obtained from at least one well-designed randomized controlled trial
Level IIa	Evidence obtained from at least one well-designed controlled trial without randomization
Level IIb	Evidence obtained from at least one other type of well designed quasi-experimental study
Level III	Evidence obtained from well-designed non-experimental descriptive studies, such as comparative studies, correlation studies and case studies
Level IV	Evidence obtained from expert committee reports or opinions and/or clinical experience of respected authorities

Remember this hierarchy of evidence relates only to how well these studies answer the question: Does it work/is it effective? It does not relate to whether quantitative research is more or less valuable than qualitative research in answering other important questions related to health care provision.

What is a randomized controlled trial?

Oakley (1989) identifies the RCT as first being used in 1946 when a controlled trial was performed to determine the effectiveness of a new drug, streptomycin, as a cure for tuberculosis. It is now recognized as the most rigorous method for assessing the effectiveness of preventive and therapeutic interventions; it focuses on answering the questions:

● does it work?
● does it lead to an improvement in patient care?
● what is the most effective treatment?

The RCT is an experimental method which tests (or trials) a particular treatment by comparing two or more groups of subjects who are allocated to these groups at random. Each group then receives a different treatment – usually one group receives no treatment and acts as the control group and the other, which is treated, is usually called the intervention group (Oakley 1989).

It is the only study design that minimizes bias because of random allocation of subjects to each study group. For example, in a study of leg ulcer treatment, subjects may be randomized either to the intervention group (those to receive a multi-layer compression bandage to treat venous leg ulcers) or the control group (those to receive single-layer compression bandages). It is the play of chance that determines the allocation, not the clinician or patient preference (Roberts and DiCenso 1999). Random allocation should mean that patient characteristics are distributed equally between the groups.

Important features of a properly conducted RCT include:

- use of an unpredictable method of randomization (e.g. computer generated, coin tossing as opposed to using date of birth or hospital number)
- the randomization schedule was concealed so that the researchers are unable to predict which treatment a subject is randomized to
- the person receiving the treatment was 'blinded' to which intervention they received and that those delivering the intervention and assessing the outcome were also blind to the intervention received by the subject.

It is important to remember, when critically appraising RCTs, that people who 'drop out' (because they are not compliant with the intervention, move out of the area or suffer adverse effects from the intervention) may be different from the remainder of the population and may have very different outcomes from the treatment. Therefore, any discrepancy between actual and intended number of patients in a study should be explained by the study authors and a table of comparative statistics should be provided for those who remain in the study and those who drop out. Furthermore, everyone should be included in the analysis, even those who are non-compliant or who did not receive the treatment to which they were assigned. This is called 'intention to treat' and gives a real-life perspective to the results (Cullum 2000).

Finally, the period of time in which participants were followed-up should be of sufficient duration to give the intervention/exposure the chance to manifest its effect (Cullum 2000). For example, if you were evaluating whether a three-layer bandage improved the healing rate of venous leg ulcers, you would need a certain time period, possibly 12 weeks, to give the intervention a chance to show whether it works.

An example of an RCT research question: does specialist nurse intervention improve the outcomes for patients with chronic heart failure (Blue *et al.* 2001)?

- Patients were randomized to usual care or nurse intervention (which consisted of a number of planned home visits and telephone support).
- Nurses involved in the study phoned an off-site office and the patient was allocated to one or other intervention group from a randomization list.
- Patients were analysed in the group to which they were assigned and were followed up for 12 months. All patients appeared to be accounted for at the end of the study.
- Researchers measuring rate of hospital admissions in each group were blind to treatment allocation of the patients.
- The results showed that home-based intervention from nurses reduces re-admissions for worsening heart failure.

Other quantitative study designs

Briefly, cohort studies are commonly used to:

- detect long-term adverse effects of interventions
- clarify the natural history of a disease
- answer questions when patients cannot be 'assigned' to an exposure group (as sometimes happens with occupational exposure), or when harmful outcomes are infrequent.

A case-control study is more feasible than an RCT when the outcome of interest is either rare or takes a long time to develop.

Overview of appropriate study design

- Questions to do with the most effective treatment/therapies/interventions/preventive strategies should be addressed by RCTs.
- Questions about prognosis/harm/risk factors require longitudinal cohort studies.
- Questions about causation require either cohort or case-control studies.
- Questions relating to the occurrence of rare events require case-control studies.

Important questions to ask when appraising quantitative study designs

- Was the design appropriate for investigating the research question posed?
- Were subjects randomly assigned to different treatments in an RCT?
- Were subjects analysed according to the groups to which they were assigned?
- Were the groups being compared as similar as possible, except for the particular difference being examined?
- Was blinding possible?
- What was the duration and completeness of the follow-up?
- Was the study large enough? (Greenhalgh 1997; Cullum 2000)

OVERVIEW OF EVIDENCE FROM SYSTEMATIC REVIEWS AND GUIDELINES

Because of the amount of time required to make evidence-based clinical decisions 'from scratch', practitioners will often not be able to review all of the original relevant research literature that bears on the clinical question they would like an answer (Guyatt *et al.* 2000). Furthermore, a high level of skill is needed to appraise original literature, i.e. primary studies, and often nurses will not have the time to acquire this.

Secondary sources, where the evidence has already been appraised by an expert(s), include evidence-based resources, such as systematic reviews, evidence summaries and clinical practice guidelines. Such resources provide the clinician with conclusions often in a format that can be more easily applied to the clinical setting. This saves the bother of extensive literature searching, quality assessments and dealing with conflicting results between different studies.

Secondary sources of evidence can help health care practitioners and policy-makers keep up with the literature related to specific topics. However, knowing which reviews and guidelines to trust still

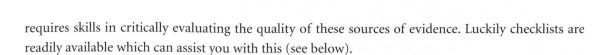

requires skills in critically evaluating the quality of these sources of evidence. Luckily checklists are readily available which can assist you with this (see below).

The most common sources of secondary evidence as outlined above are:

- systematic reviews (also known as overviews or meta-analyses) which summarize the evidence from RCTs (and less commonly other study designs)
- clinical practice guidelines (which frequently use the results of systematic reviews to underpin recommendations made about care/treatment/interventions).

What is a systematic review?

A systematic review (or overview) is:

'a rigorous summary of all the research evidence that relates to a specific question; the question may be one of causation, diagnosis, or prognosis but more frequently involves the effectiveness of an intervention.'

(Ciliska et al. *2001)*

A reviewer uses a systematic process to locate, appraise and pool (or synthesize) all relevant and methodologically sound scientific studies in a particular area. This is useful because questions about the prevention or treatment of disease may be addressed by more than one trial. The statistical combination of the result of more than one study is a *meta-analysis*. You will come across systematic reviews both with and without meta-analyses.

Systematic reviews differ from 'traditional' literature reviews in that they are developed more systematically and rigorously. Systematic reviewers will search for all relevant published and unpublished articles on the topic using predetermined criteria for study design and quality, patients, settings, interventions and outcomes. They will then appraise this research in a standardized way and be explicit about reasons for inclusion and exclusion in the review. If appropriate, they may statistically pool the results (meta-analysis). This is a far cry from including only those studies known to the writer and moves away from more opinion-driven decision-making to an evidence-based perspective which has rigorously attempted to overcome possible biases at all stages of the review process (Ciliska *et al.* 2001).

Where possible, clinical practice should be based on available systematic reviews. Basing clinical decisions on a single research study may be misleading because:

- individual studies may have inadequate sample sizes to detect clinically important differences between treatments
- the results of apparently similar studies may vary because of chance
- there are often subtle differences in the design of studies and the participants that may lead to different or even discrepant findings (Ciliska *et al.* 2001).

An example of a systematic review. In conducting a systematic review on the use of relaxation for the relief of chronic pain (Carroll and Seers 1998), the following process was followed:

- RCTs investigating the effectiveness of relaxation techniques in the management of chronic pain were sought by searching MEDLINE, PSYCHLIT, CINAHL, EMBASE and the Oxford Pain Relief Database
- nine studies met the pre-defined inclusion criteria and were critically appraised

- many of the studies had methodological shortcomings
- the review concluded that there was insufficient evidence to confirm that relaxation can reduce chronic pain.

How do you know if a systematic review is of good quality? It is important to assess the quality of systematic reviews because the proliferation of reviews in recent years has led to the following problems:

- the quality of reviews is variable
- two or more systematic reviews on the same topic may arrive at different conclusions (Hopayian 2001).

If you are reviewing whether a systematic review has been well-conducted you will need to ask (as a general rule) if:

- the review addressed a clear and focused question?
- the search for relevant studies was comprehensive and whether it is likely that important studies were missed? Reviews should provide details on the databases and other sources searched such as MED-LINE, EMBASE, CINAHL; handsearching of key journals; reference lists of relevant papers; and obtaining unpublished research by writing to key researchers/clinical experts in the area of interest
- the criteria used to select articles were appropriate and clearly stated? The authors should state their study eligibility criteria for inclusion in the review and the criteria used to assess the quality of the studies. If the 'raw material' is flawed, and is still included then the conclusions of systematic reviews cannot be trusted (Juni *et al.* 2001)
- the quality assessment and data extraction were reproducible? Having two or more appraisers and assessing the reliability (inter-rater reliability) of their judgements ensures that mistakes and biases are reduced
- variations in the studies were analysed and reported? For example, there may have been differences between the studies in terms of the types of patients included; the timing, duration and intensity of the interventions; or the outcome measures used (Ciliska *et al.* 2001)
- the reviewers' conclusions are supported by the data in the review? Have they looked at important details in the included studies that may affect the conclusions drawn? Were inferior studies included in the final summing up? Would you feel confident in applying these results to your everyday practice? In some systematic reviews the authors will sum up the implications for practice based on the results of the review. For example, Watts *et al.* (2001) sum up the practice implications for managing fever in children by stating first, that there is a lack of evidence to support the routine use of sponging in temperate climates/environments and second, that anti-pyretics should be used selectively and with caution.

In summary, systematic reviews:

- attempt to minimize bias
- provide a rigorous summary of all the available evidence about an intervention
- are useful because, if well-conducted, they provide a wealth of information that can be used in clinical practice. Often, systematic reviews are used as the basis of clinical guidelines, which often place information from research in a format that is easier to translate into clinical practice.

What are clinical guidelines?

There are many formal and scholarly definitions of guidelines, e.g.:

> 'guidelines are systematically developed statements designed to assist practitioner and patients on decisions about appropriate health care for specific clinical circumstances'.

> *(Field and Lohr 1992)*

Guidelines can be viewed as clinical recommendations for care of a particular condition that have been developed by a multi-professional team and based on the best available evidence and expert opinion where necessary (Box 7.6). The aim is to improve the quality of care delivered and patient outcomes (NICE 2001a).

Box 7.6 Differences between guidelines and systematic reviews

- Guidelines usually have a broader scope than systematic reviews, which tend to focus on an individual problem or intervention
- Guidelines may also provide a more coherent integrated view on how to manage a condition across primary and secondary settings
- Where possible, guidelines are based on the best possible research evidence (usually in the form of well-conducted and designed systematic reviews or RCTs). However, in many clinical areas, the necessary research evidence is inadequate and recommendations may have to be based on consensus expert clinical opinion (Rycroft-Malone 2001). Systematic reviews are based solely on the research evidence

Guidelines can provide evidence-based information on key clinical decisions relating to making a diagnosis; estimating prognosis; assessing relevant outcomes, including the benefits, risks and costs of alternative treatments; and finally, weighing up the various consequences of different treatment options (Eccles *et al.* 2001). Sometimes there will be a flow diagram or algorithm which identifies the key decisions and important outcomes for patients. However, guidelines will not address all the uncertainties of current clinical practice and should be seen as only one strategy that can help improve the quality of care that patients receive (Feder *et al.* 1999).

Guidelines are playing an increasing role in setting standards of care in the UK. Well-developed guidelines provide clear, concise statements of best practice that are based on critically evaluated primary research studies or systematic reviews. They are used to provide standards from which audit criteria can be derived. Although not legally binding (in the UK), they are frequently cited in courts of law as providing standards for practice which should be followed in the majority of cases, although good guidelines should also state exceptions to the case (Eccles *et al.* 2001).

The purpose of a clinical practice guideline is to:

- provide practitioners with an evidence-based guide to practice
- improve patient care
- assist practitioners and patients to make decisions about care and treatment.

Individual clinicians may use guidelines:

- to answer specific clinical questions arising out of their day-to-day practice

- as an information source for continuing professional education
- to provide an overview of the management of a condition or the use of an intervention
- as instruments for self-assessment or peer review to learn about gaps in performance (Feder *et al.* 1999).

How do I know if a guideline is good quality?

Most good quality guidelines in the UK will have been appraised and endorsed by a national body, such as NICE or the Scottish Intercollegiate Guidelines Network (SIGN). However, if appraised guidelines are not available from these sources, individuals should undertake their own appraisal because the quality of guideline development cannot otherwise be guaranteed. The best instrument to enable this process is the AGREE appraisal tool (http://www.agreecollaboration.org). Adopting recommendations from guidelines of questionable validity may lead to harm to patients or a waste of resources on ineffective interventions (Feder *et al.* 1999).

The guideline should provide evidence that there is variation in practice or evidence of harmful practice which requires the input of a guideline to correct it.

Guidelines are usually developed by multi-professional groups of health care practitioners, patients and researchers who should be listed in the guideline document. The role of the guideline development group is to formulate carefully worded recommendations based on the best available evidence that consider the relevance and likely clinical impact of the recommendations, as well as the quality of the study (or studies) on which the recommendations are based. Health benefits, side-effects and risks should be considered in formulating the recommendations.

Where possible, guideline recommendations should be based on a systematic review of all the good quality research on a particular topic or good quality RCTs. Importantly, only those guidelines that include a methods section within the guideline or supporting papers should be considered (Field and Lohr 1992). Guidelines which do not have a methods section may be invalid. Without such information it is impossible to appraise the validity of guidelines and have confidence in how recommendations were derived from the evidence.

Finally, the guideline should have audit review criteria derived from the guideline recommendations. These criteria can be used to measure your performance against best practice.

Example of a clinical guideline. The RCN clinical practice guideline for the management of patients with venous leg ulcers (RCN 1998b) is based on a systematic review (NHS Centre for Reviews and Dissemination 1997) and on other forms of evidence, including expert opinion. The recommendations on compression versus no compression and high versus low compression are based on a systematic review (Effective Health Care 1997), i.e. Level 1 evidence (see Table 7.1), while the evidence underpinning recommendations on four-layer versus other types of compression bandaging is based on two RCTs (Level II evidence). Other guideline areas, e.g. the assessment of leg ulcers and staff training and education, are based on Level III evidence (non-randomized studies).

In the case of staff training and education, RCTs were sought but none found. The research retrieved used inappropriate designs which also failed to describe in detail the education programme or baseline skill mix of the participants. However, given that surveys had shown wide variation in the clinical management of leg ulcers (cited in RCN 1998b), it was clear that education and training in leg ulcer care was urgently needed. Consequently, the ensuing recommendations were based on Level III evidence and augmented by expert consensus opinion.

OTHER HELP AND RESOURCES

There are many places where you can find evidence-based resources (Box 7.7). A number of journals and resources are specifically relevant to nurses, e.g. *Evidence-Based Nursing Journal* and the *Journal of Clinical Effectiveness in Nursing*. Many of these resources provide critical summaries of research studies.

Box 7.7 Overview of resources

- Agency for Health Care Policy and Research (AHCPR): full text versions of guidelines, quick reference guides, and versions for patients can be downloaded from http://text.nlm.nih.gov/ftrs/dbaccess/ahcpr or ordered from the AHCPR. http://www.ahcpr.gov/cgi-bin/gilssrch.pl
- AGREE Collaboration: provides a checklist for appraisal of guidelines http://www.agreecollaboration.org
- Bandolier: monthly printed bulletin published by Oxford & Anglia NHS Region, containing summaries and bullet points on treatment interventions. http://www.jr2.ox.ac.uk/Bandolier
- Biome: high quality biomedical and health-related internet resources: a search engine for quality-checked websites. http://www.biome.ac.uk/biome.html
- Centre for Reviews and Dissemination (CRD) databases: the NHS Centre for Reviews and Dissemination (CRD) at the University of York produces and disseminates reviews on effectiveness and cost-effectiveness of health care interventions and technologies from high quality health research, for decision-makers and health consumers. Also includes DARE (available on the Cochrane Library), systematic reviews, summaries of authors' conclusions and comments on practice implications; and NEED, a database of economic evaluations. http://www.york.ac.uk/inst/crd/welcome.htm
- Cochrane Library: includes the following databases:
  - Cochrane Database of Systematic Reviews (full-text Cochrane systematic reviews of health-care interventions)
  - Database of Abstracts and Reviews of Effectiveness (DARE) (abstracts of high quality systematic reviews)
  - Cochrane Controlled Trials Register (150,000+ controlled trials)
  - NHS Economic Evaluation Database
  - Health Technology Assessment Database

  Free access for NHS via National Electronic Library for Health. http://www.nelh.nhs.uk
- Current Controlled Trials: database contains over 10,000 records of RCTs provided from 20 different registers around the world and is one of the largest databases of ongoing RCTs on the Internet. http://controlled-trials.com
- Effective Health Care Bulletin: each issue addresses effectiveness of interventions on a major health care topic. http://www.york.ac.uk/inst/crd/dissem.htm
- Health Technology Assessment Programme: a national programme of research established and funded by the Department of Health's Research and Development Department to produce high quality research information on the costs, effectiveness and broader impact of health technologies. http://www.hta.nhsweb.nhs.uk/
- Joanna Briggs: an Australian website which publishes systematic reviews on a variety of nursing topics. http://www.joannabriggs.edu.au
- National Clearinghouse of Guidelines: a resource for evidence-based guidelines. http://www.guideline.gov/index.asp

- National Electronic Library for Health: a national web-based information library resource for the NHS and the UK public. It is currently being piloted and gives access to library resources including:
  - The Cochrane Library
  - clinical evidence
  - a database of full versions of clinical guidelines: http://www.nelh.nhs.uk/guidelines_databases.asp press, website and book reviews

  http://www.nhs.uk/nelh
- National Institute of Clinical Excellence (NICE): information on NICE-commissioned clinical practice guidelines that are currently being developed in the UK. http://www.nice.org.uk/nice-web/
- National Research Register: ongoing and completed research projects. http://www.update-software.com/National/
- Netting the Evidence: provides links to evidence-based links on the internet. http://www.shef.ac.uk/~scharr/ir/netting/
- PubMed: this is a free version along with MEDLINE available over the web. You can find numerous articles relating to medicine, nursing, midwifery, allied health, health management, health research via this site. http://www.ncbi.nlm.nih.gov/PubMed/
- Scottish Intercollegiate Guidelines Network: full text versions of guidelines and quick reference guides. http://pc47.cee.hw.ac.uk/sign/home.htm
- TRIP (Turning Research Into Practice): a search engine that searches for links from a wide variety of evidence-based sources, including many of those listed above. http://www.tripdatabase.com
- Other evidence publications which are useful to nursing include: *Evidence-Based Nursing*; *Evidence-Based Medicine*; *Evidence-Based Mental Health* all of which provide critically appraised summaries of research studies

The material presented here is a guide and would be fruitfully expanded by undertaking a critical appraisal skills course or consulting some of the key texts in the reference list and trying out some of the websites listed above. It is also worthwhile making contact with a good health care librarian who is aware of and can help access the evidence-based databases.

SUMMARY

The necessary foundation steps for evidence-based practice include formulating the question, critical appraisal issues and understanding the main sources of evidence.

APPLYING EVIDENCE IN CLINICAL PRACTICE

As outlined earlier, the application of research findings in practice is not necessarily straightforward. In the past, research findings were often passively disseminated in various ways, including journals, continuing professional education development and conferences, and there was an expectation that they would automatically be used in practice (Lomas 1993).

It is, however, now recognized that even the clearest research findings are not necessarily used in health care practice (Lomas 1993; Haines and Jones 1994; Bero *et al.* 1998). There are many examples of a time-lag between the dissemination of new research evidence and its use, and there are many reasons for this. As specified earlier, Hunt (1981) found that research is not always known about. There is an issue of ensuring that research is both available and placed in a format that is understandable and attractive to busy clinicians. Clinical guidelines are often useful, as the searching and appraisal work has been done for you. However, it must be recognized that clinical guidelines and systematic reviews do not always exist and that many clinical areas may be under-researched.

One of the major reasons that research findings are not used in practice, is that this would often involve *change*, and in many health care settings there may be a number of barriers to change, at an individual clinician level or a wider organizational level. Before addressing how you can go about applying research findings, it is worth giving an overview of some of the potential barriers at these different levels.

REFLECTION POINT
Think about the local barriers that you may have encountered or are likely to encounter when implementing a new clinical guideline. Make a list of these and consider ways of overcoming them.

INDIVIDUAL ASPECTS OF CHANGE

At an individual level, implementing research may involve changing the habits of a lifetime, rethinking ways of working or having to gain new clinical skills. Research has shown that individual clinicians often do not change their practice because:

- practice based on habit and ritual can be hard to change
- there may be competing expert opinion from senior clinicians. If it is the norm to practise in a certain way, then attempts at change can take time
- there is inadequate support for personal and professional development, e.g. having the opportunity to learn about and critically appraise research (Veeramah 1995; McSherry 1997)
- some practitioners see tools such as clinical guidelines as prescriptive, and as such, a threat to their clinical autonomy and to patient choice
- some practitioners may have experienced an adverse event with a certain procedure or drug and may therefore be unwilling to try it again, despite its evidence base. There may also be fears of litigation, especially if there have been previous adverse events
- some practitioners may lack the clinical skills to change practice and may not have access to the appropriate training
- there may be little time to learn and adopt new practices.

ORGANIZATIONAL ASPECTS OF CHANGE

Changes at an organizational level are often required in order to implement research findings. Implementing pain management guidelines may require new forms of documentation and, as shown in the PACE project example given below, changing practice in relation to venous leg ulcer care involved purchasing new Doppler equipment and setting up training sessions across the NHS trust.

Again, many research studies have outlined the barriers to research utilization at an organizational level, including:

- inadequate resource allocation
- too many competing initiatives
- evidence-based practice may be a low management priority (Humphris and Littlejohns 1996). In trying to implement guidelines, a process of consultation and local adaptation, which approves and endorses a certain approach, can be fundamental to the recommendations being adopted
- there may be economic disincentives to making changes, e.g. an effective drug may be more expensive
- pharmaceutical marketing can be powerful and may be contrary to research findings (Mittman *et al.* 1992; Clinical Resource and Audit Group 1993; Lomas 1993)
- there may be little multi-professional working, which has been shown to enable the implementation of change (Baggs *et al.* 1992; Johns 1992).

CONSIDERATIONS IN APPLYING RESEARCH IN CLINICAL PRACTICE

While these factors may seem overwhelming, they are not always present. Given that each context and the evidence being implemented will differ, it is essential that any plan to implement changes in practice relates to the *local context* and also to the *individual patient* being treated.

Is the evidence useful in treating my patients?

In applying the knowledge you have gained, it is important to examine whether the treatment is applicable to your patients. Regardless of whether you have retrieved a guideline, systematic review or individual study to help answer your clinical dilemma, some of the questions you should ask are given below.

Is the evidence applicable to my patients? Deciding whether the evidence is applicable to an individual patient requires knowledge about both the study and the patient. Unless the study was done on a very narrowly defined group of patients with an extensive list of exclusion criteria, the results should be generalizable to your patients and clinical setting (McAlister 2001). You will need to question whether there are reasons why the results would *not* be applicable to your patient (Greenhalgh 1997). Look for information in the study about the subject characteristics (age, sex, ethnicity, co-morbidity). Does your patient resemble those who were enrolled in the study? Greenhalgh (1997) cautions that many trials exclude patients with co-existing illness, those who do not speak English and those taking other medication.

Are the results clinically important? It is worth remembering that just because a study reports the effect of a treatment to be *statistically* significant, it does not mean that the result is *clinically* important (Cullum 2001). Ideally, recommendations made in clinical practice guidelines will be based on effects that are both highly statistically significant and clinically important. How to take into account the size of the treatment effect and whether the estimate of the treatment effect is precise is described in further detail in Cullum (2001) and DiCenso (2001).

Is the practice/intervention acceptable to the patient(s)? When critically evaluating the evidence it is important to pay particular attention to the process of care being described. Even if a study demonstrates strong benefits look for descriptions of the process and reported side-effects, as these may be unacceptable to patients. Because risks and harm associated with the treatment might outweigh the benefits, the researchers should ideally have reported both positive (improvements in health status) and any negative (mortality and morbidity rates) or unintended effects. However, this is often not done and many studies still do not collect data on patients' direct experience of a treatment and improvements/reductions in quality of life.

Although there may be a clear rationale for a certain course of treatment, patients may not always agree with it. For example, in a national audit on the management of leg ulcers, many nurses reported that while they had used three- or four-layer bandaging on patients, the patients took it off after a few days as it was uncomfortable, itchy or they could not bathe properly (RCN 2000b). This meant that the treatment was not effective. Patient education can play a key role in explaining why a certain treatment is being used and should be a central part of care. However, there may be situations where patients have their own reasons for refusing treatment and discussing this with them is essential to good care.

While these questions are fundamental to evidence-based practice, they assume that there are no further barriers to changing practice. It may be that as an individual you have answered all of these questions, but do not have the right equipment or training (for example) to continue the treatment. Often in practice settings, team-based or organizational initiatives are set up to improve certain areas of practice and as a new nurse you will be involved in them. Often such initiatives are aimed at overcoming both the individual and organizational barriers to change.

CHANGING PRACTICE: APPROACHES TO IMPLEMENTATION

So what do we know about what works? As highlighted above, changing practice involves more than passively sending out information. It is clear that people change more readily when they are involved in a process of change and are given some ownership of the process (Johns 1992; Duff *et al.* 1996). A study by Grimshaw and Russell (1993) found that nationally developed guidelines were more readily implemented when they had been adapted for local use, thereby giving clinicians a chance to assess and 'own' them. Implementation also works best when multiple approaches are used which are specific to the needs of the context (Wensing and Grol 1994). Some of these approaches include interactive education, social influence, facilitation, audit, sanctions, reminders, marketing and reminders (Clinical Guidelines Education Team 2001).

Changing leg ulcer management

The following is an example of a project which aimed to change practice across one trust. The organization of the process, the results and the lessons learnt in trying to achieve far reaching change are outlined.

PACE (Promoting Action on Clinical Effectiveness) was a 2-year programme of change management and organizational development across 16 UK sites. The aim of the programme was to support local projects to demonstrate the effective implementation of evidence-based practice. Within West Berkshire, one of these projects was established to improve the effectiveness of leg ulcer care and, in particular, to reduce the duration, variation and cost of treating leg ulcers (Dunn *et al.* 1998).

Organization of the project. The project used a multi-professional team approach. A project advisory group was convened and a project nurse was appointed to raise the profile of the project and

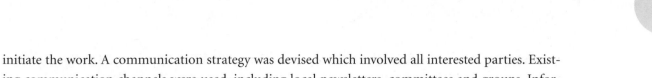

initiate the work. A communication strategy was devised which involved all interested parties. Existing communication channels were used, including local newsletters, committees and groups. Information bulletins about the progress of the project were also circulated.

The project plan included:

- clinical audit
- developing an assessment tool and protocol through a consensus process
- economic analysis
- education at three levels (specialist level, practitioner level through workshops and general awareness raising)
- patient involvement and education.

At the outset, the project group saw that to be successful it would need:

- a co-ordinated multi-professional approach (across acute and community sectors)
- use of high-compression bandaging
- the talents and expertise of a tissue viability group.

The immediate problems were seen as:

- resistance to change
- health service managers and GPs not investing in the Doppler equipment and bandaging system
- no standardized referral system to vascular surgeons
- limited communication and co-operation between hospital/community/provider units and commissioning agencies.

Results. The project ran for approximately 2 years. The clinical audit demonstrated that graduated compression was a clinically effective treatment for leg ulcers: 81% of leg ulcers had healed by more than 50%. The economic analysis showed that assessment and graduated compression could halve the treatment costs of leg ulcer care. Gaining patients' views and providing patient education was also an intrinsic part of the project.

Lessons learnt. The key lessons highlighted by the project were:

- keep on communicating. In this project they used existing channels of communication, e.g. newsletters
- there is a need for evidence-based management, such as involving budget holders who can sanction the purchase of supplies
- it is important therefore to lock into organizational priorities and develop co-operative working practices with all health care staff involved in the care of leg ulcer patients through networking
- ensure that meetings are fixed for the most likely times that health care providers can attend
- education needs to focus on experiential learning with ongoing input from a respected colleague. There is also a need for local champions of evidence-based leg ulcer care
- it is essential to keep reinforcing the change, e.g. by setting up a specialist nurse network and making available a video of leg ulcer management (Dunn *et al.* 1998).

RESOURCES FOR GUIDANCE ON IMPLEMENTATION

Duff *et al.* (2000) have developed a six-step guide which can be used as a framework for implementing evidence in practice (Box 7.8). It has been developed alongside certain guidelines including those for venous leg ulcer and pain management in children. Copies can be obtained from RCN Publishing.

Box 7.8 Six-step framework to implementing evidence in practice (Duff *et al.* 2000)

Step 1: Deciding who will lead the work
Step 2: Determining where you are now (both the context and in clinical practice through clinical audit)
Step 3: Preparing to implement the guideline
Step 4: Identifying techniques to assist
Step 5: Devising an action plan
Step 6: Evaluating your progress

Part of this approach involves clinical audit, which is about measuring and evaluating current practice within your health care setting, making the necessary improvements and then re-measuring. A comprehensive resource for conducting clinical audit is *The Clinical Audit Handbook: Improving the Quality of Care* (Morrell and Harvey 2000), which outlines how to use the clinical audit cycle to improve practice, and gives useful overviews of how to conduct an audit and some approaches to changing practice.

A further resource is a pack which has been developed and edited by the Clinical Guidelines Education Team (2001) on implementing clinical guidelines. The resource takes you through five main modules which identify:

- ways to choose guidelines
- how to promote and facilitate the uptake of guidelines in practice
- how to involve patients in the process
- how to devise an implementation plan
- how to assess the impact the implementation has had on service delivery.

The pack is designed to be suitable for individual study and also to be worked through with members of a clinical team, enabled by a facilitator.

SUMMARY

- Implementing research may require changes at an individual level but also involvement in team-based and organizational initiatives.
- Research findings are not always automatically used, even if they are disseminated to the relevant practitioners. There are many reasons for this, which include lack of knowledge and skills at an individual level and organizational constraints.
- It is well recognized that passive approaches to change are ineffective and that effective implementation relies on using a range of approaches, including continuing education, the use of change agents, and audit and feedback.

CONCLUSION

This chapter gave an overview of evidence-based practice and outlined some of the issues and limitations in practising in an evidence-based way, as well as some of the tools and techniques you will need.

The use of high-quality research has many advantages for improving nursing practice, patient satisfaction and outcomes. If research is available and appropriately applied it has the potential to:

- improve clinical effectiveness for patients
- make decision-making more transparent, thereby giving greater information to patients as well as health care professionals
- empower clinicians to make informed decisions and question practice
- enable patients to use knowledge to become more informed and involved in decisions about their care
- enable better use of resources by practitioners and purchasers by adopting more effective treatment, which can lead to better outcomes for patients.

The challenge is in knowing how to understand and appraise research studies, systematic review and clinical guidelines, and how best to apply research evidence to individual patients. Evidence-based practice requires practitioners to be open to new ideas and better ways to practice. It also requires that practitioners continually question and assess the basis of practice and know how to find, appraise and use available research. Practising in an evidence-based way requires a lifelong learning approach to training and skill development (including ongoing clinical updating, supervision, critical appraisal skills, change management, etc.). Ultimately, such an approach will help to ensure that patients are receiving nursing care based on the best available evidence.

CHAPTER

8

CARE DELIVERY: THE NEEDS OF CHILDREN

Cathy Lawrence, Faith Gibson and Judy Zur

INTRODUCTION

This chapter aims to familiarize students with the notion of competencies in children's nursing. Competency-based practice has become a fundamental aspect of care delivery in child health settings for both student and registered nurses. In terms of nursing education, a competency-based framework has been developed by the UKCC (1999a) and implemented at national level. This framework is used to structure this chapter as it reflects the recent changes in nursing education. The first part of the chapter will briefly address three key questions: What is competency-based practice? How were the competencies developed for children's nursing? Is children's nursing different?

The remainder of this chapter explores all five domains in children's nursing, providing an explanation of the importance of the identified competency in children's nursing and the outcomes to be achieved. The aim is for you to familiarize yourself with the competencies and, by reading the scenarios, which are explicit examples from children's nursing practice, you are encouraged to make the link between the reality of practice and the competency statement and outcomes. Pseudonyms are used throughout to protect the children's confidentiality (NMC 2002a). You will also be challenged to reflect upon your experiences caring for children and families in a variety of settings and to relate those experiences to the achievement of the competencies in children's nursing. Suggested reading is given to help you complete the reflection point questions in an informed way.

8

WHAT IS COMPETENCY-BASED PRACTICE?

 Competency-based practice is a relatively new concept within pre-registration nursing courses and, although competence is a term that has been widely used within nursing for a long time, the notion of competence is now central to the new pre-registration programmes as set out in *Fitness for Practice* (UKCC Commission for Nursing and Midwifery Education 1999b). Understandably, the general public expects that a qualified professional, from whatever area of work, will be competent in carrying out normal, professional tasks and duties (Eraut 1994; Chapter 2). The *Code of professional conduct* (NMC 2002a) makes explicit the need for individual practitioners to maintain and improve professional knowledge and competence. Additionally, there is a requirement to acknowledge any limitations in knowledge and competence and to decline to perform duties unless able to perform them in a safe and skilled manner. Therefore, the aim of competency-based practice in pre-registration nursing is the achievement, by the student on qualification, of the:

'skills and ability to practise safely and effectively without the need for direct supervision'.

(UKCC 1999c, p35)

HOW WERE THE COMPETENCIES DEVELOPED FOR CHILDREN'S NURSING?

The latest 3-year pre-registration programme consists of a 1-year foundation programme, which is assessed using outcomes, and a 2-year branch programme assessed using generic United Kingdom Central Council for Nursing, Midwifery and Health Visiting (UKCC) competencies. In the development phase of the new programme, it was recognized early on that the generic UKCC competencies required adaptation to reflect a child and family focus. Children are different from adults physiologically, emotionally and cognitively, and within our society they have different rights and legal status in comparison to adults (Doyle and Maslin-Prothero 1999). It can be argued, therefore, that children's needs are different and if these needs are to be met, the education of children's nurses must specifically focus upon them achieving the core skills and competencies which will meet the needs of the child and family (NBS 2000).

A project was established in anticipation of the new programme to develop clinical competencies for the child branch. Using nominal group techniques and expert panels that involved practitioners in children's nursing, the UKCC competencies have been made relevant to this specific branch. This has resulted in clinically relevant outcomes in the four domains of practice, as well as the inclusion of a fifth domain, considered by participants in the project to be essential to capture the essence of children's nursing.

IS CHILDREN'S NURSING DIFFERENT?

The specialized training for nurses caring for children has been recognized since 1888 (Bradley 1999), and the attributes required by nursing students in 1888, e.g. having acute observational skills and being able to communicate and play with children, are comparable with the competencies required by the UKCC in 1999. The continued existence of the child branch is a testimony to the fact that nurses caring for children require a different educational preparation. The routes leading to a different registration would imply that the competencies required to be entered on to the register should be different for a children's nurse when compared with other nurses: if the sphere of practice (caring for children) and the educational preparation (child branch) are different, then the result must be different in terms of outcomes and competencies. In reality this has not been the case until now. Linked to this there is an assumption that there are specific qualities, knowledge, skills and attitudes in nurses who care for children.

The development of clinical competencies in the new pre-registration programme has provided an opportunity to celebrate what is different in children's nursing. Rather than simply adding this client group to every generic competency to make them specific to the care of children, the identification of specific child health focused outcomes has helped to produce a clinical assessment document that is relevant and appropriate to assess the real world of children's nursing practice.

DOMAIN 1: PROFESSIONAL/ETHICAL PRACTICE

COMPETENCY STATEMENT 1.1

- Manage self, one's practice and that of others, in accordance with the NMC *Code of professional conduct*, recognizing own abilities and limitations (see Box 8.1 for relevant outcome criteria).

Box 8.1 Outcome criteria for competency statement 1.1

- Practice in accordance with the NMC *Code of professional conduct*
- Use professional standards of practice to assess your performance
- Identify when nursing care requires expertise beyond your own current scope of competence and consult with a registered nurse
- Consult with other health care professionals when individual or group needs fall outside the scope of your nursing practice
- Identify unsafe practice and respond appropriately to ensure a safe outcome
- Manage the delivery of care services within your sphere of accountability

The responsibility and accountability of the nurse is central to their professional practice. In terms of children's nursing, the *Code of professional conduct* (NMC 2002a) has to be applied to the context of caring for the child and family. Safety is a key concept that underpins the practice of children's nurses. Respecting the confidentiality of the child and family is crucial to the professional relationship that is built up between a children's nurse and the family.

Scenario I arrived on duty one morning and found that there were two staff nurses off sick and I was the most senior member of staff on duty. However, even as a third-year student nurse, I felt that it would be unsafe to take charge of the ward but the agency night nurse, who had been in charge of the night shift, was unwilling to stay. By applying my knowledge of accountability I contacted the senior nurse immediately and a staff nurse from another ward was sent to take charge. However, she did not know any of the children and families and I acted in a responsible manner by assisting her throughout the day as I was familiar with the care of each child and family. I also supervised a first-year student nurse so as to ensure a safe standard of practice was maintained. The staff nurse and I discussed the ward staffing problems with the doctors and they agreed to cancel admissions to the ward that day, thus demonstrating a safe collaborative approach had been taken by all the health professionals involved.

REFLECTION POINT

Reflect on your practice and consider if you have felt that on occasion you were asked to perform a task that was beyond your capability. This may have been a 'simple' task such as taking a blood pressure or recording fluids on a chart. Did you feel unsafe? Were you able to voice your concerns to the supervising nurse? Can you relate your experiences to the *Code of professional conduct?*

[Suggested reading: UKCC (1996a, 1988c); DoH (2001d); NMC (2002a, p3 and 7).]

COMPETENCY STATEMENT 1.2

- Practise in accordance with an ethical and legal framework that ensures the primacy of patient or client interest and well-being and respects confidentiality (see Box 8.2 for relevant outcome criteria).

Box 8.2 Outcome criteria for competency statement 1.2

- Demonstrate knowledge of legislation relevant to nursing practice
- Ensure confidentiality and security of information acquired in a professional capacity
- Demonstrate knowledge of contemporary ethical issues impacting on nursing, e.g. informed consent, resuscitation
- Demonstrate awareness of the complexities arising from ethical and legal dilemmas
- Uphold the primacy of the patient's or client's interests and well-being at all times

---

Ethical and legal principles are the foundations on which children's nursing practice is based. Children's nurses are legally accountable since the implementation of the Children Act (1989) and, therefore, all children's nurses need to be familiar with this Act and how it applies to the practice area. Furthermore, children are considered to be a vulnerable group and thus open to exploitation and abuse. Ethical principles require the children's nurse to uphold the rights of the child and to act as their advocate when necessary. Children's nurses must also apply ethical principles when supporting parents.

Scenario I was allocated to care for a baby whose mother was suspected of causing a physical non-accidental injury. I was aware of my professional role in terms of child protection by ensuring that I always stayed in the room with the mother when she visited her child and accurately documenting her activities during those visits. I read the hospital trust's policy on child protection and contacted the nurse specialist for child protection who was able to give me support and advice. I tried to maintain a professional and non-judgemental relationship with the mother but I found this difficult at times due to the realization that the trust between a nurse and parent is undermined by a child protection issue. I liaised with the social worker and organized a time when she could come and see the mother.

REFLECTION POINT

Reflecting on your experience, can you identify an incident from practice when you used your ethical knowledge? This may have involved upholding the rights of a parent who felt ill-informed regarding a medical or nursing decision.

Consider how 'routine' procedures, such as taking a blood sample from a child, relate to the issue of informed consent.

[Suggested reading: Dimond (1996, p1–28); DoH (1989a); Alderson (2000); Charles-Edwards (2001).]

COMPETENCY STATEMENT 1.3

- Practise in a fair and anti-discriminatory way, acknowledging the difference in beliefs and cultural practices of individuals or groups (see Box 8.3 for relevant outcome criteria).

Box 8.3 Outcome criteria for competency statement 1.3

- Maintain, promote and represent the rights of individuals or groups in the health care setting
- Act to ensure that the rights of individuals and groups are not compromised
- Respect the values, customs and beliefs of individuals and groups
- Provide care that demonstrates sensitivity to clients' diversity

The UK is a multi-cultural society where children's nurses care for children and families from a variety of ethnic and cultural groups. Thus, they need to be familiar with the cultural practices and religious beliefs of the community in which they practise. The children's nurse needs to use a non-judgemental approach to care and make efforts to understand cultures that are different from their own. Decision-making, when working with children and families, should be seen to reflect fairness and should not discriminate against vulnerable or minority individuals or groups.

Scenario While I was on my community practice placement with a community children's nurse (CCN) we visited a 7-year-old boy called Billy who had asthma. He was from a travelling family and lived in a council flat with basic sanitary conditions. The flat was very dirty and smelt strongly of urine and body odour, and throughout our visit the extended family was present. The CCN wanted to do some health promotion with Billy's main carers (mother and grandmother), so she asked me to try and develop a relationship with Billy.

I was rather anxious as to how I was going to proceed and decided to play with Billy and, by talking to him, try and understand how he lived. He told me that he did not go to school on a regular basis and felt that it was not important to be able to read or write. He told me about his family and friends and how much he liked living with all his relatives. He explained that in the summer the family 'went on the road' and gradually some of the extended family members joined in the conversation. I began to understand the importance of the extended family to Billy and how suspicious they were of authoritative figures such as us. I felt that by the end of the visit I had gained the family's trust and had begun to understand the caring beliefs of travelling families.

REFLECTION POINT

Can you identify a family that you have cared for that had a different cultural or religious background from your own? How did you feel when you were asked to care for this family? How did you develop non-discriminatory attitudes towards the family?

[Suggested reading: Richardson (1993); Dimond (1996, p35–111); Valentine and Smith (2000); Spires (2002).]

SUMMARY

- Children's nurses must always practice in accordance with the *Code of professional conduct* (NMC 2002a) and provide a safe and secure environment for children and families.
- Every nurse should be aware of their own knowledge and abilities and not practice beyond their current scope of competence.
- Children's nursing practice must be underpinned by legal and ethical principles which uphold and promote children's rights in partnership with the family.
- The same care should be delivered to all children and families regardless of their ethnic origin and the differing beliefs in relation to health, illness, diet and religion must be respected.

DOMAIN 2: CARE DELIVERY

COMPETENCY STATEMENT 2.1

- Engage in, develop and disengage from therapeutic relationships through the use of appropriate communication and interpersonal skills (see Box 8.4 for relevant outcome criteria).

Box 8.4 Outcome criteria for competency statement 2.1

- Make effective use of a range of interpersonal and communication techniques
- Ensure that verbal and non-verbal communication is compatible and appropriate, taking account of individuals/groups, gender, language, values, culture and sensory differences
- Maintain professional caring relationships that focus on meeting the patient's/client's needs
- Understand the boundaries of the professional caring relationship and how relationships are formed and maintained

The importance of effective therapeutic communication with children and families cannot be underestimated within the process of quality nursing; achievement of this competency is at the centre of every relationship the children's nurse will engage in. To communicate effectively within a relationship with children and families requires the nurse to use conversation as a goal-directed tool which is related to the health and well-being of the child. The children's nurse must use age-directed, culturally-specific language which matches the language of the child and family.

Creating a therapeutic relationship with children and their families is not always easy and requires the student to develop effective verbal and non-verbal communication skills and techniques, as well as a range of interpersonal skills. It is important to give children time; to speak to them clearly and honestly using simple language and a quiet, unhurried and confident voice; and to use transitional objects when, and if, appropriate to convey the message effectively. When communicating with families it is important to encourage them to talk and for you to listen actively, to be empathetic and to convey acceptance of the uniqueness of each family unit.

> **Scenario** On a previous shift I admitted a 4-year-old Asian girl called Saira, with her mother, for minor surgery. Saira's mother said that her English was not very good but that she did not need an interpreter. As I talked to Saira's mother I used open-ended questions and lay vocabulary which she seemed to understand. I actively listened to her and showed interest through trying to maintain eye contact. However, Saira's mother rarely looked at me when talking which I respected as being culturally-specific behaviour. From her facial expressions I could see that she was anxious and sometimes found it difficult to express herself but I tried to use silence positively to give her time.
>
> Throughout the shift I continued to build upon my relationship with Saira and her mother. Because she was only 4, Saira was initially very wary of me while she evaluated me as a stranger, but I gave her time and waited until she trusted me and then, using play with her favourite dolly, I helped to prepare her for surgery. I felt it was important that they had time together as a family, especially when her father visited.

REFLECTION POINT

From your experiences, identify your learning related to:

- greeting the child and family on admission
- communicating with a frightened child
- dealing with an aggressive/rude parent
- avoiding the blocks to communication.

Consider how differently you use your communication and interpersonal skills with the different age groups, e.g. an infant, a toddler, a school-aged child and an adolescent.

Consider the non-verbal channels of communication such as touch, proxemics, posture, kinesics, facial expression and gaze, and think of examples from your practice where the culture of the child and family has positively or negatively affected your ability to communicate using these channels.

[Suggested reading: Moules and Ramsay (1998, p272–9); Wong *et al.* (1999, p200–14); Betts (2002).]

COMPETENCY STATEMENT 2.2

- Create and utilize opportunities to promote the health and well-being of patients or clients and groups (see Box 8.5 for related outcome criteria).

Box 8.5 Outcome criteria for competency statement 2.2

- Consult with patients/clients, relevant groups and significant others to identify the whole range of needs for your patients' health and well-being

- Provide relevant and current health, welfare and economic information to patients/clients, relevant groups and significant others in a form which enhances their knowledge and acknowledges individual preference
- Provide support/education in the development/maintenance of appropriate life skills and independent living skills
- Demonstrate an understanding of the principles of education, empowerment and social inclusion

A healthy child is not simply a child who does not have an injury or a disease, but a child who is enabled to develop optimally and achieve a state of physical, mental and social well-being. As a dependent, a child is reliant on parents or carers to provide a safe environment in which they can flourish, which includes accessing the available health services and utilizing welfare and economic information appropriately. Until children become self-caring and independent, adults mediate for them between them and their environment.

As a teacher, supporter and referrer, children's nurses can promote the health of the child by focusing on health and well-being alongside clinical care. The nurse is in an ideal situation to use health education, in partnership with the child and family, as a tool to achieve health or illness-related learning. This may aim to improve knowledge and understanding, e.g. why the child's adherance with a specific diet is essential, or to facilitate the acquisition of an essential skill, e.g. suctioning a tracheostomy tube or nasogastric tube feeding.

Scenario During my community experience I was allocated to a day nursery which admitted children from 6 months to 5 years of age. While there I involved myself with learning how the health and well-being of this age group was promoted by the staff. The immunization programme was addressed with the parents and a record of each of the child's immunizations was recorded; if the child had not been immunized, the dangers of this were discussed with the family and appropriate resources and leaflets were provided.

The children were taught to wash their hands as soon as they were physically able to do so. They were taught that dirty hands had germs on them and that they had to wash their hands when they had been playing outside, before and after they had their meals and after going to the toilet. They were supervised doing this so that they were protected from the hot water. In the oldest group, the children used play to learn about healthy eating and they had cooking and baking sessions to prepare some of the food. This enabled them to learn which foods were 'healthy' and which they could eat a lot of, and others which they could only eat some of.

REFLECTION POINT

Reflect on your experiences at school and make a list of the topics of health education that you were taught. Consider this list and think about how you did/could have promoted the health of the children and families you were recently caring for in relation to these topics.

How would you increase a child or young person's ability to make choices about the things which affect their health?

A young mother cannot decide whether to breast or bottle-feed her firstborn pre-term infant. What advice would you give?

[Suggested reading: Naidoo and Wills (1994); Sriven and Orme (1996); Moules and Ramsay (1998, p167–89); DoH (2001c, p16–19).]

COMPETENCY STATEMENT 2.3

- Undertake and document a comprehensive, systematic and accurate nursing assessment of the physical, psychological, social and spiritual needs of patients/clients/communities (see Box 8.6 for relevant outcome criteria).

Box 8.6 Outcome criteria for competency statement 2.3

- Select valid and reliable assessment tools for the required purpose
- Systematically collect data regarding the health and functional status of individuals/communities through interview, interaction, observation and measurement
- Analyse, interpret, record and communicate data accurately to inform nursing care and take appropriate action

The assessment of a child is an ongoing process which commences when the child and family first require nursing care and support, and continues throughout the time the child is receiving care, whether in hospital or the community, until they are discharged (see Chapter 6). The data to be collected is directed by an assessment tool which is underpinned by the dominating concepts of the model, framework or pathway which is used in that particular setting (e.g. Casey 1988; Hutchfield 1999). Whichever assessment tool is used, the collection of information is directed towards identifying the health and well-being of the child through identifying their needs and problems.

Essentially, the assessment stage is fundamental to the planning of holistic, quality care and to assess a child effectively the children's nurse requires many skills. To collect information they require a sound knowledge base, effective interpersonal and interviewing skills, and skills of observation and measurement; to plan the care they need to have the ability to interpret the results accurately.

Scenario During a shift I admitted an 8-year-old boy called James who had suspected appendicitis. He was accompanied by both his mother and father. Using the ward assessment tool, which was formulated and underpinned by the Partnership model, I assessed James's physical, psychological, social and spiritual needs. The verbal information I collected was mainly from his anxious parents because James was very upset and in a lot of pain. I observed James's behaviour and non-verbal communication and measured his vital signs and urinalysis. I assessed his pain as being quite severe, because he looked pale and shocked, was guarding his abdomen and using a self-report pain assessment tool [Wong/Baker Faces Scale (Wong and Baker 1988)] he assessed his rating to be 8. He was being extremely brave but was very anxious and needed and received comfort from his parents.

When I felt I had collected all the essential information, I documented it on the appropriate forms and charts and discussed his plan with my supervisor. As the shift progressed I continued to observe and monitor James closely as I delivered his pre-operative care.

REFLECTION POINT

Explore the different models, frameworks, pathways you have used in practice and compare the assessment tool in each case.

From your experiences to date, consider how you welcome and greet the child and family when you first meet at the admission assessment, in order to provide a reassuring and secure environment.

List the other assessment tools (e.g. pain assessment tool) you have used for observation and measurement during the assessment of the child. Do you feel this improved the quality of your assessment data?

[Suggested reading: Casey (1995); Moules and Ramsay (1998, p596–618); Hutchfield (1999); Wong *et al.* (1999, p1148–59); Downer (2002).]

COMPETENCY STATEMENT 2.4

- Formulate and document a plan of nursing care, where possible in partnership with patients/clients/carer(s)/significant others within a framework of informed consent (see Box 8.7 for relevant outcome criteria).

Box 8.7 Outcome criteria for competency statement 2.4

- Establish priorities in collaboration with the patient/client and within the context of the multi-professional team and available resources for care/treatment, based on the assessment of an individual's or group's needs
- Formulate plans of care collaboratively with patients/clients and other members of the care network based on critical pathways and individual circumstances
- Analyse the complexity of formulating care plans within the principles of informed consent with due regard to issues that may undermine it
- Identify expected outcomes, including a time frame for achievement and/or review in consultation with patients/clients and others in the care network

Although different approaches may be taken to planning care for children, owing to the wide variety of settings in which children are cared for, care should be planned in partnership with the child (dependent on age) and the family. Whether care plans are computerized, pre-printed or hand written, collaboratively the nurse, child and family should plan individual, achievable, realistic, short- or long-term goals to enable the child to restore and maintain their optimal level of health and well-being.

The nurse is required to plan a variety of evidence-based actions in order to help and support the child to achieve their goals. Identifying appropriate actions should be undertaken in discussion with the child and family, in order to negotiate and consent to their involvement and participation in the provision of self-care/care and to promote and ensure the maintenance of the family unit. Planning appropriate, evidenced-based care can be a complex process, requiring a sound knowledge-base, and a student should undertake this in discussion with their supervisor.

Scenario During three concurrent 12-hour shifts I admitted and cared for a 2-year-old child with bronchiolitis and his resident mother. Following his admission assessment and identification of his needs and problems, David's mother and I planned and discussed his care together. The short-term goals of restoring David's usual breathing rate and oxygen requirements (Huband and Trigg 2000), as well as maintaining his optimal fluid requirements, were seen as a priority. His mother wanted to be involved as much as possible in providing care for David and agreed that initially she would continue to undertake all of his usual care, e.g. washing, toileting and comforting, as well as some basic nursing care, e.g. maintaining his position for optimal air entry. I kept her informed of the results of my observations and measurements and ensured that the doctors and physiotherapist informed her of David's progress. As she became more confident and less anxious, through teaching and support from me, she willingly undertook more of David's nursing care. Throughout the time I cared for them I continued to record and document David's progress accurately towards his identified goals and to update the care plans as required.

EXERCISE

Take a blank sheet of paper and formulate a hypothetical care plan (including problem statements, goal statements and list of actions) for one of the following children:

- 9-month-old infant admitted with acute diarrhoea
- 10-year-old boy admitted having an asthmatic attack
- 15-year-old girl admitted with an inflamed appendix.

List the difficulties/problems you have with care planning and seek advice from your mentor/supervisor/link tutor/personal tutor.

[Suggested reading: While (1991); Casey (1995); Dimond (1996, p51–66); Wong *et al.* (1999 p1325–6, p 1515–17, p1555); Huband and Trigg (2000); DoH (2001c).]

COMPETENCY STATEMENT 2.5

- Based on best available evidence, apply knowledge and an appropriate repertoire of skills indicative of safe nursing practice (see Box 8.8 for relevant outcome criteria).

Box 8.8 Outcome criteria for competency statement 2.5

- Identify and critically evaluate current interventions viewed as best practice in a range of settings
- Identify recent developments in research in practice and disseminate these to colleagues
- Ensure that current research knowledge is reflected in your own practice
- Apply a range of interventions indicative of safe nursing practice
- Identify current research in practice settings and explore your own possible contribution to this process
- Identify and discuss different forms of knowledge and methodologies applied to research
- Apply appropriately a range of skills in a number of areas, including self-management, communication, observation, technical intervention and problem solving
- Demonstrate safe application of the skills required to meet the needs of patients/clients within a range of settings

---

The primary goal of planning and delivering care for children and their families is to provide care that is underpinned by the best available evidence in the pursuit of safety and quality. Safe, quality care is dependent on best evidence and the introduction of the concept of clinical governance within the NHS is a mandate for children's nurses to access, understand, appreciate and use the best evidence in their practice.

To understand what is best evidence requires the ability to critically review evidence of all forms, e.g. primary research or clinical guidelines, appreciating the core value that best evidence is fundamental to the best interests of the child and family (see Chapter 7). Using the evidence appropriately requires a wide range and variety of skills which, once learnt, will enable the children's nurse not only to evaluate confidently and justify their own practice, but also to challenge the practice of others.

Scenario Through teaching by qualified staff and reading journal articles and ward protocols, I have learnt about evidenced-based nursing care for children with diabetes while on this placement. I have cared for several adolescents with diabetes and feel that I have been able to provide safe, quality care, based on the best available evidence. Under supervision I have been able to provide for the children's physical needs in relation to monitoring their blood sugar levels and the administration of insulin, meet their psychological needs in relation to information and adherance with treatment and help them, through discussion, cope with living with a chronic illness and their adolescent lifestyle. Using the available evidence I have been able to provide a sound rationale for the care I have given and been able to share this with colleagues.

REFLECTION POINT

Choose one aspect of care which you undertake on most shifts, e.g. tube feeding or giving parents and children information, and analyse and identify the evidence which supports your practice.

From your current placement choose one child and family and undertake a literature search on one new aspect of care which you have been involved in delivering to them and share your results with your colleagues.

[Suggested reading: Hamer and Collinson (1999); Le May (1999); Glasper and Ireland (2000).]

COMPETENCY STATEMENT 2.6

- Provide a rationale for the nursing care delivered that takes account of the social, cultural, spiritual, legal, political and economic influences (see Box 8.9 for relevant outcome criterion).

Box 8.9 Outcome criterion for competency statement 2.5

- Identify, collect and evaluate information to justify the effective utilization of resources to achieve planned outcomes of care

The provision of nursing care for children and families is a complex process and the decisions made must take a variety of influencing factors into account. Social, spiritual and cultural issues can create challenges in everyday practice, as can wider legal, political and economic forces, and when prescribing nursing care to meet the desired outcomes for the child and family a sound justification must be sought. Considering the scarcity and rationing of resources in the NHS today, a knowledgeable and thoughtful team approach should be taken in order to provide equity and fairness in the pursuit of successful outcomes of care.

Scenario Over the past few weeks on this placement I have been caring for an 18-month-old child who required tube feeding because he was unable to maintain an adequate oral intake. The mother was desperate to take the child home because she was a single mother, had another school-aged child and apart from being tube-fed there was no reason for the child to be hospitalized at this moment. Therefore, over the last week, with the help of the dietician, I have been able to teach Gavin's mother to pass a tube and tube feed him, for which she has shown her competence and is ready to go home. I contacted the community paediatric nurse who visited her in hospital, will order and provide the necessary resources for her at home and has arranged to visit her until she feels she can cope adequately. I have also contacted the GP.

REFLECTION POINT

Can you identify a situation in your community or hospital practice where decisions have been influenced by legal, political or economic forces?

On your current allocation ask your ward manager how the ward resources are managed in relation to staff, finances and equipment to enable the planned outcomes of care to be achieved.

Identify experiences from your practice where the provision of social, cultural or spiritual care for children and families has created a challenge for practitioners.

[Suggested reading: Williams (1995); DoH (1996); Dimond (1996, p101–5); Moules and Ramsay (1998, p679–82); Spires (2002).]

COMPETENCY STATEMENT 2.7

- Evaluate and document the outcomes of nursing and other interventions (see Box 8.10 for relevant outcome criteria).

Box 8.10 Outcome criteria for competency statement 2.7

- Review and monitor the progress of individuals or groups towards planned outcomes
- Revise expected outcomes, nursing interventions and priorities with respect to any change in an individual's condition, needs or other variations

As the last phase of the nursing process the aim of evaluation is to determine the effectiveness of care and to decide if the goals of nursing care have been achieved. Evaluating care is as essential as all the other phases of the nursing process and should be straightforward if all the other steps have been undertaken to the highest quality. Evaluation will enable the children's nurse either to determine the child's achievement of the goals of care or to provide them with the information required for re-assessing needs and revising the care plan. Through the continuous evaluation of the care delivered, the nurse will be able to predict that certain actions are more likely to be effective, based on experience and choice. A clearly written, accurate and unambiguous statement of the outcome of care must be documented appropriately.

Scenario While on this placement I cared for a 1-year-old boy called Ahmed who was admitted with a 2-day history of diarrhoea and vomiting. He was severely dehydrated, had a very sore bottom and was extremely miserable. The priority goals of care were to restore his hydration, retrieve the integrity of his anal skin and recover his normal, happy disposition. I delivered the prescribed actions listed in the care plan to meet the stated goals of care and, through observations, measurements and discussion with his mother, I evaluated the effectiveness of the care I had delivered and revised the care plans where appropriate, in discussion with my supervisor. I recorded my judgements of the value of the care delivered to Ahmed in relation to his predicted goals, informing the relevant team members of his progress.

REFLECTION POINT

Make a list of the sources of data which inform your evaluation of care.

From your experiences in caring for children, identify one aspect of care where you have learnt that there is more than one solution to a problem, e.g. pin site care, behavioural programmes.

When evaluating care for children who have undergone day care surgery, what would you say are the main criteria for discharge?

[Suggested reading: Campbell and Glasper (1995, p100–24); UKCC (1998c); Wong *et al.* (1999, p26–9); Downer (2001, p369–72, 386–9).]

COMPETENCY STATEMENT 2.8

- Demonstrate sound clinical judgement across a range of differing professional and care delivery contexts (see Box 8.11 for relevant outcome criteria).

Box 8.11 Outcome criteria for competency statement 2.8

- Use evidence-based knowledge from nursing and related disciplines to select and individualize nursing interventions
- Demonstrate the ability to transfer skills and knowledge to a variety of circumstances and settings
- Recognize the need to adapt and subsequently adapt nursing practice to meet varying and unpredictable circumstances
- Ensure the response does not compromise the nurse's duty of care to individuals or safety of the public

Achieving this competency is about demonstrating the ability to undertake a variety of roles, while being able to rationalize and justify safe, sound decisions. Caring for children and their families requires a wide knowledge base, ranging from physiology, child development and social care provision to the professional, ethical and legal issues which provide the basis on which decisions are made. Flexibility and adaptability are required to provide family-centred care, which upholds the best interests of the child and family and values the diversity of their beliefs and the contexts and circumstances where care is provided.

Scenario During this current placement I cared for a 12-year-old girl called Lisa who was undergoing treatment for leukaemia. She had been prescribed oral medication but hated it intensely and when I attempted to administer the drug on this occasion she refused to take it. She said she had had enough but on discussion she agreed she would take it if it could be given by another route. I was aware that she was old enough and mature enough to understand the implications of her treatment and also that it was in her best interests to have this medication. So I contacted the SHO who came to the ward and agreed to change the prescription. I feel that I fulfilled my duty of care while acting in Lisa's best interest.

EXERCISE

Make a list of the forms of consent you usually obtain from:

- a 3-year-old child
- a 10-year-old child

- a 15-year-old
- the parents.

All children and young people who are patients in hospital or in the community are owed a duty of care. What does this mean?

Can you think of any circumstances where you may feel that to promote family-centred care may not be in the child's best interests?

[Suggested reading: Dimond (1996, Chapters 6 and 13); Moules and Ramsay (1998, p651–68); Brykczynska (2000); Caulfield (2002).]

SUMMARY

- Effective interpersonal and communication skills are essential to initiate and maintain a professional caring relationship.
- Children's nurses have a key role in promoting health and they must be proactive in empowering children and families through information, support and education.
- The skills to undertake and document an accurate, reliable and holistic assessment are essential to identify the needs and problems of the child and family.
- The formulation of individual care plans/critical pathways should reflect collaboration and partnership with the child, parents and multi-disciplinary team, as should the evaluation of the care delivered.
- Research/evidence-based practice must be used to guide the delivery of up-to-date, adaptable and safe care for children and families.
- Justifying the utilization of scarce resources in the delivery of optimal care for children and families should be a priority.

DOMAIN 3: CARE MANAGEMENT

COMPETENCY STATEMENT 3.1

- Contribute to public protection by creating and maintaining a safe environment of care through the use of quality assurance and risk management strategies (see Box 8.12 for relevant outcome criteria).

Box 8.12 Outcome criteria for competency statement 3.1

- Understand and apply the principles of quality assurance to ensure the maintenance of a safe environment, physically and psychologically
- Identify environmental hazards (physical and psychological), eliminating and/or preventing them where possible
- Manage risk to provide care that best meets the needs and interests of the clients and the public

Quality assurance is now an essential aspect of nursing practice and for children's nurses its relation to safety has a particular relevance. Children are potentially exposed to more hazards within the hospital environment and community setting than adults due to their limited awareness of hazards and inability to protect themselves from harm. Policies and procedures are therefore written to protect the child and to guide safe nursing practice. Some knowledge of clinical governance is highly relevant to senior student nurses, as an understanding of how practice is managed safely within the community or hospital trust is crucial on registration.

Scenario During the course of the shift I assisted the staff nurse in the administration of an intramuscular injection to a child. I was aware of the hospital policy related to the role of students regarding the administration of drugs and the guidelines provided by the UKCC (2000b). We followed the hospital policy of checking that it was the correct drug, dose, timing, route and patient, and administered the drug appropriately. I had not seen an intramuscular injection administered before so I observed and assisted the staff nurse, and supported and comforted the child. Following the administration we signed the patient's prescription chart and I disposed of the needle and syringe safely (as stated in the ward manual), into a BioHazard sharps bin and then washed my hands. The staff nurse then discussed the risks of a needle-stick injury and how to report and document a critical incident.

REFLECTION POINT

Reflect on your own practice experience and identify a protocol or policy that has enabled you to practise safely.

Can you recall an incident during a clinical placement where you felt 'unsafe' practice had taken place? Try to explore why you felt it was unsafe and how risk management strategies may have improved quality assurance.

[Suggested reading: UKCC (1999c, 2000b); Valentine and Smith (2000); DoH (2001c); NMC (2002a).]

COMPETENCY STATEMENT 3.2

- Demonstrate knowledge of effective inter-professional working practices that respect and utilize the contributions of members of the health and social care team (see Box 8.13 for relevant outcome criteria).

Box 8.13 Outcome criteria for competency statement 3.2

- Establish and maintain collaborative working relationships with colleagues and members of the health and social care team and others
- Participate with other members of the health and social care team in decision-making concerning patients/clients
- Review and evaluate care with members of the health and social care team and others

Inter-professional care is a rapidly developing service within the arena of child care services and being able to work collaboratively is an essential skill for all children's nurses. Demonstrating an awareness of the various roles of the members of the health and social care teams, and valuing and respecting the knowledge and contribution of other professionals, is central to good nursing practice. Liaison skills are a prerequisite for all children's nurses on qualification.

> **Scenario** A 6-month-old infant called Jamie arrived on the ward from the A&E department with a suspected non-accidental injury. I admitted Jamie and gathered information from his mother about her health visitor and GP. The staff nurse in charge then suggested that I should contact the staff liaison health visitor, who liaises with the local community care teams, and the duty social worker who arranged to visit Jamie and his mother. On arrival the social worker asked the staff nurse and me to accompany her while she interviewed Jamie's mother. During the discussion the mother stated that she had been under stress and had unintentionally harmed Jamie. The social worker then explained to Jamie's mother what would happen and that the nurses would supervise her care of Jamie. The liaison health visitor contacted the family's local health visitor and GP and they both confirmed that Jamie's mother had recently sought professional help for stress. A case conference was organized for the following day and the hospital and community-based health professionals met to discuss Jamie's future. Jamie was eventually allowed home but he was placed on the at-risk register and support was given to Jamie's mother from the community care team.

EXERCISE

During the course of one day spent on a clinical placement, note how many health care professionals are involved in the care of one child and family.

Consider the information passing between the children's nurse and other members of the multi-professional team. What role does the nurse have?

[Suggested reading: Munro (1999); Soothill *et al.* (1999); Burr (2001).]

COMPETENCY STATEMENT 3.3

- Delegate duties to others, as appropriate, ensuring they are supervised and monitored (see Box 8.14 for relevant outcome criteria).

Box 8.14 Outcome criteria for competency statement 3.3

- Demonstrate the ability to co-ordinate care, taking into account the role and competence level of the staff and the delivery of health and social care
- Recognize and understand the scope of their own accountability and responsibility when delegating aspects of care to others

The ability to delegate is a complex skill and is developed over time. The ability to assess the competence of other staff demands insight and reasoning, and being able to take responsibility for your decisions and actions requires knowledge and confidence. Accountability is central to this dimension of professional practice and children's nurses are accountable, on registration, not only to the profession but also to the child and family.

Scenario During my final ward as a third-year student nurse I was encouraged by the ward sister to take charge of the ward for an 8-hour shift under the supervision of a staff nurse. I took the hand-over report from the night staff and then allocated the nurses to the children, ensuring that all of the student nurses were being supervised by a trained member of staff. I assessed the capabilities of each nurse and confirmed that each student felt able to cope with the workload. I instructed the staff to feedback details of the care they were giving and any changes that were occurring in the condition of their patients. As the day progressed I felt able to make decisions, such as contacting the doctors when a child's condition deteriorated, and I liaised with members of the multi-professional team, such as the physiotherapist and dietician.

Three hours into the shift I had to re-evaluate the workload of one student when a sick child's condition deteriorated and, following a discussion, I felt she was competent to 'special' the child; I delegated her other patients to the supervising staff nurse.

I organized the lunchtime breaks without compromising the safety of the children's care and continually encouraged the junior nurses, giving positive feedback when appropriate. By the end of the shift I felt that I had coped with running a busy ward and was in control of the care delivered to each child.

REFLECTION POINT

Reflect on your clinical experiences and consider how the care of children is organized.

Although you may not have had the opportunity to manage a ward, reflect on how you managed the care of a group of patients.

Can you identify the criteria used to delegate a certain group of patients to you? Had you cared for some of the patients before? How sick were the children and how challenging was their care? Was the presence of a parent a factor in how patients were allocated? Was skill-mix a factor and how were junior nurses supported?

[Suggested reading: Smith and Valentine (1999); Murphy (2001).]

COMPETENCY STATEMENT 3.4

● Demonstrate key skills (see Box 8.15 for relevant outcome criteria).

Box 8.15 Outcome criteria for competency statement 3.4

- Literacy: interpret and present information that is comprehensible to others
- Numeracy: interpret data and its significance for care delivery
- The application of information technology and management that takes account of legal and ethical considerations
- Problem-solving: extending to situations where clinical decision-making has to be made on the basis of limited information

Key skills underpin the practice of all nurses and for children's nurses, competence at literacy, numeracy and problem-solving are essential for safe practice. Without the skills of literacy the children's nurse would be unable to articulate clearly and concisely or to document accurately the care given to the child and family. The ability to be numerate and calculate medicines and fluids accurately is essential, and problem-solving enables the children's nurse to make clinical decisions on behalf of the child when necessary.

Scenario When caring for a patient one day I demonstrated each of the key skills. Zoe was admitted to the ward as a booked admission for routine day case surgery. I read the doctor's notes and passed on the relevant information to the nurse in charge, which included the child's diagnosis and previous admissions to hospital. I also accessed the clinical computer system to obtain Zoe's blood, urine and electrolyte results for the doctor to review on clerking. I devised a care plan, ensuring that I signed it and had it countersigned by a trained nurse, and throughout the day I made sure that the care I gave to Zoe was accurately and legibly documented. Following surgery Zoe was in pain and required the administration of analgesia. I was able to calculate the dose accurately and I administered the drug following the hospital drug policy. At the end of the day I evaluated Zoe's care and completed her discharge planning record.

REFLECTION POINT

Think about how you record the care you give to children and consider if the language you use is appropriate. Have you recorded any vague statements which give little information about the care given, and is any information missing?

Consider how numeracy is used in other areas of practice as well as in drug administration.

Explore a clinical dilemma where decisions need to be made, such as when to discharge a child and family home, or whether to carry out a clinical procedure. Try to identify the various decisions that could be made and how the final decision is reached.

[Suggested reading: Gatford and Anderson (1998); UKCC (1998c, 2000b); Baillie (2001).]

COMPETENCY STATEMENT 3.5

- Resources are appropriately managed to provide optimum patient care and safety (see Box 8.16 for relevant outcome criteria).

Box 8.16 Outcome criteria for competency statement 3.5

- Prioritize care needs and manage time effectively and appropriately
- Ensure the nursing environment is safe (hygienic and tidy) and well stocked
- By Year 3 the nurse will show an awareness and demonstrate the importance of appropriate nurse allocation and skill-mix based on the dependency of children
- Stock and equipment management skills – show an awareness of financial accountability of stock use
- Take into account knowledge as a resource

Towards the end of the child branch programme the student nurse needs to be able to understand the context in which they will be working as a qualified nurse. How to resource a ward is an essential part of a registered nurse's responsibility and for a ward to run efficiently and smoothly, a sound knowledge of skill-mix, budgeting and ordering of stock and equipment is essential.

Scenario I participated in a management day with the ward sister and she demonstrated how to order specific equipment for the ward, which was a medical ward. The majority of the admissions were babies with chest infections and, therefore, airway-related equipment needed to be ordered. The ward sister explained that during the winter months extra supplies were required and we discussed how expensive some items were and how important it was not to order too much. I enquired about the ordering of the more expensive equipment, such as IVAC machine and Kangaroo pumps, and learnt that they were funded from the directorate finances and orders were counter-signed by the clinical services manager.

For the remainder of the day we considered the staffing of the ward for the next 24 hours as there were several registered nurses off sick. With guidance from the sister I contacted the nursing agency used by the hospital and booked a children's nurse for night duty. We discussed the expense of agency staff and how the ward budget would be affected.

REFLECTION POINT

Reflecting on your experiences can you recall an incident where an item was out of stock or the equipment was faulty? What actions did the nurse in charge take?

Have you worked in a clinical area where agency staff were employed? Why were they employed? Try and find out how much a specific clinical area spends on agency staff.

Look at the off-duty rota and consider the skill-mix of grades, students and health care assistants. Ask the nurse in charge how they feel about the current skill-mix and if changes could be made.

[Suggested reading: La Monica (1990); DoH (2001f); Smith and Young (2002).]

SUMMARY

- Quality assurance and risk management strategies should be used to guide the delivery of care and the maintenance of a safe environment.
- Effective communication between children's nurses and the multi-disciplinary team should make it probable that optimal, seamless care is delivered to the child and family.
- The delegation of duties must take the roles and competence levels of staff into account because nursing activities require specific knowledge, skills and attitudes.
- Literacy, numeracy, information technology and problem-solving are the key skills which underpin the practice of nursing and the achievement of the competencies.
- Resources, both human and financial, must be managed effectively and appropriately in order to provide optimal patient care and safety.

DOMAIN 4: PERSONAL/PROFESSIONAL DEVELOPMENT

COMPETENCY STATEMENT 4.1

- Demonstrate a commitment to the need for continuing professional development and personal supervision activities in order to enhance knowledge, skills, values and attitudes needed for safe and effective nursing practice (see Box 8.17 for relevant outcome criteria).

Box 8.17 Outcome criteria for competency statement 4.1

- Identify your own professional development needs by engaging in activities such as reflection in and on practice
- Share experiences with colleagues and patients/clients to identify additional knowledge/skills needed to manage unfamiliar or professionally challenging situations
- Take action to meet any identified knowledge and skills deficit likely to affect the delivery of care within your current sphere of practice

The professional practice of children's nursing takes place in a context of continuous change. Children's nurses cannot expect to practise safely and effectively unless they engage in continuing professional development (CPD) activities to maintain and update the knowledge-base that underpins their practice. They must also facilitate the regular and ongoing monitoring and evaluation of their own practice with supervision, reflecting in and on practice, with the maintenance of a professional portfolio playing a significant part. The achievement of this competency is at the centre of lifelong learning and career development.

Scenario On a previous shift I was caring for an 11-year-old boy, James, who had been admitted that day in a sickle cell crisis: his mother was present with him, his father was at work. I was working with a senior staff nurse, who was also my supervisor for that shift.

I had never looked after a patient with sickle cell disease before and I was grateful for the comprehensive hand-over from a staff nurse. Following hand-over, the senior staff nurse and staff nurse agreed to check and administer intravenous drugs to James while I spent some time familiarizing myself with his care plan and medical notes. I popped my head in to speak to James and his mum. As I talked with them I realized that they were very knowledgeable about the treatment he was being given.

I took the opportunity early on in my shift to identify a haematology textbook in the ward library and read up what I could on sickle cell disease. On reflection, when reading about the therapeutic management during a crisis, I realized that in fact I understood quite a bit already, as I had previously cared for children receiving blood transfusions, intravenous therapy and antibiotics, oxygen therapy and intravenous morphine.

Throughout my shift I was able to observe interactions between the senior staff nurse and James' mum. On one occasion she was explaining about a new antibiotic and how this differed from the other antibiotics James had received. This highlighted to me how practice is constantly changing and how important it is to keep your knowledge up to date. This was also an example where a nurse and parent were sharing their knowledge and experience, an outcome that would benefit James and his mum, as they would have the knowledge to manage this change in his pattern of care.

REFLECTION POINT

Think about situations and the approaches you took to ensure that you had sufficient knowledge to deliver safe and effective care, such as when you were faced with caring for a child with an unfamiliar clinical condition or receiving treatments that were new to you.

Think about situations when parents/carers are very knowledgeable about their child's care and how you, as a student, can make the most of their knowledge, while remaining confident in your caring role.

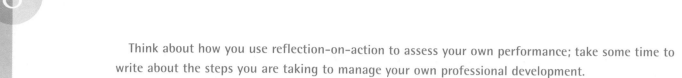

Think about how you use reflection-on-action to assess your own performance; take some time to write about the steps you are taking to manage your own professional development.

[Suggested reading: Hinchliff (1998); Johns (2000b); Rolfe *et al.* (2001, p22–40).]

COMPETENCY STATEMENT 4.2

- Enhance the professional development and safe practice of others through peer support, leadership, supervision and teaching (see Box 8.18 for relevant outcome criteria).

Box 8.18 Outcome criteria for competency statement 4.2

- Contribute to creating a climate conducive to learning
- Contribute to the learning experiences and development of others by facilitating the mutual sharing of knowledge and experience
- Act as a role model to others by demonstrating safe practice
- Demonstrate effective teaching skills
- Demonstrate effective leadership in the establishment and maintenance of safe nursing practice

Children's nurses do not work in isolation, they are part of a team and, as such, much can be gained through the giving and receiving of peer support. This is just one aspect of creating and maintaining an environment that is conducive to learning. Role modelling, teaching, preserving a questioning approach to all aspects of clinical care and seizing learning opportunities as they arise, are other facets of personal and professional development that must be kept alive throughout the career of a children's nurse. The achievement of this competency is central to children's nurses accepting responsibility for the role they play in the maintenance of safe and effective nursing practice.

Scenario I have been working on the haematology and oncology unit for 6 weeks. In that time I have been caring consistently for children receiving chemotherapy and have, as a result, observed qualified nurses and parents undertaking mouth care.

On a previous shift I admitted an 8-year-old boy called Tom. Tom was diagnosed as having acute myeloid leukaemia for which he was prescribed chemotherapy. Three days following his admission I was caring for Tom and assessed that he was now well enough to undertake his own mouth care. I discussed the mouth care Tom would require with one of the staff nurses and described the approach I would take to teaching Tom and his dad about his new mouth care regime. My plan for teaching was to be practice-based with some supporting literature. The staff nurse was able to supervise my teaching and asked if I would mind a new student joining us. Tom and his dad were happy for there to be a small group of us participating in the process.

I taught Tom and his dad about the importance of mouth care and stressed the need to clean his teeth twice a day. I talked them through the tool we use on the ward to assess Tom's mouth on a daily basis and used this to highlight the problems that Tom might experience, such as mouth ulcers, dry lips and bleeding gums. Through questioning it was clear that Tom's dad had a good grasp of the problems that may be encountered. I stressed the need to look in Tom's mouth every day and why it was important to respond to any complaints of oral problems. I observed Tom cleaning his own teeth and taking the anti-fungal agent and reinforced how good his technique was. Together we looked through the mouth care information booklet and talked about care at home and the importance of keeping up with dental checkups. I took the opportunity to talk about general oral health for the whole family and the need to use sugar-free drinks and medicines where possible. Tom's dad asked me a number of questions, all of which I was able to answer. I documented Tom's mouth care regime in his parent held record and care plan, noting that Tom and his dad had been taught oral care.

Following the teaching session we took the opportunity to talk about different children on the unit and the reasons why their mouth care regimen might be different. The staff nurse shared her knowledge and a group discussion ensued which I was able to contribute to. The staff nurse taught me and the student about the various treatments for oral problems and we discussed different approaches to teaching, e.g. with a younger child, where mouth care was not already part of daily care and where there was some resistance to undertaking the role. Our responsibility to role model safe practice and teach from an informed background was explored. I then had the opportunity to supervise the new student undertaking mouth care on another child.

REFLECTION POINT

From your experience think about situations that have challenged your abilities to teach a new skill, e.g. a frightened child, a parent who was anxious, a family whose first language was not English.

Take a few minutes to think about what supervision means to you and outline the key skills of supervision.

How do you support the colleagues you work with? Detail the approach you take in sharing knowledge.

Think about the health care professionals that you have worked with and write down the leadership skills that they have used to promote effective and efficient child health care.

[Suggested reading: Antrobus and Kitson (1999); Gibson and Nelson (2000); Chandler (2001); Rolfe *et al.* (2001, p75–98).]

SUMMARY

- Each individual nurse must accept the responsibility for their CPD and personal supervision activities in order to develop their competency within the sphere of children's nursing practice.
- Each nurse should proactively contribute to the development and progression of all team members through peer support, leadership, supervision and teaching.

DOMAIN 5: CHILDREN'S NURSING AND CHILD HEALTH

COMPETENCY STATEMENT 5.1

- Have knowledge of cognitive, social and emotional development and impact of health, illness and environment (see Box 8.19 for relevant outcome criteria).

Box 8.19 Outcome criteria for competency statement 5.1

- Identify normal and abnormal development in a comprehensive assessment
- Identify awareness of the impact of social and cultural factors on child development
- Give attention to context in completing the developmental assessment
- Create an environment that promotes development
- Understand the impact of acute and chronic illness on child development
- Understand the implications of the diagnosis of a terminal illness

Growth and development are complex processes: many changes occur during a lifetime and are influenced by numerous factors. The achievement of this competency is central to children's nurses understanding the physical changes that take place during development and the special needs generated by these changes. Ill health can have a dramatic effect on development, as can social and emotional factors. Promotion of normal development and enabling the child to realize their full potential rests on the children's nurse being fully conversant with all the stages of growth and development. Recognizing alterations from the child's norm and working with the child and family to establish realistic future goals is an important role for the children's nurse in the many areas that health care is delivered.

Scenario On a previous shift I was caring for Claire who was 8 years old and had learning difficulties. She had been admitted for a tonsillectomy and adenoidectomy. Claire's mum and dad were with her and they were both anxious about the forthcoming surgery. They had attended a pre-admission clinic where, through the use of therapeutic play, Claire had started to be prepared for the surgery. A play specialist had spent time with Claire showing her the mask and playing with syringes. Both parents were concerned about how far that preparation had helped Claire, as her learning difficulties prevented Claire from being able to express her understanding of what had taken place.

My assessment of Claire, using observation and toys, revealed that she had retained some of the information from the clinic meeting. This was confirmed when Claire recognized the play specialist who had been working with her at the clinic. Claire did not appear to be anxious, as long as both parents were present with her. I realized very quickly that I would need to spend a lot of time with Claire and her family to be able to support Claire through the procedure, allowing enough time for explanation and to use toys and pictures to encourage understanding. Through the relationship that Claire had with her parents they were able to facilitate this communication process, so it was a team approach. I was able to use the knowledge of both parents to help me to prepare Claire. We used favourite toys to help in the process and relied very much on visual descriptions. Claire had been previously admitted to hospital with a broken leg, and so with the help of her parents we were able to use that experience of how she coped to help in our preparations. I felt it was important to engage with Claire, to use myself in the process of communication, and with the help of Claire's parents and the play specialist, draw on all my creative skills as a children's nurse to ensure that Claire was prepared for surgery within the context of her developmental understanding and needs.

REFLECTION POINT

Think about a nurse that you consider to be an expert children's nurse. What makes them an expert in your eyes? Then try to share this with other colleagues so that you start to develop a picture of what it is to be a children's nurse.

Think of examples from your practice where a child's development has been affected by their health, social, emotional or environmental factors and consider the ways in which you and the rest of the health care team worked with the child and family to maximize the child's potential to progress in their development.

Spend some time focusing particularly on a chronic illness and the effect that may have on a child's developmental progress: consider how this may have an effect on the family, school, interactions with peers and future employment.

[Suggested reading: Campbell and Glasper (1995, p140–76, p369–90); Lansdown (1996); Shipton H (2000).]

COMPETENCY STATEMENT 5.2

- Demonstrate knowledge and awareness of the child in the context of the family and society (the wider context) (see Box 8.20 for relevant outcome criteria).

Box 8.20 Outcome criteria for competency statement 5.2

- Show awareness of the changing nature of the family in society
- Contribute to maintaining the integrity of the family unit
- Recognize the wider influences on child health and well-being
- Apply knowledge of child development to the care process
- Demonstrate an understanding of the potential changing family dynamics in the illness process
- Ascribe to the principles of partnership, negotiation and sharing the care

Developing a collaborative approach to working with families is necessary to facilitate them in the role as carer and to promote the health and well-being of the whole family. The achievement of this competency is central to the children's nurse delivering truly family-centred care. To involve families in their child's care requires the nurse to have an understanding of the child and family, to support the individuality of each and to be comfortable and familiar with maintaining professional boundaries (see Chapter 5).

Scenario On a previous shift I was caring for Ahmed, a 2-year-old Bangladeshi boy, who had been re-admitted with diarrhoea following a bone marrow transplant for an immunological condition (severe combined immunodeficiency). Ahmed's mother was resident with him and undertook the role of main carer. Ahmed's paternal grandmother visited daily. Although Ahmed's mother spoke English, the grandmother spoke very little English but appeared to understand a little more. On this particular day Ahmed was receiving all his care from his grandmother.

Throughout the shift I worked with the grandmother to deliver care to Ahmed. At first I thought it would have been quicker to do the care myself, as I was not sure how much the grandmother understood of what I was saying. I was busy with two other patients and did not know how I was going to remember to check on Ahmed and his grandmother. Ahmed needed frequent nappy changing, his nappies needed to be weighed and output recorded: a skin care regimen was to be followed. Ahmed's mother was confident and competent in doing all these aspects of care. I was not sure about the grandmother's role and how far she wanted to be involved in assisting in the nursing care. Yet Ahmed responded to his grandmother's involvement in a positive way, when she changed his nappy he was less distressed and much more co-operative. The grandmother was clearly an important person in Ahmed's life and her involvement in his care was natural.

We very quickly set up a way of working, with the grandmother changing his nappy. On the first occasion I showed her what we were cleaning his bottom with and applied the cream. I showed her where to store the nappies for me to weigh; the grandmother was to ring the call bell and let me know when there was a nappy there to be weighed and recorded. I observed the grandmother doing his care and was confident in her competence. I felt it was important to maintain the family structure and involve the grandmother where I could. Although negotiating roles was made complex because of the language barrier, we quickly developed a relationship using simple language and hand signs, resulting in us being able to share in caring for Ahmed.

REFLECTION POINT

Think about society today and the variety of family structures that a children's nurse works within. Reflect on your own beliefs and values and consider the different approaches you use to ensure families are involved in care through a successful process of negotiation.

Consider some of the relationships that you have witnessed in practice. Can you identify both positive and negative relationships and explore the reasons for these outcomes in relation to family structures, beliefs held by nurses and other health care professionals, and approaches to family-centred care.

Textbooks refer to professional boundaries. Can you describe what this means to you in relation to how you care for families?

[Suggested reading: Casey (1988, 1995); Darbyshire (1994); Soanes (1997); Brace O'Neill (1998).]

SUMMARY

- To enable every child to realize their full potential, every children's nurse must have knowledge of the cognitive, social and emotional development of children and the impact that health, illness and the environment may have on this.
- Understanding the child in the context of the family and a clear focus on children's services are fundamental to the achievement of true family-centred care.

CONCLUSION

The aim of this chapter has been to facilitate learning and understanding about competency-based practice in children's nursing. Following a brief explanatory background of what competency-based practice is and how the generic UKCC competencies were developed to capture the essence of children's nursing, the reality of children's nursing practice has been captured using vignettes which provide examples of how the competencies can be achieved. It is hoped that you have been stimulated to reflect on your own practice and to consider how experiences have led to competency development.

ACKNOWLEDGEMENT

We would specifically like to acknowledge the hard work undertaken by our colleagues in the Division of Children's Nursing, South Bank University, in developing the competencies for the child branch programme. Permission has been granted by the University to publish the competencies in this chapter.

CHAPTER
9

CARE DELIVERY: THE NEEDS OF YOUNG PEOPLE

Marcelle de Sousa

INTRODUCTION

This chapter aims to explore and extend your knowledge about the young people who need your care. It examines the developmental period of adolescence and the impact that illness has on this time of transition, and highlights the lack of health care provision that currently exists for this group of young people who have specific needs. It also discusses the role that health care professionals can play to help young people deal with the issues that arise from the conflict of being an adolescent and coping with illness. The chapter also discusses the current shortfall in education for nurses who care for this client group and provides some recommendations.

Health promotion is essential for young people, who need help to maintain a healthy lifestyle but discussion of this, beyond a brief look at how nurses, and particularly school nurses, can influence well-being in this population (Bekeart 2002), is beyond the scope of this chapter.

The terms adolescent, young person and teenager are used interchangeably to describe this specific group.

BACKGROUND

WHAT IS ADOLESCENCE?

WHO (1989) defined adolescence as the period between 10 and 19 years of age, but changes in the socio-economic climate may have extended this period beyond 19 years. Poor health, unemployment and lack of financial security may all contribute to this.

Adolescence is a transition from childhood to adulthood. There is change, both mental and physical, adaptation to new concepts and thinking, and great learning and preparation for a new role as an adult. Whether you agree or not that at the end of this period a mature adult emerges is a topic of endless debate.

Adolescence was not a well recognized or used term before the 19th century (Congor and Galmbos 1997). But, interestingly, Aristotle (Congor and Galmbos 1997) spoke of the young being 'passionate, irascible and apt to be carried away by their impulses'. Many would agree that this holds true today. Many theories have been put forward about this intense period of transition and development (Box 9.1). Some thought that the search for identity, that of formation versus confusion, was what the period of adolescence was all about (Erikson 1968). Elkind (1968) called the egocentric behaviour which presents itself in adolescence as the 'imaginary audience and personal fable'. Freud (Congor and Galmbos 1997) spoke about the dominance of hormonal changes and developing sexuality.

Box 9.1 Theories of adolescence

- Hall: Storm and stress/feelings and emotions
- Erikson: Search for identity formation/confusion
- Elkind: Search for self imaginary audience/egocentric
- Schave and Schave: Younger vs older adolescent thinking
- Freud: Sexual/hormonal dominance
- Piaget: Concrete/formal cognition

Schave and Schave (1989) postulated that adolescence could be separated into two distinct phases. Early adolescence, between the ages of 11 and 14, was different from late adolescence because of specific changes, including the pubertal, hormonal, social and physical changes which cause the young adolescent to 'become vulnerable to shifting and volatile states of mind' and so act differently. Young adolescents were seen as unable to accept responsibilities for their actions. The late stage of adolescence, from 15 to 18, was when 'due to a consolidation of changes in cognitive thinking, an integration of self occurs'.

Piaget's theory centred on stages of development; the two that are relevant to the period of adolescence are the stage of 'concrete operations' (7–11years) and 'formal operations' (12 years onwards). Some have argued that his work does not truly represent adolescent development (Coleman and

Hendry 1999), but the majority still find it useful in assessing how adolescents might use knowledge to make decisions.

Hall, a psychologist, was the first in the western world to theorise about a time of 'stress and storm' (Conger and Galmbos 1997). He postulated that adolescents continually fluctuate between extremes of feelings and emotions. This was a view acknowledged by many theorists, psychologists and the public, but it has been seriously challenged by the contrary view that the majority of young people do not have a stormy time but adjust very well (Offer 1981; Congor and Galmbos 1997; Coleman and Hendry 1999).

This phase of growing encompasses great physical and psycho-social change for the young person. Puberty, with its huge rise in hormonal levels, growth spurts, spots and relationships, has a profound effect on the developing adolescent. Acne, for instance, if not treated properly, can have a profound effect on the young person (Greener 2002).

Adolescence is a period when young people are often perceived as difficult. Unfortunately, this is often the view of adults who appear to have forgotten their own adolescence. The media further compounds this negative image of young people. However, the majority of young people go through this period of development without any problems and in good health. What adolescents need is information and advice given in a non-judgemental manner, which respects them as individuals with a right to confidentiality and an ability to make decisions about their lives.

Adolescence can, however, be a very distressful time for some, which may account for the high rates of depression, suicide and anxiety-related illness (Coleman and Hendry 1999). Increasing rates of attempted suicide have been reported. One of the targets of Health of the Nation (DoH 1995a) was to reduce the rate of suicide by 15% by 2000. The numbers of anxiety-induced illnesses are increasing, with very little understanding of, or resources to deal with, this issue (Mallinson *et al.* 2001).

HEALTH CARE PROVISION

The number of adolescents in the UK is growing and is projected to reach 6.5 million in 2012 (Macfarlane 1996); yet, the area of health care services specific to adolescents has largely been neglected by the government and health care providers (Ministry of Health 1959; DoH 1976). It is particularly sad that as early as 1976 the Court report stated:

'In recent years it has been increasingly evident that adolescents have needs and problems sufficiently distinguishable to warrant consideration as a distinct group for health care provision'.

(DoH 1976)

However, 20 years on, not much had been done to provide this care. Despite the UK signing up in 1993 to the United Nations Convention on the Rights of the Child (1989), children and young people have had little focus on the their rights as individuals or the care that they receive. Kurtz (1996) eloquently confirms this by commenting that:

'children and young people have always been targeted by health care programmes, more in the spirit of charity or in the interest of adult society than of entitlement by rights'.

A focus on the health care needs of young people and their general well-being is long overdue (NHS Executive 1996). Government programmes, such as those that have focused on teenage pregnancy, for which the UK has the highest rate in western Europe (Coleman and Hendry 1999), have been welcomed, but more is needed for this group with distinct needs. There is great hope that The Children's National Service Framework (NSF), which will encompasses health, social issues, education and environment and has promised a radical review of children's services, will finally address this area of gross neglect. At the time of writing (2003) England has still not appointed a Commissioner for Children's Services. What is needed is a champion for children and young people at Government level.

User views are an essential component of the clinical governance agenda in the modern NHS and it is particularly welcome that children and young people are being consulted about the service they receive in the preparation of the NSF. Perhaps adolescents, who have been at a distinct disadvantage, will finally have their voices heard and receive health care by suitably qualified professionals in dedicated clinical settings. The Hospital Standard Document (April 2003) which is the first module of the NSF recognizes the unique need of adolescents in hospital.

McKinney *et al.*'s (1977) list of development tasks that the adolescent has to achieve to reach maturity can be used as a framework to try to understand the specific health care needs of adolescents:

- achieving independence from parents
- acquiring the social skills required of an adult
- achieving a sense of oneself as a worthwhile person
- developing the necessary academic and vocational skills
- adjusting to a rapidly changing physique and sexual development
- achieving an internalized set of guiding norms and values.

RELEVANT COMPETENCIES

The relevance of the following competencies from the *Code of professional conduct* (NMC 2002a) to the care of young people will be looked at in the discussion below.

- you must respect the patient or client as an individual
- you must obtain consent before you give any treatment or care
- you must co-operate with others in the team
- you must protect confidential information.

CONSIDERATIONS IN CARING FOR ADOLESCENTS

RISK-TAKING BEHAVIOUR

Young people will experiment, take risks and take part in antisocial behaviour. Rutter *et al.* (1998) cited in Coleman and Hendry (1999) demonstrated a steep increase in recorded offences in the UK for the under 25 years (Coleman and Hendry 1999). However, in the period 1999–2001 there has been a marked decrease in the number of offences committed by young people (Coleman and Scofield 2003). They continue to comment that this may possibly be due to recent youth justice reforms. In 1992, injuries were the most common cause of death in 15–18 year olds (Macfarlane 1996). Adolescents are also vulnerable and often quite frightened. Acts of bravado are often attempts to cover insecurity. Some adolescents do consume alcohol with little regard to side-effects or long-term effects. Goddard demonstrated that 45% of young men and 35% of young women have alcohol at least weekly by the age of 15 (Coleman and Hendry 1999). Recent figures suggest the consumption of alcohol in teenagers has increased dramatically (Coleman and Scofield 2003).

Risk taking is often seen in young people who do not comply with medical regimes (Kyngas 2000a,b,c), such as taking medication or physiotherapy. Graft rejection with graft loss in young people who have had a renal transplant but do not comply with their immunosuppressive therapy is well documented and continues to be an immense problem (Watson 2002). Nurses who work in A&E departments are all too familiar with the diabetic teenager who presents with diabetic ketoacidosis, often in a coma as a consequence of not adhering to a medical regime that is seen as restrictive. The attitude of 'it won't happen to me', as well as 'I haven't taken my medicines but I feel fine', poses a challenge to health care professionals working with these adolescents (Watson 2002).

> **Scenario** Tracy is a 16-year-old girl who has been admitted to the paediatric ward from the A&E department with a fracture. She has also consumed alcohol. She needs to wait until it is safe for her to go to theatre for an operation on her fractured dislocated elbow which she sustained when she fell over in the street. You have to connect her/care for her intravenous infusion which she needs to re-hydrate her. She wants you to take way the infusion. She is angry and abusive and refuses to stop swearing. Some of the parents of the other children on the ward are beginning to complain about her language. She tells you that she has just left her foster home and was out celebrating, but now is worried about her future.

REFLECTION POINT

Take a moment to reflect on this scenario and think of how you might apply the following aspect of the *Code of professional conduct* – 'you must respect the patient or client as an individual' (NMC 2002a).

You need to make sure that Tracy is safe and that the infusion is connected and patent. You might want to move her into a side room, if one is available, away from the young children and where you can talk quietly to her, or simply stay with her until she calms down. By removing her from the main ward, you can change the atmosphere that has arisen. If no cubicles are free, then simply draw the curtains round her and sit with her until she has calmed down or has fallen asleep. When Tracy is sober you might consider giving her advice on the dangers of binge drinking. There is a need to involve social services and the expertise of the multi-professional team if you happen to work with one.

INVOLVING PARENTS

Parents must be involved and informed of all aspects of care. They must also be educated, supported and encouraged to help their child towards achieving independence, taking ownership of their disease and becoming autonomous in decision-making.

CONSENT AND DECISION-MAKING

The issue of consent continues to be an item of great debate. The Family Law Reform Act (1969), Section 8 allows a young person who is 16 years of age to consent to treatment. This consent applies only to treatment and does not include consenting to blood or organ donation (Dimmond 1996);

however, adolescents under the age of 16 may consent to treatment if they are deemed to be Gillick competent, i.e. 'have sufficient maturity and understanding' (Frasier 1986). Young people cannot refuse treatment as this can be overruled by their parents or the courts. Practitioners need to be aware of the differences in age of consent across the UK: 16 in England and Wales, 12 in Scotland and 17 in Northern Ireland. The Department of Health has produced an excellent document for 'good practice in consent' (DoH 2001n).

REFLECTION POINT

Thinking back to the scenario described above, can you think of anything else you might do for Tracy in accordance with the *Code of professional conduct* ['You must promote the interests of patients and clients. This includes helping individuals and groups gain access to health and social care information and support, relevant to their needs' (NMC 2002a)]. Would you obtain her consent for the infusion? Do you need to? Do you think you will see her on the ward again?

The subject of how children learn, think and make decisions, can be traced back to ancient Greece (Wood 1998). How children develop this ability and are encouraged to make decisions is varied and dependent on child-rearing patterns, culture and the society in which they live (Nash 1984).

As health professionals we often seem unable to respect the decisions young patients make about their treatment or their lives. Young children are deemed incompetent and even those over the age of consent may have their decision overruled by the courts. However, article 16 of the United Nations (1989) convention states that 'young people have a right to information'. Nurses can play an important part in decision-making by acting as advocates for the young person. They are in the unique position of ensuring that the young person receives the correct information and has the time to reflect on it prior to making a decision.

Piagetian theory (Lefrancois 1992) suggests that children are unable to make logical decisions until they are adolescents (formal operational). However, several studies suggest that even infants can display sophisticated powers of reasoning and understanding of human relationships (Alderson 1996). Children, by the age of 5, are developing a sense of identification with parents and a sense of responsibility for their own actions (Erikson 1987).

The Children Act (1989) states, 'children and young people must be consulted and kept informed about actions taken and participate in decisions about them'. Children who have been seriously ill for a long period of time have been shown to have a 'profound and mature understanding and can cope with and discuss complex and painful knowledge' (Alderson 1996). The author has personal experience of this. A teenager who had been ill for a long period of time decided quite calmly and clearly that she did not wish to continue with treatment. She was 18 years old. The only people who initially had difficulty accepting her decision were the members of the medical and nursing team.

Children in Western society are usually seen as being dependent on their parents, probably until they leave home or go to university. However, this view is changing, e.g. the current climate has seen a change in the grant status for students and so dependence continues. How difficult it must be to try and make truly independent choices while you are still financially dependent on your parents for your education, even though you may be living away from home?

REFLECTION POINT

How do young people who are dependent on their families for care achieve independence? Think about further education, relationships and careers.

An example of young people who have the burden of responsibility are young carers who care for a parent who is chronically ill or disabled at home. They have to assume great responsibility for caring but are not asked if this what they want to do and often have no voice in the decision-making processes, either about themselves, their quality of life or their sick parent (Dearden and Becker 1998). Many of these young people find it difficult to visualize an independent care-free future.

Alderson (1996) cites cases of children becoming more responsible for their actions, where they are either called as witnesses in criminal cases or where they are on trial for the crime. Remember the case of the murder of the toddler Jamie Bulger? The two persons found guilty of his murder were children.

If we are to believe what the theorists say about the cognitive abilities that are beginning to blossom in a child from the age of 7, then adults should listen closer to what they say. Do parents of well children do this? At best a child's view is listened to, but in the end the adult makes the final decision in 'the best interest of the child'. Adults assume that it is their right to make the decision because they know best.

'The need for adults to feel in control can also serve as a barrier to listening to children.'

(Alderson 1996)

Alderson (1996) considers adults fear that listening seriously to children will commit them to supporting unwise choices that the child might make, or worse let children 'run rings round them' or 'stop respecting them'. She sees setting limits as a licence for adult power. This is a powerful statement and is one that the majority of adolescents would agree with but which a large number of adults would find offensive. This is summed up well by the quote, 'What is best for the child is often only best understood 20 years after childhood' (Lansdowne 1998).

REFLECTION POINT

Think about adolescents who have survived because their parents made treatment decisions when they were children. There is no right or wrong but there is a debate about decision-making.

Erikson (1987) reminds us that development takes place because of the experiences a child gains through a series of conflicts. Piaget alludes to the infant's world here and now, i.e. whoever feeds and keeps them warm will be the most significant. This of course develops into the next phase, when a baby is able to identify their mother. So, when do children begin to decide? The familiar scenario of a toddler having temper tantrums because they cannot get their own way, may not be acceptable to many adults as being an indication that the toddler is making up their own mind. However, it must represent the start of the decision-making process which will get more finely tuned with the acquisition of knowledge. Erikson (1987) puts forward the theory that from the age of 18 months children learn that they can be autonomous and that their intentions can be realized. This stage progresses until about the age of 3, and then the child begins to develop a sense of self and a responsibility for their own actions. Does this imply that children who fall ill at this age worry that they may be responsible for their illness?

Nurses can also become emotive when difficult decisions have to be made for their patients, and they need to be familiar with the law governing this area. It is not easy to find the answers to some questions that arise when caring for young people in a clinical setting. How do you measure competency? Who is available to do so? Why can you consent but not refuse?

Consider the case of Re W (1992) (Dimmond (1996), which concerned a young girl who had a long history of being in care and had developed anorexia. She was being tube fed. The local authority decided that she needed specialist treatment and that she should be moved to a specialist unit. At the age of 16, she consulted her solicitor and decided that she should not be moved to a specialist unit for treatment without her consent. The court overruled her, stating that she was not able to make a competent decision as she had anorexia, which would impair her mental capacity, and that unless she had the specialist treatment at the new unit her condition would deteriorate.

Now consider the case of Mrs Gillick who challenged the health authority about her daughter getting contraceptives without her permission. The law lords upheld for the health authority and gave us 'Gillick Competent', whereby a young person under the legal age of consent, can consent on their own if they are competent and mature enough to be able to understand. This represented a milestone for all health care professionals who care for young people, but remember a young person under the age of 16 can consent to treatment but they cannot refuse treatment as they can be overruled by their parents or the court. This is always done in the best interest of the child or young person.

> **Scenario** Neil is 17 years old and has just been diagnosed with non-Hodgkin's lymphoma. He needs to start chemotherapy and the doctor has given him and his parents all the information about the drugs, their side-effects and why he must commence treatment soon. He has been told that he has a good chance of making a complete recovery if he has treatment. Neil, after some deliberation, decides that he will not consent to the treatment. His parents, though very upset, are determined that he must consent for treatment to commence.

REFLECTION POINT

Consider the above scenario. Do you think Neil has made the right decision? What has influenced or guided your answer? Why do you think his parents are not making the decision to treat, after all he is still a minor? Do you think that Neil is competent to make the decision? What can you do to help Neil and his parents?

Neil has an illness that has a good prognosis if treated. He is worried about the side-effects. He is still in shock after hearing the diagnosis. He has cancer. He needs time and someone to talk to both him and his parents. His parents need support to help Neil make the right decision. Giving them all time and more information informs their decision. Young people also have a right to advocacy services and to have legal representation in matters relating to decisions that they have made. Where a patient has refused a particular intervention, you should ensure that the patient realizes they are free to change their mind and accept treatment later. Where delay may affect their treatment choices, they should be advised accordingly (DoH 2001n).

ATTITUDE TO DEATH AND DYING

Young people often have a curious attitude to dying and death. This might relate to themselves dying, or anyone close to them. A belief in the personal fable can be damaging as adolescents may be reluctant, or refuse to accept, that they may have a potentially life-threatening disease (Eiser 1993). Adolescents often avoid or are reluctant to know about long-term effects of disease.

The author works with young people who attend a late effects clinic. These teenagers were treated with chemotherapy and radiotherapy for oncological problems when they were children. They have survived and now have issues that are important to them. Some mention that they were never really involved in the decision to have treatment. They talk of 'not owning their cancer'. Most are glad to be alive and extremely grateful that their parents made all the decisions, but some say that the treatment was so painful and unpleasant that had they known beforehand 'they would not have agreed to it'. This is said even with the knowledge that without the treatment they would have died. Many of these teenagers are sterile, impotent and short in stature and have the added onus that they may develop a secondary malignancy (Wheeler *et al.* 1998). Many of these side-effects were not made clear when treatment options were offered. This action is defended by the argument that there is a limit to what you take in when you are in shock. However, practice is changing to accommodate the questions that young people have. Today young people do not have to rely on adults 'telling them things'. Information can be accessed via the Internet, television and magazines that cater to the teenage market.

DEVELOPING A RELATIONSHIP AND TRUST

A predominant preoccupation with self often irritates all who come into contact with adolescents and this can make it difficult to have a relationship with them. This unfortunately can apply equally in the health care setting, making it problematic for young people to access health care.

Adolescents take time to form relationships with health care providers. A common complaint from both parents and other adults is the adolescent who 'grunts' or who is monosyllabic. Team working to deliver a comprehensive package of care is often difficult when caring for young people who often appear not to want help.

Adolescents who are asked questions about themselves rarely answer truthfully. Trust has to be established before real information is divulged. So, if a young person is asked whether they smoke, they will often say no. This has potential risks if the adolescent is being admitted for surgery. It is vital that the nurse gets the right information and achieving this is a skill that comes with practice. Treating the adolescent with respect and dignity enables the nurse to gain the adolescent's confidence.

> **Scenario** You have been asked by the nurse in charge to admit and carry out an assessment for care planning on a 15-year-old girl, Kirsty. She is being admitted for investigations. Her mother has had to return home but will be in later to answer any questions. Kirsty tells you that she smokes 'only a few' when she is with friends. Her mother does not know and 'will kill her if she finds out'.

REFLECTION POINT
How will you carry out your task? Do you think you will receive the information you need? What will you do about the information that Kirsty gave you that is sensitive and which she does not want her mother to know? What advice will you give Kirsty?

In the one dedicated adolescent medicine service in the UK, information obtained during the admission process by nurses is shared with the multi-professional team at the weekly meeting. The issue of a young person smoking is taken on board not only by their nurse but also the school teacher, youth worker, doctor and play specialist; each has a different approach and advice. The team does not always divulge information to parents unless it is in the best interests of the young person. This is where the crucial difference between paediatric and adolescent care lies.

REFLECTION POINT

Is there a difference between caring for a child and an adolescent? Why is there a difference? When do you break a confidence?

CONCERN WITH IMAGE

It is interesting to note that adolescents are less concerned with issues around smoking, drugs and alcohol intake (Coleman and Hendry 1999) than they are about their image – weight, acne, how they interact with peers and form relationships. Adolescents who have had renal and endocrine disease may be very concerned by their short stature; teenagers who have diabetes find the high calorie diets difficult to adhere to because of the weight gain they experience. Nurses who care for young people have a professional duty to offer health advice and information which deals with all these issues.

REFLECTION POINT

Think about an adolescent who is physically disabled. What do you think are the issues for them? Is it easy for them to form relationships with able-bodied peers? Do they challenge boundaries?

ADDRESSING THE HEALTH CARE NEEDS OF ADOLESCENTS

As discussed above, adolescents have been ignored as a client group with specific care needs; this applies not only in clinical settings, but also in the community. Young people often receive post code care in the community. This is dependent to some extent on current resources but more on who should deliver care to whom, and up to what age care is received. Health visitors will usually provide a service to children up to the age of 12. District nurses usually care for adults and rarely have the time for adolescents who are at home. In some areas where there are paediatric community nurses, they provide the care that young people at home need. School nurses have always been the providers of care and health advice to adolescents. They probably are the most important group as they have contact with large numbers of teenagers. Practice nurses are an underused resource for meeting health care needs in young people. This deserves investment.

The impact of disease on normal development is illustrated by Figure 9.1. Young people find medical regimes restrictive and they interfere with daily living. Frequent hospital admissions, clinic visits, therapy and blood tests, which are essential to maintaining health, may hamper socialization with peers and school life (Eiser 1993). Clinics that are held after school, less frequent hospital visits, more shared care with local clinicians, and a negotiation with young people about therapy can have two positive outcomes: less emphasis on the sick adolescent and more on being normal; and perhaps a better adherence with medication and therapy. Adolescents have been shown to favour drop-in clinics where anonymity is assured to their family GP.

Adolescents like being seen by the nurse they know (Norwich Union 2002). Nurse-led clinics and nurse specialists or practitioners can develop good relationships with young people and help them prepare for transition and transfer to adult services (see below).

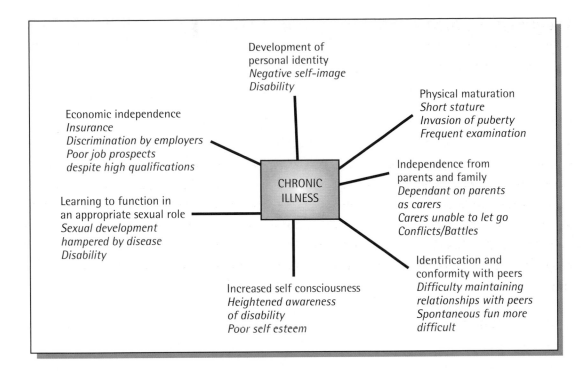

Figure 9.1 Impact of disease on development

Much work is needed to change current methods of treatment which are often paternalistic. Involving the young person in negotiating treatments, giving them ownership and encouraging decision-making is a way forward.

DEDICATED CLINICAL AREAS

Teenagers continue to be cared for in inappropriate clinical settings (e.g. adult or paediatric wards) despite their views on how and where they should be cared for (Norwich Union 2002). When health authorities were surveyed about current and future provision for adolescents, the majority had no plans for separate provision (Viner and Keane 1998).

Henderson *et al.* (1993) analysed admission rates in the Oxford region of adolescents between the ages of 10 and 19 years. Most admissions were for surgical rather than medical reasons. The single most common reason for male adolescents to be admitted was head injury and for female adolescent, it was to give birth or have a termination of pregnancy. These admissions were significant in that with increasing age, the adolescent was likely to be admitted to adult speciality areas such as obstetrics. This confirmed the view held by the National Association for the Welfare of Children in Hospital (NAWCH 1990), now called Action for Sick Children, that it may be difficult to place these patients according to age in a suitable ward. A dedicated clinical area is the answer.

The argument that there are insufficient numbers of adolescents in any hospital to warrant separate facilities is one that is convenient but not true (Audit Commission 1993; Viner and Keane 1998). A recent survey demonstrated that nurses find it difficult to care for young people and respect their individual needs when they are surrounded by either young children or old people (Norwich Union 2002).

Clinical settings dedicated to adolescents would be able to address the most important areas of care:

- privacy
- confidentiality
- promoting autonomy
- dignity and respect
- holistic approach to care
- education
- leisure
- information and advice.

It could be argued that all patients deserve this. The only dedicated adolescent medicine service unit in London that has addressed these needs for young people, despite the obstacles, deserves praise. If a unit is to cater to the needs of young people, it must incorporate their views (de Sousa 1999). Adolescent units must have a charter, so that young people know what to expect from the team which cares for them, and house rules so that they know what is expected of them as inpatients (Baker 1996).

THE MULTI-PROFESSIONAL TEAM

Teamwork is essential for an holistic approach to health care. The ideal multi-professional team for adolescent care consists of:

- a doctor (dedicated to adolescent medicine)
- nurses (both child and adult trained, and mental health as a bonus)
- psychologists/psychiatry/psychotherapy
- teachers
- youth worker
- activity co-ordinators
- dedicated physiotherapy and occupational therapy

All members of the MDT should be able to contribute to the care of the adolescent.

When working as a member of a team, you remain accountable for your professional conduct, any care you provide and any omission on your part (NMC 2002a).

DISCLOSURE OF INFORMATION

The *Code of professional conduct* instructs us that the health care record must be used as a tool of communication within the team and that it should be written with the involvement of the patient whenever this is practical (NMC 2002a). At the one specialist unit in London, mentioned above, nurses have devised a questionnaire and assessment tool that is completed by the adolescent and then checked by the nurse. It has been found to be extremely useful in getting difficult information from young people. The adolescent then signs a contract of care which has been jointly planned by the team and young person.

Where there is an issue of child protection, you must act at all times in accordance with national and local policies. Unfortunately, there will always be occasions when an adolescent discloses information which must be shared with people outside the immediate team. This may happen in the acute situation in A&E or on the wards. There is a direct association between self-harm and abuse, including sexual abuse (Coleman and Hendry 1999). Therefore, any adolescent who presents to an A&E department with self-harm needs to have counselling and psychiatric help to find out if there is any history of abuse. Abuse, whether it is sexual or physical, must be investigated further. There is mandatory training for all staff who care for young people so that they can recognize signs, help the young person and know when to refer on. Also, as young people are vulnerable, police checks on all staff who care for them are mandatory.

This is where inter-agency working comes into its own. A hospital-based nurse will never have the information that is held in the community. Sharing of essential information, while not breaking the rules of confidentiality, is now mandatory (Laming 2003).

The sexual act is illegal under the age of 16, and when a young person discloses they are sexually active, the nurse must seek advice to help clarify the situation. All NHS trusts, both hospital and community based, must have a designated child protection contact.

REFLECTION POINT

Are you aware of local and national policies about child protection? Why do you think it is important for all nurses to be aware of policy regarding child protection?

TRANSITION FROM ADULT TO PAEDIATRIC SERVICES

The American Society of Adolescent Medicine defines transition as:

'the purposeful, planned movement of adolescents and young adults with chronic and medical conditions from child centred services to adult oriented health care systems'.

(Blum et al. 1993)

Adolescents who live with chronic illness such as renal disease or cystic fibrosis face a further hurdle: making the transition to adult services (Viner 1999). Greater numbers of children now survive such illnesses, often with a disability or signs of long-term effects of medication. Transferring these young people to large adult services, which often have scant resources and in some areas a lack of expertise in paediatric disease processes (Viner and Keane 1998; de Sousa 1998; Esmond 2000), is sometimes a daunting task.

All of these young people will have been cared for by expert paediatric teams, with few financial constraints. Patient numbers are small in paediatric practice compared with adult. Paediatric teams focus on growth and education, and adopt an holistic approach to care, but as Viner (1999) points out, neglect the development of autonomy and increasing adult behaviour. In contrast, adult services focus on reproduction and autonomy, but not on growth and family concerns.

The report of the House of Commons Health Select Committee (1998) concluded that:

'services for adolescents should be given greater priority. The transfer of young people, particularly those with special health needs, particularly from child to adult services requires specific attention'.

Transition is now an issue and various programmes for preparation for transition have been developed. Greater resources and training of all health care professionals is needed to ensure that transition is a smooth successful process for young people and their families. The issue of transition needs to be part of nursing, medical and allied profession education so that helping, and supporting children, adolescents and young adults to make the transfer becomes part of care.

Adult doctors are perceived to be reluctant to accept adolescents with chronic disease into their services, and paediatricians may be reluctant to let them go (Viner 1999; White 1997; Schidlow and Fiel 1990). There may be several reasons for this: many adult doctors may be unfamiliar with the pathology of congenital diseases; or there may be a reluctance to accept patients who have expensive treatment regimes and medication, e.g. frequent physiotherapy or growth hormone replacement therapy injections. Adult nurses may feel uncomfortable in the presence of questioning parents who have greater understanding and knowledge about the disease process and treatments than they do.

Walford (1996) accused paediatricians of, in the process of making life easier for their patients and families, putting their patients at risk of potential problems and failing to adapt to the long-term effects of their illness. Adult physicians have the resources and ability to discuss fertility and genetic issues which paediatricians do not offer to the adolescent. Post-transition groups who were interviewed indicated that they found it easier to talk to adult doctors about contraception, children and marriage (Pownceby 1996).

INFLUENCE OF SCHOOL

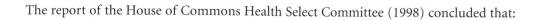

Adolescents with a chronic disease may spend long periods in hospital and this can interfere with normal development; they are isolated from their 'well' peers at school and home, and missing school can impede the development of independence and autonomy. McGinty and Fish (1996) point out that of the many transitions that an individual makes in a lifetime, the one from school through adolescence is the most important.

Adolescents who are moved to adult care while still in full-time further education may not be able to access teachers and tutorials, as the staff who provide education are not part of adult health care systems. Primary school teachers may often extend their role to covering secondary education when a teenager is a patient on a paediatric ward. This is despite the recommendations from the Department of Education and the National Health Executive (1994) which 'stressed the need for continuity in education for the sick or injured child'. Parents may also have negative views about education in the light of chronic life-threatening illness; in a study of chronically ill children, parents expressed serious concerns about their children's prospects for successful adult roles following interrupted periods of schooling (Luft and Koch 1998).

'The importance of school for children with chronic disease cannot be underestimated, it is often the yardstick by which the impact of the disease is assessed.'

(Eiser 1993, p46)

Fiorentino *et al.* (1998) reviewed the importance of schooling for disabled teenagers. Many viewed their school as their main source for socialization. This study commented on the abrupt end of this important part of their lives when they reached school-leaving age. Unlike their non-disabled peers, teenagers with special needs continue to have these needs in adulthood. Stevenson *et al.* (1997) reported on the lack of continuation of this service. Very often there is no provision for normal adolescent activity for teenagers with a disability and, as a result, many are often not only less mature, but also less confident and not equipped to deal with adult-orientated dilemmas (Eiser 1993). In addition, teenagers with a disability or chronic disease often miss out on work experience, as treatment regimes and lack of mobility may prevent them from taking part in this (White 1997).

HEALTH PROMOTION

'You must promote the interests of patients and clients. This includes helping individuals and groups gain access to health and social care information and support, relevant to their needs.'

NMC (2002a)

Smoking, drinking alcohol and teenage pregnancy continue to be issues among young people (Coleman and Hendry 1999). The government has promised to provide more education and advice in order to reduce and prevent adolescents from indulging in behaviours which pose a risk to their health. Nurses have a crucial role to play in helping adolescents maintain a healthy life style. Nurses who work in the community, particularly school nurses and nurses in general practice, are best placed to address the health needs and risk behaviours of young people. Good practice, like the drop-in clinics service for schools (Stansfield 2001), must be supported and replicated.

The Adolescent Health Forum of the Royal College of Nursing calls for nurses in the primary sector to:

- recognize the unique difficulties young people have in accessing services and seek creative alternatives for its provision, ensuring youth friendly environments
- ensure public health and health promotion activities are inclusive of diversity, i.e. gender, ethnicity, disability, sexuality, refugee status and socio-economic status
- support multi-agency partnerships
- receive training that explores attitudes, develops skills and knowledge of this age group relevant to the school, home or practice setting.
- support the development of health and social care research that identifies gaps in service provision and 'best practice' (RCN 2002).

Unfortunately, health promotion is largely planned by adults with little reference to adolescents and little understanding that the concepts of health for adolescents are not the same as for older people (Coleman and Hendry 1999).

NURSE EDUCATION IN ADOLESCENT CARE

Current nursing curricula do not address adolescence. In the author's own practice, only nurses who have undergone the Mental Health (RMN) programme are well equipped to care for adolescents.

The author constantly meets nursing students and newly registered nurses who do not understand the issues that arise when caring for adolescents. Perhaps, the time is right for institutes of learning to look at this omission and address it. Nurses who have trained on the adult branch often care for adolescents in the A&E department, but they do not receive any formal education or training that focuses on adolescence. There is also an opinion that all health care professionals may need specific training so that they can care for this distinct group (de Sousa and Needham 2002).

Many universities have developed modules which do address this gap in nurse education. This is not the answer, however, as these modules are costly and difficult for nurses to access, particularly if the trust they work for does not view such training as a priority. Adolescent development, and its related issues, must be included in the curriculum for both child and adult branch education. A pathway to the first adolescent health degree in the UK has been launched. This is good news for nurses who wish to focus on the care of young people.

CONCLUSION

This chapter has tried to engage the reader in the interesting world of adolescents. It is hoped that after reading this, young people will not be dismissed as non-adherent or difficult. They have distinct health care needs which have largely been ignored. Adolescents should not be cared for inappropriately on paediatric or adult wards, they deserve dedicated clinical settings. They deserve nurses who have had specific training to recognize their needs and development. To understand their concept of health, this intense challenging period of development must be taken into consideration. Young people need to be respected, and given more information and time so that they can become autonomous and make sensible decisions about their health and lives. Nurses need to recognize the legal aspects of caring for young people. This area of caring is dependent on a multi-professional team approach and services must be seen to be accessible, friendly, non-judgemental and confidential.

CHAPTER 10

CARE DELIVERY: THE NEEDS OF THE MATURE ADULT

Jacqueline Elton

INTRODUCTION

Pre-registration nurses are required to care for people of all ages and nationalities. They experience a wide range of health and illness. Following registration, nurses may decide to specialize in one particular field of nursing; this is often determined by either medical pathology or age. This chapter explores some of the fundamental issues which influence the care delivered to mature adults.

Three patient vignettes are used to consider not only physical care but also the psycho-social and cultural factors, which impact on care. It should be noted that many of the themes which arise – communication, confidentiality, consent and lifestyle – will be common to any age range, and as such you should not limit yourself to thinking the issues discussed only apply within the narrow age range covered here.

The chapter will also demonstrate how the guiding principles and competencies of the United Kingdom Central Council for Nursing, Midwifery and Health Visiting (UKCC 2001a) requirements for pre-registration nursing programmes have direct application in clinical practice.

The mature adult is, for convenience, considered to be an adult between the ages of 40 and 60. Every mature adult, regardless of age, is unique, having different life experiences, different care requirements and different expectations of their care in the event that they come into contact with the health and social care services.

It should be noted when caring for individuals within this age range, that many junior nurses may be caring for patients the age of their parents, friends or even themselves. In the past, the need for professional detachment was much discussed. We now talk in terms of holistic care, of becoming more involved in the patients' experiences. However, the need for a degree of detachment is still as relevant. If we over-identify with patients it may not always be possible to give the best advice or treatment, as we can become too close to the problem. Professional distance is not to say nurses do not care; it is about being able to engage in and then disengage from an appropriate therapeutic relationship which will benefit both the patient and the nurse, as noted in competency 2.

CHANGING PATTERNS OF HEALTH CARE

Ideally, the provision of health care within the NHS is both equitable and equal. In other words, all people, irrespective of who they are and where they live, will have the same level of, and access to, high quality services. Unfortunately, this is not always the case. The inverse care law (Tudor Hart 1971) postulates that the greater the need for care within a given population the poorer the provision and access.

The *Independent Inquiry into Inequalities in Health* (Acheson 1998) noted that death rates have fallen among men and women over the last 20 years across all social groups. However, the difference between class 1 and class 5 (see Table 10.1) has widened, with shorter life expectancy for both men and women in social class 5 compared to social class 1. It also noted that premature mortality (before age 65) is higher among individuals from lower social classes. The report identified that people from many ethnic minority groups have higher than average mortality rates, e.g. they are twice as high in infants of mothers born in Pakistan and the Caribbean Commonwealth as compared to the national average. The *National Service Frameworks for both Coronary Heart Disease* (DoH 2000d) and *Diabetes* (DoH 2001o) also clearly indicate inequalities in both mortality and morbidity.

Table 10.1 Registrar General's classification of social class (OPCS 1980)

Class	Example
I Professional	Doctor
II Managerial	Senior manager
III Skilled manual/non manual	Secretary
IV semi-skilled	Assembly line worker
V unskilled	Labourer

In addition to these clear inequalities, there is the demographic shift, which must inevitably affect the service. Put simply, the demographic shift refers to the ageing population within the UK. In 1961, around 12% of the population was aged 65 or over and 4% was 75 or over. By 1997, this had increased to 16% and 7%, respectively (Office for National Statistics 1999). The ageing population, with more people living to a greater age outside the extended family, will increase demands on health and social care services. At the same time, the percentage of the working population, and thus those paying taxes towards health and social care services, becomes proportionately smaller. By the year 2021, 20% of the population will be over the age of 65.

Health care is also becoming more technological, with interventions that would have been impossible 20 years ago now being seen as mainstream. An example is surgery to correct cardiac abnormalities *in utero*; such advances are costly and are an additional pressure for health care providers.

GOVERNMENT INITIATIVES

The NHS Plan (DoH 2000a) is the most recent major plan for investment in, and reform of, the NHS. It outlines a long-term vision for UK health care provision in the 21st century and highlights a number of key initiatives, which will impact on the care nurses and medical staff are expected to deliver. Some of the key areas are listed in Box 10.1.

Box 10.1 Key initiatives identified in *The NHS Plan* (DoH 2000c)

- Extra beds in both hospital and primary care
- New hospital build programme
- Modernization of GP premises
- Introduction of the modern matron – a visible assertive figure who supports ward sisters in delivering services and to whom the public can turn for help and support
- Better hospital food – this is in response to the public request for better hospital food coupled with research indicating that malnutrition can occur when patients are in hospital (Wise 1997)
- More nurse training and medical school places to meet the current shortfall in trained nurses and doctors
- Modern information technology (IT) systems – the NHS currently runs a wide variety of information technology systems, many of which are incompatible with one another. By having modern IT systems, the plan anticipates that service delivery will be both faster and more convenient for patients. This includes electronic booking of appointments (to save the current paper trail), electronic prescribing (the GP surgery links directly to the dispensing pharmacy) and electronic patient records in 75% of hospitals and 50% of primary care trusts by 2004
- New skills and roles for nurses, this includes the new nurse consultant role, the introduction of the 'modern matron' and the Chief Nursing Officer's 10 key roles
- Initiatives to standardize and raise services to a minimum acceptable level, e.g. *National Service Framework for Mental Health* (DoH 1999c), *Coronary Heart Disease* (DoH 2000a), *Older People* (DoH 2001e) and *Diabetes* (DoH 2001b), with more in the pipeline
- Greater public and patient involvement in health care; this means the establishment of patient advocacy and liaison services (PALS) in all trusts, which will act to advise patients if they are having difficulty using health care services

Within *The NHS Plan*, the National Institute for Clinical Excellence (NICE) is a recently established body which has the remit to examine the evidence for the efficacy and efficiency of NHS treatments and to recommend their use, or otherwise, within the NHS. This should address the inconsistencies within, for example, prescribing patterns. One of the inconsistencies within prescribing is the so-called postcode lottery: if you live in one area of the country, it is possible to get certain forms of treatment, whereas if you live in another nearby area, treatment may not be available.

EXERCISE

How would you address the issue of a patient, or patient's family, wanting to know why they could not receive a treatment which medical staff have indicated would be beneficial but are unable to pre-scribe within your geographical location?

The nurse is not in a position to prescribe. If the health authority has taken this decision about the treatment, there is nothing the nurse can do to alter the intervention. Instead concentrate on advising the patient of both their rights and avenues of influence which may be open to them, such as pressure groups and the community health councils. Also consider who would be most appropriate to speak to the patient.

The NHS Plan includes the Chief Nursing Officer's 10 key roles which all relate to expanding the role of the nurse better to meet the needs of patients (see Box 1.3). As a nurse, it is important to consider the possible implications of these changes for the patterns of health and illness. However, in the majority of cases, patients are unlikely to consider these aspects of society, health and illness. They will be more concerned with the more immediate effects of their illness. They will wish to have access to services when they become ill and to be treated in comfortable, clean surroundings by staff who have time for them, their problems or anxieties. They will want to be cared for by nursing and medical staff who have good technical knowledge, good inter-personal skills, can engage with them and have the ability to 'do a good job.'

SUMMARY

- Nursing is delivered within an ever-changing environment. Key changes within society are the demographic shift and changing public expectations.
- The key government documents which will guide service change over the next 5–10 years are *The NHS Plan* (DoH 2000a) and the National Service Frameworks (NSFs).

CASE STUDIES

Three case studies are presented. Each considers, in broad outline, the physical care requirement and then, in more detail, the core elements that determine the patients' experience. These cases have been selected to represent a range of 'typical' yet diverse patients and their families. By considering both acute and chronic illness in the hospital and in primary care, a wide range of issues can be examined. However, it should be noted that most of the issues examined will have a degree of application in all the cases outlined and also to many of the patients a student will care for in the course of qualifying as a registered nurse.

CASE STUDY 1: MRS PATEL

Scenario Mrs Patel is a 56-year-old Asian lady, who has lived in the UK for the past 5 years in a traditional household where she has very little contact outside the family and local Asian community. She speaks no English, although she is fluent in three Asian languages. She is married, lives within an extended family, which consists of her husband, grandparents and three children.

She has been admitted to the coronary care unit (CCU) and is diagnosed as having had an anterior myocardial infarction (MI). She has no previous cardiac history. Her recovery is uneventful and she is transferred to a general medical ward after 48 hours and discharged home at 7 days with follow-up by a cardiac rehabilitation nurse.

What is a myocardial infarction?

An MI is one type of coronary heart disease, commonly referred to as a 'heart attack'. Although the heart may stop beating during a heart attack (cardiac arrest), this is often not the case, although some patients believe that a heart attack and a cardiac arrest are the same thing. Coronary heart disease kills more than 110,000 people a year in England; of these 41,000 are under the age of 75. Around 300,000 people have an MI each year (DoH 2000d). Death from coronary heart disease is three times more likely in unskilled working men than in men in professional or managerial occupations. As such, coronary heart disease can be seen to reflect the inequalities in health outlined above. There is also ethnic variation in the incidence of heart disease, with people from the Indian sub-continent having a disproportionately high mortality: the death rate is 38% higher for men and 43% higher for women than for the UK as a whole.

An MI causes tissue within the heart to be damaged due to an interruption of the blood supply to that area of the heart. This results in the heart beating less effectively while recovery takes place. If the damage is extensive, scar tissue forms in the muscle of the heart so it may not regain its former efficiency.

Predisposing factors. These are believed to be the increasingly processed, high sugar, high fat diet and increasingly sedentary lifestyle which can lead to obesity, and smoking. The new *Coronary Heart Disease National Service Framework* (DoH 2000d) sets out clear targets to help individuals who wish to give up smoking.

Symptoms. The symptoms at onset will typically be pain in the central chest, which radiates down the left arm; the pain may be described by the patient as crushing. Signs of shock, with a rapid irregular pulse, falling blood pressure and shortness of breath may accompany this. For a diagnosis of MI to be made, there will also be changes in the patient's electrocardiogram (ECG) and raised cardiac enzymes. At least two of these three symptoms need to be present for the diagnosis to be confirmed and, importantly, it is possible for some people to be having an MI without complaining of any central chest pain. Sometimes they report feeling as though they are suffering from indigestion.

Physical care

The key points for the immediate physical care of an individual being admitted with an MI are analgesia, stabilization of the condition, possible thrombolysis and rest to relieve the work of the damaged myocardium. Diagnostic tests include:

- electrocardiogram (ECG) (Box 10.2): indicates where the cardiac damage has occurred and gives an indication of the degree of damage; however, it is not 100% effective and changes may not occur until sometime after the event

- cardiac enzymes: these are enzymes released when cells are damaged and they increase markedly when an MI has occurred. It is noteworthy that some cardiac enzymes are less specific and will be elevated in the event of other trauma, including bruising or knocking oneself. Cardiac enzymes are typically assessed on admission, at 6 hours and again at 24 hours. The troponen T test is more cardio-specific and will only show an increase in the event of the myocardium being affected

- urea and electrolytes, and full blood count (normal ranges listed in Table 10.2): these are standard blood tests where the levels of the various components within the blood are measured. Variation in these may give information about the cause of a cardiac (or other) irregularity.

Box 10.2 The electrocardiogram

The 12-lead ECG is carried out on the ward or the coronary care unit in the event of suspected MI or a patient developing chest pain. An ECG is a graph of the electrical activity within the heart. As the muscles of the heart contract, a small electrical current is detectable. This is what is recorded by the ECG. To perform an ECG the leads are attached to the limbs and chest as shown. It is important to ensure good adhesion of the electrodes, otherwise a poor quality trace will result; for the same reason it is important that the patient remains still and is as relaxed as possible as muscle activity from anywhere in the body will be detected by the ECG.

The position of the leads give a trace which is a two-dimensional representation of the three-dimensional heart; this requires skill to interpret. The trace illustrated here is a normal heart rhythm, and the key features that the non-specialist would look for is regularity, i.e. does the trace look the same all the way through?

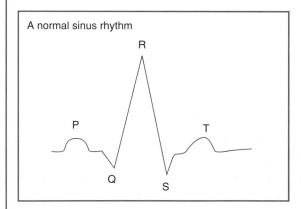

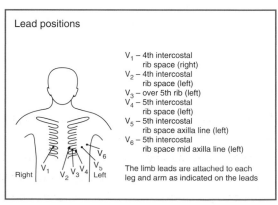

Each part of the trace indicates electrical activity within the heart; this electrical activity results in muscle activity, so for depolarization read contraction.

P wave: depolarization of the atria

QRS wave: depolarization of the ventricles

R wave: repolarization of the ventricles (getting ready to contract again); the repolarization of the atria is masked by the QRS complex

Table 10.2 Normal ranges for full blood count and urea and electrolytes

Full blood count	Urea and electrolytes
Hb 11.5–18 g/dL	Sodium (Na) 133–142 mmol/L
White cells 4–11 × 10^9/L	Potassium (K) 3.3–5.3 mmol/L
Platelets 150–400 × 10^9/L	Urea 2.5–6.5 mmol/L
Neutophils 40–75% × 10^9/L	Creatinine 60–120 mcmol/L
	Glucose 3.5–5.5 mmol/L

As a nurse, it is important to have knowledge of the typical values of the commonly used blood tests in a given clinical area. The nurse is usually with the patient more than the medical staff and is in a better position to observe changes in physical condition, which can then be related to the investigations. It could be argued that such knowledge is part of the medical remit rather than that of nursing, since it will typically require a medical intervention to initiate treatment. However, it can be argued that such knowledge is actually an illustration of competency 2 h, noting the need to be able to use and recognize knowledge from other disciplines – for the benefit of patient care.

In the immediate period post-admission, a number of interventions are likely:

- rest
- constant monitoring of heart rate and rhythm
- analgesia
- oxygen.

Analgesia is important and is likely to include an opiate, such as diamorphine, in the first instance, to give rapid pain relief; this is often paired with an antiemetic. Glyceryl trinitrate (GTN) may also be given to reduce cardiac workload, thus reducing pain. If not already receiving it, patients are often given aspirin on arrival in A&E or the CCU, not as an analgesic, but because of its antiplatelet activity – typically the dose would be 300 mg.

Psychological care

It can be argued that to consider physical and psychological care separately is unreasonable, given that nurses strive to achieve an holistic approach to care. Here they are separated to allow the development of themes, but in the case of a real patient they are inextricably linked.

It is noteworthy that psychological adjustment to a diagnosis of coronary heart disease is often problematic: 15–25% of patients remain depressed for long periods post MI (Lewin 1997) and 20–58% have relationship and sexual problems (Lewin *et al.* 1998).

When Mrs Patel arrives in the hospital, she is likely to be in pain. She has never been in hospital before, so the pain, the new environment and being unable to speak English will increase her level of anxiety and possibly that of her family. To care adequately for Mrs Patel, it is vital for the nurses to be able to communicate effectively. Without communication how do you obtain her consent for procedures, how do you provide access to rehabilitation and, at the very basic level, how does she make her needs known and how do you determine if she is in pain or not?

EXERCISE

How would you facilitate communication with Mrs Patel and how would you obtain her consent for a procedure such as insertion of a peripheral cannula?

Communication. The need to communicate is central to effective delivery of healthcare and is implicit within all the competencies for entry to the register (UKCC 2001a). Without communication many aspects of assessment, planning and evaluation of care are impaired. Without communication how is it possible to know if the nurse is respecting the patient's cultural and spiritual needs? Communication can be both verbal and non-verbal. Verbal communication is the spoken word, but even this may not be straightforward. It is important to take note of someone's background when considering the language which is used. An example would be the contrast between professional language and everyday language, e.g. asking a patient if they have 'passed stool' may not be understood as asking them if they have opened their bowels. It is important to identify the patient's first language. Even if the patient appears to understand some English, it would be inappropriate to assume full and clear understanding.

Non-verbal communication should also be considered, as this component often has more meaning and significance than the spoken word. An example would be to ask a patient if they are feeling well or if they have any problems. They may say, 'Yes, I feel fine nurse, no problems', but if they are sitting with arms and legs tightly crossed, avoiding eye contact with you and growling the response, there is a clear difference between their verbal and non-verbal cues. Generally, non-verbal cues are regarded as being the accurate indicator of what a person feels.

EXERCISE

With a partner face each other and have a short conversation (the subject matter is irrelevant – it can be your next holiday if you wish). Get a third person to watch the conversation and keep notes of the body language displayed by both participants. At the end of the conversation feed this back. Repeat the exercise switching roles.

Next repeat the exercise using inappropriate body language, i.e. avoiding eye contact, shuffling. Afterwards discuss how the different body language made you respond to one another.

Another good exercise is to observe someone you regard as a good communicator, to see how they use body language to put someone at ease, i.e. eye contact, placing themselves on the same level as the patient, reflecting back the patients' statements. It is also interesting to watch a poor communicator and see what it is that makes their communication skills poor.

In Mrs Patel's case it is necessary to gain access to an interpreter. Interpreter services may not be readily available in the language required, and even if they are accessible, they are unlikely to be available 24 hours a day at short notice, e.g. if Mrs Patel wants a cup of tea or to visit the bathroom. In such cases there is a temptation to use either family or other hospital staff as interpreters. However, this may create difficulties in terms of both confidentiality and consent.

Confidentiality. As a nurse you have a duty to respect the confidentiality of patient information gained. Clause 5.1 of the *NMC Code of professional conduct* (NMC 2002a) sets out the nurse's duty of confidentiality (see also Chapter 4). There have been a number of cases of nurses losing their registration for divulging patient information inappropriately.

EXERCISE

Which, if any, of the following three circumstances represent a breach of confidentiality by the nurse?

- Mrs Patel's son asks you to explain his mother's condition and prognosis.
- You discuss Mrs Patel's case with a friend who is also a nurse.
- In an unrelated case, a former patient of yours is arrested and charged with an offence which the police believe he may have discussed with you. They request information from you which you gained in the course of looking after the patient?

It could be argued that a breach of confidentiality has occurred in all three cases. Mrs Patel's son has no right to access information about his mother's condition – unless she gives her consent. In the event that Mrs Patel has given consent for her son to receive information, how has that consent been obtained? If the nurse has asked Mrs Patel, via her son, if she minds information being given out, what certainty is there that the translation and its feedback have been accurately relayed by her son? At ward level practicality often means that family members are used to interpret, but this needs always to be approached with a degree of caution.

If the nurse in the second circumstance is working in the same area and you are discussing professional management issues, it may be argued that this is a continuation of care for Mrs Patel. However, any discussion of a patient with an individual not related to their care is a breach. Thus, a discussion of who did what for whom on the bus on the way home is wholly unacceptable.

The third circumstance is less clear cut. Referring back to the *Code of professional conduct*, confidentiality can be broken 'if it is in the public interest or by a court order'. Some nurses are not best placed to decide what is in the public interest and the safest course of action may well be to refer the issue, e.g. to your senior manager or the trust's legal department.

Informed consent. Consent can be verbal, non-verbal or written. Implied consent may be assumed if, for example, the patient holds out their arm for a blood sample to be taken. However, even in such circumstance care needs to be taken – had the patient been expecting to have their blood pressure checked? Guidance from the Department of Health identifies the following factors as being required for a patient's consent to be valid (see also Chapter 4):

- patient must be competent to take that decision
- patient must have sufficient information to take that decision
- patient must not be acting under any duress (DoH 2001n).

An important point to emphasize is that a signature on a consent form is evidence that the patient has given consent, but not proof of valid consent.

In obtaining consent from Mrs Patel for any intervention, as noted earlier, in the absence of a professional interpreter, family members or other members of hospital staff are commonly used. The guidance from the Department of Health (DoH 2001n) states that it is inappropriate for children to act as interpreters. As discussed above, the use of a family member could violate the duty of confidentiality, although if Mrs Patel assents to the use of a family member, it could be argued she has given implied consent to the practice. However, when using a family member, there is no form of quality control, and as such, you are unable to establish whether translation is accurate.

When considering consent, it is important always to remember that 'any competent adult has the right to refuse treatment' (DoH 2001n) and that if the nurse is to advocate effectively for the patient, they may need to support the patient in this refusal, sometimes in the face of criticism from other health professionals.

Rehabilitation. As Mrs Patel recovers from her MI she will benefit from access to a cardiac rehabilitation programme. These vary widely around the country, but generally such a programme will include information on regaining former activity levels, preventing a further MI and general health education relating to diet and exercise. The World Health Organization (WHO 1993) recommends that cardiac rehabilitation programmes should include exercise training, relaxation and secondary prevention, and pay attention to the patient's psycho-social adjustment; the patient's partner and other family members should be included.

There is evidence that individuals from ethnic minorities are less likely to access cardiac rehabilitation programmes (Thompson *et al.* 1997) and that a lack of interpreter services, among other factors, means that the needs of patients from some ethnic minorities are not fully met (Tod *et al.* 2001). To be most effective such interventions need to be tailored to the needs of the individual patient and to their understanding of illness. For some people illness is seen as fate; it may be viewed as a punishment from a higher power, or it may be seen to be the result of a poor lifestyle. Unless the nurse becomes familiar with the implications of transcultural nursing and understands the meaning of illness for that patient, it will not be possible to provide optimal care.

SUMMARY

- Communication is central to care and where communication is impaired by, for example, a language barrier, the patient can be disadvantaged.
- Consent is a complex issue and the nurse must always be aware that *any competent adult* has the right to refuse any intervention.
- Illness can mean different things to different people, this being determined by experience, culture and background.

CASE STUDY 2: MRS SMITH

Scenario Mrs Smith is a 42-year-old lady with long-standing asthma who works in a textile factory. She smokes 5–10 cigarettes per day and has done since the age of 15. Over the past 5 years her asthma has worsened and chronic bronchitis has been diagnosed. She is currently taking inhaled steroids in addition to regular bronchodilators. She is a single parent with a 12-year-old son.

She has not previously required hospitalization, but has been admitted to a general medical ward, via the medical admissions unit, with an exacerbation of her chronic obstructive pulmonary disease (COPD) due to a chest infection. On arrival from the admissions ward she is receiving 40% oxygen with humidification and has regular nebulizers prescribed. She is expectorating thick yellow–green sputum and is receiving intravenous antibiotics.

What is airways disease?

Asthma is a chronic condition, where narrowing of the airways occurs in response to a stimulus, e.g. infection, allergy, exercise or unknown. When the airways narrow, breathing becomes increasingly laboured with expiration being particularly difficult; there is a typical wheezing sound on expiration. In the early stages, this narrowing is reversible using bronchodilators such as salbutamol. However, if the condition progresses, the airways become permanently thickened and narrowed. The next line of treatment is the addition of an inhaled steroid, e.g. beclomethasone, which reduces inflammation and makes the airways less sensitive to the stimulus, thus reducing the likelihood of an asthma attack.

As the condition progresses the degree of reversibility decreases and the loss of function becomes permanent. This is COPD – you may also hear it referred to as chronic obstructive airways disease (COAD).

Causes:

- Smoking (main cause)
- certain occupations, e.g. miners, furnace workers or grain workers
- childhood respiratory tract infections
- low birth weight
- low socio-economic status
- airway hyper-reactivity
- passive smoking (GOLD 2001).

It is estimated that smoking causes approximately 12,000 premature deaths per year (HEA 1998), of which a quarter are from lung cancer and around a fifth from COPD. COPD is rare in non-smokers and approximately 80% of the deaths from this disease can be attributed to cigarette smoking (HEA 1998). The prevalence of COPD in men in the UK appears to have peaked but the incidence in women continues to increase, which is probably linked to the continued increase in smoking among women. It has also been noted that children of patients who smoke have more respiratory diseases than those of non-smokers (Cook and Strachen 1997).

The NHS Plan (DoH 2000a) includes a major expansion of smoking cessation services with the aim of widening the availability of help to give up smoking. This includes making nicotine replacement therapy more widely available and requesting NICE guidance on the most appropriate and cost-effective prescribing regimes for smoking cessation. The target is that by the year 2010 at least 1.5 million people will have given up smoking. There is evidence that active interventions from health care professionals can increase smoking cessation rates (Lancaster *et al.* 2000).

Physical care

Mrs Smith will require humidified oxygen until her condition improves. High percentage oxygen is given as both the COPD and the super-imposed infection compromise oxygen exchange. It is possible for her to become hypoxic which would potentially impair mental functioning and cause further tissue damage. Oxygen needs always to be prescribed, since it is not without potential hazards, especially in individuals with COPD. Humidification of the oxygen keeps secretions loose to aid in their expectoration. If high percentage oxygen is not humidified, drying of the upper airway can result, leading to mucus plugs, which make for poorer gas exchange and impaired respiration.

When assessing Mrs Smith's breathing, a number of observations can be made.

- Respiratory rate – a healthy individual will generally have a respiratory rate of 12–14 breaths per minute; a much higher rate (over 20 is not uncommon) can be an indication of serious respiratory distress. The rate needs to be checked regularly, possibly 4 hourly to begin with, as an increase in rate could indicate that Mrs Smith's condition is deteriorating.

● Saturation – this is measured using a pulse oximeter and indicates the level of oxygen in the blood by means of an external probe. A healthy non-smoker will generally have a saturation of 96% or higher; if it is below this, monitoring is required. Some individuals with COPD will have saturations in the mid-to-high 80s and be quite well on this as their physiology has adapted to being chronically hypoxic.

● Are the accessory muscles being used to support respiration? If the patient is finding it particularly difficult to breathe, they may adopt the orthopnic position; this is sitting forward with arms resting on their knees or possibly the bed table. This position increases the available respiratory volume.

As part of the assessment of her physical needs, it is important to establish how Mrs Smith sleeps, not only in hospital, but also at home. Many patients with chronic respiratory difficulties sleep with three or more pillows in an upright position. While Mrs Smith is acutely short of breath, she will certainly benefit from being nursed sitting upright.

EXERCISE
Using a basic anatomy text, identify the locations and insertion points of the accessory muscles. This will enable you to recognize if the accessory muscles are being used in your assessment in any patient with respiratory difficulties.

A central part of the assessment process will be to determine what degree of help Mrs Smith needs with her activities of daily living. It is important to remember that a large part of her energy is going on the physical act of breathing and therefore she will not be able to function as she did before this acute episode of the illness. She is likely to require assistance with hygiene and elimination in the short term, as any exertion may exacerbate her breathlessness.

Since Mrs Smith has a chest infection she is receiving antibiotics. She may be pyrexial, in which case paracetamol will help to lower her temperature and keep her more comfortable. There are various non-pharmaceutical methods for lowering temperature: reducing the load of the bedclothes, ensuring good ventilation (not always easy in a ward bay where other patients may be feeling cold) or providing a fan. Tepid sponging is a possibility in the event that her pyrexia becomes more pronounced. It is worth noting that often when patients have a temperature, which is increasing, they will report feeling cold, or may even have rigors. This is because the part of the hypothalamus (the body's thermostat) that regulates body temperature has been temporarily 'reset' to a higher than normal temperature. This means the body will activate the mechanisms to raise temperature, e.g. muscle tremors, to reach the temperature dictated by the brain. The patient will only report feeling hot when the hypothalamus has been set back to normal temperature and the body recognizes that the temperature is too high. At this point the patient will state they feel hot, sweat and look flushed.

Monitoring of Mrs Smith's temperature indicates if the infection is beginning to settle. Regular monitoring of the respiratory rate gives early indication of any change. Observation of the sputum is also important as changes in its appearance and/or volume can indicate changes in condition. In some cases of severe chest infection, there may be blood in the sputum. Infected sputum can appear viscous and yellow–green in colour. Care should always be taken when handling any body fluid, due to the potential risk of infection. A sputum pot should always have a lid on, which is only removed briefly to observe the contents, and should be changed at least daily and the used pot disposed of according to the hospital's clinical waste policy. It is probable that sputum will be requested for culture and sensitivity (C&S). This laboratory test checks which antibiotics the infective organism is sensitive to, so as to ensure the patient is prescribed the correct antibiotics.

Monitoring peak flow readings or spirometry may also give an indication of both the degree of lung reversibility and overall function. A peak flow recording gives a measure of the lung elasticity, as it requires the individual to exhale as rapidly as possible, giving a reading in litres/minute exhaled.

As the infection resolves, Mrs Smith will come off the oxygen and hopefully revert to her normal medication with a view to returning home as soon as she is well enough. During this recovery phase it is important not to push Mrs Smith to do more than she is physically capable of. She is likely to be keen to go home as soon as possible, as she has a child and her job to return to. In many cases patients simply want to go home because hospitals are usually noisier than their own home, the food is not what they are used to and, as they recover, there is often very little for them to occupy themselves with.

Psychololgical care

As with Mrs Patel, the factors discussed here are inextricably linked to the physical care outlined previously.

Dignity and privacy. This is one of the benchmarks covered in *The Essence of Care* (DoH 2001f). This document aims to promote improvement in the delivery of the fundamentals of care. Mrs Smith is normally an independent woman, but for at least a few days she will need help washing, dressing and going to the toilet. There is an unfortunate tendency to regard the privacy curtains around hospital beds as being sound proof; they are not. Not only will Mrs Smith's neighbours hear everything you say to her (see the above discussion on confidentiality), but they will also hear when she uses the commode. In some individuals this can, unsurprisingly, lead to constipation as they will not be able to open their bowels when they know others can hear everything. If her breathlessness permits, it is far preferable that she is wheeled to the toilet. In either case, it is important to remember to give her the opportunity to wash her hands afterwards. It may be helpful to prescribe laxatives to prevent constipation, as straining to open her bowels could increase her breathlessness.

Mrs Smith is producing a large amount of sputum and expectoration may also be a cause of embarrassment to her. As a minimum she will need access to a clean sputum pot which is disposed of frequently (not forgetting to examine it first).

Health education. A number of areas of health education can be considered in the case of a patient with a chronic chest condition – some are more practical than others.

As Mrs Smith smokes, you can recommend strongly that she stops, but you cannot force her to. If she wishes to stop it is possible to obtain nicotine replacement patches or gum to reduce the stress of withdrawal; support is also available from the smoking cessation advisers now based in a number of hospitals and health centres. Many hospitals are now non-smoking areas, with very limited areas available for smokers to use (and possibly quite inaccessible when the patient is still unwell). It can be argued that the stress of being hospitalized makes it a particularly difficult time for someone to give up smoking. However, if no facilities for patient smoking are available, then very firm advice needs to be given as to the inadvisability of lighting up on the hospital ward. There is a clear risk management problem if a patient does smoke around oxygen, since it is highly flammable.

The involvement of the multi-professional team is vital for Mrs Smith, as she may benefit from pulmonary rehabilitation, which is run in some centres. A pulmonary rehabilitation programme enables the individual to move towards the best possible health condition and maximize their potential. Self-management education for individuals with asthma improves their health outcomes (Gibson *et al.* 1998).

Everyone admitted to hospital has an individual lifestyle. It is important not to judge this lifestyle or to expect that you can make them change their way of living. Nurses can advise on areas that may be deleterious to health and encourage change, but that is all. There are a number of aspects of Mrs Smith's lifestyle where health education may improve her health.

Mrs Smith works in a textile factory. This is likely to be a high dust environment which is not helpful for an individual with COPD. It may be that you discuss the possibility of changing job with Mrs Smith, as this may improve her health. However, Mrs Smith is a lone parent and probably needs to work to support both herself and her son. It may be that she is unqualified for a job elsewhere. If she has worked in the one area for some years it is probable that the majority of her friends and social acquaintances also work there. By recommending she change her job, you could be asking her to lose her social support network. Leidy and Haase (1999) describe the challenge to patients with COPD of maintaining their personal integrity given the changes in lifestyle and health forced on them by the disease.

Moving to a warm dry climate helps many chronic chest conditions; you can certainly suggest this to Mrs Smith and her son, but then all the previous concerns about losing her social network would apply. The expense of moving house and emigrating with a young child who is in school may not be feasible. In such cases, the best advice for health may be unachievable, even if the patient wishes to follow it.

The UKCC (2001a) competencies clearly identify the need to utilize appropriate opportunities to promote the health and well-being of patients and clients. The dilemmas presented by Mrs Smith's case are very real. Health education and suggestions for lifestyle changes can be clearly seen as being in the patient's best interest, but they are not always practicable and nurses need to be aware of these potential limitations and conflicts.

 Changes in self-image. Mrs Smith will have certain perceptions about her own self-image. That she has an acute-on-chronic condition must impact on this. She has seen her condition deteriorate over the past 5 years to the point where it is not curable and she has had to learn to live with it. Given the deterioration, it is likely she will be asking herself the question: 'What next – will I get worse?' These questions are not easy to answer; the nurse can say, 'Yes you are likely to get worse', but then what? The nurse needs to be able to offer something more constructive and, importantly, if asked a question of this type and unsure of the answer, needs to refer it to someone more senior. Far more damage will be done by providing an inaccurate or badly handled answer than by saying, 'I don't know but I will get someone else to come and talk to you'. The *Code of professional conduct* (NMC 2002a) and the registered nurse competencies (UKCC 2001a) both refer to 'recognizing one's own abilities and limitations'.

It is possible that Mrs Smith may undergo a form of bereavement reaction. Consider the four stages of grieving (Parkes 1986): shock and alarm; searching, anger and guilt, and gaining a new identity (see also Chapter 13). These stages identify a possible model to understand the phases an individual goes through when they, or a loved one, are dying. This can be applied to chronic illness where the loss of function and abilities are beyond the control of the individual or their family.

Once again, the answer may lie in accessing another member of the multi-professional team, a psychologist or counsellor, who can help Mrs Smith to accept changes in her body image.

Effects on children. Mrs Smith's son will perceive that his mother is different from other children's mothers if she becomes breathless when they play, or if she is unable to run with him. As Mrs Smith is a single parent her son will have to be cared for by someone else while she is in hospital. This may be a friend from work, another member of her family or even foster care via the social services. For any child this must give a degree of uncertainty: 'Will this happen again?', 'Is my mum going to be all right?' Zahlis (2001) found that the child of a mother with breast cancer does try to understand the situation and wonders what may happen in the future to them and the rest of the family. Brandt and Weiner (1998) studied families where one of the parents had multiple sclerosis and found that children in households with less adequate finances and more discord were at greater risk of mental ill-health than those in families with better finances and better relationships.

The nurse will need to facilitate Mrs Smith's son visiting if his mother is unable to arrange this. From a risk management point of view it would not be appropriate for ward staff to fetch her son. However, it would be entirely appropriate for nursing staff to liaise with friends, relatives or even the voluntary sector to facilitate visiting.

Community concerns. Within competency 1 (professional and ethical practice), the need 'to recognize one's own abilities and limitations is noted'; competency 3 (care management) notes the need 'to utilize contributions of the health and social care team' (NMC 2002a). Both these competencies clearly apply in relation to Mrs Smith's future planning, in that it may be advisable to ask Mrs Smith if she wishes to access a social worker. If her condition is likely to force her to alter her employment or affect how she is able to care for her son, the social worker is the member of the multi-professional team who has the greatest knowledge as to the available benefits or services.

Although it may not yet be required, there is the possibility that Mrs Smith may require home oxygen at some point in the future. This is usually ordered via the GP and can take the form of either cylinders (if oxygen is for fairly short periods each day) or an oxygen concentrator (if required for longer periods). Mrs Smith would need to be educated in respect of the dangers of smoking and oxygen. Support would also be required, as patients on home oxygen therapy can experience physiological and psychological difficulties (Ring and Davidson 1997).

SUMMARY

- In chronic illness, the effects on the individual extend beyond a single episode of care.
- Chronic illness can change how both the individual, and others, regard themselves.
- Health education should always be offered, but may be refused or ignored.
- The effects of parental ill health on children should always be considered.

CASE STUDY 3: MR JONES

Scenario Mr Jones is a 45-year-old married man who lives with his wife. They have no children. They live in a two-bed bungalow. Mr Jones gave up work as a policeman 18 months ago and Mrs Jones has just given up work to care for her husband.

Mr Jones was diagnosed with motor neurone disease (MND) when he was 43; he is now wheelchair bound and has an electric chair which he controls himself around the house and garden. He has an adapted car that will take him and his wheelchair, so he and his wife still go out together into the local town. They are supported in the community by a private home care daily who helps him to wash and dress.

The community nurse visits twice weekly to check his bowel movements. He is alert and fully orientated but has lost the use of both legs and has marked weakness in both arms; speech and swallowing are still unaffected.

You are visiting him with the community nurse who is making an additional visit to assess him for an upgrade in his pressure-relieving mattress.

EXERCISE

Using the activities of daily living (Roper *et al.* 1996; see Table 6.2) assess this patient. What key problem areas do you identify?

Caring for a patient like Mr Jones crosses all the boundaries of health and social care. It requires nursing skills of the highest order to provide not only physical but also emotional support to the family.

What is motor neurone disease?

MND is one of the most common neurodegenerative diseases of adult onset. There is currently no treatment that substantially slows the progression of the disease and the average survival period from the start of symptoms is about 3 years. The mean age of onset is 55 years (Shaw 1999). There are about 5000 people in the UK with the disease at anyone time (BBSF 2000).

MND causes progressive degeneration of the cells and nerves in the spinal cord and brain which control the muscles. Although the motor system is affected, the rest of the brain remains unaffected.

Symptoms. The commonest are:

- muscle weakness
- muscle wasting
- fasiculations – involuntary twitches of the muscle just under the skin
- muscle spasms
- difficulty in swallowing
- difficulty with speech.

As the symptoms are progressive they will often first be noted in one part of the body or one limb, but will spread with time. Death is usually the result of respiratory failure due to the weakness of the ventilatory muscles (Shaw 1999).

If Mr Jones is assessed using the activities of daily living (Roper *et al.* 1996), deficits will be identified in most areas, with both he and his wife needing physical and psychological support.

Physical care

Skin integrity. As Mr Jones is wheelchair bound, the sacral pressure areas will be at high risk when he is seated. Also, as he has marked weakness it is unlikely he will move himself a great deal in bed. This means that in the pressure area re-assessment, both seating and bed-relief need to be considered.

The Waterlow score (Waterlow 1985; see also Chapter 6) is a commonly used scoring system based on a variety of indicators which influence the chance of an individual developing a pressure sore. There is some debate as to its accuracy, with some authors claiming it over-estimates the risk of a sore developing (Wardman 1991). It should be noted that a pressure sore risk assessment tool is not intended to be used in isolation but in conjunction with other documentary evidence and the nurse's own clinical judgement (Waterlow 1994).

Depending upon the risk assessment outcome, appropriate preventative equipment will be ordered by the community nurse. The prevention of pressure sores is both a financial and care necessity. It has been estimated that to heal a single Grade 4 pressure ulcer in hospital can cost £40,000 (Hibbs 1988); the patient will also suffer additional discomfort. A wide variety of preventative equipment is available, which Mr Jones may already have in his home. Hospital beds can be supplied to patients in the community, both for their own comfort and that of those caring for them. There is a clear need to eliminate and prevent environmental hazards where possible. The height of a typical divan may be as little as 60 cm, which is a very low height to nurse someone at and as such a risk to both patient and nurse.

Pressure-relieving mattresses and cushions come in a variety of grades, from low risk for an individual who has intact skin and the ability to move independently, to very high risk for patients who have no ability to move themselves and/or with existing sores. There is clear evidence that products designed to prevent or cure pressure ulcers are more effective than a standard hospital mattress, but less clear evidence as to which is the most effective (Cullum et al. 2000). By visiting Mr Jones to re-assess his needs for pressure-relieving equipment, the nurse will be addressing competency 2 which relates to care delivery. It must be noted that in some areas the availability of pressure-relieving equipment is sub-optimal (Jones et al. 1999), so even if the assessment indicates a need for an increased level of equipment, there may be a delay in obtaining it.

It is important to be sure that both Mr Jones and his wife and the private home carers are aware of interventions to prevent pressure sore formation. Mrs Jones and other carers need to taught safe and effective moving and handling techniques. If Mrs Jones were to become injured, Mr Jones may no longer be able to remain at home.

Pain management. This may be an issue for Mr Jones, as muscle spasm can be a symptom of MND. Drugs such as baclofen are used to control spasticity and quinine sulphate can be used to treat muscle cramps. Some people find that tonic water is effective in relieving muscle cramps as this contains small amounts of quinine. Pain may also result if Mr Jones becomes constipated which is one reason why good bowel management is important. For patients with MND it is important to remember that, although they have a degenerative neurological condition, it is the motor nerves that are affected, not the nerves of sensation, so there is not normally loss of sensation.

Elimination. The ability to urinate and open the bowels can be affected by MND. Mr Jones has a long-term indwelling catheter and twice weekly visits by the community nurse to maintain his elimination functions. The indwelling catheter puts Mr Jones at increased risk of urinary tract infection. The risk can be reduced by ensuring good intake of fluids, at least 2000 ml per day. Catheter hygiene is also important; a daily shower ensures the area is well washed and limits the risk of infection. If Mr Jones is unable to do this, then twice daily catheter toilet with clean water is satisfactory. This is likely to be undertaken by his wife, so again there is the need for the community nurse to ensure the procedure is being safely performed.

Mr Jones is likely to become constipated due to a number of factors:

- immobility
- possible change in diet
- medication
- weakened pelvic floor muscles.

Realistically, nothing can be done to increase his level of mobility, but the nurse and other members of the multi-professional team can encourage both him and his wife to make the most of the mobility that he does have. Similarly, nothing can be done to strengthen weakened muscles in the pelvic floor. A high fibre diet, e.g. plenty of fruit, vegetables and wholemeal bread, and good fluid intake both help towards regular bowel functioning. The dietician would be able to advise on such matters.

Useful aids. Other adaptations/pieces of equipment which are available include:

- a hoist if Mr Jones becomes unable to transfer, e.g. from bed to chair, without help
- adapted cutlery
- bath aids
- hand rails and ramps to ease access to the house
- stair lifts
- communication aids, including speech synthesizers.

EXERCISE

People who use wheelchairs report that when they are out shop assistants talk over them to the person pushing the chair and that many places are not accessible. If possible, borrow a wheelchair and get pushed around the hospital or your local shopping area and observe how strangers respond to you? Is it any different from how they respond to you normally?

Psychological care

The psychological care is for the whole family. Mr and Mrs Jones will have seen a major change in their lifestyle over the past 2 years: Mr Jones had to give up work due to his illness and Mrs Jones has just given up work to care for her husband. This is likely to have a financial impact on the family and advice from a social worker is helpful to ascertain what social care help or financial assistance is available. The involvement of the social worker is a clear case of getting the best for the patient by utilizing inter-professional working practices, as noted in competency 3 (care management). Since the social worker, the GP, the community nurse, the physiotherapist, possibly the occupational therapist, dietician and psychologist will have input to Mr Jones' care, the need for accurate care planning and documentation cannot be over-emphasized. It is possible that at some point Mr Jones will be admitted to hospital. Good documentation following him into hospital is more likely to get his care needs addressed in a timely manner, rather than all assessments being repeated, which may take until he is ready to be discharged again.

As in Mrs Smith's case, both Mr and Mrs Jones are likely to be experiencing a bereavement reaction. Since Mr Jones was diagnosed 2 years ago, a period of adjustment may have taken place as both try to come to terms with the diagnosis. Even if both now accept the illness, they will be aware that further deterioration is inevitable. To this end, the possibility of involving the palliative care team should be considered. Palliative care is often referred to in relation to cancer, but it must be noted that MND is also a disease with a terminal prognosis. Much of the support required by terminally ill cancer patients is equally applicable to patients with this type of rapidly degenerative neurological disease. In many cases, in the later stages of the disease, hospice input in either an inpatient or outpatient capacity is helpful.

Although Mr Jones' physical needs – to be kept clean, to eat, to drink – are being met by carers, the impact on him of having these intimate and basic tasks performed by others must not be overlooked. It is also important that other friends and acquaintances realize that his hearing, sight and mental faculties are unaffected. The possibility of a psychologist having input to Mr and Mrs Jones may be worth considering if they are willing, as once again health care staff can only offer help, it cannot be forced on people.

When considering the psychological difficulties which are likely to be faced by Mr and Mrs Jones, it is worth noting that the multi-professional team also faces stress caring for individuals with rapidly progressive debility (Carter *et al.* 1998) and needs to ensure it has its own support mechanisms.

EXERCISE

You are caring for a patient where both you and they are aware that they are terminally ill. The patient asks you to promise not to tell anyone and then informs you of their intention to commit suicide upon discharge from hospital. They intend to do this because they wish to die with dignity at a time of their choosing rather than risk pain and loss of dignity. How would you respond?

SUMMARY

- To provide effective care the multi-professional team needs to work across health and social care boundaries.
- When caring for patients with a terminal prognosis (or any other), the nurse must remember their own needs for support.
- Ethically it is not always possible to meet the requests patients may make.

APPLICABILITY OF THE COMPETENCIES TO PRACTICE

Each of the competencies has applicability to each of the three cases discussed above; what follows makes the relationship between practice and the competencies explicit.

Competency 1 (professional and ethical practice)

This requires that a nurse acts in accordance with the *Code of professional conduct* (NMC 2002a) and recognizes their own limitations. The case studies clearly show that there is a need to hand elements of the patient's care over to other professionals when the knowledge required is not that of nursing. Also apparent in the cases is the necessity of acknowledging limitations within nursing practice or knowledge. No damage will be caused to the patient by saying 'I don't know, but I'll find out', whereas mishandling a communication or a procedure can do irreparable harm. The need to maintain confidentiality and act in the patient's interest appears clear-cut when written down, but as demonstrated in Mrs Patel's case, the situation can be less clear in real life.

The need to practice in fair and anti-discriminatory ways, while acknowledging differences in belief and culture, can also be more difficult with a real patient. The majority of trained nurses within the NHS are white, but in some areas of the country the patient caseload can be very different – 27% of the population is non-white in the city of Leicester. To this end it is important that nurses take the opportunity to study the culture of the communities they care for.

Caring for a patient like Mr Jones can raise difficult ethical issues. The recent case of Diane Pretty, who had advanced MND and who took her case to the European Court of Human Rights to gain permission for her husband to assist her to commit suicide, is a case in point (see Chapter 4). Mrs Pretty lost her case and has since died, but the ethical dilemma remains – the patient was quite clear she wished to die, but legally her wishes could not be granted.

Competency 2 (care delivery)

This has eight interdependent categories. The need to develop a therapeutic relationship is central to all three case studies. In some cases, the nurse may find that an effective therapeutic relationship eludes them. It would be wrong for the nurse automatically to assume they are a poor nurse, rather they should consider if they could have tried a different approach and review if other patient interactions are more effective. (If none of the nurse's interactions lead to an effective therapeutic relationship then, possibly, the problem lies entirely with the nurse and some urgent clinical supervision or guidance needs to be sought!)

The need to promote well-being and health is central to Mrs Smith's vignette. It is important to remember that a patient has a life both before and after they leave your care. Sometimes the choices that the patient makes do not meet the recommendations of the nurse. However, this is the right of the patient, providing they have been given all relevant information so they can make an informed choice as to whether or not to take the advice. If the nurse has provided the information in a form the patient is comfortable with, and can understand, then whatever the patient's decision, it can be argued that the nurse has discharged their responsibilities appropriately. All the nurse can do is to advise, not compel.

By providing a supportive non-threatening environment when caring for the patient, by building up the therapeutic relationship and by providing practical help (i.e. advice on how to obtain nicotine replacement patches), advice for health promotion is more likely to be positively received.

The need for accurate assessment, care planning and documentation is central to effective care delivery in all the patients. Accurate documentation not only facilitates the effective delivery of care by the members of the multi-professional team, but it also permits retrospective assessment of care provision for audit/research purposes or to facilitate investigation of a complaint.

The use of evidence-based nursing practices and an ability to have sound clinical judgement, is also a key element within the case studies, since without the evidence base and the clinical judgement, how is it possible for the assessment and care planning process to take place?

Competency 3 (care management)

The four elements within this category are interdependent. The case of Mr and Mrs Jones identifies the need to utilize risk management tools in the assessment of Mr Jones' pressure areas, as it ensures that Mrs Jones has received appropriate training in manual handling. The provision of accurate documentation across inter-professional boundaries is another example of risk management.

Demonstration of the key skills of literacy and numeracy is also central to effective communication. The best care plan in the world is of no use if the nurse taking over care provision cannot read it!

Competency 4 (personal and professional development)

Although these areas are not explicit in the case studies, for a professional nurse such ongoing development should be implicit in all interactions in the workplace. Nursing is about dealing with people and each person is unique, which makes each interaction slightly different. Because of this uniqueness, there is opportunity to learn and reflect – could that situation have been handled any differently? Much of this reflection is informal, but nonetheless it provides an opportunity to develop.

The utilization of a clinical supervisor is to be recommended, as this provides the option of more formalized reflection, while still maintaining the confidentiality of the patient–nurse interaction.

Leadership does not mean the ward sister or the senior nurse. Leadership is a characteristic that every registered nurse can display. The nurse provides leadership and learning opportunities to the patient, if that is what the relationship requires, and to the health care assistants and students in a team, and helps to create an environment conducive to learning and caring.

CONCLUSION

As can be seen from the vignettes, caring for the mature patient has many challenges, not only those presented by the physical condition of the patient, but also those by the psychosocial condition of the patient and the demands of differing cultural expectations. The chapter has examined how the nurse meets the needs of these patients, and related this to the competencies required for entry to the nursing register. Each of the competencies applies in each of the vignettes either implicitly or sometimes explicitly; the competencies act as a framework within which practice develops.

Although the competencies inform and underpin the practice of every registered nurse, it is the unique personal and professional characteristics of that nurse, their interpersonal skills, their enthusiasm and their ability to care about the work they do that patients will respond to. In short, it is about wanting to do a good job and enjoying the work.

CHAPTER 11

CARE DELIVERY: THE NEEDS OF OLDER PEOPLE

Jacqueline Elton and
Jane Valente

INTRODUCTION

This chapter considers the care and treatment of the older adult, defined here as being over the age of 60. However, it should be noted that, as with the mature adult (see Chapter 10), the older adult is not a homogeneous population. Some individuals are running marathons at the age of 70, others may be requiring total nursing care due to multiple disabilities. Age is just one factor that needs to be taken into account when assessing and caring for any individual.

A series of linked vignettes follow an older couple (Mr and Mrs White) and their family over 2 years. Through this family the chapter examines how government policy affects the service these individuals receive, as well as examining the physical and psychological care they require. Their care needs are linked to the competencies required of the registered nurse (UKCC 2001a).

WHY DO WE AGE?

Evidence indicates that the maximum human lifespan is about 110 years (Wynsberghe *et al.* 1995). There is a range of biological theories to explain why we age and these divide into the whole organism theories and cellular theories (Rudd and Millard 1988). It is important to note that these are all theories, but that there is no one accepted theory; the only thing we know for certain is that we do age!

The whole organism theories are:

- wear and tear: ageing is the result of the gradual wearing out of non-replaceable parts
- accumulation: ageing is the result of the accumulation of waste products within the body
- neuroendocrine changes: ageing is thought to be due to changes in hormone levels
- immunological: there is evidence that with age the body is less able to mount a normal immune response, coupled with increasing autoimmunity.

The cellular theories are:

- random error: this considers that errors occur in the deoxyribose nucleic acids (DNA) due to either mutation or damage and this leads to the genetic material deteriorating
- error catastrophe: incorrect coding of DNA leads to deterioration of genetic material
- Hayflick phenomenon (Rudd and Millard 1988): it has been demonstrated that tissue cultures of fibroblasts undergo a set number of replications before dying. From this Hayflick suggested that there is a cellular clock controlling ageing
- free radical theory: free radicals are produced in greater numbers with increasing age and these cause damage by reacting with nucleic acids and proteins
- programmed theory: we have a programme controlled by our genes which dictates our ageing.

GOVERNMENT POLICY AND THE OLDER ADULT

As noted in Chapter 10, the population within the UK is ageing with the number of older people making up an increasing percentage of the population. Since the 1930s, the number of people over the age of 65 has more than doubled. Today, 20% of the population is aged over 60 and between 1995 and 2025 the number of people over the age of 90 will double (DoH 2001i). Older people also make up the largest single group using the health service: those over 65 account for two-thirds of hospital patients and 40% of all admissions (DoH 2000a). It is against these pressures and those identified in Chapter 10 that *The NHS Plan* (DoH 2000a) and the *National Service Framework for Older People* (DoH 2001i) have been produced to improve and raise the standards of care and service to older people.

The NHS Plan (DoH 2000a) notes the need to ensure dignity, security and independence in old age and intends to do this as follow.

- *Assuring standards of care.* The National Care Standards Commission targets standards of care within domiciliary and residential care, while the *National Service Framework for Older People* sets out standards for services, including stroke, falls and mental health problems.

- *Extending access to services.* This includes individuals being able to access extended health screening, such as a retirement health check to identify any potential problems. It also includes the introduction of the single assessment process. This means that for individuals who have complex needs, which include both health and social care requirements, only one joint assessment will be required, thus, in theory, streamlining and speeding the process whereby the person's needs are addressed. There will also be greater involvement of carers in the care planning process where appropriate and the personal care plan will be held by the patient/client or their carer. It will detail the health and social care details. For nurses, the extension of clinical leadership, with potential nurse consultants and nurse specialists for older people, is identified as an area for exploration.

- *Promoting independence in old age.* The plan identifies the need for people to be able to maintain independence with good quality ongoing support at home rather than needing to move into institutional care. It also identifies the need to extend intermediate care and rehabilitation services and what this will cost. Intermediate care is non-acute care where the patient has no acute illness requiring medical intervention, but requires intensive nursing or therapy interventions over a short period to enable them to regain an improved level of functioning. It is typically nursing or therapy-led. Such interventions can reduce so-called 'bed blocking', which is when a person (usually elderly) is occupying an acute bed when they have no acute medical or nursing requirements and are waiting for, possibly, equipment to be fitted at home or a place in a residential home or in a community hospital.

- *Ensuring fairness in funding.* If an individual needs to go into a nursing or residential home the situation with regard to funding (i.e. who pays for the care) has long been confusing and complicated. For example, a person receiving nursing care in an NHS hospital does not pay for it, but would have to pay for the same care in a nursing home. The plan will make the system fairer by ensuring that nursing care is funded, although individuals will still have to fund personal elements of care.

The *National Service Framework for Older People* (DoH 2001i) is a key document, which will enable elements of *The NHS Plan* (DoH 2000a) to become a reality. It specifically addresses those conditions which are significant to older people and have not been addressed by the other national service frameworks (NSFs). However, it should be noted that conditions such as stroke and falls are not limited to older people. The framework has eight standards (Box 11.1).

Box 11.1 Standards identified within the *National Service Framework for Older People* (DoH 2001i)

- *Standard 1: Rooting out age discrimination.* NHS services will be provided regardless of age, on the basis of clinical need alone. Social care services will not use age in their eligibility criteria or policies to restrict access to services.
- *Standard 2: Person-centred care.* NHS and social care services treat older people as individuals and enable them to make choices about their own care. This is achieved through the single assessment process, integrated commissioning arrangements and integrated provision of services, including community equipment and continence services.
- *Standard 3: Intermediate care.* Older people will have access to a range of new intermediate care services at home or in designated care settings. This will promote their independence by providing enhanced services from the NHS, and local authorities, to prevent unnecessary hospital admission and to provide effective rehabilitation services. This will enable early discharge from hospital and the prevention of premature, or unnecessary admission, to long-term residential care.

- *Standard 4: General hospital care.* Care in hospital is delivered for older people through appropriate specialist care and by hospital staff who have the right set of skills to meet their needs.
- *Standard 5: Stroke.* The NHS will take action to prevent strokes, working in partnership with other agencies where appropriate. People who are thought to have had a stroke have access to diagnostic services, are treated appropriately by a specialist stroke service, and subsequently, with their carers, participate in a multi-professional programme of secondary prevention and rehabilitation.
- *Standard 6*: Falls. The NHS, working in partnership with local authorities, takes action to prevent falls and reduces resultant fractures or other injuries in their populations of older people. Older people who have fallen receive effective treatment and, with their carers, receive advice on prevention through a specialist falls service.
- *Standard 7: Mental health in older people.* Older people who have mental health problems have access to integrated mental health services, provided by the NHS and local authorities to ensure effective diagnosis, treatment and support for them and their carers.
- *Standard 8: Promotion of health and active life in older age.* The health and well-being of older people is promoted through a co-ordinated programme of action led by the NHS with support from local authorities.

AGE DISCRIMINATION

The first standard of the NSF concerns non-discriminatory delivery of services and the nursing competencies are clear that care must be delivered in a non-discriminatory manner. However, it can be argued that a core of discrimination runs through much of the care we deliver to the older person (see also Chapter 12). As noted earlier, 14,000 people die prematurely from a fractured hip – there was no public outcry when this fact became available.

EXERCISE

You are a manager in a hospital, you have a quantity of money to allocate which will allow you either to: treat 10 children with juvenile arthritis so they can walk without pain; or treat 10 older people who require hip replacements so they can walk without pain. How would you allocate the money and why?

CASE STUDY OF AN OLDER COUPLE

Scenario Mr and Mrs White have been married for 60 years. Mr White is a retired bus driver and is 79 years old. Mrs White is 78 and used to work as an ambulance driver in the Second World War, but has not had regular paid work outside the family home since then. Mrs White has always done all the housework and cooking, with Mr White believing that such tasks are the woman's and declaring that he is unable even to boil an egg! They own their two-bed semi-detached house that has the bathroom and toilet upstairs adjacent to the master bedroom.

They have two children: Tony White (53), who lives 40 miles away, is married with a 10-year-old daughter and works in sales. Their daughter, Grace (55) is also married and lives locally (a 20-minute drive away). Grace and her husband have three children.

The vignette is an amalgam of many individuals the authors have nursed rather than a specific individual. The progress of the family over 2 years will enable you to appreciate the complexities that can ensue as illness becomes chronic and the ability of the family unit to function is impaired or ceases. As nurses we generally see a person in one setting (e.g. hospital) for a fixed period of time, at which point either they or the nurse moves on. It is important to realize that patients have a life both before we meet them and, hopefully, continue to have a life after leaving our care.

> **Scenario** Month 1. Mrs White collapses one evening while doing the washing up. Several hours before collapsing she had complained to her husband that she felt dizzy with a headache, but had put the symptoms down to getting a cold. Mr White called an ambulance and Mrs White was admitted to the stroke unit at their local hospital following assessment in the A&E department where a left cerebrovascular accident (CVA) was diagnosed, resulting in a right-sided hemiplegia. Mrs White's speech and swallowing are unaffected, but on arrival at the stroke unit, she is incontinent of urine, has no movement at all in her right arm and only a small amount of movement in her right leg.

WHAT IS A STROKE?

A stroke or cerebrovascular accident (CVA) occurs when the blood supply to part of the brain is interrupted, causing damage and death to an area of the brain. There are two major types: ischaemic and haemorrhagic. In an ischaemic stroke, the blood supply to part of the brain becomes occluded or blocked due to either thrombosis or embolism. In a thrombotic ischaemic stroke, the blood vessel within the brain becomes blocked, often due to atherosclerosis. In the embolic stroke the blood clot travels from elsewhere in the body and blocks the vessel in the brain. For example, the patient may have a pulmonary embolus and part of the embolus breaks off from the main clot and travels to the brain causing the stroke.

The haemorrhagic stroke occurs when a vessel within the brain ruptures causing leakage of blood into the brain (intracerebral haemorrhage) or into the membranes surrounding the brain (subarachnoid haemorrhage).

Stroke is the biggest single cause of severe disability and the third most common cause of death in the UK (DoH 2001i). Each year, in England and Wales, 110,000 people have their first stroke and 30,000 go on to have further strokes. Although CVA affects predominately older people, it also affects a significant number of younger people: 10,000 people under the age of 55 and 1000 people under the age of 30 have a CVA each year (DoH 2001i). The degree of damage and eventual disability caused by the CVA depends on which area of the brain has been affected. It is important to remember that the right side of the brain controls the left side of the body and vice versa.

Risk factors

A large number of factors increase the risk of having a stroke, including:

- atherosclerosis
- hypertension
- transient ischaemic attack
- atrial fibrillation
- diabetes
- previous stroke

- age
- positive family history
- smoking
- obesity (Hickey 1992).

DIAGNOSIS

The diagnosis of stroke will be made by the medical staff. When Mrs White arrives in A&E she will have her baseline observations taken, i.e. blood pressure, temperature, respiratory rate and pulse, plus routine blood tests, such as urea and electrolytes (U&E) and full blood count (FBC), and an electro-cardiogram (ECG) performed. She will be given a complete physical examination by the doctor to reveal the extent of the neurological deficit and give the initial diagnosis of stroke. The National Clinical Guidelines for Stroke (RCP 2000) recommend that brain imaging (computerized tomography or CT scan) should be undertaken within 48 hours of the onset of the symptoms in order to confirm the diagnosis and to determine both the location and the extent of the damage. The guidelines further note that the CT scan should be carried out more urgently if:

- the patient's condition deteriorates
- a subarachnoid haemorrhage is suspected
- hydrocephalus secondary to intracerebral haemorrhage is suspected
- trauma is suspected
- the patient is being anticoagulated or has a known bleeding tendency
- there are other unusual features.

It should be noted that on some occasions the CT scan will not detect the stroke, in which case a magnetic resonance imaging (MRI) scan may be undertaken.

ASSESSMENT AND PHYSICAL CARE

The only medication routinely prescribed in the case of first stroke, and if the medical staff decide the stroke is unlikely to be haemorrhagic in origin, is 300 mg of aspirin. In the early stage of the admission much of the assessment and care is aimed at stabilizing the patient's condition and establishing the degree of disability. The nurse will need to assess Mrs White's needs fully using a recognized assessment tool or set of criteria.

Mrs White's condition is assessed by the nurse on the stroke unit using the Roper, Logan and Tierney (1996) activities of daily living (ADL) model (see Chapter 6). Her assessment is summarized in Table 11.1. Following this assessment the nurse will need to ensure that both Mrs Smith's nutritional status and risk factors for pressure area breakdown are formally assessed. The pressure area assessment should be completed as part of the initial admission process, with the nutritional screening tool being completed within the first 12 hours.

The Waterlow score (Waterlow 1985) is a widely used tool for pressure area assessment (see Chapters 6 and 10). By assessing the risk of Mrs White developing pressure ulcers, appropriate interventions, including correct preventative equipment, e.g. mattresses, can be employed to prevent pressure area breakdown. Assessment of nutritional status allows the formulation of interventions in the event that Mrs White is assessed as being at risk (see Chapter 10).

Table 11.1 Mrs White's admission assessment

Activity of living	Usual routine	Problems (actual/potential)
Communication	Says usually wears glasses and that her hearing is excellent	Mrs White is alert and orientated, is responding to questions appropriately, speech does not seem slurred
Breathing	Says sometimes has a touch of bronchitis in the winter. She is a non-smoker	Respiratory rate 12 per minute, no coughing, does not appear at all distressed
Eating and drinking	Says she has a good appetite, cereal for breakfast, sandwich at dinner and cooks hot meal for her and her husband in the evening. No alcohol. She is not overweight	Her speech and swallowing are unaffected as this was formally assessed in the A&E department
Eliminating	Usually fully continent, has to get up to go to the toilet to pass water twice in night, has bowels open three or four times a week	She is incontinent of urine although she says she is aware of needing to go to the toilet. The routine ward urine test is negative for signs of infection
Personal cleansing and dressing	Has a shower every morning at home	The condition of her skin is good with the skin over all pressure areas intact
Body temperature	Reports her hands get very cold in the winter, otherwise no difficulties	On arrival on the ward her temperature was 36.8°C
Mobilizing	Usually walks independently around her house and upstairs. Uses no walking aids and walks to the local shops twice a week (approx. ½ a mile each way)	Mrs White has no movement in her right arm and only minimal movement in her right leg, she is able to flex her hip and knee slightly, has no movement in her ankle and toes. She is unable to lift the leg from the bed. Her sitting balance is also poor, she is flopping to the right
Working and playing	Usually plays bingo once a week when she goes to the local shops. Enjoys 'pottering around the garden'	Worried she will not be able to help her husband with the garden
Expressing sexuality	Mrs White has been married for 60 years	Mr White is with his wife and she is expressing concerns about how he

(Continued)

Table 11.1 (*Continued*)

Activity of living	Usual routine	Problems (actual/potential)
		will cope at home as he is 'useless in the kitchen' and they have not spent a night apart since 1982
Sleeping	Usually has a broken night as gets up to pass water a couple of times overnight. Does not take any night sedation. Usually goes to bed at 10 pm and gets up at about 6 am	Is worried that her husband will not get to sleep with her away from home. She is concerned that the hospital will be too noisy for her to sleep
Dying		She says her friend, Mrs Mullins, had a stroke and died a few months later

Continence care

Mrs White had no continence problems prior to her stroke. It is important that a full assessment is carried out to identify the type, and if possible, the cause of her incontinence, in order that it is treated appropriately. The National Clinical Guidelines for Stroke (RCP 2000) state that management of both bowel and bladder problems should be seen as an essential part of the patient's rehabilitation. It recommends that all registered nurses should be able to assess incontinent patients, and know who to contact for advice and support. This problem needs to be addressed promptly, as there is considerable evidence that incontinence has a negative effect on a person's social and emotional well-being (Norton 1986; Grimby 1993; Harris 1999).

When a patient is admitted it is usual to test their urine. This is because many potential or actual problems can be detected. When the nurse obtains the sample it needs to be checked visually – is it clear or cloudy, pale or dark? If urine is cloudy it may indicate infection; if it is very dark it may indicate very concentrated urine, which can be due to dehydration or poor renal function. Does the urine smell – is there the typical 'fishy odour' which is a good indication of infected urine? The urine is usually tested with a urine dipstick which changes colour in the presence of, among others, glucose (possible diabetes), ketones (possible diabetes or prolonged fasting), protein (possible infection) and blood (possible infection, although for women it is important to ask if they are menstruating before assuming infection). In the event that potential infection is indicated, a sample (midstream sample of urine or MSU) is sent for culture and sensitivity. This means the microbiology department attempts to grow bacteria from the sample and in the event that they do grow, identify them and check which antibiotics they are sensitive to, in order to facilitate effective treatment.

Mrs White's urine sample did not indicate any infection, neither did she report any discomfort on passing urine (another potential indicator of infection). As she knows when she needs to go to the toilet, it is probable that the loss of mobility, which is preventing her from getting to the toilet, is causing her incontinence. This type of difficulty is referred to as functional incontinence, in that the problem is the physical act of getting to the appropriate place and removing clothing to urinate appropriately, rather than a problem with the urinary tract itself. As with any other form of incontinence, a complete assessment to establish the cause of the functional incontinence is required (Vickerman 2002). It is worthy of note that an Audit Commission report (1999) identified that the standard of assessment for incontinence is variable and often poor.

Once it has been clearly established that the difficulty is due to the loss of mobility, then steps need to be taken to manage the problem in a way that is acceptable to both Mrs White and her family. There are a number of ways to manage urinary incontinence: catheterization, pads and bladder retraining.

Catheterization. This involves passing a thin tube or catheter into the bladder (usually via the urethra). Such a device can be temporary and removed as soon as the bladder has been emptied, or it can be longer term and held in place by a small balloon at the tip of the catheter, which when inflated stops the catheter from falling out. Catheterization is common practice in hospitals with up to 12% of patients being catheterized during their time in hospital (Mulhall *et al.* 1988). Between 10 and 20% of catheterized patients develop bacteriuria and, even more alarming, of the 1–4% of catheterized patients with urinary tract infection (UTI) who develop bacteraemia, 13–30% die (Ward *et al.* 1997). As such catheterization should be avoided wherever possible for stroke patients; if it is required, the use of aids such as flip flow valves which retain bladder tone should be considered.

Pads. Absorbent pads can be worn inside adapted underwear and hold both urinary and faecal soiling. Many have a gel core which draws the fluid away from the skin and contains both odour and fluid. They come in a wide variety of sizes and absorbencies. If the smaller sizes are used, they are relatively unobtrusive.

Bladder retraining. This can be used if the problem is one of habit or muscle weakness and as such is less relevant in the case of functional incontinence.

In Mrs White's case the cause of incontinence is lack of mobility; thus, it would not be appropriate to pass a catheter, since if her medical condition is stable she can be assisted out of bed onto a commode or toilet, using the hoist until her mobility improves. A case of least intervention is the best.

EXERCISE

You are a student on a general medical ward. The staff nurse you are working with tells you she is going to catheterize a patient who is being incontinent because this is going to be easier than taking her to the toilet. How might you respond? What evidence could you use to try to persuade the staff nurse that there is another option?

Mobility

Mrs White will have a full manual handling assessment carried out by the ward nursing staff. This addresses issues of safety for both Mrs White and the nursing staff. If Mrs White is not moved appropriately, it is possible to cause further injury to the affected limbs, e.g. subluxation of the shoulder joint. Also, inappropriate manual handling can cause injury to the nursing staff – back injury being particularly prevalent with 30% of nurses reporting work-related back pain each year (RCN 1999c).

The physiotherapists and occupational therapists will be involved as part of the multi-professional team from the start of her admission. The physiotherapists work on mobility issues such as sitting balance, standing, transferring and walking. The occupational therapist will be working with Mrs White and her family to help Mrs White re-learn the everyday tasks of self-care and establishing alternative techniques to allow her to care for herself. Both will order equipment and adaptations for Mrs White prior to her discharge. Some aids are readily available, e.g. most hospital physiotherapy departments would be able to supply Mrs White with a walking stick to take home, but if she needed a stair lift fitted, the involvement of social services would be required and the process would be much more time consuming.

The role of the nurse looking after Mrs White is to continue with the therapeutic regimes the physiotherapist and occupational therapist have initiated. For example, the occupational therapist assessed

Mrs White for washing and dressing and has found she can wash her front with minimal assistance, but requires help to wash her back and legs. If the nurse has a considerable workload in the morning it can be tempting for them to wash Mrs White as it is quicker. This is wholly inappropriate since both the nursing competencies and the *Code of professional conduct* (NMC 2002a) are explicit in the need to work as part of a team and to act in the patient's best interest. If the nurse takes away the independence the patient is attempting to regain, this is in clear breach of the spirit and the word the document.

PSYCHOLOGICAL CARE

Mrs White and her family require a great deal of support after a stroke. As can be seen from her assessment, her previous experience of stroke relates to a friend who died from it. She is facing spending time apart from her husband and is worried about his ability to cope in her absence. Section 1.2 of the *Code of professional conduct* states that:

> 'As a registered nurse or midwife, you must: protect and support the health of individual patients and clients, and protect and support the health of the wider community'.

> *(NMC 2002a)*

It could be argued that this stipulation means that the nurse also has a duty to ensure that Mr White's needs are met. The nurse will need to liaise with Mrs White's family to see if they will be able to assist Mr White at home while his wife is in hospital. In some cases where it is the main carer who is taken ill, the nurse will need to ensure that social workers become involved to arrange emergency care for individuals. In Mr White's case, Grace is happy to come and check on her father each day and check he has food in the house which he can prepare. It is important for Mrs White's psychological wellbeing that she is confident that her husband will manage without her at home.

Although Mrs White has not asked directly if she will die, she will require reassurance that everything that can be done is being done. This need for information extends to the rest of her family, but the nurse must remember that their duty of confidentiality lies with the patient. Thus, it would be appropriate to gain Mrs White's permission before speaking, in depth, to relatives. The need to ensure that patients and relatives receive accurate information in a form they can understand is also explicit within the competencies.

For Mrs White communication is not an issue, as her speech has not been affected by the stroke, but for many individuals the ability to communicate is seriously impaired and this can further increase their isolation. It is important that the nurse does not assume that a patient who cannot speak, cannot hear or cannot understand. A patient who has a stroke can develop expressive and/or receptive dysphasia. A patient with receptive dysphasia cannot understand what is being said to them, although they know what they want. A patient with expressive dysphasia knows what they want to say and understands what is being said to them but cannot find the words to respond appropriately. Mitchell (2002) describes graphically the experience of being aware but unable to make herself understood.

THE MULTI-PROFESSIONAL TEAM

Following her admission, Mrs White's physical and psychological needs will be addressed by the multi professional team working with her and her family. The standard within the NSF identifies the need for care to be provided within a specialist stroke unit by appropriately trained individuals. The National Clinical Guidelines for Stroke (RCP 2000) identify the need for a co-ordinated team and for staff with specialist expertise in stroke and rehabilitation. These guidelines are based on evidence of the effectiveness of specialist care within stroke units (Stroke Unit Trialists' Collaboration 1998). The multi-professional team within such a setting would typically consist of the stroke physician, nurses, physio-therapists, occupational therapists, speech and language therapist (SALT), the dietician, the social worker and possibly the clinical psychologist. The nurse has a central role within the team as they have most contact with the patient, but all members of the team are equally as important. Although a small scale study, Pound and Ebrahim (2001) noted that while patients in stroke units have better outcomes than those in general ward areas, they received less personal care than in a unit caring for older people. A possible explanation for this is that the members of the multi-professional team did not see themselves as equals, thus creating tension. The care management competencies note the need for effective inter-professional working practices and risk management strategies, both of which can be seen in the care Mrs White and her family receive.

REHABILITATION

Rehabilitation applied to older people is increasingly viewed as re-enablement; this means that people are helped to adapt to changes in their life circumstances, its ultimate goal being to maximize the social well-being of the individual and enabling them to regain their maximum quality of life. The concept of rehabilitation as re-enablement can be applied to an individual of any age. According to the Royal College of Nursing (RCN 1997), rehabilitation needs to involve all an individual's daily activities and has three main focal points:

- enhancing and maintaining quality of life
- restoring physical, psychological and social functioning by recognizing the health potential of each individual
- preventing disease and illness.

In addition to these focal points, the RCN (1997) identifies five role functions that the nurse engages in while working with older people in a re-enabling setting:

- supportive functions, i.e. providing psychosocial and emotional support
- restorative functions aimed at maximizing independence
- educative functions – teaching self-care
- life-enhancing functions, i.e. relieving pain, ensuring adequate nutrition
- team functions – the range of administrative and supervisory functions of the nurse.

For rehabilitation to be effective, the various members of the multi-professional team must work with the patient to determine realistic and shared goals for the rehabilitation process. If shared and realistic goals are not agreed, then disappointment for the patient is the likely outcome. For example, the multi-professional team may believe that to transfer independently from bed to chair is the greatest level of mobility the patient will achieve, but the patient is expecting to walk into the local village unaided!

As mentioned above, of the members of the multi-professional team, the nurse is typically the one with the greatest contact with the patient and, as such, is in a unique position to facilitate understanding and agreement with the patient on what they hope realistically to achieve. Mrs White was fully independent prior to her stroke: her intention and that of her family is for her to return home with suitable support.

The National Clinical Guidelines for Stroke (RCP 2000) advise that early discharge from the stroke unit back into the community should only be considered if there are specialist community stroke rehabilitation teams and if the patient is able to transfer safely from bed to chair. They also state that:

- carers should have received all necessary equipment and training in manual handling so they can safely transfer the patient at home
- patients and families are prepared and fully involved in the discharge
- GPs, the primary health care team and community social services are fully aware
- all necessary equipment and support is in place
- any continuing community-based treatment continues uninterrupted after discharge
- the patient and family have information about appropriate statutory and voluntary agencies.

In a Canadian study, Mayo *et al.* (2000) found that stroke patients who were discharged early with appropriate home-based rehabilitation had better physical health and re-integration into the community at 3 months than patients who continued with hospital-based rehabilitation. However, Anderson *et al.* (2000) found that early discharge with home-based rehabilitation did not improve (or worsen) health or quality of life for stroke patients in a study in Australia. Griffiths (2000) argues that both these studies required participants to be relatively independent and, as such, the results cannot be generalized; also, both studies were relatively small scale. Further work needs to be undertaken to examine both the effects on carers of early discharge and how best to deliver the co-ordinated multi-professional rehabilitation which clearly does improve outcome for stroke patients.

Scenario Month 2. Mrs White is discharged home following an 8-week stay on the stroke unit. Her family has arranged for private home care to visit twice daily to help Mrs White get up in the morning, and again to put her to bed in the evening. Mrs White still has a fairly dense right hemiplegia affecting her arm more severely than her leg. While she has no useful function in her right arm, she is able to stand with the aid of her stick and can walk around the ground floor of her house and in the garden. She has a hospital bed downstairs in the front room and a commode. Her husband helps her by adjusting her clothing when she needs the toilet. She is happy to be home and says she will teach her husband to cook!

It could be argued that this phase of care for the White family has been successful: Mrs White is back home, she has identified a goal for herself and adequate support appears to be in place. Careful planning for discharge is an important part of attempting to limit readmission to hospital. Munshi *et al.* (2002) studied readmission of older people to acute medical units and noted that about 40% were avoidable and that unresolved medical and social problems accounted for 62% of all readmissions. They also identified that intermediate care provision may play a crucial role in preventing readmission to acute medical services.

Scenario Month 11. Grace visits two or three times a week and checks the freezer is well-stocked with meals that Mr White can prepare with minimum effort, as Mrs White has been only partially successful in teaching him to cook. As she is getting out of bed, Mrs White falls to the floor and she complains of severe pain in her left shoulder. Mr White calls an ambulance and Mrs White is admitted to A&E. She is admitted to the hospital with a suspected fractured humerus; however, the diagnosis is severe bruising but no fracture. She is unable to use her left arm due to the bruising and pain, and her right arm has been affected by the stroke. Mrs White is admitted to an intermediate care facility for rehabilitation.

FALLS

Standard 6 of the NSF aims both to prevent falls and to treat them effectively when they do occur. Falls are a major problem in the UK; they are a significant cause of both disability and death in people over the age of 75. Up to 14,000 people a year die in the UK as a result of osteoporotic hip fracture (DoH 2001i). To give that figure a sense of proportion it is the equivalent of approximately 35 fully laden jumbo jets crashing and killing all passengers each year. If that were to happen it seems likely there would be a public outcry with questions being asked in parliament and the press!

Nursing care

Mrs White does not have a fracture, but she has fallen and is unable to use her one good arm. Intermediate care is covered by Standard 3 of the NSF (DoH 2001i) and would be ideal for Mrs White under these circumstances, as she is not medically unwell, but requires further rehabilitation following her fall. Equally as important, she is likely to have lost confidence as a result of this fall and this may prevent her from regaining her former level of mobility.

Within the intermediate care setting Mrs White will receive intensive nursing and therapy input to facilitate her return home as soon as possible. There are a variety of programmes or aids to prevent falls and injury. Robertson *et al.* (2001) identified that a home-based, nurse-delivered exercise programme, concentrating on muscle strengthening and balance retraining, was effective in reducing falls and serious injury in people over the age of 80. In the evaluation of a nurse-led falls prevention programme, Lightbody *et al.* (2002) found that patients receiving the nurse-led interventions had fewer falls and hospital attendances, and spent less time in hospital. They were also more functionally independent 6 months after the original fall. Hip protectors have been found to reduce the level of hip fractures in elderly people living in institutional or supported home care environments (Parker *et al.* 2001; Campbell 2001).

The rehabilitation dilemma

Mrs White requires rehabilitation to regain her maximum level of functioning in order to return home if at all possible. This can, however, present the health care team with a dilemma. Rehabilitation has a certain level of risk: Mrs White has fallen once, if the physiotherapists, nurses and medical staff encourage and enable her to walk, there is a danger she may fall again and sustain further injury. If the health care team were to prevent Mrs White from undertaking or attempting activities independently, then the risk of falling may be reduced, but at what cost? The patient will be hindered in their recovery and thus may not regain the maximum possible level of independence.

EXERCISE

You are approached by the relatives of an elderly lady who has been admitted for rehabilitation. She has fallen and fractured her hip while walking to the toilet, unaccompanied by a nurse. The woman is usually fully mobile using just her walking stick. When admitted to the ward, she was unable to transfer from the bed to the chair without the help of two nurses; she is now able to walk independently the length of the ward using a walking frame and is fiercely determined fully to regain her independence. The family is very angry that she is allowed to walk around the ward without a nurse and are demanding that the nurses on duty are disciplined for negligence. How might you respond in such a situation?

The nurse has, as their first duty, the need to address the patient's requirements. In the above case the patient is very clear she wishes to regain her independence. A risk assessment as to her mobility will have been completed indicating she is safe with the frame – it is vital such points have been documented. If the nurses are operating in the best interests of the patient and with completed documentation, there should be no question of any disciplinary action. In which case, talking to the relatives needs to be sensitively handled and these facts need to be reflected. A relatively junior nurse may wish to approach a more senior college for support. The relatives always have the option of accessing the trust's complaints procedure, and the nurse may find it useful to facilitate their access to this.

> **Scenario** Month 13. Following the fall, Mrs White's mobility has become more restricted. Both Mr and Mrs White were determined that she return home, so after 4 weeks intensive re-enablement she has returned home. She is able to walk around the house but does not feel able to go into the garden. Grace is now visiting daily, except at the weekend when Tony visits. Tony's wife is complaining that he is out working all week and she does not see him at the weekend now that he is visiting his parents. The home care continues twice a day. Mr White confides to Tony that he finds it difficult because he is afraid his wife will fall again if he lets her out of his sight. Mrs White tells Grace that she feels her husband does not trust her anymore as he is always watching her.

CARERS

The strain on carers is often not fully recognized and, if the family is being nursed holistically, the needs of the whole family should be taken into account. Although all practical aspects of providing for Mrs White have been addressed, it could be argued that the less tangible need for support for her family unit have not been taken into account. Both the NSF (DoH 2001i) and the Clinical Guidelines for Stroke (RCP 2000) note the need for contact with local voluntary and statutory agencies. This does not seem to be the case here. If Mr White had been invited to the local carers' support group he could meet others in the same position as himself and gain support. If Mrs White were to access a day centre that would give Mr White a day to himself. Possible information the family could receive includes:

- local service directories
- local day centre information
- stroke association leaflets
- social security benefit leaflets
- local carers group information (Exall and Johnston 1999).

Hall (2002) notes that carer support groups provide a focus for health education and should be an integral part of service delivery, while acknowledging that such groups do have limitations.

Informal carers provide an estimated 80% of community-based long-term care. There are around 6.8 million carers in the UK (OPCS 1990) and approximately 13% of carers are over the age of 65. For carers, there are lifestyle implications, not just from the act of providing the care, but also the financial implications of such caring. Tony is driving 80 miles a week to visit his parents, which is potentially expensive in addition to being time-consuming. As Grace is visiting her parents once a day the possibility of her taking paid employment is greatly reduced. There are also implications in terms of the care she can provide to her own children. In the future, the house may be sold to pay for long-term nursing or residential care, thus any expected financial windfall from their parents' will is lost.

Scenario Month 17. Grace is concerned that Mr White is becoming muddled at times. She has visited and found that he has switched the gas on to reheat food and forgotten to light it. She has also found that he is forgetting things that he has been told or asked. He is also neglecting to lock the front door at night. She takes him to visit his GP. The early stages of Alzheimer's disease are diagnosed. Grace increases her visits to twice a day. Mrs White is still fully alert and orientated and believes she can watch her husband and remind him to do things.

THE MENTAL HEALTH STANDARD

Standard 7 of the NSF (DoH 2001i) concentrates on the need for early detection of mental health problems and access to specialist teams. The need to support carers is also noted. The goals within this standard are longer term than many of the others, with health and social care having until April 2004 to put the necessary interventions in place.

LIFESTYLE CHANGES

The social functioning of both Mr and Mrs White has undergone great change over their lifetimes. They have moved from worker to retired person, from parent to care recipient, from active member of the local community to being outside due to physical and mental disability. In the same way, the roles of Grace and Tony have reversed; they have moved from care recipient as children to care providers to dependent parents. There is also the possibility that Grace, as the local carer, may find the social stigma of mental illness will affect how others act towards her.

As noted earlier there is a wide range of voluntary groups that can give carer support; however, it is probable that groups of this type will not prove effective for all individuals.

Scenario Month 24: Mr and Mrs White are not coping at home. Mrs White has fallen twice in the past 3 weeks, although she has not injured herself. Mr White is forgetting to help his wife to prepare food and to help her when she needs the toilet. He has been found wandering down the street at night and is becoming more confused and aggressive towards his wife and Grace. The social worker, district nurse and GP do not feel it is safe for them to remain at home together. Mrs White agrees that she cannot remain in these circumstances and wants them both to move into residential/nursing care so they can remain together. Social services arrange for emergency placement in a local nursing home while a more permanent solution is sought.

Mrs White has made the decision that she and her husband will go into care together. This is not always possible, e.g. only one partner may require care. For couples who have been together for many years separation is difficult. In a small scale study, Sandberg *et al.* (2001) identified four stages in the process of separation:

- pretending – the carers tell themselves this is just a trial separation and not permanent
- dawning – a growing awareness that the placement is permanent
- putting on a brave face – exactly what it sounds like, showing the world that everything is alright
- seeking solace – attempting to discuss feelings with friends or relatives.

A theme which runs through all the stages of the separation is that of trying to keep the relationship with the spouse. It is important that the nurse, in such a situation, does not underestimate the effect of the separation for a couple who may have been together for 60 years.

CONCLUSION

To care effectively for older adults the nurse needs clinical and interpersonal skills of the highest order. All of the competencies for entry to the register are applicable and, coupled with the NSF, provide a clear indication about how care for older people in both acute and primary care should be provided. Lifestyle changes can and do affect people of any age, but the case study of the White family illustrates the profound changes that can occur in health status, social position and living arrangements. In the space of just 2 years they have gone from healthy, independent older people, fully integrated into their local community, to needing care to be provided by relative strangers.

It can be argued that a society is judged by how it deals with its poorest and most disadvantaged members. In the same way it can be argued that nursing will be judged by how it addresses meeting the needs of the older adult with dignity and respect.

CHAPTER 12

A RELATIONSHIP-CENTRED APPROACH TO WORKING WITH OLDER PEOPLE AND THEIR FAMILIES

Sue Davies and Mike Nolan

INTRODUCTION

This chapter aims to consider the range of health and social care needs commonly experienced by older people and their family carers, and to suggest how these might be met most appropriately within a variety of care settings. Recurrent concerns about the quality of care received by older people will be highlighted, together with policy initiatives aimed at ensuring acceptable standards of care across a range of care environments. To achieve these standards, nurses working with older people need access to more explicit frameworks to help with the assessment, planning and evaluation of care. The chapter concludes by outlining one such framework, which has been developed by the authors, following a number of research studies. It will demonstrate how the framework can be used to help to articulate goals of care for nursing older people, and to identify subsequent interventions for older people and their family carers. The importance of supporting staff and providing them with a stimulating and challenging work environment is also highlighted.

Within the UK older people are the main users of health and social care services (HAS 1998; DoH 2001i), and consequently most nurses will come into regular contact with older people in their day-to-day practice. The complexity of health need, which often accompanies advanced old age, means that many older people require the help and support of formal and family carers to ensure that they experience the best possible quality of life. However, it is important to remember that most older people lead independent and fulfilling lives and contribute a great deal to society in a variety of roles.

The term 'older' is, of course, relative and, given that we are all living longer, people termed older will span more than a generation. The needs of older people are therefore very diverse and heterogeneous, and it is just such heterogeneity that makes working with older people such an exciting and challenging career. For example, older people may require support to meet a wide variety of needs, ranging from health promotion advice to palliative care, and this demands a range of well-developed skills on the part of those working with them.

This idea of 'working with' older people, rather than simply providing care to or for them, is an important concept and marks a change in emphasis in health and social care towards empowering older people to take greater control of the services they receive (Bernard and Phillips 2000). Nurses, therefore, need to work in partnership with older people and their family carers, who provide 80% of the care that older people require (Walker 1995).

It is clear that nursing roles with respect to older people and their family carers are constantly being redefined as a result of both demographic and social change. As a consequence, the boundaries of gerontological nursing have become increasingly blurred (Wade 1996). Such changes require that new models of working with older people and their family carers are developed and evaluated, which recognize that all parties have an important contribution to make. This chapter describes one such model, based on the idea of relationship-centred care, which can inform nursing practice with older people and their family carers within a range of care environments. However, to set the scene, the implications of the demography of ageing for nursing practice is first considered.

DEMOGRAPHIC CHANGES AND CHALLENGES

Consistent with countries across Europe, the average age of the population of the UK has been steadily increasing. The long-term trends of lower birth rates, improvements in health status and rising longevity have combined to produce a constant growth in the proportion of the population who are aged 60 years and over (Royal Commission on Long Term Care 1999). Importantly, however, these changes have not been consistent across different age groups, with the most rapid recent changes being apparent among those aged 80 and over.

It is this latter group, who generally have far higher levels of disability secondary to multiple chronic diseases and who are most in need of care and support, that presents potential challenges to health and social care systems.

Despite this, it is important to recognize that even among very frail older people only a minority require institutional care, with the majority continuing to live in the community, often with family support (Walker 1995). The chance of living in a long-stay hospital or care home, for example, is currently estimated at 5% for people aged 75–84 and 21% for those aged 85 and over (Laing and Buisson 2000). Furthermore, the development of new technologies is likely to allow older people to remain in their own homes for longer (Fisk 1999). Nonetheless, an ageing population does present a series of challenges for health and social care practitioners, partly because of the association between disability (including dementia) and advanced old age, and partly because of changes in the household situation of older people.

As Sundstrom (1994) points out, the ways people live together have fundamental implications for patterns of giving and receiving care. The growth in solitary living, the decline in co-residence between generations and the increase in women's employment outside the home are all impacting on families' ability to provide informal networks of support for older people who need help to remain in the community (Commission of the European Communities 1996). Most importantly, the trend towards smaller family size has resulted in a reduced number of potential carers compared to those needing care. Changes in family structure, resulting from increased geographical mobility and the impact of divorce, are also influencing the availability of family support (Victor 1991; Coleman *et al.* 1993). Consequently, families are facing the prospect of caring for older relatives for longer, with fewer potential family members to help. Without adequate support these caring relationships are likely to break down, resulting in increased demand for formal care services. Developing more effective ways of working in partnership with family carers is therefore crucial, and is an area in which nurses can make a significant difference.

In response to these demographic changes, services for older people and their families have been continuously reconfigured over recent years. For example, the drive towards providing health care in the community wherever possible has resulted in the creation of new roles for nurses working with older people in such settings. Health visitors and practice nurses have been encouraged to expand their role in health promotion and screening activities with older people (Ellefsen 2001; Iliffe and Lenihan 2001). In addition, community health development activities, which encourage consumer participation in the identification of health need and the development of services to meet that need, are increasingly involving older people as active participants (Fisher *et al.* 1999; Davies 1999). Other initiatives, such as intermediate care schemes intended to reduce hospital admission and length of stay, also involve an important role for nurses in a range of hospital and community settings. Simultaneously, during the past 15 years, long-term care for older people has been relocated within the independent sector and there are now very few continuing care beds within the NHS.

From the above it is clear that an understanding of the situation of older people in the UK today is important if nursing is to respond to the current challenges, and completing the AGEIN quiz (Figure 12.1) gives you a chance to 'check out' what you know.

This quiz was developed as part of a 3½ year project funded by the English National Board for Nursing Midwifery and Health Visiting which explored the ways in which nurses are prepared to work with older people. The questions are all based upon facts about the situation of older people in the UK. Do not be too concerned, however, if you get many of the answers wrong, as the study indicated that most students and registered nurses have only limited knowledge about the situation of older people (Nolan *et al.* 2002). Furthermore, this study also suggested that nurses have considerable potential to improve the care that older people receive, but this area of work must be given a higher status if this potential is to be realized, as work with older people has often not been valued.

	I think this figure is:		
	Too High	**About Right**	**Too Low**
1. The percentage of people currently over the age of 65 in the UK is about 17%	☐	☐	☐
2. The percentage of people in ethnic minority groups who are currently over the age of 65 years in the UK is about 10%	☐	☐	☐
3. Between now and 2034 the percentage of people over the age of 85 is expected to increase by about 60%	☐	☐	☐
4. By 2016 the number of people aged over 100 will treble	☐	☐	☐
5. Of women over the age of 75 about 60% live alone	☐	☐	☐
6. The percentage of people between the ages of 60–74 living in residential or nursing homes is about 5%	☐	☐	☐
7. People aged 75 years and over are 3 times more likely to die an accidental death than the general population	☐	☐	☐
8. Of people aged 75 years and over about 50% report long-term illness or disability	☐	☐	☐
9. The percentage of people over the age of 65 who need help with the following activities is about:			
a) Washing all over — 20%	☐	☐	☐
b) Dressing — 12%	☐	☐	☐
c) Using the toilet — 10%	☐	☐	☐
d) Climbing steps/stairs — 30%	☐	☐	☐
e) Hearing someone talk — 20%	☐	☐	☐
f) Reading a newspaper even with glasses — 15%	☐	☐	☐
10. The percentage of people between the ages of 65–74 in some form of paid employment is about 5%	☐	☐	☐
11. In any one year the percentage of people aged 75+ who have an in-patient stay in hospital is about 30%	☐	☐	☐
12. On average people aged over 75 spend about 15% of their income on heating and lighting	☐	☐	☐

Answers: Q1 – about right. Q2 – too high (correct figure 3.2%). Q3 – too low (correct figure 89%). Q4 – too low (correct figure quadruple). Q5 – about right. Q6 – too high (correct figure 1%). Q7 – too low (correct figure 6 times). Q8 – too low (correct figure 66%). Q9a – too high (correct figure 12%); Q9b – about right; Q9c – too high (correct figure 4%); Q9d – about right; Q9e – about right; Q9f – too high (correct figure 10%). Q10 – too low (correct figure 9%). Q11 – too high (correct figure 20%). Q12 – too high (correct figure 8%).

Figure 12.1 AGEIN Project questionnaire

SUMMARY

- Within the UK older people are the main users of health and social care services.
- Most nurses will come into regular contact with older people in their day-to-day practice.
- Demographic changes and challenges mean that new models of care must be continually developed and evaluated.
- Practitioners need explicit frameworks to help them to develop partnerships with older people and their families.

OLDER PEOPLE'S EXPERIENCES OF NURSING AND HEALTH CARE

The potential for nursing to 'make a difference' to the care experiences of older people and their family carers has been recognized for nearly half a century, with some of the earliest nursing research studies stressing the importance of the nursing contribution (see, for example, Norton *et al.* 1962; Wells 1980). However, despite this, several subsequent studies have provided substantial evidence to suggest that nursing has failed fully to realize this potential (Nolan *et al.* 1994). For while there are examples of excellent nursing practice with older people (Davies *et al.* 1999), the picture is variable with a number of studies over several decades demonstrating that 'routine' rather than individualized care predominates within many care environments (Wells 1980; Evers 1981; Reed 1989; Kitson 1991; Waters 1994; Nolan *et al.* 1995).

More recent studies and reports continue to identify a number of difficulties in providing older people with the quality of care they desire. For example, there have been recent concerns about the poor standards of care that older people receive when they are admitted to acute hospital wards (HAS 1998; Help the Aged 1999). In particular, older people and family carers have expressed their dissatisfaction with the extent to which their nutritional and hygiene needs are met, and with the lack of attention to their psychological well-being and mental health needs (SNMAC 2001). While financial constraints act as an obvious barrier to the development of acute services, studies have shown that older patients are able to identify small improvements that would not be too demanding but that could make a considerable difference to the quality of care they experience (Davies *et al.* 1999; Meyer *et al.* 1999). The challenges of providing high quality care to older people in a range of care environments (such as community settings, continuing care and palliative care, in addition to those with learning difficulties or mental health problems) have also been described (see Nolan *et al.* 2001 for a review of literature in relation to each client group).

ETHNIC MINORITY GROUPS

Of particular importance in an increasing multi-cultural context are the needs of older people from ethnic minority groups. In 1991 approximately 6% of the population in the UK was from an ethnic minority background (OPCS 1991b). By 2001 this figure had grown to 7.9%. As people from ethnic minority groups grow into old age, nurses must be able to provide care which is culturally sensitive

(RCN 1995a). Particularly in relation to personal care and nutritional care, practitioners should be aware of cultural preferences and ensure that these are respected. Yet a number of studies have found that nurses often feel ill-prepared to meet the needs of older people from different ethnic minority groups (Gerrish *et al.* 1996; Davies *et al.* 1999). A review by Thomas and Dines (1994), for example, found that many health professionals were unaware of any specific needs that older people from ethnic minority groups might have; and yet ethnic minority elders may be multiply disadvantaged by relatively low income, urban living and poor health (Askham *et al.* 1995). Not surprisingly, older people from ethnic minority groups frequently find it difficult to access relevant health services, often as a result of poor communication and lack of information. There are also suggestions that they may delay seeking care, fearing discrimination on racial grounds, and there is some justification for this (Chadda 2001). These challenges have led to calls for specialist services for ethnic minority elders to operate alongside mainstream services.

SUMMARY

- Recent studies and reports continue to identify a number of difficulties in providing older people with the quality of care they desire.
- The challenges of providing high quality care to older people in a range of care environments, including community settings, continuing care and palliative care, in addition to those with learning difficulties or mental health problems, are significant and require the development of frameworks to guide practice.
- Of particular importance in an increasingly multi-cultural context are the needs of older people from ethnic minority groups.

POLITICS OF AGEING, CHRONIC ILLNESS AND DISABILITY

Issues of power and control are fundamental to understanding experiences of ageing, chronic illness and disability within our society. To a large extent, social policies shape experiences of ageing. It is therefore essential that nurses develop the skills to identify and critique the key values underpinning policy initiatives and determine their impact for service users and for formal and informal carers. With this is mind, some of the important policy initiatives affecting health care for older people and their families at the time of writing this chapter are outlined: however, it is important to recognize that the policies which shape services for older people and their families are constantly changing and it is necessary to keep up to date with the most recent developments. One way to do this is to access the government's website at http/www.gov.uk, where current policy documents and short summaries can be found. Alternatively, the professional nursing press publishes succinct summaries, usually within a few weeks of publication of important policy documents.

Possibly the most significant development in recent years was the publication in March 2001 of the *National Service Framework for Older People*. This comprehensive document aims to improve and standardize the quality of care for older people across care environments in England (DoH 2001i), and is underpinned by four main themes: respecting the individual, intermediate care, providing evidence-based specialist care and promoting an active and healthy life. Standards are set in eight key areas, as discussed in Chapter 11 (see Box 11.1).

The national service framework (NSF) embraces the principles of dignity, personhood and self-determination within its recommendations and has already done much to raise the profile of older people. However, it is important that the broad goals of care outlined within the NSF are translated into practical and measurable objectives and interventions, in order to guide nursing and health care practice. A further publication released at the same time as the NSF attempted to do this in relation to nursing care for older people in acute hospital settings (SNMAC 2001). This report identified that greater attention needs to be given to the fundamental aspects of care, such as nutrition and hygiene. A series of standard statements were developed (Box 12.1), accompanied by a set of precise indicators designed to enable older people and practitioners to recognize when each standard had been achieved. The value of these indicators lies in the fact that they were developed in consultation with practitioners, researchers and organizations representing older people and family carers.

Box 12.1 Areas covered within standard statements for nursing older people who are acutely ill (SNMAC 2001)

- Respect for, and maintenance of, the older person's dignity
- Promotion of choice, involvement and independence of older people and carers
- Facilitation of communication with older people and their carers
- Individualized care and its management
- Specific clinical aspects:
  - continence
  - dementia and confusional states
  - mental health needs
  - mobility
  - nutrition and hydration
  - pain management
  - palliative care for people with degenerative disease
  - palliative care for people who are dying
  - pressure damage prevention and management

New proposals for intermediate care, which were also outlined in *The NHS Plan* (DoH 2000a), are aimed partly at avoiding crisis admissions to long-term care by providing a period of ongoing assessment and rehabilitation. It is anticipated that a proportion of this intermediate care will be provided in care homes as well as in people's own homes.

For those needing full-time care, initiatives aimed at standardizing structure and process within care homes are currently being established. The Care Standards Act (2001) (DoH 2001j) introduced a range of minimum standards which proprietors and managers of care homes must achieve from April 2002. These include minimum standards for building specifications, room occupancy, staff training and management. However, there are concerns that many homes within the independent and voluntary sectors will be forced out of business as a result of these requirements, resulting in compulsory relocation for some residents. This is likely to have important implications for residents and their relatives who have settled in a particular home.

ANTI-DISCRIMINATORY PRACTICE

Central to the aims of the NSF is the desire to 'root out' ageism and age discrimination in health and social care in particular, and in society at large in general.

An awareness of all forms of discrimination, including discrimination on the basis of age and disability, is a prerequisite to the development of effective nursing practice. Given the high proportion of older people using health services, it is essential that nurses develop the skills to challenge ageist practices in all contexts and settings. Unfortunately, ageist practices which discriminate against people purely on the basis of their age are fairly widespread within the UK health service (HAS 1998; DoH 2001i).

According to Butler (1969), ageism is a process of systematic stereotyping of people on the basis of age. Wade (1996) suggests that such stereotyping allows younger people to see older people as different:

'thus they subtly cease to identify with their elders as human beings.'

(p30)

Wade differentiates three types of ageism.

- *Compassionate ageism* emphasizes the problems of old age which, Wade suggests, promotes an image of older people as weak, dependent and burdensome.
- *Conflictual ageism* attempts to limit the resources available to older people, who are seen as 'avaricious consumers of health care' (p31) who conversely contribute little to society.
- *Medical ageism* perpetuates practices whereby older people do not benefit from advanced technology and medical interventions (Grimley Evans 1994).

Ageist attitudes and discriminatory practices are often prompted by misinformation about older people and the demands they place upon society. Recent research found that both nursing students and registered nurses knew very little about the demography of ageing in the UK and about older people's need for support and use of services (Nolan *et al.* 2002). Furthermore, responses to a knowledge quiz (see Figure 12.1) suggested that they tended to overestimate the numbers of older people within the UK and their use of resources and services such as residential care and hospital beds.

REFLECTION POINT

Think back to the quiz in Figure 12.1. Were you surprised by the correct figures? What do your responses suggest about your own perceptions of older people?

SUMMARY

- Social policies have an important impact on experiences of ageing and it is essential that practitioners in health and social care appreciate these influences.
- Current policies within the UK emphasize respect for the individual, providing evidence-based, individualized care and promoting an active and healthy life.
- It is particularly important that nurses develop the skills to challenge ageist practices in all contexts and settings.

CHALLENGES FOR ENHANCING QUALITY OF LIFE FOR OLDER PEOPLE AND THEIR FAMILIES

As will be apparent by now, a complex range of factors interact to shape the way that we view older people and influence the health care that they receive. Moreover, despite the fact that older people often have complex needs and require skilful nursing, gerontological nursing is still not accorded high status and value. Ford and McCormack (1999) identified a range of attributes required of a gerontological nurse specialist (Box 12.2), but despite this, gerontological nursing is still often seen as being less demanding than other forms of nursing.

Box 12.2 Key attributes of a gerontological nurse specialist (Ford and McCormack 1999)

- *Holistic knowledge and practice:* ability to synthesize a diverse range of knowledge to provide person-centred holistic care aimed at enhancing quality of life
- *Saliency:* ability to identify key issues of relevance to the older person and select models of care that are interdisciplinary, holistic and person-centred
- *Knowing the patient:* use of in-depth knowledge of individual and family biographies to help forge partnerships
- *Moral agency:* should respect and promote dignity, choice and autonomy to empower older people and their carers
- *Skilled know-how:* delivery of expert care in an holistic, proficient and fluid way

Therefore, there is still some way to go before all older people and their families can be assured that they will receive the highest standards of care, whatever their needs and circumstances. One of the biggest challenges facing practitioners caring for older people is the need to change entrenched care practices, which are often based on inappropriate attitudes and beliefs. In particular, routinized care practices are the norm in many institutional care settings. Nevertheless, awareness is growing that the way to improve care for older people in a range of care environments is to create a culture of positive care which values older people and the staff working with them. Research by Davies *et al.* (1999) and Davies (2001), for example, suggested that the most positive culture of care was associated with staff who felt well supported and appreciated, and benefited from effective leadership. However, these findings still 'beg the question' of how to create such positive cultures, particularly in situations where staff feel undervalued and demoralized.

A significant challenge for the future of gerontological nursing is, therefore, to consider how it can respond to the health care needs of older people, while at the same time promoting work with older people as valuable and important. In 1998 a workshop was held by the Royal College of Nursing and Agenet (Agenet/RCN 1999) to explore areas in which there was a need for further research in relation to gerontological nursing. It identified the following five areas as being of a high priority:

- *increasing health expectancy:* developing appropriate models of service delivery, exploring organizational barriers, evaluating technology and understanding individual expectations
- *person-orientated quality of life:* measures that reflect subjective experience
- *user and carer involvement:* intergenerational working, accessing the views of people with dementia, methods of determining user expectations

- *effectiveness of therapeutic interventions:* use of artistic expression; effectiveness of specific interventions; the nursing contribution to the compression of morbidity
- *new roles:* the need for registered nursing, models of service co-ordination, nurse practitioner roles.

These sorts of new roles are being promoted in the gerontological nurse specialist and the consultant nurse, but just what such practitioners will or should do is not quite so clear. The remaining four of the above five points will be used below to consider important aspects of gerontological nursing, whether care is provided by a care assistant or a nurse consultant. Recent government policy will be considered and a critical review provided of recent trends and developments.

INCREASING HEALTH EXPECTANCY

Helping older people to remain healthy and independent is one of the government's main aims for health and social care (DoH 2001i), and lies at the heart of the NSF. It is also an important focus of research in gerontology, with Wetle (1998) arguing that research into reducing disability and increasing healthy lifespan are two of the main goals for gerontological research over the next few decades. He stresses the need to explore more fully how to promote the health of older people by giving attention to a range of lifestyle factors, e.g. exercise, diet, smoking and alcohol use, combined with improvement in screening and early diagnosis. Helping older people to live for as long as possible, as healthily as possible, is termed 'compressing morbidity', so that people are as free of disability, and hence the need for help and support, for as long as possible.

Of course, all of us would like to be healthy for as long as possible and the humanitarian arguments in favour of such an approach are powerful. However, some commentators suggest that the main motive for wishing older people to remain healthy is economic, and is driven by a desire to reduce the cost of the health service (Hanford *et al.* 1999). For example, in presenting evidence to the Royal Commission on Long Term Care, Prophet (1998) argued that a fall in morbidity among older people of just 1% per year would, by 2030, result in a 30% reduction in the costs to the welfare state, a saving of some £6.3 million annually. In exploring how services respond to health promotion agendas, the Joseph Rowntree Foundation (1999) identified two broad approaches:

- strategies that prevent or delay the need for more costly services
- strategies that maintain and improve quality of life.

However, there was great variation across the UK in the services designed to meet either aim, with evidence of ageist attitudes towards the benefits of, and possibilities for, health promotion among older people.

The Joseph Rowntree Foundation (1999) argues that if a preventative culture is to flourish, then a number of structures have to be developed, including:

- cross-agency and cross-sector commitment
- engaging older people in service design and delivery
- locally-based initiatives
- institutional commitment at a senior level
- dedicated budgets and staff.

However, this will be difficult to achieve unless ageist attitudes that perpetuate the belief that older people have neither the desire nor the capacity to participate fully in their care can be countered. Such attitudes are very evident in the literature on health promotion.

While it is widely recognized that the main goals of health promotion with older people are to maintain independence, delay dependency and disability, and improve quality of life (Nolan 2001), these aims are rarely realized. For, despite the growing literature on health promotion, very little of this focuses on the needs of older people (Victor and Higginson 1994). Consequently, there is little evidence for the effectiveness of health promotion programmes with older people, who, Greengross *et al.* (1997) argue have often been patronized or 'neglected' by the health promotion movement. Ageist assumptions about the limited benefits of promoting the health of older people (Victor and Higginson 1994) have resulted in a poor understanding of their health status and the factors which might influence it (Greengross *et al.* 1997; Poxton 1998). For example, studies focusing on younger age groups are often applied to older people when the relevance of the results is questionable. Furthermore, despite the recent policy of health promotion, many government documents have ignored, or given limited attention to, the needs of older people (Young 1996; Dalley 1998). However, despite this, there is growing interest in the potential benefits to older people of a variety of lifestyle changes, such as:

- increased exercise and physical activity
- giving up smoking
- better diet
- reducing alcohol consumption (Nolan 2001).

In addition, Evandrou (1998) suggests that there is a need to consider a number of other potential threats to health, such as stress, pollution and food contamination.

However, while potentially important, preventative measures alone are unlikely to be fully effective; if older people are to have a healthy and active retirement then a range of other factors, such as housing, income and using technology, also need to be considered (Alford and Futrell 1992; Evandrou 1998). In promoting a broader view of what constitutes prevention, Prophet (1998) cites the work of Wistow and Lewis (1997) who outline a number of strategies aimed at:

- delaying or reducing the impact of biological processes
- minimizing socio-economic differences
- helping older people build social networks in the community
- informing attitudes and expectations of older people
- addressing environmental factors.

Environmental factors are particularly important in enabling frail older people to remain in their own homes, and the wider application of technology has considerable future potential.

Clearly then, health promotion with older people is one area in which gerontological nurses have an important, if as yet largely unrealized, role to play.

However, it is also important to look critically at some of the ideas underpinning health promotion. Some argue that it is one example of the move towards 'successful ageing', which is now the subject of international interest (Grundy and Bowling 1999). Visions of successful ageing are often based on the idea of maintaining health and wellness and of remaining physically and mentally fit and able. In an ideal world this would be the way that we would all age, but we do not live in an ideal world and, as has already been noted, the incidence of disability rises sharply with advanced older age. Minkler (1996) argues that while there is nothing wrong with the idea of successful ageing *per se*, it rather depends on how success is defined, and who defines it.

Scheidt *et al.* (1999) contend that current definitions of successful ageing are based largely on the absence of disease and high levels of physical and mental functioning, and create a vision of 'super-ageing' based on physically fit, creative and active older people (Feldman 1999). Although this might reflect the situation for many older people, it seriously disadvantages others, especially those who are frail or chronically ill (Minkler 1996). The danger is that an increasingly narrow view of successful ageing is likely to result in thinking which oppresses and stigmatizes older people who do not meet the criteria for success (Feldman 1999). This 'idealization' of ageing fosters an image against which many people would fail, with potentially serious consequences:

> 'In the West we inhabit a youth-centred and a youth-dominated culture … to be old in the 1990s might (therefore) be a worrying prospect. To be old, dependent and ill could be a terrifying one'.
>
> *(Garner and Ardern 1998)*

Therefore, while we would certainly not argue against the benefits of producing optimal health in older people, this vision should not be based simply on being physically fit and able. Rather the goal should be to promote an optimum quality of life, and this, as will be demonstrated below, is not based solely on people's objective circumstances.

CREATING PERSON-ORIENTED QUALITY OF LIFE

Quality of life, or more specifically, health-related quality of life (HRQoL), is now one of the most important indicators used to judge the success, or otherwise, of health care interventions (O'Boyle 1997). However, the ways in which HRQoL is defined and measured suffer from many of the limitations noted above, with regard to 'successful ageing'. It is now widely accepted that prolonging life at any cost is not as important as the quality of life that is lived (Clark 1995), and this has resulted in increasing attention being given to what we mean by quality of life (Haas 1999). Along with successful ageing, many measures of quality of life are underpinned by ideas such as interdependence and autonomy (Carson 1995), which is often reduced simply to being able to perform a number of activities of daily living (Clark 1995). To make matters worse, many of the questions in quality of life scales have been developed with younger people and are of questionable value for older people (O'Boyle 1997). Furthermore, it is often the researcher who decides which questions to include, with the views of patients and carers rarely being considered (Chesson *et al.* 1996). It is, therefore, suggested that many existing approaches to the measurement of quality of life rely too much on 'statistical sophistication' (Bowling 1995) and as a consequence they 'lose the human being' in the process (Kivnick and Murray 1997).

We do not, as yet, have any definitive theories which explain why some individuals 'navigate the last chapter of their lives with equanimity', whereas for others 'ageing represents as a wound to the self-esteem' (Garner and Ardern 1998), or why:

> 'Some old people seem able to maintain their dignity and spirit despite terrible adversity, while others who experience apparently minimal discomfort are able to enjoy nothing'.
>
> *(Evans 1998)*

However, there is growing evidence that such differences cannot be explained simply by variations in independence and autonomy. Several authors have commented on the fact that subjective quality of life can often improve, even as disability increases (Brändstädter and Greve 1994; Johnson and Barer 1997). Two recent theories offer some potential explanation for the complex factors which influence the way older people judge the quality of their lives, and the factors that they use to define 'successful' ageing. First, Steverink *et al.* (1998) propose that quality of life in older age comprises two key components: physical well-being and social well-being, with two physical and three social goals determining the overall level of well-being (Box 12.3).

Box 12.3 Physical and social goals that determine overall well-being (Steverink *et al.* 1998)

Physical:
- Comfort: basic needs are met, absence of fear and pain
- Stimulation: absence of boredom, presence of challenge

Social:
- Behavioural confirmation: performs important roles or tasks adequately
- Affection: loved by self and others
- Status: feels valued

They argue that the relative importance of these goals varies over time and is influenced by cultural and other factors, such as gender. However, they believe that an acceptable quality of life requires that at least one goal be met within each domain. As a minimum the authors argue that individuals must experience comfort and affection.

Second, from a more sociological perspective, Nilsson *et al.* (1998) conducted in-depth interviews with over 30 older people, ranging in age from 82 to 92 years, and identified six 'types' of old age, ranging from successful to miserable. Box 12.4 contrasts what makes for a 'successful' old age with a 'miserable' one.

Box 12.4 Criteria for successful vs miserable older age (Nilson *et al.* 1998)

Successful:
- Does not feel old, even if disabled
- Feels independent, even if reliant on others
- Lives for present/future
- Strong beliefs about life

Miserable:
- See themselves as old
- Not satisfied with efforts
- Has poor relationships
- Little meaningful activity

The authors conclude that a successful old age is underpinned largely by: a feeling of being embedded in social relationships, usually but not exclusively, within the family; being able to pursue meaningful activity and feeling needed; having a positive view of the past, the present and the future; and having a philosophy of life based on religious or other personal beliefs. Lawton *et al.* (1999) proposed that the 'valuation' people place on various aspects of their lives is the key to understanding not only their quality of life, but also their continued desire to live.

Issues of personal identity and meaning should, therefore, figure more prominently in debates about the goals of health care in an ageing society, raising difficult questions about the ways in which 'success' is judged, and the evidence we use to judge it:

'An understanding of illness that reunites the psychological with the experiential will ... require a far richer and more varied conception of evidence than that previously at stake in 'evidence-based' medicine, taking more seriously patients' conceptions of their own values and goals'.

(Evans 1999)

This challenges us to think about the sort of health care system that is appropriate for the 21st century. Van de Plaats (1997) outlines three models: the curative; the situational and the transformative. The curative can be likened to the traditional medical model, where the aim is to remedy faulty physiology, with cure being a goal to which we would all aspire if possible. Situational interventions concern themselves with the environments in which people find themselves, and therefore include not only restorative and compensatory health care but also efforts to address a range of societal obstacles, which inhibit the full participation of people with disabilities. Such interventions are also essential for all individuals, older or not, who experience chronic illness and disability. However, notwithstanding the importance of situational factors, there is a need to move beyond 'compensation and remediation' (Kivnick and Murray 1997). 'Transformative' interventions can be thought of as addressing what Trieschmann (1988) has called 'I am' questions concerning what gives life value and meaning and what is necessary to sustain or recreate a sense of identity (Minkler 1996; Phillipson and Biggs 1998). It is these concerns that must be more fully incorporated into definitions of 'success' and measures of HRQoL if a more holistic and balanced perspective is to emerge. Such a perspective is essential if person-centred care is to become a reality.

ENHANCING USER AND CARER INVOLVEMENT

One manifestation of the move towards person-centred care is the priority now given to user and carer involvement. According to Bernard and Phillips (2000), the 1990s saw the emergence of a new 'language' of social policy, prompting the more active involvement of service users. Certainly the terms 'participation' and 'empowerment' feature heavily in current policy rhetoric aimed at ensuring that services are more responsive to the needs of users, including older people. However, the means for ensuring that older people are able to participate in service planning and delivery, and furthermore feel empowered, are more elusive, with the attitudes and practices of health care practitioners often acting as an important barrier. Walker and Warren (1996), for example, call for a change in professional values and attitudes within the formal sector so that co-operation and partnership with older people is regarded as a normal activity. They identify a number of organizational principles and structures which militate against user-participation in service planning and delivery, in particular those which encourage professionals to regard themselves as 'experts'.

Participation in care necessarily involves a change in relationships between professionals and lay people, whether they are patients, residents of care homes or family carers (Kirk and Glendinning 1998). This requires a sharing of professional knowledge which professionals may find threatening (Trnobranski 1994). Some recent work has attempted to access user views and feed these directly into the commissioning process for older people's services (Mitchell and Koch 1997; Raynes 1998; Reed *et al.* 1999). However, for many older people and family carers, conditions do not yet exist which would facilitate active participation in decision-making in health care. This can often result in a tokenistic approach to user participation which fails to realize the true potential for either service users or providers.

EXERCISE

Imagine that you are the manager of a care home for frail older people with continuing care needs. What steps could you take to ensure that the views of older people and their carers contribute to planning services within the home? What difficulties might you encounter? The references cited by Reed *et al.* (1999) and Burton Jones (2001) might be particularly useful in helping you think about this.

As suggested above, many of the difficulties in actively promoting and achieving participation and empowerment turn largely on who is seen as the 'expert'. Traditionally, it is the professional, and in the medical model the 'patient' adopts a largely passive role in the process of diagnosis and is then expected to 'comply' with the treatment that is prescribed. Such a view has, however, been under increasing challenge, especially in chronic illness, where the patient or carer is often more expert than the professional. Indeed, a recent Department of Health (DoH 2001k) policy document states that there is a need for greater recognition of the 'expert' patient, who should be seen as a full and active partner in the delivery of health care:

'The era of the patient as a passive recipient of care is changing and being replaced by a new emphasis on the relationship between the NHS and the people whom it serves – one in which health professionals and patients are genuine partners seeking the best solution to each patient's problems – one in which patients are empowered with information and contribute ideas to help in their treatment and care'.

(DoH 2001k, p9)

Fuelled by the realization that the greatest future health challenges faced by modern societies are chronic illnesses, the aim is to recognize and build upon the 'expertise' of patients themselves and to harness this to forge new partnerships with health professionals. This, we are told, will require a 'fundamental shift' in ways of working. Indeed, this is only one of many such 'shifts' that have been promoted in a series of recent documents, such as *The NHS Plan* (DoH 2000a) and the NSF (DoH 2001i).

The idea that there are complementary sources of expertise held by individuals, particularly those with chronic illness, is not new and has been noted in the sociological literature for some time. Indeed, in highlighting the knowledge potentially held by frail older people, the literature on chronic illness provides important insights, having long argued that 'top down' models of professional practice (Strauss and Corbin 1988) fail to recognize the differing types of 'work' required in managing long-term illness, thereby ignoring the genuine expertise held by lay people (Strauss *et al.* 1984, Strauss and Corbin 1988). This can have a profoundly detrimental effect on the quality of communication between professionals and disabled people.

A number of nursing authors have suggested that if communication between older people and health care practitioners is to improve, then in addition to the usual 'knowledge' which underpins professional practice, there is a need to recognize and draw upon other ways of 'knowing', which help practitioners better to understand individual responses to illness. For example, Liaschenko (1997) argues that, particularly in chronic illness, practitioners need to draw upon knowledge that helps them to appreciate what it is like to live a particular kind of life. She identifies three broad types of knowledge that can be used to inform nursing practice (Box 12.5).

Box 12.5 Types of knowledge for nursing older people (Liaschenko 1997)

- *Case knowledge:* this comprises biomedical, disembodied knowledge of a particular condition, e.g. stroke
- *Patient knowledge:* this is best viewed as a 'case in context'. In other words, information about a person's social circumstances, level of support, etc, to provide a better understanding of the impact of the 'stroke' and the resources that can be mobilized
- *Person knowledge:* this is based on understanding 'biographical life' which comprises three components: agency, the capacity to initiate meaningful action; temporality, which is related to an individual's pattern of life rather than 'clock time'; space, in terms of how an individual relates to their physical, social and political environments so as to create a sense of 'belonging' somewhere

Liaschenko (1997) argues that patient and person knowledge are decidedly different and that for 'interventionist' disciplines, i.e. those which aim to do things to, for, or with people, person knowledge is often essential in order to promote and maintain individual integrity. However, she believes that person knowledge is not appropriate in all contexts.

Eliciting person knowledge takes time and trust and thus case and patient knowledge may be more relevant in situations where the primary aim is to cure a condition and 'move a person out'. Person knowledge is not therefore intrinsically desirable and may be unacceptably intrusive in certain contexts. Conversely, person knowledge is usually essential where there is an ongoing relationship, e.g. in the case of older people with learning disabilities, and its value – but also its potentially resource-intensive and time-consuming nature – has to be recognized. For Liaschenko (1997) this raises political questions, not only for professionals but also for society more generally, about the type of health care that we 'envision'. Person-centred care cannot be manifest unless the skills required are seen not only as legitimate but also important. Liaschenko (1997) doubts that this is the case as:

'the kind of attentiveness this (person) knowledge demands is increasingly being seen as fluff, not essential to a vision of health care in which people are cared for only on the basis of case and patient knowledge'.

Clearly then, if user involvement is to become a reality, there is a need to recognize and actively draw upon 'person knowledge'. The idea that there are other forms of 'expertise' does not only relate to people with chronic illness, but also extends to family carers – who after all – provide 80% of all the care needed by older people (Walker 1995). Harvath *et al.* (1994) argue that professionals have what they term 'cosmopolitan' knowledge, i.e. a generalized understanding of a condition, e.g. stroke. Carers, on the other hand, have 'local knowledge', based on their unique understanding of the person having suffered a stroke. Using Liaschenko's (1997) framework, cosmopolitan knowledge would equate to case knowledge and local knowledge largely to person knowledge. It would seem that the two might most meaningfully come together in helping to shape patient (or client) knowledge. In other words, both cosmopolitan and local knowledge are needed in order to understand fully the needs of an older person within a particular context.

REFLECTION POINT

Think about an older person you have nursed recently. Make brief notes about the way in which the three types of knowledge identified by Liaschenko (case knowledge, patient knowledge and person knowledge) combined to enable you to make an assessment. Did you draw upon all three types of knowledge? Did you prioritize any particular type of knowledge within your assessment? What were the consequences?

Nolan *et al.* (1996) argued that it was important to see 'carers as experts' and they developed a model and a set of assessment indices for helping professionals to recognize carer expertise. This has been shown to be very useful in helping professionals to gain new insights into the world of carers (Qureshi *et al.* 2000). However, many professionals see the 'expert' carer (or older person) as a threat and difficulties can arise, leading to conflict, unless care is taken (Allen 2000).

Therefore, while the idea of user and carer involvement is actively promoted, making it happen is not easy and will require changes of attitude and new ways of working among professionals. For example, the way in which the assessment of need is approached will have a profound effect on subsequent interventions and the support that is offered.

The complexity of need commonly associated with ageing, chronic illness and disability is an important consideration in planning appropriate care for older people and their families. A wide range of assessment tools has been developed which can assist in identifying need and suggesting appropriate interventions for service users and family carers, e.g. the RCN assessment tool for older people (Wills and Ford 2001). However, practitioners must be discerning in their use of these tools and be confident that any assessment tool is appropriate for an individual, is valid (i.e. it assesses the factors which it was designed to assess) and is reliable (i.e. it assesses these factors consistently). It is also necessary to keep in mind that many assessment tools, e.g. tools designed to assess general health, anxiety, depression, and quality of life, have not been developed and tested specifically for use with older people.

The importance of involving older people, and, where appropriate, their family carers, in the assessment process cannot be overestimated. As noted above, many older people with chronic health problems and their carers have built up a wealth of expertise in the management of their condition, and it would be extremely foolish not to build upon this expertise in devising and implementing a plan of care.

The points in Box 12.6 have emerged in discussions with successive groups of students and practitioners and are offered here as experience-based pointers for practice.

Box 12.6 Experience-based pointers for assessment

- For general assessments, guidelines for assessment may be more useful than rigidly structured tools and checklists
- It is important to assess the need for each aspect of assessment rather than applying a blanket approach
- The accuracy and value of assessment is likely to be increased if service users and carers are involved as fully as possible

To involve older people and families in the assessment processes, Smale *et al.* (1993) argue that we must move away from the 'questioning model', in which the professional is the expert who asks the questions to which the older person/carer passively responds, and the 'procedural model', in which there is a checklist of questions determined in advance. Instead we must adopt an 'exchange model'. This is based on the belief that good assessments require the exchange of differing forms of knowledge and expertise and that all these ways of knowing are essential in reaching 'a mutual understanding' of the issues involved. This is a very important consideration, because without such a mutual understanding, it is difficult to identify the type of therapeutic intervention required, or to judge its effectiveness.

DEVELOPING THERAPEUTIC INTERVENTIONS WITH OLDER PEOPLE AND FAMILY CARERS

Tensions about the appropriate goals and outcomes for the health and social care of older people have been apparent since the early days of geriatric medicine, going back to the 1950s. In acute conditions the goal is fairly obvious, with the intention being to 'cure' the condition. It is here that the traditional 'medical' or 'curative' model (Van de Plaats 1997) is most relevant. All of us want, of course, to be 'cured' if we are ill but this is not always possible, especially with many of the conditions that affect older people. For example, it is not possible to 'cure' a stroke *per se*, but it is possible to help the person regain as much function as possible. Therefore, in the early days, geriatric medicine replaced 'cure' as the major goal of care by rehabilitation; the latter was based on a functional model of health in which the ability to perform the main activities of daily living (ADL) became the criterion of success. Indeed, some authors argue that this has resulted in an 'ADL research and practice' tradition (Porter 1995), in which 'success' is viewed only in such terms. As noted earlier, this rather limited view of success is still evident in many current visions of successful ageing. Such a development had a particularly negative effect in long-term care settings where the application of a curative or restorative model (Reed and Bond 1991) made it very difficult to define appropriate indicators of success. Reed and Bond (1991) argue that when neither cure or restoration is possible, then nurses tend to gauge the quality of their work in terms of 'good geriatric care', the aim of which is to have patients clean, comfortable and well fed.

More recently, however, there has been much talk of 'new cultures' of care, especially in fields such as dementia, where the idea of 'person-centred care' (Kitwood 1997) has had a very positive effect, by providing staff with a set of meaningful goals to aim for. Indeed, so influential has the idea of person-centred care been that it now underpins the NSF for older people, which is about, we are told, 'care which respects them [patients] as individuals and is arranged around *their* [authors' emphasis] needs'.

It can be argued that, while the idea of person-centred care has been very useful in raising awareness and providing a sense of direction in certain areas of care (e.g. dementia), it has limitations. First, exactly what it is and how it is achieved is difficult to define (see, for example, Packer 2000). Moreover, focusing on individuals and their needs runs the risk of overlooking the role of 'communitarian values' (Evans 1999) and the delicate interdependencies that characterize the best caring relationships (Brechin 1998).

More recently, commentators have highlighted the relevance of relationship-centred care as a concept to guide practice (Nolan *et al.* 2001). It has been argued for some time that caring can only be fully understood within the context of a relationship (Nolan *et al.* 1994; Brechin *et al.* 1998), and yet the important dimensions of caring relationships have yet to be fully understood. Brechin goes further to argue that care is primarily about relationships and any account which fails to consider these relationships will 'only reveal part of the story'.

> 'If we want to understand 'good care' in the sense of care which brings positive consequences for those who are involved, then we must take account of the person and the relationships itself and not just see care as an instrumental means to an end'.
>
> (Brechin 1998, p177)

Brechin believes that care can only be seen as 'good' if it is good from the perspectives of all parties involved. This requires a construction of care which recognizes and acknowledges different perspectives, but which is underpinned by relationships based on mutual respect and a sense of equality.

The idea of 'relationship-centred', as opposed to 'person-centred', care was suggested following the discussions of a Task Force in the US in the early 1990s, which concluded that the notion of relationship-centred care should underpin all health interactions. The argument was made that a focus on relationships should underpin curricula across the caring disciplines (including medicine), with the following definition being provided:

'Relationship-centred care is health care that values and attests to the relationships that form the context of care, including: those among and between clinicians and patients; individuals as they care for themselves and one another; clinicians and the communities in which they practice; health care clinicians across various professions; and administrators and managers as they set the environment and resources for care'.

The report of the Task Force (Tresolni and Pew-Fetzer Task Force 1994) provides further detail, including an indicative set of knowledge and skills upon which to base a relationship-centred approach. The importance of this is summed up as follows:

'The phrase 'relationship-centred care' captures the importance of the interaction among people as the foundation of any therapeutic or teaching activity. Further, relationships are critical to the care provided by nearly all practitioners and a sense of satisfaction and positive outcomes for patients and practitioners. Although relationships are a prerequisite to effective care and teaching, there has been little formal acknowledgement of their importance, and few formal efforts to help students and practitioners learn to develop effective relationships in health care'.

(Tresolni and Pew-Fetzer Task Force 1994, p11)

While the document provides a well-constructed set of arguments for such an approach, it also admits that there is a need for further research to explicate 'the dimensions of a relationship-centred approach to care'.

THE SENSES FRAMEWORK

This chapter concludes by describing an approach to relationship-centred care, based on what is termed the 'senses framework', which has been developed following a number of research studies in which the authors have been involved over the past 5 years.

Concerned with the lack of a therapeutic rationale for work in long-term care settings with older people, Nolan (1997) identified six 'senses' which he believed might both provide direction for staff and improve the care older people received. The term 'sense' was chosen deliberately to reflect the subjective and perceptual nature of the important determinants of care for both older people and staff. These 'fundamentals' were termed: a sense of security, belonging, continuity, purpose, achievement and significance. These senses have now been refined and developed within a series of research projects exploring the needs of older people and family carers within a range of contexts (Box 12.7) (Davies *et al.* 1999, 2001; Nolan *et al.* 2001, 2002). Although still in need of further refinement and empirical testing, the authors believe that the senses have application beyond long-term care settings and can help to inform service development across a range of care environments.

Box 12.7 The six senses

A sense of security: to feel safe

Older people:

- To receive competent, sensitive and consistent care in a supportive environment enabling them to feel safe and free from threat, harm, pain or discomfort
- To acknowledge and reduce unnecessary risk while encouraging informed risk-taking

Staff:

- To have the physical and emotional demands of work acknowledged and minimized
- To work in a supportive, enabling but challenging environment, free from rebuke and censure
- To have secure conditions of employment
- To be able to raise and discuss concerns in an open and honest manner

Family carers:

- To feel able to say 'no' to care if they want to
- To have their own needs recognized and acknowledged
- To feel that they have the knowledge and skills to provide good care without detriment to their health
- To have appropriate, sensitive and timely support
- To recognize the existence of differing viewpoints within caring relationships

A sense of belonging: to have a 'place' and to feel part of something

Older people:

- Having a place or personal space
- To be able to maintain and form meaningful, valued and reciprocal relationships
- To feel part of a community or group if desired
- To be an equal partner in a caring relationship

Staff:

- To feel part of a team or group with a recognized and valued contribution
- To have a sense of professional/work 'identity'
- To have a say in the way in which things are done

Family carers:

- To be able to maintain/form meaningful, valued and reciprocal relationships
- To have someone to turn to if they need to talk things over
- To feel that they are not 'in this alone'
- To feel an active and equal partner in caring

A sense of continuity: linking the past, present and future

Older people:

- To have their personal biography acknowledged and used as a basis for planning and delivering individualized care
- To receive consistent care delivered by known people within an established relationship
- To receive seamless care at key transition points such as hospital discharge and admission to care

Staff:

- Positive experience of work with older people, exposure to good role models and standards of care
- To work as part of a stable team
- To work in an environment where there are consistent expectations and standards of care which are clearly communicated

Family carers:

- To be able to maintain shared pleasures and interests with the person they care for
- To be able to ensure consistent standards of care, whether given by themselves or others
- To be actively involved in care across care environments when desired/appropriate

A sense of purpose: to have direction

Older people:

- To have the opportunity to do something that is meaningful and stimulating
- To pursue personal goals and challenges
- To be able to exercise choice

Staff:

- To have a clear rationale and direction for the care you give
- To be able to pursue personal career goals and aspirations

Family carers:

- To ensure the dignity and individuality of the person they care for
- To ensure that the person they care for receives the best possible care
- To be able to achieve a balance between caring and other important parts of their life

A sense of achievement: to feel you're getting somewhere

Older people:

- To feel satisfied with efforts
- To feel that they are making progress towards meaningful and valued goals
- To feel that they are making a recognized and valued contribution

Staff:

- To feel that you are able to give the best possible care
- To be able to use your skills and abilities to the full
- To have your contribution acknowledged and valued
- To meet personal career goals and aspirations

Family carers:

- To know that they are providing/have provided the best possible care
- To develop new skills and abilities
- To be able to meet competing demands successfully
- To have their caring abilities and expertise acknowledged and valued

A sense of significance: to 'matter'

Older people:

- To feel that they are recognized and valued as a person
- To feel that their actions and existence are important
- To feel that they 'matter'

Staff:

- To feel that gerontological practice is valued and important, that you and your work 'matter'

Family carers:

- To feel that they are recognised and valued as a person
- To feel that their actions and existence are important
- To feel that they 'matter'

While Box 12.7 includes a broad definition of the senses for older people and for family carers, the way in which each sense can be achieved will vary according to the context and caring situation. Box 12.8 provides some suggestions for achieving the senses for older people living in care homes and their family carers. These are based upon group discussions with nurses, care assistants, older people and family carers undertaken within the context of the AGEIN project (Advancing Gerontological Education in Nursing) (Nolan *et al.* 2002). This 3½-year project was commissioned by the English National Board for Nursing, Midwifery and Health Visiting (ENB) to explore the effectiveness of education in preparing nurses to meet the needs of older people and their carers within a multi-professional, multi-agency context. Data was collected from a number of groups, including student nurses, educationalists, registered nurses, older people and family carers using a variety of techniques, such as individual face-to-face and telephone interviews, focus groups, workshops, observation and documentary analysis. The following scenarios provide an opportunity to consider how the senses might be achieved for individuals in other caring situations.

Box 12.8 Factors creating each of the senses for older people, family carers and staff within continuing care settings

Sense of security

Older people:

- Staff being aware of your life story so that they really know you
- Effective communication
- Introducing all staff so that you know who is who
- Encouraging visitors – people who know you really well, to be involved in your care
- Encouraging residents to bring in their own possessions – again to create a sense of familiarity
- Rearranging furniture if necessary
- Comprehensive assessment of needs on admission, including risk assessment
- Ongoing assessment and evaluation
- Allocation of key workers

Staff:

- Effective teamwork and communication
- Effective leadership
- Accurate record-keeping
- Mutual respect – knowing you will be respected as an individual
- Appropriate staffing levels
- Adequate human and mechanical resources
- Training
- Open and approachable management
- Flattened management system
- Confidentiality
- Up-to-date records
- Compassion and understanding

Family carers:

- Approachable teams/management
- Effective communication
- Feeling safe to complain without fear of recrimination

- Keeping appropriate people informed
- Advocacy
- Involving the multi-professional team
- Staff being able to mediate between patients without taking sides
- Keep relatives informed of changes in care plan

Sense of belonging:

Older people:

- Opportunities to visit the home prior to moving in
- Own room/belongings/privacy
- Wait until invited into resident's room
- Open visiting
- Own place in dining room
- Clarify expectations on admission
- Respect personal choice wherever possible
- Residents' groups with nominated chairperson

Staff:

- Important for all grades of staff
- Responsibility based on defined roles
- Opportunity to share
- Feeling valued, trusted and competent
- Thanking staff for their contribution
- Work towards common goals to deliver high standards of care
- Having a sense of camaraderie
- Not working in isolation
- Important for care assistants to have a sense of professionalism

Family carers:

- Important but difficult
- Make relatives feel welcome
- Encourage to take a more active part
- Ensure that staff are there for relatives and residents, physically, mentally and financially
- Encourage involvement in all aspects of care and decision-making
- Value relatives' ideas
- Use appropriate terminology – avoid jargon
- Create care partnerships
- Educate relatives in promoting independence and optimizing opportunities to enhance quality of care
- Make sure that relatives are informed of all changes
- 'Be there' for relatives and encourage them to talk
- Individual service planning to create social activities and opportunities

Sense of continuity

Older people:

- Life history sheet – developed with relative if possible/appropriate
- Consistency in key worker/associate nurse/support worker
- Visit hospital prior to discharge and ensure a familiar face on admission

- Comprehensive information on discharge from hospital and admission to hospital
- Involve activity co-ordinator in helping resident to continue with enjoyed pastimes

Staff:

- Monthly newsletter
- Regular staff meetings
- Clinical supervision and appraisal
- Audit
- Quality standards
- Follow policies/procedures

Family carers:

- Residents/relatives meetings
- Being involved in caring
- Involve relatives in reviews of care plans
- Update relatives with information regularly
- Opportunities to go on outings

Sense of purpose

Older people:

- Create personal profiles including hobbies and interests
- Assess actual and potential abilities
- Identify targets and goals
- Establish a residents' committee
- Considering potential for discharge

Staff:

- Team nursing
- Care plans
- Standing orders
- Induction and training available
- Assessments of quality of care

Family carers:

- Establish a relatives' committee
- Involvement in care planning and delivery (based on relative/resident choice)
- Communication

Sense of achievement

Older people:

- Promoting independence (where possible) in relation to activities of daily living
- Promoting mental well-being and motivation
- Setting individual goals and needs
- Recognizing own capabilities
- Multi-professional approach

Staff:

- Seeing clients improving and gaining confidence in their ability to achieve goals
- Keeping knowledge updated/sharing knowledge
- Regular appraisals/constructive criticism and practice development

- Written evidence of learning/acknowledgement of achievement
- Audit/quality control
- Support of manager/back-up

Family carers:

- Family carer interview on admission – identify expectations
- Open visiting
- Communication from care staff
- Opportunities to assist in providing care
- Support systems for relatives
- Acknowledgement of and help to deal with guilt
- Information about services and benefits
- Addressing conflicts and concerns

Sense of significance

Older people:

- Find out how clients wish to be addressed
- Involve fully in care planning
- Individualized care planning in identifying individual needs
- One-to-one/forming relationships
- Show an interest in the individual and their family
- Social care assessment identifying family relationships
- Use of photographs

Staff:

- Feedback from clients and relatives (either verbally or evidence of contentment)
- Feedback from the local community – knowing you have a good reputation
- Feedback via letters and cards
- Sense of pride in the quality of care provided
- Having opportunity to feedback to education providers

Family carers:

- Opportunity for family to give positive and negative comments about the service provided
- Annual quality control (opportunity to make comments about services anonymously)
- Service user forum
- Choices about involvement in the care of a resident
- Welcoming atmosphere

Scenario Agnes Smith, a 94-year-old lady who lives alone at home, is physically frail and needs assistance in many activities of daily living. She receives a package of care which includes three visits a day from paid carers to help with washing and dressing, and meals on wheels. She is partially sighted and hard of hearing. However, she retains her sense of humour and enjoys conversation and watching television. Her daughter Sue visits every day. Once a week, Agnes attends a local day centre.

Scenario Ron James is a 65-year-old married man with Alzheimer's disease receiving respite care in a specialist ward of a local community hospital. Ron is fully mobile but has a poor short-term memory and needs direction in the activities of daily living. His wandering is a threat to his safety. His wife Sarah, who cares for him at home, is on holiday with their son, daughter-in-law and grandchildren.

Scenario Audrey Collins, a 74-year-old woman admitted to her local hospice for pain and symptom control, is a spinster but is well supported by members of her local church. She is in the advanced stages of lung cancer with widespread bony metastases. Her main problems are breathlessness and severe pain. These symptoms are affecting her ability to be independent in the activities of daily living.

EXERCISE

Consider the senses framework in Box 12.7 in relation to each of the above individuals. Write down as many actions/interventions that you can think of that could help you to make sure that each 'sense' was achieved for each person.

Next, think about the senses framework in relation to the family carers. Again, write down actions for achieving each 'sense' for these individuals.

SUMMARY

- Health promotion with older people is one area in which gerontological nurses have an important, if as yet largely unrealized, role to play.
- The goal of person-centred care for older people should be the promotion of an optimal quality of life.
- Involving older people and their families in their health and social care involves creating a mutual understanding of the issues involved.
- The relevance of relationship-centred care as a concept to guide practice with older people and their families is beginning to emerge.
- The six senses of security, significance, belonging, purpose, continuity and achievement provide a logical framework for beginning to articulate the goals of care for older people and their families and for implementing the philosophy of relationship-centred care.

CONCLUSION

In many ways, the future of gerontological nursing appears brighter than it has for some time. The recognition that older people now form the major proportion of users of health care services, together with the articulation of goals of care within a range of care environments, provides a clear impetus for further developing the knowledge-base for practice with older people and their families, and for ensuring that gerontological nursing is perceived as a positive career choice. New roles and opportunities are being created as services are reconfigured better to meet the needs of older people and their carers. Simultaneously, practice models and frameworks, such as person- and relationship-centred care, and the senses framework outlined within this chapter, are beginning to reveal the fundamentals of care for older people and are helping to define the nature of gerontological nursing.

The next challenge is to ensure that all older people and their family carers have access to the highest possible standards of care, whatever their circumstances and in whatever caring environment. As argued within this chapter, this will require that everyone involved in helping older people to meet their health and social care needs – staff, family members and older people themselves – are able to participate and contribute in mutually fulfilling ways.

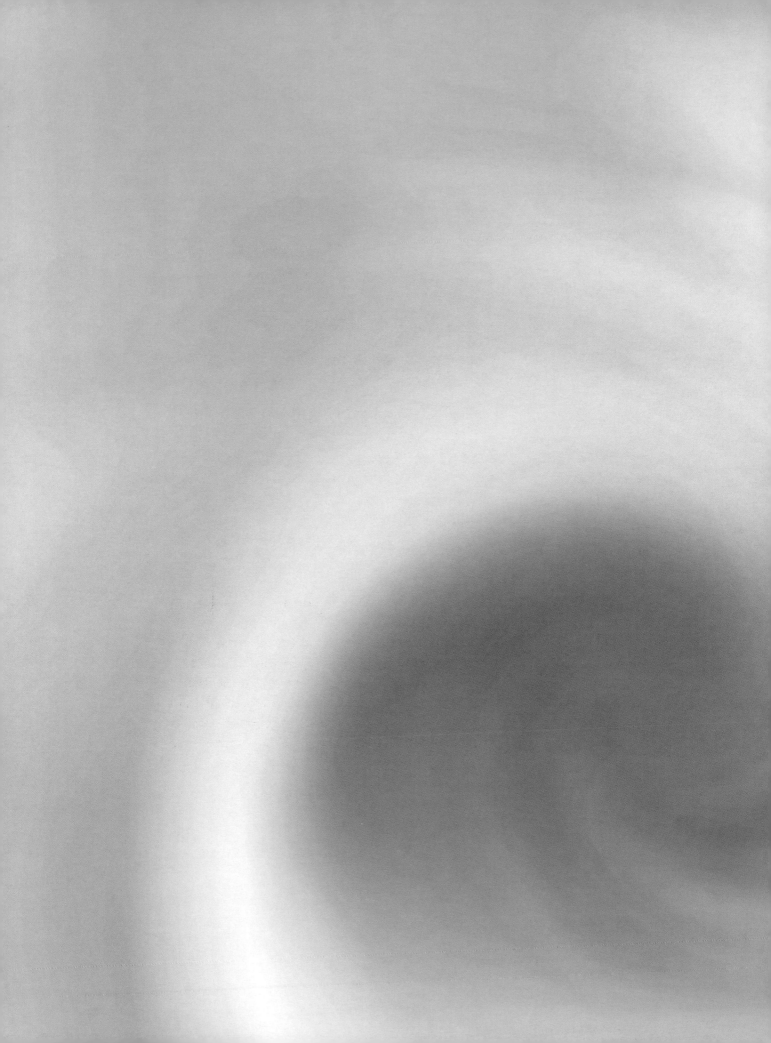

CHAPTER

13

COPING WITH EXPECTED AND UNEXPECTED DEATH

Kieron Thayre and Ian Peate

INTRODUCTION

The aim of this chapter is to introduce you to a variety of issues surrounding the care of dying patients, their relatives and people who are bereaved. This will help you understand the complexities of caring for dying patients and their relatives when death is expected or if death occurs suddenly and unexpectedly. When attending to the care of the dying patient and their relative(s), and people who are bereaved, after expected or unexpected deaths, you will have to assess, plan, implement and evaluate care based on the four care domains: professional/ethical practice, the delivery of care, care management and your own personal and professional development. It must be noted that all domains are inter-related and aspects overlap.

UNDERSTANDING BEREAVEMENT AND LOSS

Coming to terms with loss and bereavement is one of life's most painful, distressing and fragmenting experiences. The expected or unexpected death of someone who is clearly loved brings emotional pain and grief as the temporal bonds between them and those who remain are severed (Raphael 1984, p3). It is also one of the most difficult aspects of your personal and professional development because of the quality of care and support that distressed patients and their relatives will need you to give. While the term 'relatives' is used throughout this chapter, it is implicit that friends and partners of either sex are included.

From a predominantly western Caucasian perspective, grief is viewed as a person's response to any loss that they perceive as emotionally significant.

'Grief is essentially an emotion that draws us toward something or someone that is missing.'

(Parkes 2000, p326)

Bereavement is the period of time encompassing the duration of the emotional and physiological disequilibrium that follows a loss; or as Willis (1979) suggested, it is the time for bereaved people to regain their 'emotional homeostasis'. The 'grieving process' describes the complexity and extremes of psychological and physiological reactions which many people experience during, after or when facing loss. Initially it is the raw feelings and emotions that are at the centre of the process that engages the individual(s), or family, in adjusting to their changed circumstances. Latterly, the process surrounds the difficulty and pain of having to say goodbye, and assimilate and come to terms with their loss as they gradually begin to 'let go' and 'move on' with the rest of their life. In its widest sense, the fundamental issues of grief and loss centre on the 'cost of loving', the power and degree of commitment to people, places, objects, goals and ambitions. The grieving process surrounds *having* to come to terms with enforced change(s) versus current and future needs, hopes, dreams, goals and aspirations. Part of the difficult legacy of bereavement is that many losses are (or are perceived to be) irreparable and irreplaceable, with fear of the unknown taking their place.

The type, intensity and duration of a patient's/relative's reactions depends on many variables. Parkes' (1972) classic studies on grief identified a number of determinants which contribute to the individual's grieving process and eventual resolution:

- circumstances surrounding the death and how the patient died
- type and nature of the relationship and attachment
- historical antecedents, e.g. the person's previous experience(s) of loss and their learned coping mechanisms
- personality variables, e.g. age, sex, ethnicity, cultural and religious background
- social variables, such as the degree of additional help and support that is available.

REFLECTION POINT

As you prepare yourself to face distressed parents and relatives, reflect on the concept of a 'good' or 'bad' death [refer to Bradbury (2000)]. Consider the degree of dependence on, or independence from, or the ambivalence of, the relative's relationship with the dying patient or the person who has died.

Reflect on people's internal and external, positive and negative coping mechanisms and link this to your developing understanding of psychology; stress and health and defence mechanisms. Reflect how these variables may impact on people's reactions and coping styles. What other ethnic, cultural and religious needs will you have to respond to and know how to respect?

Reflect on your advocacy role. What other sources of help, e.g. friends, specialist practitioners or support groups, do you need to be aware of and be able to access?

The 'stages' or 'phases' of grieving and the potential reactions associated with the fundamentals of grief and loss are well described in the literature (Parkes 1972; Raphael 1984). Kübler-Ross's (1969) pioneering work described a series of stages as dying patients and their families moved towards an accepted, and hopefully, more peaceful death: denial and isolation, anger, bargaining, depression and acceptance. The problem with this early terminology is that it implies a successive and orderly progression, whereas the dying patient, their relatives and people who are suddenly bereaved oscillate between a vast range of feelings and emotions, widely differing in intensity and duration. You will find that there is a broad acceptance of a general pattern of behaviour, succinctly summarized as initial *shock and disbelief,* followed by a period of intense *sadness and pining,* with gradual *re-organization and re-integration* (Katz and Sidell 1994). However, there is no consensus over the use of appropriate labels or over any typical chronology of the component thoughts, feelings and behaviours.

The fundamental principle is that any reaction that you may have to respond to, attributed to any particular phase or stage, should not be expected to occur in any set order; a particular reaction may not occur at all, may recur several times or aspects of several may occur simultaneously. A crucial element, underpinning your care, is your appreciation and empathic sensitivity to the patient's/relative's unique perception of their loss, its magnitude and its meaning to them as an individual. It is essential that you recognize that no one person's grieving process or reaction is the same as another's, no matter how similar the cause or situation may appear. Comparisons are meaningless. No one can predict how a patient/relative will react. Many will not react in the way(s) we expect, feel appropriate or understand. In essence, they will react in whatever way is the most acceptable or familiar to them. The skill is to adapt your responses accordingly and to remain non-judgemental.

The pain and manifestations of grief are more universal. The range of emotions, reactions and behaviours that you may encounter is vast and largely dictated by cultural background and familiarity. Reactions you may see are listed in Box 13.1. Later on, if you were to visit during a community placement, other components that you might find include difficulty in eating, sleeping and concentrating, weight loss, palpitations, anger, depression, apathy, gradual resolution and re-integration.

Box 13.1 Initial reactions to grief (Kübler-Ross 1969; Parkes 1972; Raphael 1984; Thayre and Hadfield-Law 1995)

- Shock and numbness
- Withdrawal and lack of response
- Silence
- Denial and disbelief
- Confusion and agitation
- Anger and resentment
- Tension and frustration
- Restlessness

- Disorganization and repetition
- Frantic questioning and searching behaviours
- Distress and crying
- Keening and pining
- Cathartic behaviours
- Distressed silence
- Relief
- Guilt
- Remorse and acceptance

Another important issue that nurses need to be aware of is the length of time or warning period that the patient/relative has had to prepare themselves. The period of 'anticipatory grief', as part of the dying process, is often intensely stressful and distressing but the 'worry work' undergone can facilitate and maximize preparation time, as the painful reality is gradually acknowledged and accepted. Many patients and families may cope by maintaining a 'closed awareness' and choose not to talk about it; however, the converse is equally true. As painful as it is, many people choose to use the time they have left together to 'mend bridges' and make amends for 'sins of omission and commission'; to say, and therefore hear, what they need to and to finish otherwise 'unfinished business'. It is important, however, for you to appreciate that anticipatory grief does not necessarily occur automatically (Wright 1996). Wright (1996, p11) also supports Fulton and Gottesman's (1980) conclusion that:

'the usefulness of anticipatory grief is not determined by its duration … it is the manner in which it is experienced and responded to by those concerned'.

Although a death may be expected, do not make the assumption that it may not also be perceived as sudden. Relatives may be distressed, shocked and angry that the death occurred 'so soon' – 'we had so little time', and deeply regret that they did not use their time well. Even though there is an acceptance, there is frequently a preference to use 'distancing and avoidance' tactics to continue to hold out hope and to shield and protect everyone from exacerbating further upset and distress. Relatives will frequently say, 'even though I knew she was very ill I didn't realize she was that ill', or 'I knew she was dying but I didn't expect it so soon'. Quietly acknowledge how much their loved one's death hurts.

CONCEPT OF HEALTHY GRIEF

Grieving is an emotionally and physically draining and exhausting 'active' process. Many of the psychological and physiological manifestations are frightening and overwhelming at times, but according to the concept of 'healthy grief', it is the process by which people heal. Using a wound-healing analogy, the initial raw and acutely painful wound must eventually heal, but to a greater or lesser extent a scar will always remain, as the experience, for good and bad, will have irrevocably changed the life of those who were bereaved.

Bereavement is a life transition – or a series of psychosocial transitions – as a process of adaptation to change(s) (Parkes 2000). Resolution must occur to enable the person to gain acceptance, integrate the experience and eventually recover. The focus of nursing with expected and unexpected deaths usually involves responding to intensely painful emotions – the initial raw face of grief when all is lost. It is strengthening and empowering to hold fast quietly to the knowledge that, with resolution and healing, remarkably positive change(s) may accompany bereavement in the longer term. Zisook *et al.* (2001) report that:

'individuals often comment that bereavement prepared them well to face many of life's challenges … [often emerging from their losses as] vital, hopeful, autonomous and more capable individuals.'

Many models of grief have been described in the literature. Worden's (1991) distinctive contribution is his analysis of the Harvard bereavement study 'Omega Project' and his suggestion that four 'tasks of mourning' must be completed for grief resolution: accepting the reality of the loss; being able to feel and express pain and distress, which in turn allows a gradual adjustment (to the environment in which the deceased is missing); being able to 'let go' and move on; re-investing in further relationships and finding renewed meaning in life.

All members of the health care team are important contributors to the patient's/relative's overall quality of care; our multi-professional role is often as a co-ordinator to ensure that needs, which may be explicitly or implicitly expressed, are met. Our role within the nursing care team is vital to ensure the highest quality of care and support is given to dying patients, their families and the people who are bereaved after expected and unexpected death.

Effective personal qualities that your patients/relatives will need from you as you develop self-confidence and competence in all four domains of caring (UKCC Nursing Competencies, Appendix 2) are listed in Box 13.2.

Box 13.2 Effective personal qualities in a nurse

- Warmth
- Compassion
- Caring and calmness
- Acceptance
- Trust and genuiness
- Understanding and empathy
- Insight and emotional intelligence
- Strength and encouragement
- Courtesy
- Respect and commitment

Effective professional helping strategies that you will need to develop include your abilities to listen, acknowledge, empathize and legitimize. Reflecting upon, and sensitivity to, your own reactions allows you to hear and feel; slowing down enables you to allow emotions to be expressed and shared; using open-ended questions, paraphrasing, summarizing and 'supportive confrontation' facilitates clarity, understanding and acceptance. For example, a substantial period of time may be needed as the patient/relative acknowledges deterioration(s).

REFLECTION POINT

- What have you needed when you were very anxious, upset or frightened/had just been given bad news?
- What personal and professional strengths do you have to give?
- What personal and professional limitations do you have?
- What personal and professional resources do you need to develop?
- Who do you need to help you develop these?

SUMMARY

- Grieving patients and relatives typically experience a wide and complex range of emotions and reactions as they have to come to terms with enforced change(s).
- Grief resolution is a slow, lengthy and painful process. All members of the health care team are important contributors to helping patients/relatives deal with the difficult realities they face.

EXPECTED DEATH

Caring for the dying patient requires astute, high quality nursing care. The *Code of Professional Conduct* (NMC 2002a) states that each registered nurse and midwife is personally accountable for their own practice and that all patients must be treated as individuals.

Within the professional/ethical practice domain, the nurse will need to consider some issues that are currently controversial, and have the potential to provoke an emotional response. For example, the associated ethical and moral dilemmas concerned with the complexities of euthanasia, the question of advanced directives and 'do-not-resuscitate' orders.

The second domain concerns the implementation and the delivery of informed care. This domain considers care for both the patient and their relatives – caring for the 'whole being', promoting dignity, providing physical comfort and consideration of the patient's spiritual needs. Social care, such as help with personal issues, demands that you act as an advocate. Care management involves teamwork and effective leadership skills. Care delivery needs to be monitored and evaluated; and you will have to make the best use of all the resources available.

Unless death occurs suddenly, as described later in this chapter, there is usually a 'terminal phase' associated with it. Costello (2001) describes terminal care as care of people in the final stages of their lives. At this stage the nurse is aware that death is certain. However, this phase has the potential to last for days, weeks or even months. If it is long, the multi-professional team may decide to reassess the treatment options previously planned for the patient. The team may have come to the conclusion that the primary cause of the patient's illness, e.g. an infiltrating carcinoma, is less important than the provision of palliative care. Unfortunately, when previously set goals are adapted to reflect the terminal phase of a patient's life, the multi-professional team may neglect to inform the patient's relatives of this. Effective and honest two-way communication is vital throughout. The patient's relatives may have the impression that we have given up on the patient (and also on them). We have a duty to help them understand that we are now focusing on control of the symptoms and the provision of psychological support.

How might you feel if a loved one of yours had their care dramatically altered due to a change in their condition?

PALLIATIVE CARE

Mills *et al.* (1994) reported that the care of the dying patient is often neglected in hospitals and there is evidence to suggest that there are inadequacies in hospital provision of care, in particular poor communication and poor standards of nursing care (Copp 1999). Many government directives have sought to ensure that the provision of care nationally is of a consistently high standard (DoH 1997, 2001i; Scottish Executive 2000a; Department of Health and Social Security and Public Safety 2002).

Palliative care includes terminal care (Field and Copp 1999) and aims to promote both physical and psychological well-being (Husband and Henry 2002). The provision of palliative care is, according to Moss (2002), often demanding, complex and challenging.

The European Association for Palliative Care (1989) suggests that palliative care is:

'…active total care of patients whose disease is not responsive to curative treatment. Control of pain, of other symptoms and of psychological, social and spiritual problems is paramount'.

This definition will help nurses to understand the complex needs of dying patients and their families. An understanding of what palliative care means and the ethos underpinning it will help patients to achieve a more peaceful death (Henderson 1966).

PROFESSIONAL AND LEGAL PERSPECTIVE

The death of a patient can be surrounded with legal and professional issues that may have ramifications for both the nurse and the patient (see also Chapter 4). It is acknowledged in law that patients have a right to die, but they also have a right to have their lives protected. Indeed, article two of the Human Rights Act (1998) states that everyone's life shall be protected by law. However, article three says that no one shall be subjected to torture or to inhumane treatment or punishment (Wilkinson and Caulfield 2000).

Euthanasia

No legislation allows for euthanasia – to kill another person intentionally is murder. The charge of manslaughter will be brought against a nurse who assists another person to die, if it can be proved that the nurse's intervention which caused death was unlawful.

Advanced directives

These are often called living wills and they have become increasingly popular in the past decade (Fairweather and Border 2001). The legality of a 'living will' is recognized as common law, i.e. law made by a judge rather than an Act of Parliament. In 1992 the Terrence Higgins Trust (a charity concerned with HIV/AIDS) compiled a form that would allow a person to make provision for future health care in the event of their suffering permanent mental impairment or incurable physical illness. The 'living will' is unlike an 'ordinary will' (which only takes effect on the death of the person), as the advanced directives are designed to take effect at some point during the person's life.

There are advantages and drawbacks to advanced directives. They have the potential to maximize the patient's autonomy by allowing them some control over their care and may also enable discussion and debate between the patient and the care team. However, Grey (2000) is of the opinion that people may grossly underestimate their desire to have medical intervention if they become ill. Patients should be advised to draw up their directive with appropriate nursing or medical advice.

The current legal situation surrounding advanced directives remains undetermined. However, there is every reason to believe that, in principle, the contents of such a document would be enforceable in the courts and, as such, would be binding on health care professionals (Korgaonkar and Tribe 1992). The 'living will' is signed by the patient and witnessed by another person. Its contents set out what the patient wishes to happen in the event of them becoming incapacitated or requiring other treatment or care, such as resuscitation. If the doctor is of the impression that the contents of the document reflect the patient's wishes then they can rely on its provisions as defence if any action were to be brought against them for their failure to treat the patient. It is important that you are aware that the 'living will' can be withdrawn by the patient at any time, and as developments in medical technologies occur; the 'living will' should be reviewed on a regular basis.

In English law an adult can, and has the right to, consent to or refuse treatment. The person must, however, be able to demonstrate that:

- they have the capacity to make that decision (i.e. is free from the influence of drugs, or not suffering from a mental illness)
- their decision was not influenced by a third party
- they understand in broad terms the nature and effect of the treatment that is being consented to or refused
- the refusal must cover the actual situation in which the treatment is needed.

A court will recognize the patient's wishes in the form of an advanced directive so long as all four criteria have been met.

Nurses, confronted with a patient who has made an advanced directive, should seek advice from their regulatory body and other colleagues with regards to the validity of such a document.

REFLECTION POINT

Can you identify any areas that may cause you concern surrounding the use of advanced directives?

Do-not-resuscitate orders

Patients who are coming to the end of their life should receive the same treatment and care as any other patient, which includes making every effort to resuscitate them should this be needed. However, in some instances the patient may feel that this is not appropriate, and as such, their wishes must be respected (Sutherland 2000).

ACTING IN THE PATIENT'S BEST INTERESTS

Many of the above issues can provoke strong emotional responses and some nurses may find themselves confronted with ethical dilemmas. It is difficult to begin to provide answers, as often these situations are context-dependent but, in order to act in the patient's best interests, you will need to consider many issues. At all stages of the patient's care you must ensure that they are involved in treatment decisions. It is imperative that nursing documentation is accurate, detailed and up-to-date. All appropriate discussions with patients, families and other health care professionals must be recorded (UKCC 1998c).

REFLECTION POINT

Reflect on your clinical experiences and try to think about the documentation that may be needed when the patient's life has ended.

MANAGING THE CARE OF THE DYING PATIENT

Hill (1993) advocates an inter-professional approach to palliative care, using a multitude of health care professionals and volunteers. The palliative care multi-professional team has its roots embedded in the hospice movement, which supports a non-authoritarian or non-hierarchical approach (Husband and Henry 2002), enabling those health care professionals with a specific area of expertise, i.e. a clinical specialist in palliative care, to contribute to the patient's total care. The palliative care team works within the multi-professional team in an advisory, educative and supportive capacity (Moss 2002). A good team will work well if it respects the contribution that each member makes. A good leader is vital and the team must set objectives which are realistic and achievable (Smith 1998).

EXERCISE

When caring for the dying patient many health care professionals are often involved in the holistic care of the patient. Can you list them?

Many authors consider that the management of the patient who is dying will only be as good as the team caring for them (Moss 2002; Husband and Henry 2002). The palliative care team will have to communicate effectively in order to make difficult and appropriate clinical decisions. Although a multi-professional approach should be employed, the nurse, acting as the patient's advocate, should also be prepared to challenge any decisions that they consider are not made in the patient's best interests. Working as a team member is reinforced in the *Code of professional conduct* (NMC 2002a). The *Code* demands that nurses work in a collaborative and co-operative manner with health care professionals and others. In palliative care, nurses work collaboratively, not collusively, with other team members.

Hospital-based multi-professional teams consist of nurses, doctors and other allied health professionals, e.g. radiographers, physiotherapists, speech and language therapists, social workers, religious and spiritual advisers.

Palliative care teams work in acute hospital settings and are evident in areas such as day care centres and home care environments. The *Hospice and Palliative Care Services in the United Kingdom and the Republic of Ireland* directory (Anonymous 2000) provides details about palliative care teams and hospice units across the UK (Table 13.1).

Table 13.1 Palliative care teams in the UK (Anonymous 2000b)

	Home care	Day care	Hospital support teams	Hospital support nursing services
Total	433	243	226	123

The nurse is at the centre of a co-ordinated approach for the provision of effective palliative care. The key principles of palliative care are outlined in Box 13.3. For these key principles to come to fruition, the nurse has to co-ordinate the activities of the multi-professional team, which is a complex process requiring many skills. The way this is managed will depend on where care is being delivered, i.e. in an acute hospital setting or in the patient's own home. In home care settings, Bosanquent and Salisbury (1999) state that the greatest burden of care often falls on the patient's family.

Box 13.3 Primary principles underpinning palliative care (adapted from National Council for Hospice and Specialist Palliative Care Services 1999)

- Focus is the quality of the patient's life
- Symptom control is vital
- Patient is seen as a whole being and the team must take into account the current situation and the patient's past experiences
- Paramount consideration is given to patient autonomy and choice. This includes issues such as where care is given (i.e. at home or in a hospice) and treatment options
- Effective two-way honest communication is instigated between all members of the palliative care team and the patient

The most effective way of managing care is to promote an environment where communication flourishes. Equally important is the notion of support. A supportive attitude towards one another is vital if the team is to function in a competent manner.

The nurse has a responsibility to monitor and evaluate the care that has been delivered. This can be done either internally via audit, or externally (in England and Wales) by statutory bodies, such as the Commission for Health Improvement (CHI), which was introduced in 1998, and charged with the task of monitoring clinical governance.

REFLECTION POINT
How is care monitored and evaluated in the clinical areas you have been allocated to?

Delivery of palliative care

The patient who is dying, or approaching death, has increasing physical, psychological and emotional needs, all of which must be met.

Spiritual care

Spiritual care must be carefully considered. It is important that nurses do not confuse spiritual needs with religious needs; while they may be similar they are not the same. Spiritual needs are often based

on an individual's values and beliefs and a search for meaning. Patients who are members of some religious groups will hold specific spiritual values that must be assessed and goals must be set to enable these needs to be attended to (Kemp 1999). Spiritual needs are often a difficult issue to assess (Carpentino 1997) and the nurse, as co-ordinator of care, may find it helpful to contact the chaplain or religious faith representative for help and advice.

Social needs

Social issues focus on the practical aspects of life, e.g. questions concerning finance, employment and social benefits. Social care agencies may provide financial and physical support, but patients and relatives may not be aware of their entitlements. You will need to contact those who are more knowledgeable about such issues, i.e. social workers, voluntary organizations and trades unions. However, you can continue to have an important role to play here by providing relatives with practical support; this may be something commonplace, e.g. a 'fold away' bed for a relative.

Physical care

As the patient deteriorates and their abilities decline, much of the emphasis will be on the physical aspects of care. It is most important that you do not address these aspects of care in isolation, as they are all inter-related, each having an effect on the other. Roper *et al.* (1996) consider the delivery of nursing care as having five influential factors (physical, psychological, environmental, socio-cultural and politico-economic) and 12 activities of living that must be assessed when providing care for any patient (see Table 6.2).

REFLECTION POINT

Think of a patient you may have nursed in the terminal stages of their life. How many of the activities of living listed in Table 6.2 did you need to consider?

Hill (1993) uses seven headings to categorize the physical needs of the dying patient and notes that some physical aspects will also impinge on the psychological aspects of the patient's life, i.e. depression (Box 13.4).

Box 13.4 Needs of the dying patient (adapted from Hill 1993)

- *Breathing:* dyspnoea (pleural or rib pain), infection, coughs (productive or non-productive) and Cheyne Stokes breathing (death rattle)
- *Nutrition:* anorexia, dysphagia, nausea, vomiting and oral problems
- *Mobility:* weakness, lethargy, muscle and joint pain, pressure sores, paralysis, fractures, pain and lymphoedema
- *Elimination:* urinary retention, urinary incontinence, dysuria, infection, haematuria, constipation and faecal incontinence
- *Hygiene:* inability to self-care, diaphoresis and incontinence
- *Skin integrity:* pressure sores and fungating lesions (i.e. fungating breast cancers)
- *Rest:* anxiety, nightmares, hallucinations, confusion and depression

Many patients with a terminal illness will be experiencing pain. As the disease process progresses, patients may complain of pain with increasing frequency. There are many strategies you can employ in order to minimize pain and suffering. The key to adequate pain management is assessment (Kitson 1994), as accurate and astute assessment of pain allows problems to be identified and immediately addressed.

Having difficulty in breathing is unpleasant and frightening; fear and anxiety exacerbate the experience, and it is therefore distressing for both patient and relatives. Smith (1998) states that 30% of patients with cancer and 65% of patients with lung disease will experience breathing difficulties. You should approach the dyspnoeic patient with a calming and reassuring attitude. It is vital that the cause and effect of the breathlessness is assessed and identified so that appropriate interventions can be implemented, e.g. positioning of the patient, administration of prescribed oxygen and diuretics, ventilation of the room/area and help with expectoration with the assistance of the physiotherapist. Corner *et al.* (1996) suggest that nursing interventions, such as breathing retraining, counselling, relaxation and teaching coping adaptation strategies, will help the dyspnoeic patient.

Peate (1993) suggests that oral hygiene should be a central part of nursing care, and a recognized tool should be used to assess the oral cavity (see Chapter 6). Careful oral hygiene is of paramount importance when caring for the terminally ill patient, as a clean, healthy mouth will improve the patient's feelings of self-esteem.

The oral cavity can very quickly become dry and sore in the terminally ill patient, which is further compounded if the patient is dehydrated as a result of anorexia. Where the oral cavity is left unclean, this will provide an ideal breeding ground for bacteria. The bacteria begin to die and the patient is left feeling uncomfortable and may suffer with halitosis, which is an unpleasant condition and can lead to social withdrawal and isolation.

The production of saliva can be stimulated by giving the patient frequent sips of water, or offering boiled sweets or pineapple. In some cases there may be a need to give the patient prescribed artificial saliva. Complementary therapies, such as tea tree oil, may help the patient but should be used with caution.

In people with advanced cancer, anorexia is a common issue. It is compounded by the fact that the patient may be nauseous and vomiting due to prescribed medications, or they may be constipated, which is a frequent side-effect of analgesic medication, causing additional discomfort.

Vomiting must be controlled, as hyperemesis can result in an electrolyte imbalance. Feeling nauseous can last for a period of time before the patient actually vomits. The nurse can help by ensuring that the patient's bed area or room is well ventilated and any odours that provoke nausea are reduced as much as possible. The patient should have their call bell, a receiver, tissues and mouth-wash solutions within easy reach. During vomiting the patient must have their dignity and privacy maintained. Prescribed antiemetics should be given on a regular basis. Continuous assessment of the situation is needed and the effects of antiemetics should be noted.

Constipation is frequently exacerbated by immobility, changes in diet and reduced fluid intake and, in addition, the side-effects of medication; patients may also be bloated, have abdominal cramps, complain of headache, become confused and be at increased risk of urinary tract infection (Nazarko 1997). Diet is an important feature in the prevention of constipation; high fibre and increased fluid intake is advised. Small, appetizing meals may encourage the patient who does not feel like eating. Finally, prophylactic administration of laxatives is advocated.

Emotional support

Emotional needs will vary considerably and often focus on the patient's ability to adapt to, and to cope with, the immense issues surrounding loss, and to deal with their worries and apprehensions. Losses experienced in illness have been described by Hill (1993) and are listed in Box 13.5.

Box 13.5 Losses associated with illness (Hill 1993)

- Independence
- Status
- Self-image
- Family roles
- Social activities
- Work responsibilities and rewards
- Money
- Mobility
- Plans for the future

People who are facing death may find it difficult to express their needs and may have strong and conflicting emotions. You need effective communication skills to listen and support the patient and family actively in making their needs known. Equally, it is important that you are aware of your own limitations and are able to refer, for example, to the clinical psychologist, counsellor or social worker as appropriate.

WHEN DEATH OCCURS

Care for the patient does not stop at death. Immediately, you have the responsibility to care for the patient's body and their relatives. A GP or hospital doctor must certify that the patient has died. If the patient dies at home, the body cannot be removed until the death certificate has been issued.

Washing the body, straightening limbs, closing eyes, ensuring dignity and removing invasive appliances (as required by the local coroner and local policy) are often referred to as 'last offices' and you should adhere to local policy when carrying this out. You need to be aware of the person's various cultural/religious values and beliefs, as it may not be appropriate for you to carry out last offices – the family or a religious representative may be preferred. Different families have different ways of dealing with their bereavement and this should be recognized and respected.

EXERCISE
Consider and familiarize yourself with the hospital/community policy concerning 'last offices'.

Nurses should be available to sit and stay with relatives if they wish you to. You may also need to contact the mortuary technician so that the family can view the body in the chapel of rest. A nurse should always escort the family and relatives to the mortuary. Relatives should not be rushed during this difficult time as this may be the last opportunity to say goodbye. The memory which we create at this time is a lasting one.

You may also be called upon to assist the patient's relatives if they ask for advice in organizing funeral arrangements, how to register the death and/or the role of the coroner. Many hospitals have a bereavement officer or bereavement adviser whom you may need to involve.

SUPPORTING THE NURSE

Nurses need to have support systems in place that will help them deal with the immense emotional and psychological issues associated with working so close to patients who are dying. There are many ways in which these support systems operate. Each nurse needs to know in themselves when they are beginning to feel the pressure and are becoming stressed.

Nurses not only have a duty to care for their patients but they also have a duty to care for each other and the other members of the care team. Support can be offered in many ways and the team leader should promote a mutually supportive environment in situations where nurses are faced with death and dying on a daily basis. The provision of quality care to a patient and their family has the potential to take its toll on the nurse, emotionally and/or psychologically. Counselling skills should be developed and a degree of reflection and self-awareness will be needed.

REFLECTION POINT
Think about ways in which nurses can be supported when caring for a dying patient.

SUMMARY

- Nurses who care for dying patients will deal with issues that may provoke emotional responses. Ethical and moral dilemmas exist. Excellent clinical and leadership skills are needed. It is vital that nurses communicate in an honest and open manner with patients and their relatives.
- The provision of effective palliative care is complex. It aims to promote physical and psychological well-being.
- There are many legal, professional and ethical issues that confront nurses when caring for dying patients: euthanasia, advanced directives and do-not-resuscitate orders must be considered if the nurse is to act in the patient's best interests.
- An inter-professional approach towards palliative care is advocated when attending to the needs of the patient and their family. The nurse acts as co-ordinator of care and the patient's advocate. Often, towards the end of life, nurses will concentrate on the physical aspects of care but they must not ignore spiritual and psychological aspects of holistic palliative care.
- After death has occurred the nurse still has a duty to care for the patient's body and their relatives.
- Support mechanisms for nurses are vital if they are to continue to cope with the immense emotional and psychological issues associated with caring for the dying patient. Strategies should be in place that encourage nurses to speak of their anxieties and managers need to accept, support and respect this when needed.

UNEXPECTED DEATH

A further series of challenges that you will have to learn to face is responding to the needs of relatives who are suddenly bereaved. With good teaching, mentoring and support from professional colleagues and academic staff you will learn the skills needed to gain confidence in your role within the resuscitation team and how to give distressed relatives compassionate and effective initial bereavement care.

The majority of sudden deaths occur in high dependency and acute care areas, such as A&E, intensive therapy units and critical care. Therefore, when a sudden death occurs on the ward it is frequently a shock for staff, too, especially if it happens without warning and when the patient had been responding to treatment and progressing.

WHY DEALING WITH SUDDEN DEATH IS SO DIFFICULT

Although it is the only inescapable truth of all our lives, there is a huge variation in contemporary western society's perceptions of, and subsequent attitudes to, death. The issues surrounding the dynamics of sudden death may compound the difficulties experienced. Advances in pre-hospital care, medical and nursing interventions and technology have created an increased life expectancy and perceptions of expertise and skills. The sociological implications of our increasingly urbanized and non-secular society need to be appreciated, as does the impact of different models of family life. Many individuals may not have experienced a close death or even seen a dead body, apart from news reports or portrayals in the media. Consequently, many individuals' perceptions of, and attitudes to, death have evolved to the extent that, although death is the natural outcome of life, many people tend to treat it as if it were a myth. There is a tendency for many to speak about '*if* something happens to me' rather than '*when*', and a dichotomy appears to exist between an understanding and acceptance of death in the abstract, as universal and eventually inevitable, and a contemporary cultural preference to deny its existence. Contemplating the sudden death of a loved one is so painful that many people prefer not to think about it as if it might be tempting fate. Emotionally unprepared for, sudden bereavement frequently confronts relatives with some of the worst stressors they may have ever encountered.

Dynamics of sudden death

In essence, sudden death is unexpected, unanticipated and unprepared for. Those who are bereaved are often left with lost opportunities and painful 'if onlys' – 'If only I had insisted he'd worked shorter hours'; 'If only I had made her go to the doctor'; 'If only I had told him I loved him'.

Sudden death cheats people out of their 'assumptive world' – what was supposed to happen in the pattern, order and planned structure of their lives. Compounded by unfulfilled intentions, anguish and regret, their life and plans are left suspended. Consequently, their pain, anger, guilt, frustration and helplessness are often multi-factorial and may be, rightly or wrongly, misdirected and displaced. A key element is that they are left powerless to change the situation; they will have had no time to say goodbye or to finish their 'unfinished business'. This may lead to anguish and bitter regrets, with many people desperately searching for meaning, understanding and answers. There is a need to make sense of the death before they can start to rebuild their shattered lives (Thayre 1985).

The sudden death of a loved one who was central and integral to the relative's shared life, is potentially one of the most stressful major life events and is recognized as one of life's most difficult transitions.

Sudden death leaves those who are bereaved with no or only minimal emotional preparation time or 'anticipatory grief'; the difficulties are exacerbated if they face the death of a loved one without ever having discussed the possibility. It is our individual problem-solving abilities and coping mechanisms that enable us to develop effective strategies to maintain a relative balance or degree of control in our lives. The sudden shock and intensity of the emotional turmoil, however, may create a degree of initial emotional crisis for the relative.

According to Willis (1979):

'the long process of restoring emotional homeostasis can either begin or be delayed, be facilitated or frustrated by the care they [relatives] initially receive'.

All team members, including emergency services responders, need to respect and value the impact of their collective and individual contributions to the relatives' care, however brief or prolonged, or at whatever point in time they come into contact with them. Caring is the foundation if not the essence of our therapeutic practice. If we cannot openly, honestly and sensitively respond to distressed relatives' needs, and cannot listen, our behaviour and responses deny the relatives care. We become part of their problem rather than potentially valuable sources of initial strength, support and direction. Learning to give care in these emotive and difficult situations is not easy. Responding to distressed relatives is never easy. For example, by being party to or actually giving bad news, we may feel and be perceived to be part of both the cause and its effect. At the very least, as Wright (1991) noted, we are:

'witness to an event that cannot be equalled in its ability to impose emotional pain and distress on another person'.

To a certain extent we are all vulnerable to the fear of sudden death, particularly if the situation or the relatives' distress triggers an insecurity or unresolved personal conflict. It is important to appreciate the inherent stress for staff of dealing with bereaved relatives; feelings of responsibility, anxiety and incompetence can result. Buckman (2000) presents the medical perspective in palliative care, describing a number of reasons why some colleagues may have difficulties. Several of these elements are universally applicable (Box 13.6). Additionally, the exigencies of the clinical situation, competing and conflicting priorities, lack of time, shortages of staff, variable skill mix, minimal nursing education and pressure to be professional and say the 'right thing', further compound the difficulties. It is crucial for you to gain supported and supervised experience, by accompanying trained staff. However, you may find that staff, whom you respect as positive role models, are sometimes hesitant or reluctant. This may be because they consider it is intrusive for others to witness the privacy of grief. Our inadequacies are exposed in other's eyes as well as our own, particularly if we feel impotent to be able to help in the face of such distress.

Box 13.6 Fears staff face in palliative care (Buckman 2000)

- Fear of causing pain
- Fear of being blamed
- Fear of not knowing the answers

- Fear of unleashing and having to respond to strong reactions
- Fear of expressing personal feelings
- Fear of having to confront own fears of illness and mortality
- Fear of reaction from peers (who are not always supportive)

CONTACTING AND NOTIFYING RELATIVES

In many situations, where the police are not involved, your first contact with the relatives may start with having to notify them of their need to come to the hospital. Although the first step in the process of breaking bad news is crucially important, there is disagreement as to how this should be done. It can present a real dilemma. Do you tell the family over the telephone, to avoid a futile and panicked rush to the hospital? Or should you withhold full information until they reach the hospital to allow the news of the death to be broken in a more controlled environment?

Jones and Buttery's (1981) small scale, but seminal, research involved asking people who were bereaved about their experiences. They concluded that *whatever* is said, it is crucial that the person making the initial contact sounds 'warm and supportive … confident and competent'. This is important later, as it appears to reduce relatives' anxiety and may dissipate anger about the care their loved one received. Suggestions for this difficult first step are listed in Box 13.7.

Box 13.7 Suggestions for your initial contact with relatives

- Identify yourself and your hospital slowly and distinctly, verify who you are talking to and their relationship to the patient
- Explain that the person has either been brought into the department, e.g. A&E, or has suddenly deteriorated on the ward
- Reassure the family that *everything possible* is being done. This implies the seriousness of the situation and therefore gives relatives marginally more time to prepare
- If you want the family to come in, suggest that they come with someone, as this also implies that the situation is serious

It is essential to emphasize the importance of exercising caution when travelling to the hospital. However, you need to understand that the relative may become angry when they arrive, then to be told that their loved one has *just* died. What we are then saying, in effect, is: 'you are too late … you took too long to get here … he has just died'. Information withheld, or the '*kind lie*' used on the telephone initially, may cause greater distress later. Unless the relative is told the truth, a vicious destructive cycle of guilt, anger and self-recrimination can occur. This may be minimized if the relative is gently, but directly, told the truth, e.g. 'he was dead when I called you but I did not want to tell you over the telephone'. Stay with their anger, if there is any. Acknowledge it and their distress. Be calm and gentle and explain *why* you felt this was the best way to handle the situation. However, be prepared to apologize if, in their view, it was wrong.

A situation that may occur when you telephone is a relative demanding to know and challenging you directly, 'He is dead, isn't he nurse?', which may cause a personal and professional conflict for you. To begin to cope many relatives have an overwhelming need to know the truth, *there and then*. However, the concern, particularly if you do not know anything about the relative's current or past mental and physical health, is not knowing what might be happening if they hang up abruptly. You will have to be guided by your trust/hospital/department's policy, but a coping strategy that avoids having to lie is to say, 'My role is to care for you, as his relative, and to help you get here safely, the team is caring for him and doing everything they can'.

REFLECTION POINT

Consider whether there is ever a place for lying to patients and/or their relatives.

If the family lives some distance from the hospital, or if the relative is elderly or immobile, you must consider whether it is appropriate to ask them to come in. If you do want them to, you must be able to give them clear travelling directions.

As they are trying to take the news in and struggle with their emotions, they may need you to be gently but firmly directive. Try to discourage the relative from driving themselves. Give your name and number if they want to stop and call you during their journey. It is very supportive to tell them who will be waiting for them when they arrive.

When a sudden death occurs on the ward a team decision should be taken as to who should call the family. So, you may be asked to care for the family on their arrival, but may not have been the nurse who telephoned them. Alternatively, they may have been brought in with the ambulance crew or by the police. Before going in to meet them, try to establish:

- the relatives'/friends' identities
- their involvement and what they already know
- what they may have been told and by whom.

The majority of A&E and critical care departments now have specifically designed and suitably furnished relatives' rooms. Privacy can be difficult to obtain on the ward.

Further discussion on breaking bad news can be found in Wright (1996) and Dolan and Holt (2000).

REFLECTION POINT

Do you have these skills? Who can you access to help you develop these?

MAXIMIZING PREPARATION AND TRANSITION TIME

Interventions for this difficult first step focus on helping the relatives deal with the reality of the death or the seriousness of the patient's condition and maximizing their preparation for the most likely outcome:

- introduce yourself by name and tell them why you are there and your role in their family's care
- irrespective of any information you may have been told, *always* try and establish for yourself who is who and what *their* understanding of the situation is.

The fundamental principles underpinning quality care include being a good listener, having the personal and professional strengths to be able to respond effectively to intense and often escalating distress, flexibility to be able to adapt to the unexpected and the ability to grasp the dynamics of the situation.

The key to moving towards people's pain and distress, and knowing where or how to start, is your ability to get behind their perception of the event. Start from a basis of knowledge rather than assumption.

Supportive eye contact should be maintained, conveying feelings of caring and sensitivity rather than professional distance. Sitting down with the family reinforces the message that you are 'there for them'. To remain standing may be perceived as being aloof and detached.

Use sensitive and active listening as this may give you a good indication of the diversity of their needs. A key determinant at this stage, is the relatives' perception of the event and its individual meaning for them. Insight and sensitivity are essential to help you employ any intuitive tactic that you sense will best meet their needs.

Allow time for those relatives who need space and privacy. No matter the degree of rapport you may have established, and how supportive you are, they may be inhibited by your presence. On the other hand, many relatives resent being left alone, uncared for and seemingly forgotten for long periods.

If the relative is alone, help them to access friends and support, so that they can be supported when you are not able to stay with them. Use any available support, or start the process of accessing other support, e.g. hospital chaplain, relevant religious faith representative or team social worker.

Many relatives will display varying degrees of intense anxiety and emotions, shock or numbness, possibly using denial as a temporary mental defence mechanism. They may need information repeated several times as they struggle to assimilate the events and face their emotions. Encourage relatives to ask questions as these may disclose any misunderstandings which can easily occur due to shock and distress.

It is essential that relatives have frequent assessments of the patient's condition and the reality of what the team is trying/having to do. Allowing the relatives to begin to accept the events, as they unfold, is an important determinant of their grieving process. Continue to be open, honest and explain the seriousness of the situation, preparing them for the outcome. It is important that they are informed, as soon as possible, of any sign of the patient's deterioration or failure to respond to the team's efforts.

Some relatives will try to get you to 'collude' with them, 'But he *will* be all right won't he?', 'She isn't going to die is she?' While hope for a positive outcome should not be totally excluded, the family should *never* be given false hope or expectations. It can only complicate the situation further if you try to shield them from the truth. Empathize with them, help them acknowledge their pain, reflect back their emotions as you share their pain, but gently and supportively confront the reality: 'The waiting and not knowing is like a nightmare'; 'It's so *terribly hard* isn't it?'; 'Right now it would be wrong for me to give you any false hope'; 'I am afraid that you need to begin to prepare yourself for the worst'.

Particularly for the silent, numb and withdrawn relative, assess and focus their awareness by gentle but *supportive confrontation*, 'I need to know you understand how *badly* injured or how desperately ill your husband/mother is'. Helping the relatives by encouraging them to *retell* their story or relive the events of the patient's sudden injury or this last illness, helps them begin to make it real for themselves.

However, do not be afraid of periods of silence. It is not always necessary or desirable to say anything; your quiet presence can be very helpful. During periods of 'distressed silence' resist the temptation to do or say something; under pressure it is easy to begin to speak without thinking and end up by responding inappropriately. Stay calm and wait for the relatives to indicate their needs. Allow them time to absorb and process the situation as it gradually sinks in. Allowing them this space, but being there and sharing the burden, can be very powerful.

Continuing to respond to the relative who is numb, or withdrawn and showing little emotion is a balanced process of careful timing, repeating information and supportive affective exploration. The ability to remain 'in control', for some relatives, may be crucial to their perception of coping. Respect this but do not compound the situation by a pretence of cool detachment which may be interpreted as evasion and disconcern.

In our multi-racial society we must recognize different socio-economic, cultural, ethnic and religious needs. An information file should be developed, containing the essentials of different religious death rituals and customs. It can be devastating to a family if an important ritual has not been adhered to. Information should also be held about how to contact religious ministers and/or interpreters, particularly out of hours, and also about the role that specific local or voluntary support organizations are able and willing to play.

BREAKING THE NEWS

The process of actually breaking the news is another difficult stage with many inherent stressors. No matter how strong a rapport you may have established with the family, there is no easy way. We cannot protect those who are bereaved or ourselves from the distress; it *hurts* to break bad news.

Traditionally, it has tended to be the doctor's role and not the nurses' to inform relatives of the death, but there is a degree of shared responsibility in multi-professional teams. The focus should not be on professional background but on the individual's ability and skills. The *when* and *how* and *what* is said is crucially important; *who* actually does the telling is not. Whoever assumes the responsibility, role and seniority does *not* necessarily equate with ability.

Facial expression, eye contact, sitting down and reaching out conveys the seriousness of your message. Feelings of inadequacy and our anxiety at having to give bad news and deal with its reactions can cause us to make long drawn out statements; these may gain us time but only increase the relatives' anxiety and tension. Use a gentle, straightforward approach with clear terminology. If this is done thoughtfully, showing concern, it will not appear cold and detached, which contributes to the relatives' overall perception of care.

There is no magic recipe; start with a short general warning statement, 'I am afraid I have some very bad news for you', or 'I am sorry to have to be the one to tell you this'. The relatives may react by saying 'He's dead, isn't he?', or in some other emotional way, screaming 'No!'; do not be afraid to use the word 'dead'. It is not being insensitive or unkind; it is the truth and it is important to help them to confront reality. The use of the words 'dead' or 'died' may sound shocking and final, but they leave no doubt as to the intended message. The use of euphemisms such as 'gone', 'passed on' or 'passed away' are often used to protect the deliverer of the news rather than the recipient and may lead to potential confusion. Relatives do not need vague, statements, full of cliché. To say 'I am sorry, Mrs Smith, but your husband is no longer with us', may give relatives, desperate for good news, the impression that their relative has been transferred to another hospital.

Reinforce your message, 'We did everything we could. I am so sorry that he has died'. It is important to reassure the family that everything was done that could have been. Confusion and misperceptions are very common because of the intense emotion, e.g. saying 'There was nothing more we could have done' may imply other personnel, or other hospitals, *could* have done more.

If you have broken the news you must involve the doctor. They need to talk to the relatives and to answer their questions, particularly as this demonstrates a conclusion of the medical involvement.

There must, however, be effective communication between you and the doctor, *before* they come in to see the relatives. You must brief the doctor. Medical colleagues need to know their role, what is expected and needed from them.

A further aspect to consider is the advantage of having two people with the relatives when the news is broken, i.e. one saying the words and leaving the other to act as 'the supporter'. In situations of intense and volatile anger, relatives may turn against the person breaking the news. If you are trusted by the relatives, it may be prudent for you to take on the role of 'supporter', so the one doing the telling and at whom the relatives direct their anger can leave once the message is given, allowing you to remain with the family.

Reaching out to people in distress involves a degree of risk, e.g. saying the wrong thing or being rejected for trying to help. Knowing the 'right thing' to say is often very difficult, particularly if you do not know the family. If you realize that you have said the wrong thing, stay calm and be gentle with yourself, take a slow breath and acknowledge the situation; continue to be warm, open and honest, e.g. 'In not knowing you and in trying to find the right things to say, that was obviously the least helpful thing I could have suggested. I am sorry'. The key point is to carry on and stay available as you do your best. There is a tendency to want to withdraw from the situation, particularly if you are feeling anxious because you temporarily made a difficult situation worse, but this only denies the relatives further care.

There will be times when your offers of help and support may be despairingly or angrily rejected. Try to remember that nothing that anybody can do is good enough. Responding to cathartic and angry reactions is very challenging but do not respond defensively. Never allow yourself or others to be put at physical risk; assess whether it is safe to stay. Continuing to be calm and gentle may help.

Relatives may have cause to be angry, e.g. if they are unhappy about the care given or if a mistake had been made. In these instances there may be personal, professional, legal and ethical implications, but it is the authors' view that relatives should be told the truth by the medical staff or by a 'risk manager' rather than being left to discover it by default; most people can eventually find ways to forgive a mistake but they will never forgive arrogance, collusion, perceived indifference or cover-up. Do not be afraid of not knowing or not having all the answers to some of the difficult questions that can arise. A distraught wife screaming at you or begging you to answer 'Why?' can feel overwhelming: stay 'present' and share their burden.

Although various social and cultural factors influence the appropriateness of touch, physical comfort or a hug may be greatly appreciated, provided you feel comfortable, too. Be sensitive to the cues about when to continue or to withdraw. Overall do not be afraid to show you care. Relatives often gain comfort when staff show emotion, as functional responses can both hurt and offend. It is important to be aware that the relatives may have all their senses heightened or sharpened. Several studies have found that relatives tend to have very vivid and definite recollections of their experience. Fraser and Atkins' (1990) respondents could relate 'specific conversations, incidences and the names of physicians, chaplains and nurses'. It is the authors' experience that relatives either remember nothing at all, or every detail, look and gesture.

Having friends and family members with them enables relatives to draw on each other for emotional support and may encourage open expression of grief, initiating steps towards Worden's (1991) second task of mourning.

REFLECTION POINT

How would you feel and respond, personally and professionally to a relative's anger?

VIEWING THE BODY

Irrespective of the need for a formal identification of the body (typically in A&E), the next immediate ordeal for the relatives is deciding whether or not to see the body. Some express this need immediately, others have neither the strength nor the desire to, and some may be frightened of seeing the body.

The degree of encouragement that some relatives may need is a difficult but important judgement to make: gently encourage the relatives, but wait for *them* to be ready. The key is to give them supported opportunities to see the body and to change their mind. A well-meaning friend or relative may want to try and shield or protect them from seeing the body. Assisting relatives, as they view the body, is difficult.

After appropriate liaison and negotiation with the coroner's officer who may be involved (see Box 13.8), staff accompanying the relatives should give 'permission' for them to be able to touch, hold, kiss and talk to the body: to be able to begin to say their 'first goodbye'. Some relatives may wish to have the opportunity, time and privacy to lie beside their loved one and hold them in a last embrace, without the stress of feeling hurried. This may be very upsetting for you. The pace and pressure may make it difficult to find the time and facilities to accommodate this. It is salient to remember that if this is what the relative would have done, had the death occurred at home, then the hospital routine should *not* dictate their behaviour. However, this has to be balanced against any actual or potential criminolegal investigations arising from the coroner's jurisdictional imperatives. Continue to be as supportive and discreet as possible. A relative may need to hold on to you physically, or may forget you are there.

Box 13.8 Criteria for a coroner's investigation

- Deceased person had not been attended by a doctor during the last illness or had not seen the patient within the previous 14 days
- Cause of death is unknown or uncertain
- Death was sudden, violent or occurred in suspicious circumstances
- Death occurred while the patient was undergoing an operation or recovering from an anaesthetic
- Death occurred in prison or while in police custody
- Death was caused by an industrial or notifiable disease

CONCLUDING CARE

The time it takes for you to conclude your care is very variable. Some relatives require care to the extent that they look for 'permission' to leave; they almost need confirmation that there is nothing more for them to do. Conversely, some relatives need to 'flee' because they must reach the privacy and sanctity of their own home and they need to get away from everything *we* and the hospital represent. A principle of best practice is that no one should be allowed to leave alone if at all possible.

Most people are totally unprepared for, and unfamiliar with, the bureaucracy of death and encounter it when they are least able to cope. Therefore, they may need information about what to do next. Fraser and Atkins (1990) highlighted the increased need for giving and receiving information. Ewins and Bryant's work (1992) illustrates the value of formalized follow-up for bereaved relatives.

Extending supportive care and providing any appropriate referral can vary. For example, would the relatives like you to contact the family doctor for them; for you to give them your name and work number and the days you will be available should they like to talk to you again; or for you to offer to call them in a few days or weeks time. Telephoning the family shortly after their arrival home, to ensure their safe arrival, is a small but effective demonstration of care and compassion and can be a therapeutic conclusion of your care. Wright (1996, p49) illustrates the value of relatives being offered the opportunity of returning to discuss any outstanding issues. He emphasizes the importance of careful and detailed record-keeping as some people only re-contact the hospital many months later.

SUMMARY

- Sudden death can be an unexpected shock which leaves the majority of relatives emotionally unprepared and powerless. Eventual resolution is one of life's most difficult transitions. Nurses are important sources of initial strength, support and direction.
- Always verify who you are talking to. Develop your communication skills over the telephone and face-to-face, as relatives need you to sound warm and caring, supportive and confident.
- Flexibility will help you to adapt to the unknown and the unexpected. Use sensitive listening to assess relative's diverse needs. Access support early. Do not collude with relative's desperation but acknowledge the difficulty of not knowing. Develop your ability to be comfortable with the distressed silence.
- Use a gentle but straightforward approach with specific terminology. Do not be afraid of not having all the answers. Learn to be comfortable with cathartic distress.
- Give relatives supported opportunities to see and spend time with their loved one and to change their minds. Accommodate relative's needs/requests after liaison with the coroner's officers who may need to be involved.
- Give relatives an information sheet/booklet if available. Avoid sending them home alone, if possible. Telephoning relatives to ensure their safe arrival home is a caring and compassionate conclusion of your role.

DEVELOPING PERSONAL AND PROFESSIONAL CONFIDENCE THROUGH REFLECTIVE PRACTICE

The pace and demands of the clinical situation and of the service we give frequently requires us to repress our personal feelings, thoughts and reactions, 'to get through the work'. This may be a necessary and appropriate coping mechanism when we are busy. However, one of the challenges in evaluating the quality of care given, requires us to acknowledge our feelings and attitudes. Only by doing this can we *learn* from them. We can only recognize our individual strengths and weaknesses by being open and honest with ourselves; allowing them to *teach* us and enable us to be open to change.

Taking time to reflect is important. Reflection allows us systematically to appraise experiences given and received, promoting an atmosphere of enlightenment through understanding, empowerment through focus and emancipation through transformation (Fay 1987).

REFLECTION POINT

Think of a bereaved relative you have been in contact with. What do you need to do or say, advocate on their behalf or refer them to, to help them deal with the reality? What do you have to do, say or listen to, to help them feel or express their pain and distress? What personal and professional skills do you need to develop to enhance your practice?

Be aware of and sensitive to the personal needs or issues that you may have which may increase your vulnerability. Be prepared for the 'personal growth work'/support which you may need, from time to time, and specifically in relation to critical incidents. Set realistic and appropriate personal limits/boundaries that will enable you to continue to meet patients'/relatives' needs for support.

Dolan and Holt (2000) illustrate the importance of maintaining a healthy balance between work and your life outside, in addition to developing ongoing support mechanisms. Support systems need to be in place to deal with the emotional and psychological issues associated with working so closely with expected and unexpected death. Suggestions include clarifying individual, team and organizational roles and responses, establishing a standard setting/quality audit group and creating favourable and positive working conditions. Constructive coping strategies, such as establishing formal and informal peer and mentor support, defusing, debriefing, critical incident stress debriefing and supported access to continuing professional development, are also important.

REFLECTION POINT

What personal and professional support mechanisms do you have in place?

SUMMARY

- You need to evaluate the quality of the care you have helped to give. Recognize and acknowledge your feelings, attitudes, strengths and weaknesses.
- Use reflection to facilitate your development.
- Develop and maintain personal and professional support networks to empower your care.

CONCLUSION

Responding to dying patients, their relatives and people who are bereaved is demanding and frequently challenging. Developing and maintaining personal and professional effectiveness, in all four domains, requires compassion and commitment, confidence and competence.

CHAPTER
14

QUALITY IN
HEALTH CARE

Alison Norman and Jane Brown

INTRODUCTION

This chapter looks at the policy background to the focus on quality in health care, and at how quality is achieved, measured and monitored in NHS organizations. The four countries of the UK are developing policies on quality of health care. However, for clarity of focus, references have been confined to policies for England. It also explores the important concept of professional accountability in nursing, midwifery and health visiting, and the role of the statutory regulatory body for these professions in helping practitioners to apply professional accountability in their daily practice.

POLICY BACKGROUND TO QUALITY IN HEALTH CARE

Health professionals have always been concerned with the quality of the care they give. So too have their individual employers, and the health care system within which they work. Also, of course, patients, carers and relatives of those receiving health services have always wanted to know that the level of care provided, and the skills of those providing it, are of the highest quality. Many significant steps have been introduced in the past to try to ensure quality of care:

- registration of doctors in 1865, to ensure that only suitably qualified practitioners could practise medicine
- registration of midwives in 1902 and nurses in 1919, bringing standardization and quality assurance to the education required to enter these professions
- establishment of medical, nursing and midwifery royal colleges with remits to foster high quality practice
- setting up of four national confidential enquiries to monitor outcomes in four key areas (see below) and ensure that lessons are drawn from findings
- development of post-registration courses for nurses and midwives, designed to confer additional skills and knowledge for practice
- changes to pre-registration nursing courses to reflect changes in the nature of nursing
- introduction of mandatory re-registration associated with standards for post-registration education and practice.

So, it would be inaccurate to identify any particular government policy statement or document as the starting point for concern with quality in health services. Here only a few of the more recent policy documents and initiatives that are focused on improving the quality of care in the health services can be identified.

THE NEW NHS, MODERN AND DEPENDABLE

This white paper (DoH 1997), set out the new Labour government's agenda for the health services. It placed considerable emphasis on quality, e.g.:

> '[The new NHS] will work to new standards of quality and efficiency that will guarantee better services for patients'.
>
> *(DoH 1997, para 3.1)*

Specifically, it introduced three major new initiatives on quality which are now embedded in the health service:

- introduction of the concept of 'clinical governance' for NHS organizations
- national service frameworks (NSFs) for particular conditions or care groups – evidence-based standards which were intended to ensure consistent access to services and quality of care across the country

- setting up of the National Institute for Clinical Excellence (NICE), to give a lead on clinical effectiveness and cost-effectiveness.

These quality initiatives were further explained in *A First Class Service – Quality in the New NHS* (DoH 1998).

CLINICAL GOVERNANCE

Clinical governance is the framework through which NHS organizations are accountable for continuously improving the quality of their services and safeguarding high standards of care (see also Chapter 7). The Health Act (1999) gave chief executives of NHS trusts a statutory responsibility for clinical governance, in addition to their statutory financial responsibilities. In practice, clinical governance is an umbrella term for all the activities and information that support quality improvement in an NHS organization. The elements of clinical governance are listed in Box 7.1 and examples of clinical governance activities are given in Box 14.1.

Box 14.1 Clinical governance activities (DoH 1998)

- Work to identify and build on good practice
- Work to assess and minimize the risk of untoward events
- Work to investigate problems as these arise and ensure lessons are learnt
- Work to support health professionals in delivering quality care

Although the statutory responsibility for clinical governance lies with the chief executive of an organization, the day-to-day activities that support clinical governance need to be built in to the practice of everyone in the organization. Managers cannot minimize risk to patients if, for example, nurses fail to wash their hands adequately or if they undertake tasks beyond their competence. Clinical governance is an excellent example of the way in which some policies have no impact until they are translated into practice: 'policy' is not something remote from, and irrelevant to, the practitioner. On the contrary, it is an example of a policy that only happens through the medium of health professionals.

NATIONAL SERVICE FRAMEWORKS

National service frameworks (NSFs) set common standards across the country for the treatment of particular conditions. They are descriptions of the service required for a condition or a care group which:

- set national standards and define the service models
- put in place programmes for implementation
- set the performance measures against which progress will be measured.

They are developed by a national reference group of experts in the field, including health professionals, service users, carers, health service managers and other relevant groups. The content of an

NSF is listed in Box 14.2. To date NSFs have been published on coronary heart disease, diabetes, mental health and care of older people (DoH 1999c, 2000d, 2001i,o) and implementation of the services, and measurement against the targets set, is under way. NSFs to come include those on long-term medical conditions and on midwifery and child health.

Box 14.2 Content of national service frameworks (DoH 1998)

- Definition of the scope of the framework
- The evidence base
- National standards and timescales for delivery
- Key interventions and associated costs
- Commissioned work to support implementation, e.g. R&D, benchmarks, outcome indicators
- Supporting programmes, e.g. workforce planning, education and training
- A performance management framework, which enables monitoring of progress

NATIONAL INSTITUTE OF CLINICAL EXCELLENCE

NICE was set up in 1999 to promote clinical effectiveness and cost-effectiveness by producing guidance and audit tools for front-line staff. It does this by:

- advising on best practice in the use of existing treatment options
- appraising new health interventions
- advising the NHS how these interventions might fit alongside existing interventions.

NICE is a special health authority, with membership drawn from the health professions, the NHS, academics, health economists and patient interest groups. As well as undertaking new work, NICE brings together and oversees the four national confidential enquiries into perioperative deaths, stillbirths and deaths in infancy, maternal deaths and suicide, and homicide by people with mental illness.

MAKING A DIFFERENCE

In addition to these NHS-wide policies on improving quality, the issue of the provision of high quality care is explicitly addressed in *Making a Difference* (DoH 1999d), the government's strategy for nursing launched by the Prime Minister in 1999.

'We want nurses, midwives and health visitors to play a full part in every aspect of our plans for quality improvement'.

(DoH 1999d, para 7.2)

It acknowledges existing mechanisms and activities for the attainment of professional standards of care, and for quality improvement, and suggests that nurses need to build on them, rather than starting again with a different system:

'These activities [professional self-regulation, clinical supervision, continuing professional development] need to be developed, strengthened and integrated into the wider clinical governance development programme and linked to annual appraisal and personal development planning'.

(DoH 1999d, para 7.5)

It promised two key initiatives to help front-line nurses deliver high quality care:

● an exploration of the potential benefits of 'benchmarking' (i.e. identifying agreed best practice standards so that care can be measured against them) for eight fundamental and essential aspects of nursing care (see Box 3.1; DoH 2001f)
● the development of a strategy to influence the research and development agenda, to strengthen the capacity to undertake nursing and midwifery research, and to use research to support practice (DoH 2001p).

This explicit integration of developments in nursing practice with the delivery of quality brings nursing to the forefront of policy on quality in the health service. Not only must nursing practice be of high quality, but it must take place in the context of a high quality service, delivered to nationally defined standards, and for which NHS organizations will be held accountable.

THE NHS PLAN

The NHS Plan is the government's 'blueprint' for the NHS, published in 2000 after the allocation of significant new resources to the health service, and setting out how the funding should be used to achieve the policy aims of the government in relation to health care (DoH 2000a). These aims include speeding up patients' access to parts of the health service, cutting waiting times, recruiting more doctors and nurses, and changing some of the traditional professional roles. It also focuses specifically on the quality of the service, and the standards of care provided. It allocates funding to infrastructure improvements – such as refurbishing some doctors' surgeries and buying new equipment – as well as to improving basic conditions by investing in cleaning hospitals and improving hospital food. *The NHS Plan* also heralds the appointment of 'modern matrons' – senior sisters with responsibility across a group of wards for ensuring that standards of cleanliness and basic care are reached and maintained.

THE POLICY PICTURE

With these few examples of policy-led quality initiatives in the NHS and in nursing, it is clear that the individual responsibility for professional accountability that each nurse assumes on registration, is matched by a responsibility shared with the team of people they work with, and the organization that employs them, continually to improve the quality of care for patients. The need for day-by-day attention to standards, questioning of ways of working and reflection on practice is illustrated by some of the high-profile tragedies in which patients have been injured, or their care badly compromised, such as the paediatric heart surgery case in Bristol (DoH 2001d). Whatever the focus of the enquiries into such cases, the lessons described and recommendations made are applicable to all the professions. High quality nursing care, protecting patients from both major disasters and more minor failures in the care they should expect, cannot happen solely because of the policies in place to support it. High quality care is a product of the daily attention to the implementation of those policies, and the practice of individual nurses, midwives and health visitors, and a continual focus on quality services by the organization.

QUALITY IN THE ORGANIZATION

'The new NHS will have quality at its heart. Without it there is unfairness. Every patient who is treated in the NHS wants to know that they can rely on receiving high quality care when they need it. Every part of the NHS, and everyone who works in it, should take responsibility for working to improve quality. This must be quality in its broadest sense: doing the right things, at the right time, for the right people and doing them right – first time. And it must be the quality of the patient's experience as well as the clinical result – quality measured in terms of prompt access, good relationships and excellent administration.'

(DoH 1997)

TECHNICAL ASPECTS OF QUALITY

During the 20th century 'quality' developed different meanings and, despite its importance, there is no universally accepted definition. This lack of agreed definition leads to different interpretations of how quality should be measured. The first systematic attempts to measure and improve quality used statistical methods to reduce the variation in processes and hence improve quality by reducing the variation in the output of the process. As quality ideas developed the emphasis shifted to concern for the integration of organizational activities to improve quality. In particular Feigenbaum (1963) argued that quality improvement should include the inter-dependent activities throughout the organization. At the time, particular emphasis was being placed on the role of the customer in determining quality and this idea that quality is determined by the customer became stronger as the century progressed, leading to definitions of quality such as 'meeting the needs of customers' (Kearns and Nadler 1992). As part of this development 'internal' customers were identified as a way of internalizing the final external customer into the organization and its activities.

Thus, two different types of quality can be identified: technical (or mechanistic) quality, involving an objective aspect or feature; and humanistic quality, involving the subjective response of people, which is likely to vary between individuals. For example, when making a cup of tea, the technical quality may be related to the design of the teapot and the humanistic quality to the quality of the drink. Clearly, the personal, subjective aspects of quality are of vital importance in health care but the technical aspects are important, too (Donabedian 1980).

QUALITY IN SERVICES

During the last quarter of the 20th century the attention being paid to quality in manufacturing industries extended to service industries and the public sector. The aspects of quality emphasized in manufacturing sectors were insufficient to understand service quality, for which four aspects of services need to be appreciated:

- services are intangible. Often the delivery of the service is a more significant aspect of quality than the design of the service. Because of this intangibility it is difficult for the quality of the service to be measured, tested or verified before the delivery of the service
- by their nature services tend to have a high people content. This leads to a variation of service quality from practitioner to practitioner, client to client and day to day. Consistency of service is difficult to assure and may not even be desirable in quality terms
- it is difficult to separate production of the service from its consumption. Quality is therefore the outcome of the interaction of the practitioner and client as the service is delivered. In circumstances where input from the client is high, the customer's input is critical to the quality of the service. For example, when visiting the hairdressers the resultant cut may be highly dependent on the instructions that the client has given to the hairdresser
- a service is an activity or series of activities, which contain interactions with the client, where the client–provider interaction during service delivery occurs as a series of 'moments of truth'. The implication is that quality assurance in such circumstances is difficult since poor service quality cannot be hidden from the client.

REFLECTION POINT
Think about the varying quality of services that you have accessed and how the 'perceived quality' was dependent on the attitude and actions of the person delivering the service.

An influential approach to the definition and measurement of service quality is the gap model (Parasuraman *et al.* 1985; Box 14.3).

Box 14.3 The gap model (Parasuraman *et al.* 1985)

This model considers the discrepancy or gap between the service quality the client expects to receive and the perception of the client of the service quality they actually receive. This overall gap is the result of several other gaps in the service delivery process. This gap model has been simplified in the case of professional services to consist of three gaps:
- client expectations – client experiences
- client expectations – practitioner perceptions of client expectations
- client experiences – practitioner perceptions of client experiences.
From gap models a multiple item scale for measuring service quality has been developed (Parasuraman *et al.* 1988) called SERVQUAL. It consists of five interrelated dimensions intended to assess a client's perceptions:
- empathy – the caring, individualized attention that the organization provides to the client
- assurance – the knowledge and courtesy of service personnel and their ability to inspire trust and confidence

- responsiveness – the willingness to help clients and provide prompt service
- reliability – the ability to perform the promised service dependably and accurately
- tangibles – the peripheral aspects of the service (e.g. physical facilities, appearance of staff) that are not a primary part of the service but are indicators of the quality of the service

Maxwell (1984, 1992) suggests there are six components of health service quality:

- effectiveness – for individuals, including technical competence
- efficiency – relating outcome to costs and resource use
- equity – availability to all in relation to need
- access – ease of accessing the system, physical accessibility and length of waiting time
- acceptability – including physical and interpersonal aspects, and the ethical nature of treatment procedures
- appropriateness – for the whole community and its health care needs.

Moss (1998) suggests that other components could be added:

- respect – to the client from the service provider
- choice – providing more than one option and the appropriate information to allow the client to make an informed choice
- availability of information – in a style that is easily understood by all users.

Klein (1998) further suggests that in the wake of the Bristol cardiac surgery case, 'technical competency' could also be added, thus resulting in the 'Ten Commandments' of NHS quality.

DEFINITION OF QUALITY IN HEALTH CARE

The publication of *The New NHS, Modern and Dependable* (DoH 1997) and *A First Class Service* (DoH 1998) clearly identified the importance of quality within the Labour government's 10-year modernization agenda for the NHS. The message for modernization is clear: services are to be equitable across the country with users encouraged to contribute to the planning and criticism of services. The structure of modernization is:

- national standards for service set by NICE and NSFs
- local delivery of services through the structures of clinical governance and clinical effectiveness
- monitoring of the delivery of standards by:
  - Commission for Health Improvement (CHI), a statutory body set up to provide independent scrutiny of improvements to quality and assist in addressing any identified serious problems in service provision
  - national framework for assessing performance
  - national survey of patient and user experience.

SETTING STANDARDS

The setting of standards within the 'new NHS' is undertaken primarily by NICE (see above). Standards for individual services, or care groups, will be set by NSFs (DoH 1998; Box 14.2).

DELIVERING STANDARDS: CLINICAL GOVERNANCE

Health care professionals often criticize their organizations for only paying lip service to quality improvement. They further identify that quality management consists of two interrelated tasks – doing the right thing and doing things right. The government agenda now makes it clear that the NHS needs to focus on the variation in practice of practitioners and geographical regions.

Wilson (1998) suggests that clinical governance will have an important part to play in the restoration of public confidence in care delivery of the NHS by ensuring that treatment is up to date, clinically- and cost-effectively applied by staff whose skills have kept pace with evidence-based practice and up-to-date techniques.

The structure of clinical governance in the NHS require organizations and individuals to monitor and improve the quality of the services provided, ensuring that there are clear lines of responsibility and accountability for the quality of clinical care. Each organization must have an identified, comprehensive programme of quality improvement activities supported by clear policies for risk management and procedures for all professional groups to identify and remedy poor performance.

Implementation of clinical governance should be underpinned by the key principles of:

- patient focus – ensuring improvement of patient services throughout all patient pathways
- transferability – good practice systematically disseminated across all organizations of the NHS
- partnership – between clinicians, managers and patients
- user/patient involvement – in planning and monitoring of services
- nurse involvement and leadership – in improvement of patient care quality
- culture of continuous quality improvement – which celebrates success and learns from mistakes rather than seeking to attribute blame
- clinical risk reduction – programme with adverse incidents, near misses and incidents detected and investigated. Poor clinical performance dealt with appropriately to minimize harm to patients and staff
- lifelong learning – should be learner centred, relevant, problem based, built on learners' experience and lead to further study
- openness – staff need to understand the importance of clinical governance to all aspects of their work
- clinical frameworks – as a complement to professional self-regulation and individual clinical judgement by providing an operating framework.

Essentially, clinical governance is a linking together of activities in which nurses are already involved within a framework that facilitates reflection and action planning to improve the quality of NHS services.

REFLECTION POINT

When developing a framework for clinical governance questions need to be posed which will evoke reflection and action from individuals that will hopefully result in an improvement in the quality of patient care. Table 14.1 provides an opportunity to assess aspects of your organization and identify actions required to improve the service.

Table 14.1 Assessment of clinical governance in your organization

Elements	Is a structure in place?	Does the structure work?	Improvements	Action points
Multi-professional clinical audit				
Evidence-based practice				
Clinical supervision				
Annual personal appraisals				
Clinical leadership development				
Risk management systems				
Clinical incident reporting systems				
Patient feedback systems				
Multi-professional teamwork				
Information sharing and networking				
Open culture for learning from mistakes				

DELIVERING STANDARDS: CLINICAL EFFECTIVENESS

Clinical effectiveness is based on a triangular framework (Figure 14.1). 'Inform' means ensuring that clinicians, patients and managers know of, and can access, the best available evidence of clinical effectiveness and cost-effectiveness. It is important too that nurses use critically appraised research to help to develop their own critical appraisal skills (see Chapter 7). Mulhall *et al.* (1998) identify four prerequisites to the effective appraisal of evidence in the practice setting:

- creation of a 'can do' culture
- provision of the skills and knowledge to critique research

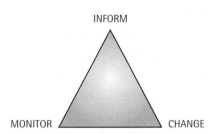

INFORM

MONITOR   CHANGE

Figure 14.1 Triangular framework for clinical effectiveness

- recognition of the range of research approaches that may inform nursing practice
- exploration of the constituents of evidence and how evidence other than empirical evidence should be critiqued.

'Change' means using the information concerning clinical effectiveness and cost-effectiveness to review, and where necessary, change routine clinical and managerial practice. Individuals must accept the need for making changes in clinical practice. Changes are more easily facilitated by development of strategies, organizational commitment and skilled facilitation of the process. There are, however, a number of barriers to the changes that need to be addressed for clinical effectiveness to be fully embraced, including competition for resources, time for clinicians to develop research pilots, unsophisticated IT systems and access to protocols and evidence on which decisions can be made.

'Monitor' means ensuring that changes are implemented, resulting in improvements in the quality of health care services. Monitoring of the delivery standards at national level will mainly be the responsibility of the CHI (see above). Walshe (1999) outlines the work of, and relationships between, the various statutory, semi- and non-statutory inspection bodies of the NHS. It will be important that the CHI fits into the existing complex system and learns from the existing inspection bodies.

ORGANIZATIONAL MEASUREMENT AND ACCREDITATION

Internal organizational measurement of the quality of services provided can be undertaken in a number of ways:

- clinical audit
- accreditation
- user satisfaction/dissatisfaction, e.g. complaints, user involvement.

Clinical audit

The collection and analysis of information regarding clinical practice by means of clinical audit has been undertaken in England for a number of decades following the establishment of similar activities in the US. Clinical audit is the measurement of the performance of a service against predetermined standards. The formal introduction of clinical audit followed the government white paper *Working for Patients* (DoH 1989b) and resulted from the development of the audit cycle (Fowkes 1982).

The importance and commitment to clinical audit has often been questioned. Johnson *et al.* (2000) consider that clinical audit has progressed despite meagre financial support and a lack of dedicated time for staff to participate, often resulting in conflict between the demands of treating patients and participation in clinical audit. However, significant evidence can be found to illustrate that clinical audit is well established and a valuable contributor to the quality improvement of health care in the UK. Many lessons have been learnt during the first decade of clinical audit but some important lessons are still to be addressed. The geographical variations identified by Fowkes and McPake (1986) still cause concern today, although it is hoped that the national initiatives of NSFs, NICE and the CHI will soon address these inequalities. Professional isolation and secrecy (Gabbay *et al.* 1990) should be reduced by the emphasis on multi-professional clinical teams working together to develop integrated care pathways and plans of care which will facilitate audit of the whole patient experience.

Accreditation

Accreditation is a system of external peer review for determining the compliance with a set of predetermined standards. The development of accreditation has a long history in the US, Canada and Australia, with a recent explosion of activity internationally. The King's Fund Organizational Audit programme was set up in 1989 in an attempt to introduce this approach to quality improvement. To date most of the accreditation within health services has been in the secondary, rather than primary, care environment.

The main purposes of accreditation are quality improvement, informing of future decision-making regarding prioritization of activities and professional accountability. The critical questions to be considered before an organization embarks on an accreditation programme are listed in Box 14.4.

Box 14.4 Questions to be asked about accreditation

- Purpose – of the accreditation and what it will achieve for the organization
- Participation – what participation will be necessary and what are the incentives?
- Costs – how much and who pays?
- Standards – level, content, derivation and measurability
- Appropriateness – is the accreditation appropriate for the organization?
- Assessment – how will the organization be assessed and by whom?
- Results – presentation and publication
- Impact – what is achieved and what follow-up is required?

During the accreditation process the following activities are undertaken:

- review of performance
- external involvement
- review of standards
- measurement against standards
- report of results.

Accreditation is not, however, free:

- direct cost of fees – to the accreditation body which vary widely
- indirect cost of time and effort in the preparation, assessment and follow up activities.

Several accreditation bodies or systems are used by the NHS:

- Clinical Negligence Scheme for Trusts (CNST) – by achieving the standards set by CNST, trusts can reduce the premium of their insurance against clinical negligence
- Investors in People – accreditation related to how an individual organization cares for the employees in terms of family friendly policies, training provision and annual performance appraisals
- medical royal colleges, e.g. Royal College of General Practitioners – GP practices are assessed against accreditation standards both in self-assessment and by a visiting team.

The most recent development in accreditation is self-assessment models, which aim to identify and continuously improve aspects of service. For example, the European Foundation for Quality Management (EFQM) model examines what an organization has achieved and how. It facilitates the organization to undertake benchmarking both internally and externally with other organizations deemed to have best practice in a specific area.

ISO 9000 is the international equivalent of the British Standard BS5750. It was originally written for the manufacturing industries but can be used for most organizations as it is cast in such general terms. The essential idea is that the processes by which goods or services are produced should be clearly specified and documented, ensuring that audit of the system is easily undertaken. The requirements for ISO 9000 are complex with heavy emphasis on documentation, e.g. the organization must demonstrate that it is able to:

- identify 'control documents', i.e. manuals, protocols, etc.
- only issue control documents that have been checked by designated staff
- ensure availability of control documents to everyone that needs them
- ensure removal and updating of control documents
- maintain a master list of all who are to receive control documents.

ISO 9000 has been adopted by several NHS organizations, e.g. some general practices, biomedical engineering departments and directorates of NHS trusts.

REFLECTION POINT

Consider your own knowledge of accreditation processes within the organizations where you have had clinical placements.

COMPLAINTS

The demands of the Patient's Charter (DoH 1991b) and the difficulties people were experiencing when raising concerns about NHS services resulted in a new complaints procedure for the NHS in 1996. While it was recognized that there would always be causes of dissatisfaction in a service as complex and diverse as the health service, there was also a demand for more accountability for those within the NHS. The purpose of the new complaints procedure, which is currently under review, was first to standardize the process and second to facilitate the improvement of the quality of services provided within the NHS (see also Chapter 15).

The complaints procedure specified that the first stage of the process should involve 'local resolution'. Verbal or informal complaints should be resolved by front-line staff immediately, if possible, or within 2 days. Written or formal complaints should be investigated and the complainant should receive an initial response from the chief executive of the organization within 4 days.

Local resolution provides an opportunity for the practitioner to whom a complaint is made to attempt to correct any practice which is causing concern to the complainant. Any action at this point can resolve the issue, prevent a further, more formal, complaint being made and reinforce confidence in the service. Perhaps a more useful way of thinking about this stage of the procedure is one of feedback or comment from a patient to a person who can do something about it.

Failure to correct any deficiencies in the service will almost certainly result in a formal complaint and investigative procedure. Findings and recommendations resulting from an investigation are reported to the manager of the service involved and an action plan is formulated which will address the immediate problem and prevent further problems occurring.

Should a complaint remain unresolved a short screening process will determine whether or not it is to proceed to stage 2 of the process – 'independent review' by a 'convenor', a non-executive director for an NHS trust. A decision is then made whether to establish a review. If the complaint is to be reviewed, a panel is convened within 6 months, with a lay chair appointed by the Secretary of State for Health.

The 1996 complaints procedure has been successful in dealing with complaints and identifying them as a positive source of information to be used in the maintenance and improvement of standards of service provision, e.g. following a complaint from a patient kept without food and minimal drink during a 6-hour wait in an A&E department the hospital changed its approach to the needs of such patients (Evans 1998).

REFLECTION POINT

Consider your clinical placements to date and anticipate issues that patients could complain about and what actions you could take to avoid complaint and improve the service.

USER INVOLVEMENT

Public, user and carer involvement is an important aspect of the quality improvement cycle highlighted in the government's modernization agenda and includes involvement in the following areas.

Research

Users may be involved at all stages of research (see Box 14.5), including:

- identification and prioritization of topics
- commissioning
- design, managing and performing projects
- analysis and interpretation of results
- dissemination of results
- evaluating the research process.

Box 14.5 Example of user involvement in research planning

Researchers at Mount Vernon Hospital in Middlesex designed a research protocol to address the problem of waiting times in breast cancer outpatient clinics. This proposed a shift to primary care as a solution to problems. Following consultation with users they found other solutions were more acceptable, including making access to consultants easier.

Identification of quality indicators and criteria

It is important to gain the user perspective on what is good service quality as users can be the only true commentators. Box 14.6 shows how a panel of health professionals and users/carers met to identify the standards of care required and guidelines regarding the delivery of care.

Box 14.6 Example of user involvement in the identification of quality criteria

Wensing *et al* (1996) involved users in the development of indicators of good quality GP care for people with chronic illnesses. A panel of 37 patients with a range of chronic conditions and 24 GPs with expertise in the conditions were recruited. The process had three stages:

- focus groups separately with GPs and users to identify quality criteria
- an anonymous survey 1 month after focus groups to assess if criteria were deemed to be extremely relevant, very relevant, moderately relevant or of doubtful relevance for the improvement of quality in health care
- an anonymous survey 3 months after focus groups in which four aspects which were controversial in the first survey and five new aspects were rated. A total of 41 aspects of care were included in this written consensus procedure.

GPs and patients expressed different priorities: patients stressed the importance of 'knowing the most recent developments in medicine'; GPs stressed 'working according to protocol'. Patients valued involvement in decisions whereas GPs thought that patients' capacities should not be overestimated. Problems arose in assessment of categories such as availability, accessibility and organization of services.

Monitoring of services

Users and carers are an integral part of many of the organizations and processes that determine service quality. NICE includes two lay members on its board and has several members on the 'Partners Council' which assesses the 'objectivity of the appraisal process performed by the Institute'.

All NSFs are being developed with the assistance of an External Reference Group that includes users and carers. The group responsible for the development of the NSF for coronary heart disease included four users and carers. They emphasized the need for clear information, support and reassurance for the patients diagnosed with this disease (DoH 2000d).

Independent national surveys of audit committees have confirmed that there is also often user involvement in clinical audit projects. The CHI has a lay chair and a majority of lay members on the board. It includes lay representatives as part of local reviews and will investigate the ways in which users and carers are being involved by trusts. Clinical governance committees should have lay representatives with a senior individual responsible for overseeing the development and implementation of a public and user involvement strategy. Users and carers, as well as community representatives, are also formally involved in the service planning and review of some specific areas of the health service: maternity services, cancer services, community care plans and health improvement programmes.

CROSS-ORGANIZATIONAL ISSUES

Care pathways

The clinical governance agenda ensures that management and measurement of quality of services within single organizations or services is relatively easy; however, patients rarely receive services from one organization, department or team during an illness. The likelihood is that they receive care from their GP and at least one secondary care provider of services. Despite the fact that individual professionals may meet to discuss the care of a patient, a common plan, which includes the input of all the professions, is rarely evident, particularly across organizational boundaries. It is therefore important that systems are developed that facilitate continuity of good quality care.

The importance of the planning of care pathways and related protocols is that all stakeholders are identified and involved in the process, which can at times prove to be difficult. One model of care, which potentially facilitates continuity of quality services, is that of 'pathways of care'. The philosophy behind this is that a planned journey carries less risk than an unplanned one and knowledge of the journey's steps and stages reduces anxiety for the traveller (Layton *et al.* 1998). The development process for a pathway of care has first to identify the milestones that patients with a specific illness will pass through. These milestones need to include evidence-based standards (e.g. discharging patients post myocardial infarction with aspirin unless contraindicated), critical steps in the pathway and priorities for each participating organization.

One criticism of the model is that care may become prescriptive and not individualized. However, the pathway should be seen as milestones which have to be met and the exact route can vary as long as identified protocols are adhered to. The benefits of introducing structured pathways with protocols have been reported to be:

- quality assessment and better use of evidence-based care
- reduction in the duration of hospital-based stay
- reduction in staff time recording information
- improved staff attitudes
- improved risk management
- optimum clinical and management financial planning (Layton *et al.* 1998).

Managed clinical networks

Managed clinical networks, introduced in 2000, are an additional vehicle for managing the cross-organizational issues which can impede a patient's care during an illness. However, rather than being restricted to an NHS district or region, clinical networks often cross these boundaries and mirror the treatment pathways of patients with specific conditions, e.g. cancer (Box 14.7). Thus, they have the potential to break down the barriers that exist between primary, secondary and tertiary care, as well as those between health and social care. There is no single structure or model for clinical networks and diversity both within and across specialties exists. However, the networks are funded by their partner organizations with all partners having equal standing within the organization of the network.

Box 14.7 Network features

- A leadership team with a minimum of network manager and clinician
- Lead nurse or health professional
- Inclusion of public, private and voluntary partners
- Flexibility, ensuring that networks change with need
- Service development plans
- Documented clinical governance arrangements with participating organizations
- Information and user/patient involvement
- Ensuring that national standards are met across the clinical pathways of patients by the introduction of site-specific clinical groups to plan and develop care across the network

PROFESSIONAL ACCOUNTABILITY

Professional accountability is a formal phrase that is often associated with the negative concepts of blame, guilt and punishment. 'Because I am accountable for my actions, I'll get blamed if something goes wrong, and I could be struck off.' These concerns can lead to defensive practice, failure to report errors or problems in practice, and poorer quality care for patients. To avoid these undesirable outcomes, it is essential that nurses understand the wider concept of professional accountability, and what it means in practice, so that they can use it as a positive framework for practice.

WHAT IS PROFESSIONAL ACCOUNTABILITY?

Professional accountability means that every professional nurse, midwife or health visitor is held to account for their actions (and omissions) by the regulatory body of the profession, which has a statutory responsibility in law to do so. Specifically, nurses are accountable for ensuring that their actions and their practice meet the standards set for the profession. As nursing is a self-regulated profession, the regulatory body is a nursing one: since April 2002, the Nursing and Midwifery Council (NMC), consisting of 12 elected practitioners (one nurse, midwife and health visitor from each of the four countries of the UK).

Two important points arise from this understanding of professional accountability:

- it is continuous – it covers a nurse's actions at all times, not only when something goes wrong, or a complaint is made
- it covers a nurse's actions outside of their professional practice as well as when they are working in a professional capacity.

This is illustrated by the fact that the regulatory body considers two factors when holding to account a nurse who has been referred to it: their professional conduct and their fitness to practise. A health problem, a criminal offence or a demonstrable lack of a necessary competence are all factors which might arise at work or in a nurse's personal life, and which might affect their ability to practise at the standard expected.

THE REGULATORY BODY

The main responsibility of the regulatory body, the NMC, is to protect the public by:

- maintaining a register of registered nurses, midwives and health visitors
- setting standards for the preparation of these practitioners (its 'registrants')
- considering cases of registrants who have been referred to it because of concerns about their health or their professional conduct.

By fulfilling these roles, the NMC ensures that practitioners who qualify as nurses, midwives and health visitors have reached a specific standard before they begin to practise; and that they are recorded individually in a central register so that a person who has not reached the standard, or who has not undertaken the appropriate preparation, cannot successfully pass themselves off as a nurse, midwife or health visitor. This individual registration is signified by the personal identification number allotted to each practitioner when their name is recorded in the register. The periodic (3-year) re-registration, which is a prerequisite for continuing to practise, ensures that the standard reached for registration has been maintained (see Box 18.1).

The third function of the regulatory body is to hear cases of alleged professional misconduct, or unfitness to practice due to health problems. Before considering this function, it is worth reflecting on how the first two functions are put into effect. Once a student has qualified as a nurse or midwife, and their name has been recorded on the professional register, there is not a professional vacuum until they are required to re-register 3 years later. Instead, the UKCC, during its period as the regulatory body for nurses, midwives and health visitors, drew up guidance for practitioners to help them to practise to the expected standard. The key document which sets the standard for professional practice for nurses, midwives and health visitors is the *Code of professional conduct* (NMC 2002a). These standards provide the framework for professionally accountable practice.

It lists the expectations that the regulatory body has of registrants, starting with the general requirement that: 'Each registered nurse, midwife and health visitor shall act, at all times, in such a manner as to:

- safeguard and promote the interests of individual patients and clients
- serve the interests of society
- justify public trust and confidence
- uphold and enhance the good standing and reputation of the professions'.

The *Code* goes on to list those standards of behaviour which the regulatory body requires of members of the professions 'in the exercise of your professional accountability'.

The significance of this document cannot be overstated. It sets clear boundaries for professional conduct and practice. It makes explicit the behaviour and ways of working expected of nurses, midwives and health visitors – 'professionally accountable' means that a nurse's actions and omissions are measured against these standards. On a day-to-day basis, this assessment is made by the nurse themselves: 'Is my care in the best interests of patients?', 'Am I protecting public confidence in the profession?', 'Do I need additional knowledge or a new skill before I take on that task?'

Nurse managers and senior nurses in organizations are also applying the same standards to their nursing workforce, ensuring that the patients or clients receiving services from the organization receive appropriate professional care.

Only on a rare basis – and never for most practitioners – does the regulatory body itself consider the professional conduct of an individual registrant (see below). So, the responsibility for ensuring that practice is maintained at the professional standard lies first and foremost with the individual: this is the most fundamental meaning of professional accountability.

It is important to realize that these standards do not say that a nurse must never make a mistake or a poor decision. While the individual is accountable for such actions – as for all their acts and omissions – such actions would not of themselves constitute professional misconduct or unfitness to practice, if the *Code of professional conduct* (NMC 2002a) or other professional guidance was not breached.

Professional conduct procedures

The great majority of nurses will never enter the professional conduct proceedings of the regulatory body. In 1999–2000, 1142 practitioners were reported to the UKCC for allegations of misconduct. This is only 0.2% of approximately 600,000 practitioners on the register. Of these, 642 cases were closed without further action, and 164 were referred to the Professional Conduct Committee. Ultimately, 27 registrants were cautioned, and 96 were removed from the register. The commonest reasons for referral to the preliminary proceedings committee of the Council were:

- physical or verbal abuse of patients/clients (31% of allegations), including serious physical assault
- unsafe clinical practice (12%) such as failing to call medical assistance when appropriate, or failing to examine a patient after a fall.

Other reasons for referral include criminal convictions, failing to disclose convictions when applying for a post as a nurse and fraud.

PROFESSIONAL ACCOUNTABILITY IN PRACTICE

It should be clear from the above that a number of mechanisms are in place to prepare nurses for, and support them in, their professional accountability for their practice. These include:

- pre-registration education (for which standards are set by the regulatory body)
- registration (entry onto the professional register)
- PREP (continuing professional development and practice standards)
- professional conduct proceedings (to measure practice against standards when concern has been formally expressed)
- reflective practice/clinical supervision.

All these measures are designed to ensure that practitioners know what is expected of them, and can practice to a standard that both protects the public and offers the professional opportunities to develop and mature in practice. Professional accountability becomes a positive act: the individual reviews their practice against this framework and confirms that their practice continues to meet these standards on a day-to-day basis. It is not always easy to protect and maintain these standards, as a number of common factors, both structural and personal, can challenge the professional:

- shortage of resources (equipment, time, space)
- shortage of staff

- lack of training opportunities
- pressure of work
- inadequate facilities
- lack of leadership
- poorly functioning team
- demotivation/boredom
- 'burn out'
- health problems
- personal problems or stress.

Given that professional accountability is constant (in all circumstances, all the time) and permanent (from registration onwards), what can an individual nurse do to ensure that their standards of practice are not compromised when these circumstances arise? For structural factors which cause barriers to high quality practice it is important to:

- recognize the problem – is it really an underlying shortage of staff, or staff sickness, or the fact that some staff will not work together?
- report the problem – to the senior person close to the problem initially, in objective and preferably measurable terms
- record the problem in an appropriate place(s), the fact that it has been reported and any response to the report – the appropriate place might be the accident book, a patient's record, the ward or clinic record, or in a letter, depending on the problem and the circumstances
- try to remedy the problem – take any steps possible to prevent a detrimental effect on practice or patient care
- take advice, e.g. from professional organization advisors, occupational health, a mentor or supervisor, if the problem continues.

The key is that the practitioner will be held accountable, not for the structural problems if they were not of their making, but for maintaining the standards of their practice in the face of the problems.

Personal factors can be harder to tackle than structural ones; it is almost always easier to find and blame external causes than to acknowledge personal issues. But it is important to recognize and acknowledge the real problem. Reflective practice and clinical supervision sessions are key opportunities to examine personal aspects of practice and identify both problems and potential solutions (see below and Chapter 17).

Again, it is important to stress that professional accountability does not require the practitioner to be exemplary at all times. But it does require the practitioner to use the frameworks set out by the regulatory body to protect the standards of their practice by tackling any deficiencies that may threaten those standards.

TOOLS FOR THE PRACTITIONER

In addition to the formal framework described above of professional regulation, education and guidance that helps nurses reach and maintain the required standards of practice, there are other 'tools' that the practitioner can use to deliver, and to measure, high quality practice.

It is easy to identify books, guidelines and other tangible resources as tools to support practice. They may exist in hard copy form in the clinical setting, or be accessed using information technology (Box 14.8). A key issue for busy practitioners, however, is the difference between having and using such tools. The provision of access to the internet, or a set of 'Essence of Care' benchmarks (Box 3.1) on a ward, will not automatically improve care. It is the use and application of the knowledge, evidence, research findings or audit tools to be found in these resources that improves practice. Alongside the provision of such resources, practitioners will need time and, in some cases, relevant skills to access them. It is the combination of these factors that has the potential to improve practice.

$$\text{Information resources} + \text{time/skill to access} + \text{understanding/application} = \text{potential for practice improvement}$$

Box 14.8 Resources to support high quality care

- Research evidence, e.g. that published in reputable academic and professional journals
- Guidelines for treating particular conditions e.g. those published by NICE or professional bodies such as the British Hypertension Society
- Consensus 'benchmark' standards, e.g. *The Essence of Care* benchmarks (DoH 2001f)
- Patient information from reputable sources
- Authoritative factual information, e.g. drug tariff, *British National Formulary*

Some of the most important tools for achieving high quality practice are less visible, and less reliant on provision by the organization, or training and opportunities to access: communication, preceptorship/mentorship, professional support such as clinical supervision, and reflective practice.

Communication

Communication is such a routine concept that its impact on the quality of nursing care provided to patients is easy to overlook. But failures in communication – written or verbal – are the most commonly cited cause of many of the avoidable tragedies and failures in the health service.

Verbal communication is a common, frequent and fundamental part of practice within a nursing team. Box 14.9 gives an example of two contrasting verbal communications about the same incident, to illustrate the need for a high standard of communication. To support high quality care, it should be:

- accurate – avoiding meaningless phrases and idiosyncrasies
- clear – using accepted terms and measurements rather than generalizations or jargon
- objective – focusing on the facts
- professional – avoiding irrelevant value judgements, or derogatory comments, about the patient.

Box 14.9 Example of unclear and clear communication

Unclear/inaccurate/subjective:
'He didn't have a bad night, though he spiked a temp at one point and his output is not so good. But he's a stubborn old so-and-so and he hasn't been drinking nearly enough.'

Clear/accurate/objective:

'His temperature was up from 37 to 38.4°C when it was checked at 2 am, but it was down to 37.5°C at 6 am. His urine output in the last 24 hours has been 1200 ml, and we need to encourage him to drink more fluids.'

It is useful in considering all of these tools to refer back to the *Code of professional conduct* (NMC 2002a) to check whether the tool does in fact help deliver the standard. Ensuring that verbal communication takes place as described above reflects the requirements of sections 1 and 7 of the *Code*, which state:

'Act always in such a manner as to promote and safeguard the interests and well-being of patients and clients.'

'Recognize and respect the uniqueness and dignity of each patient and client, and respond to their need for care, irrespective of their ethnic origin, religious beliefs, personal attributes, the nature of their health problems or any other factor.'

(NMC 2002a)

Written communication is equally important to nursing practice. The UKCC's *Guidelines for Records and Record-Keeping* (UKCC 1998c) make clear that the activity of making and keeping records is an essential and integral part of care, and not a distraction from it (Box 14.10). Failures in the adequacy of nursing records are a common finding of investigations into poor patient care, or allegations of professional misconduct. But the purpose of good record-keeping is not solely to make a historical record of what happened to the patient, or to document clinical decision-making, though these are vital functions. During an episode of care, the written record is an essential element of the communication between members of the clinical team – a tool for communication in 'real time'. In terms of the *Code of professional conduct*, it allows the team to, 'act always in such a manner as to promote and safeguard the interests of the patient', and to 'ensure that no action or omission on your part or within your sphere of responsibility, is detrimental to the interests, condition or safety of patient and clients' (NMC 2002a).

Box 14.10 UKCC guidance on record keeping: essential elements (UKCC 1998c)

Records must:

- Be written legibly and indelibly
- Be clear and unambiguous
- Be accurate in each entry as to date and time
- Ensure that alterations are made by scoring out with a single line followed by the initialled, dated and timed-correct entry
- Ensure that additions to existing entries are individually dated, timed and signed
- Not include abbreviations, meaningless phrases and offensive subjective statements unrelated to the patient's care and associated observations
- Not allow the use of initials for major entries and ensure that local arrangements for identifying initials and signatures exist
- Not include entries made in pencil or blue ink, the former carrying the risk of erasure and the latter (where photocopying is required) of poor quality reproduction

Clearly, if something written in the patient record is not clear, or if care given is not recorded, then the potential for duplication, omission, or mistake is greatly increased when other professionals rely on that record to plan their actions. The quality of care is reduced and the patient may be put at risk – breaching the *Code of professional conduct*.

The fact that both verbal and written communication are such everyday parts of nurses' practice makes them susceptible to the development of bad habits over time. An essential part of maintaining high quality practice is constantly to review such important elements of practice, checking back against the standards, and correcting any deterioration. Clinical supervision sessions, or reflection of practice, provide ideal opportunities to do this (see below and Chapter 17).

Preceptorship and mentorship

Preceptorship is a system which aims to help the newly-qualified nurse build confidence in practice in the early months following registration, by allocating a more experienced nurse to provide guidance. Mentorship is sometimes defined as a similar system for nurses during training, but the term is more commonly used to refer to the linking of a less experienced with a more experienced professional at any stage during their career.

The role of the preceptor or mentor can be described as:

- listening – to issues, concerns, successes and dilemmas
- reflecting – helping to show the situation or concern in a different light
- challenging – allowing the 'mentee' to find their own solutions or approaches
- signposting – to information, contacts and different ways of thinking about an issue or problem.

Preceptors may be allocated to a newly registered nurse and often work in the same clinical area. Their role may include more teaching and practical guidance than that of a mentor. They are key to helping the inexperienced nurse to identify good practice and to consider the quality of their practice as a whole – rather than simply the correct performance of tasks. The preceptor helps to set the habits of practice for which the newly qualified nurse is accountable throughout their career. It is therefore a very responsible role and one that ideally benefits both parties by helping them both reflect on what constitutes high quality patient care.

Mentorship is not always such a formalized system and a nurse is much less likely to be allocated a mentor than a preceptor. But many nurses do approach someone to act as a mentor and choose voluntarily to use this tool both to support their practice and develop their career. In doing so they need to be prepared to explain:

- why they want mentorship
- what they hope to achieve from it
- how they have identified the prospective mentor.

It is also important to be prepared for the commitment of time, energy and effort to the relationship, at least for a trial period. This means, for example:

- agreeing to meet at regular intervals for a specified period of time
- prioritizing mentorship meetings and protecting the time from interruptions
- participating fully in the mentoring: talking, listening, exploring and accepting challenges and opportunities.

Mentors frequently provide their mentees with very practical benefits as well as the chance for discussion and reflection. These include access to their own professional networks and contacts, opportunities for job swaps or to shadow key individuals who can provide relevant experience, and direction to literature, projects, individuals or sites which provide new ideas or examples for the mentee's work.

Referring back to the *Code of professional conduct*, it is clear that preceptorship and mentorship are key tools to help 'maintain and improve your professional knowledge and competence' (NMC 2002a, section 3) and 'work in a collaborative and co-operative manner with heath care professionals and others involved in providing care' (section 6). In addition, for the mentor or preceptor themselves, providing this kind of support for less experienced colleagues fulfils the requirement of section 14, to 'assist professional colleagues … to develop their professional competence, and assist others in the care team … to contribute safely and to a degree appropriate to their roles'.

Clinical supervision

Professional support can take many forms, of which preceptorship and mentorship are examples. In recent years, a more formal system of providing professional support has become more widespread under the general title of 'clinical supervision'. The concept was proposed in the Department of Health's first strategy for nursing, *A Vision for the Future* (NHS Executive 1993). It is a formal process of providing opportunities for support, learning and reflection on practice to practitioners in the clinical setting. The UKCC produced a position statement on clinical supervision in 1996, setting out some key statements about what clinical supervision is and does (Box 14.11; UKCC 1996b). Importantly, the position statement stresses that clinical supervision is not a managerial control system and this understanding is key to the idea of such professional support as a tool to use in ensuring high quality practice. Only if it is not seen as an imposed management process can it be fully used by the practitioner to test out for themselves how their practice measures up to standards set, and to improve and develop their practice skills.

Box 14.11 UKCC guidance on clinical supervision: Six key statements about clinical supervision (UKCC 1996b)

- Clinical supervision supports practice and aims to maintain and promote standards of care
- Clinical supervision is a practice-focused professional relationship to assist guided reflection
- The process of clinical supervision should be developed by practitioners and managers according to local circumstances. Ground rules should be agreed so that practitioners and supervisors approach clinical supervision openly, confidently and aware of what is involved
- Every practitioner should have access to clinical supervision. Each clinical supervisor should supervise a realistic number of supervisees
- Preparation for supervisors can be effected using 'in-house' or external education programmes. The principle and relevance of clinical supervision should be included in pre- and post-registration education programmes
- Evaluation of clinical supervision is needed to assess how it influences care, practice standards and the service. Evaluation systems should be determined locally

---

Clinical supervision takes many forms and is usually adapted by an organization to suit the needs of its staff. In organizations that provide different forms of care, e.g. ward- and community-based care, quite different forms of clinical supervision may be implemented for different groups of staff. Ideally, staff can choose or design the form that best suits them – and adapt it over time in the light of experience. Some of the commoner forms are:

- one-to-one supervision – between an individual practitioner and an individual supervisor
- group supervision – led by a trained facilitator to ensure that everyone has the chance to be heard, and that issues are explored appropriately
- peer supervision – in a group without a designated facilitator, or where the role of facilitator rotates around members of the group.

What happens in the supervision sessions also varies according to the needs of the practitioners and the model used. Sometimes the focus is on learning, sometimes on support and sometimes on standard setting. The key factor which distinguishes clinical supervision from other discussions or relationships is the existence of a set of 'ground rules' about behaviour, participation and the confidentiality of proceedings.

Using clinical supervision as a tool to achieve high quality practice supports section 3 of the *Code of professional conduct*, 'maintain and improve your professional knowledge and competence'.

Reflective practice

Reflective practice is a technique which may be used as part of clinical supervision sessions, or separately from the formal process. It involves consciously and systematically thinking about professional actions and experiences, in order to learn from them and maintain or improve high quality practice. There are many different ways to 'action' the internal process of reflection – including making notes, drawing and producing mind maps – and different models for incorporating reflection into the development activities of a team or clinical supervision group. Keeping a reflective diary is one way of both undertaking and recording this process – but the way that the learning, insight and understanding is used to change and develop practice is more important than the way it is written down or recorded.

It is important not to confuse simple recall of events with reflection. Remembering and describing what happened in a situation is not necessarily reflection. Reflection would involve, for example, in addition to the description:

- thinking about why it happened in the way that it did
- considering the professional issues and consequences
- being aware of the impact on the patient and on other professionals
- measuring events and professional responses to them against the standards expected of the profession
- identifying lessons to be learned – both the good practice to be continued and instances where better practice could be substituted in future.

Reflective practice should not just improve the practice of the individual nurse; it should also at times identify ways in which the organization of care, or the functioning of the team, could be changed to improve the patient's experience.

Combining tools

The tangible and intangible tools summarized here are not of course the only ones available to nurses to maintain and improve the quality of care. There are many others, from many sources. Nor are they intended as alternatives for the nurse to choose from. The undertaking of accountable professional practice as a nurse, midwife or health visitor requires the ability to use all of these tools in combination on a day-to-day basis. Maintaining the standard of practice required is not an automatic ability conferred on a practitioner by registration. Nor does it happen in fits and starts when the practitioner attends another course or reads a new book. High profile cases of failures in practice, as well as the day-to-day experience of most nurses, confirms that it is not always easy to provide the quality of practice expected. Registration as a nurse following qualification is only the starting point for a process, often described as 'lifelong learning', which requires the practitioner to use the tools available, in a pragmatic and practical way, to support their practice on a daily, even hour by hour, basis.

CONCLUSION

This chapter has considered a number of health care policies that have brought a focus to quality in health care. Clinical governance provides the framework through which organisations and individuals can focus on the clinical aspects of care and their continual improvement. A key component of the quality of care patients experience is the practise of those caring for them. Professional accountability and regulation to protect the patient through ensuring standards and behaviour are part of the whole quality picture. This chapter has attempted to show how policies, organisations and individual practitioners combine to focus on making the patient's health care experience a good one.

MANAGING RISK IN A HEALTH CARE ORGANIZATION

Sally M Taber

INTRODUCTION

Risk management is about practising safely. It aims to develop good practice and to reduce the occurrence of harmful or adverse events (RCN 2000a). Learning from mistakes and changing the culture is essential to take this agenda forward. Adverse clinical incidents need to be managed systematically but within a blame-free culture.

The first part of this chapter will describe the integration of risk management to ensure quality improvement and in particular how standards can help reduce risk. Later, issues such as complaints management, health and safety – including the decontamination agenda and coping with the challenge of variant Creutzfeldt Jakob disease, and the management of abuse and violence will be covered, all of which are essential components of a risk management programme. The need to ensure the integration of risk management into everyday work will be explained; continuing professional development is also integral to taking the agenda forward. The structures responsible for delivering the education and training agenda will be examined.

The subject of risk management relates to specific NMC requirements for pre-registration nursing programmes (UKCC 2001a) and these will be identified throughout the chapter.

WHAT IS CLINICAL GOVERNANCE?

The Department of Health's definition of clinical governance is:

> 'a framework through which NHS organizations are accountable for continuously improving the quality of services and safeguarding high standards of care by creating an environment in which excellence will flourish'.

(DoH 1998)

This definition has also been encompassed by independent health care organizations, but for organizations under the social care agenda, the concept of 'best value' has been added, which addresses value for money issues, including the quality agenda.

REFLECTION POINT

What do you understand by clinical governance, as it is practised where you work?

Effective clinical governance should ensure:

- continuous improvement of patient services and care
- a patient-centred approach that includes treating patients courteously, involving them in decisions about their care and keeping them involved
- a commitment to quality, which ensures that health professionals are up-to-date in their practices and properly supervised where necessary
- a reduction of unacceptable variations in treatment
- a reduction of the risk from clinical errors and adverse events, as well as a commitment to learn from mistakes and share that learning with others.

An adverse event is when a series of issues are identified, such as the series of events surrounding the mistakes in giving intrathecal injections, when lack of training was identified as a causal factor and where there was no possibility of junior staff being supervised.

The main components within NHS trusts, independent sector hospitals and primary care organizations required to make clinical governance operational are:

- clear lines of responsibility and accountability for the overall quality of clinical care, which includes care delivered by nurses, allied health professionals and medical staff
- a set of systems, such as peer review and incident reporting arrangements, to improve quality. Peer review can take place in both formal and informal settings, when a group of professionals, such as nurses, discuss a patient's care and how a particular change could improve quality. It should be possible to raise incidents in a blame-free culture
- education and training plans; this includes the importance of all student and registered nurses having their own individualized development plans
- clear policies for managing risk, e.g. a policy for managing violent patients
- integrated procedures for all professional groups to identify and remedy poor performance (Wilson 2002).

The Department of Health in England made a commitment in 1997 that trusts would have to produce a comprehensive statement – the Controls Assurance Statement – on the controls they had in place to manage risks. Controls assurance has historically been concerned with financial and organizational control matters. The Department of Health sees controls assurance and clinical governance as being complementary. This is obviously a sensible step, as risk management cannot be addressed without financial input and the right management structures. The re-introduction of the 'matron' (known as the 'modern matron') is an example of addressing the agenda, as is the Chief Nurse's strategy for the *Essence of Care* (DoH 2001f).

Scotland, Wales and Northern Ireland follow a similar model for the implementation of clinical governance, which includes risk management.

DEVELOPING AND MONITORING AN EFFECTIVE RISK MANAGEMENT STRATEGY UNDER CLINICAL GOVERNANCE

We are all exposed to risks every day, such as crossing roads or catching a cold, but in the health care environment a strategy is needed to manage these risks and this must be addressed as part of the quality agenda. To do this, the questions in Box 15.1 need to be taken into consideration.

Box 15.1 Questions to be answered in developing a risk strategy (answers are given in italics)

- Why develop a risk management strategy? *Patient and staff safety is paramount*
- What should be included in the strategy? *Policies and procedures that are in place*
- How do you ensure risk management is integrated with quality improvement? *This requires a complete change of culture throughout an organization, whether it is a hospital, community setting or a care home*
- How do you monitor and benchmark the strategy? *This requires an audit programme to be introduced to measure key performance indicators, e.g. the incidence of falls across a medical unit, identified infections occurring within a surgical unit, or the frequency of the utilization of restraint within a mental health setting, which can be benchmarked, e.g. month by month or across the organization. An example of an audit mechanism, Safecode, will be explained in the text*
- How do you obtain commitment to risk management? *Again, this requires a cultural change to ensure that there is both commitment from the top of the organization to the shop floor and vice versa*
- How do you communicate a planned approach to risk management across complex and geographically widespread organizations? *To do this it is essential for a communications strategy to be introduced*
- How do you provide a central focus for a number of initiatives aimed at risk control? *Again, this must be part of the organization's communication strategy; if the incidence of, say, infections is not reported on, then how can it be a central focus and hence the risk control addressed?*

Whether in the NHS or the independent sector, it is important to communicate the risk management strategy to stakeholders/regulatory bodies (see Box 15.2). To integrate the strategy with quality improvement, it is important to identify the mechanisms of implementation. Examples are given in Box 15.3.

Box 15.2 Stakeholder/regulatory bodies

- Quality management initiatives:
  - Controls Assurance
  - Health Quality Service
  - Healthcare Accreditation Programme
  - ISO series (British Standards Institute)
- National Care Standards Commission. The Care Standards Act (2000) was enacted on April 1 2002 to regulate and inspect the independent sector. The Care Standards Commission is the body that carries out this task. However, plans are already in place to set up a new structure, the Commission for Healthcare Audit and Inspection (CHAI), which will include the Commission for Health Improvement (CHI) and the value for money part of the Audit Commission. This is proposed to inspect both the NHS and the health care part of the independent sector. A separate Commission is planned for the social care division which will include the Social Services Inspectorate and the social care services of the National Care Standards Commission; however, this will include all care homes. This is the agenda proposed for England and Wales; Scotland has a similar agenda involving the Clinical Standards Board for Scotland
- Private medical insurers
- Primary care trusts which will buy NHS services via a contracting process
- And most importantly, patients

Box 15.3 Mechanisms of implementation of the risk management strategy

- Risk Management Committee
- Clinical Governance Manual
- Clinical Effectiveness Committee – clinical effectiveness is about doing the right thing in the right way and at the right time for the right patient (RCN 1999b)
- Health and Safety Manual
- Consultant/Junior Doctor Handbook
- Incident reporting procedures
- Clinical risk assessment policy

All health care professionals must ensure that risk management is a process for identifying the risks that have adverse effects on the quality, safety and effectiveness of service delivery; assessing and evaluating those risks; and taking positive action to eliminate or reduce them.

Key components in effective clinical risk management include:

- applying and monitoring risk management standards
- having a clear risk management strategy with an action plan
- undertaking focused risk reviews in a systematic way across all specialities and departments, and having effective near-miss and incident reporting systems.

Near-misses are occurrences which, but for luck or skilful management, would in all probability have become an incident. However, on a future occasion it may be that a near-miss becomes an actual incident or occurrence. Reporting near-misses can prevent avoidable adverse clinical incidents which could affect patient safety or, for example, in the case of a wrongly administered intrathecal injection, a fatality.

Safecode is a software system that aids the collection of meaningful data with regards to incident reporting, such as slips, trips and falls, needlestick injuries and manual handling. It can monitor increased stay costs caused by slips, trips and falls by department, time of day, age and environmental factors. The cost of needlestick injuries in disposal against cost of retractable needles or improved sharps bins, or the cost of manual handling incidents against cost of improving lifting aids/devices/systems or improved training, can also be measured.

Best practice through continuous improvement from using Safecode in reducing all types of incidents, as well as year-on-year reduction in cost of incidents and reduction in sickness absence, is evident.

MODIFYING RISK: TAKING POSITIVE ACTION

The Health Act (1999) for the NHS and the Care Standards Act (2000) for the independent sector require the entire health care sector to implement quality and risk standards. Health care professionals, including registered nurses, student nurses and managers, need to be proactive in ensuring that risk and quality management stay at the top of their agenda by undertaking clinical risk reviews to demonstrate clinical effectiveness and compliance. Consumer pressure is also ensuring that this actually happens. Recent high profile cases such as the Kennedy inquiry (DoH 2001d), the Ledward case (NHS Executive 2000) and the O'Neale case have described problems, both in the NHS and the independent sector, and lessons need to be learnt.

Lessons learnt from these cases include the importance of ensuring that professionals maintain and update their competence, that poor practice is reported and addressed and that having an open culture allows problems both to be communicated to senior management and addressed (Wilson 2002).

The importance of eliminating or controlling risk has been recognized by health care professionals for many years. The key issue is not to dissuade anyone from risk taking, as we all take risks with everything we do – such as when we cross the road or go on holiday. The key is to try to change behaviour to take account of risk, which is difficult, as it often takes cultural, individual and management changes to alter practice, so as to modify behaviour and reduce risk. This can be actioned through identifying risk and raising risk-awareness, reviewing and changing practices, and ongoing evaluation.

The process of awareness and evaluation, education and implementation, integration and support is all about developing ownership, control and action around the issues. Teaching staff to analyse their concerns and potential problems helps to minimize risk, modify practitioners' behaviour and integrate quality and clinical audit into daily practice.

The multi-professional team can begin to apply risk management to its own health care setting and achieve risk reduction/modification in three steps.

- *Awareness and evaluation:* an in-depth assessment of the organization's services and practices, and the costs related to each, provides data for identifying potential risk areas. This assessment should cover both clinical and non-clinical components. An example of this is a safer patient handling policy; the costs involved are ensuring that the ward/unit/home has the correct manual handling equipment.
- *Education and implementation:* development of processes and interventions that begin to change undesirable practices is the second phase of risk modification. This combines specific structural

and procedural changes with an educational process for all involved. All safer handling policies require training prior to implementation.

- *Integration and support:* once changes and interventions are decided upon, a system for monitoring their integration into the organization is needed to determine whether the change has actually modified the risk. Data collection, analysis, measuring, monitoring and re-evaluation constitute the third element of risk reduction/modification. Analysis, monitoring and re-evaluation are part of a safer patient handling strategy, ensuring that the policy and education is making a difference, in particular to the staff involved and the comfort of the patient/resident/service user.

A risk management strategy provides the framework for developing a rigorous risk management process throughout a health care organization. The strategy will acknowledge that while health care is, by its very nature, a risky activity, it is of considerable concern that a wide range of risks can occur by accident, mishap and mistake. Even more worrying are incidents that result from deficiencies caused by a lack of clear policies, procedures, protocols or pathways of care, deficient working practices, poorly defined responsibilities, inadequate communications or other systems failures.

The challenge for some managers and all health care professionals is to eliminate, or at least reduce, the potential for such misfortunes by being more positive in the future management of risk. The key components of a successful risk management strategy are summarized in Boxes 15.4 and 15.5.

Box 15.4 Key components of a risk management strategy

- A risk management policy statement
- An assessment of organizational requirements for managing risks
- Management of attitudes to cultural changes towards risk within the organization (Changing cultural attitudes is not an easy process)
- Processing for identifying and assessing risk
- Identification of key clinical, environmental and other risks, e.g. the decontamination agenda
- Implementation of systems to prevent, contain and control risk
- Training and education to make the risk management process effective
- Setting risk and quality management standards
- Involving staff in identifying and managing risk
- Near-miss and incident reporting systems
- A system to manage complaints and legal claims
- Monitoring the risk management process

Box 15.5 Creating the awareness for a risk management strategy

- A rigorously organized framework to co-ordinate and oversee risk management activities
- An open and honest, learning and participative organizational culture
- Managers, clinicians and staff who are aware of their risk management responsibilities
- Inter-professional working through integrated care management and seamless care, which follows patients across the different sectors of care into their home environment
- An effective communication strategy supported by good documentation of policies, procedures, multi-professional pathways and clinical guidelines. Multi-professional care pathways are good practice standards for commonly performed operations and treatments to ensure that patients receive the best possible care. A care pathway is when an agreed standard is set for each stage of patient care and treatment, from

before admission to discharge, and in some cases beyond, including how the patient is expected to respond and recover

- Collection and analysis of information from risk assessments, audit data, incident reporting and user feedback
- Subsequent review and development of operational practices and systems

Risk management must be seen as an essential component of the organization's continuous quality improvement programmes, embracing good working practices, processes and systems. A key to successful risk management is to embed within the organization routine collection of information, its analysis and subsequent feedback and appropriate action by health care professionals and managers. Positive outcomes for risk management processes are only possible where staff are engaged in the process and are given time and opportunity to reflect on their practice and take any necessary action to improve it. At the heart of the process is the organization's desire to create services that minimize risks to patients and clients, and provide a healthy and safe environment for staff.

REFLECTION POINT

Take some time to think about your own workplace in relation to what you have read and try to identify the risk management strategies that are in place.

ADVISORY AND REGULATORY ORGANIZATIONS

Two organizations need to be considered in England and Wales when reviewing the agenda for taking positive action to manage risk. First, The National Clinical Assessment Authority was set up in April 2001 to provide a central point of contact for the NHS when concerns about a doctor's performance are raised. The authority will give advice to NHS hospitals and health authorities to make sure the performance of doctors is checked and action taken to ensure they are practising safely (DoH 2001l).

Building a Safer NHS for Patients, published in April 2001, set out a blueprint for a national reporting system (DoH 2001h) and The National Patient Safety Agency (NPSA) was established in July 2001. It is currently implementing a new national mandatory system for reporting, analysing and learning from clinical and non-clinical adverse incidents, and near-misses across the NHS, as part of the government's drive to improve patient safety and quality through reducing the risk of harm (DoH 2001m). The NPSA is founded on the following principles:

- reporting is mandatory for individuals and organizations
- confidential but with open access
- generally blame free and independent
- simple to use but comprehensive in coverage and data collection
- systems are in place for learning and change at local and national level.

The system it is implementing comprises five linked key components:

- *identifying* and *recording* reportable adverse events
- *reporting* by individuals to local sites and to the national system, and by institutions to the national system

- *analysing* incidents, including root cause analysis, and trends
- *learning lessons* from analysis, research and other sources of information, and disseminating them
- *implementing* change at local and national level.

The independent sector's involvement in these two organizations is currently being discussed with the intention of it becoming involved.

RELEVANT COMPETENCIES

 'Manage oneself, one's practice, and that of others, in accordance with the *Code of professional conduct,* registering one's own abilities and limitations.'

(UKCC 2001a)

This is an important competency that you should reflect on, in particular the sub-component 'identify unsafe practice and respond appropriately to ensure a safe outcome'. Earlier, accountability to ensure safe practice has been emphasized.

Even more appropriate to risk management is the following competency:

'Contribute to public protection by creating and maintaining a safe environment of care through the use of quality assurance and risk management strategies.'

(UKCC 2001a)

The three sub-components 'use appropriate risk assessment tools to identify actual and potential risks', 'communicate safety concerns to a relevant authority' and 'manage risk to provide care which best meets the needs and interests of patients, clients and the public' are particularly relevant.

It is important having read the above, that you mirror these competencies and take on board the importance of a risk management strategy.

SUMMARY

The components of a successful risk management strategy, particularly analysing incidents, learning lessons from the analysis and implementing change, have been described.

HANDLING PATIENT COMPLAINTS

Complaints range from grumbles about the standard of food right through to accidents and patient deaths. Often they arise as a result of poor communication. This may reflect verbal failures, e.g. not telling a relative that a patient has moved wards, or written ones, e.g. failure to keep adequate or accurate records. However, a complaint can provide a measure of patient satisfaction, support quality improvement, provide an early warning indication of risk exposure, meet control assurance objectives and meet accreditation bodies' requirements.

The importance of complaints handling cannot be overemphasized. Most people do not make complaints lightly and an assurance that something is being done to ensure it does not happen to others is sometimes all that is required. Complaints properly handled offer the opportunity to learn and improve the quality of care.

The NHS Ombudsman issues an annual report on complaints referred to the Ombudsman's office. It details the issues surrounding the complaint, how the stages have been handled and lessons learnt. Issues raised in past reports include poor communications, inadequate records, lost records and systems and process failures.

It is helpful to reflect on the following statistics:

- the prime motivation of 90.4% of complainants is to ensure that the issue of the complaint will not happen again; only 8.9% are motivated to seek financial compensation
- 60% of patients are dissatisfied with the care they receive from the NHS but fail to complain due to: fear of retribution, lack of 'know-how', feelings of gratitude and deference towards health professionals
- medical error results in 40,000 deaths per annum in the UK. It is the third most likely cause of death after cancer and heart disease (Vincent 2000)
- in the NHS, 280,000 patients suffer non-fatal clinical incidents per annum and spend, on average, 6 extra days in hospital at a cost of £730 m per annum (Vincent 2000).

Maintaining an efficient and practical patients' complaints procedure requires effective communication between the various functions and tiers of staff within hospitals/clinics/care homes, and between management, professionals, clinicians and patients.

EXERCISE

Try to find out how complaints are handled in the area/unit where you work. Look through the complaints over the last year – what is their main focus?

The NHS complaints procedure is currently under review having undergone extensive consultation (see Chapter 14). However, whatever the outcome of the review, effective systems for the management of complaints help address patient safety and identify system failures. As previously stated, complaints provide an opportunity to examine hospital/clinic/care home service and clinical practice and to ensure that a culture of quality improvement and risk reduction exists in the overall clinical governance framework.

The skills required for handling complaints are:

- clear communication – verbal and written, including report writing
- eliciting views of service users, e.g. interviewing techniques
- a calm, open approach
- ability to reduce anxiety in someone who is making a complaint
- making the person feel heard and taken seriously
- handling conflict.

EXAMPLE OF A COMPLAINTS POLICY: THE INDEPENDENT HEALTH ASSOCIATION'S CODE

The following describes the independent sector's implementation of a complaints policy, *Handling Patients' Complaints – A Code of Practice for Members of the Independent Healthcare Association (IHA)* (Independent Healthcare Association 2002). It is based on recommended good practice described by the British Standards Institute (1999) and the Mental Health Act (1983) Code of practice (DoH 1999a).

The IHA's Code has three stages: local resolution, internal appeal and independent external adjudication. At the local resolution stage, it is the responsibility of the IHA member hospital concerned to look into and to respond to the patient's complaint. The aim is to try and sort out any problems as quickly and informally as possible. In some cases a word with an appropriate member of staff is all that is needed to put things right. If a patient feels anxious about making a complaint themselves, then a friend or relative can do so on their behalf. The IHA member hospital will ask the patient's relative or friend to confirm in writing whether they have permission to do so. By taking this course of action the patient is waiving their right of confidentiality regarding their own clinical information by sharing this with the person acting on their behalf.

If the patient is not happy with the way the compliant has been dealt with at a local resolution level, then they may request an internal appeal within 20 working days of the date of the final written response. The internal appeal stage is the responsibility of the chief executive (CEO) or managing director (MD) of the organization (when the hospital belongs to a group), or in the case of independent hospitals, a non-executive director or trustee. They will consider the complaint and may undertake a review of the correspondence and the handling of the issue at local hospital level. The CEO/MD will then confirm the decisions and actions of the hospital manager or offer an alternative resolution.

The independent external adjudication process is for patients who are not satisfied with the results of a hospital's internal process and is therefore only available once the internal process is exhausted. A separate third stage has been established in the independent sector, as the sector does not currently have access to the NHS Ombudsman.

The Code applies to acute and mental independent health hospitals and is currently being extended to care homes. It was initiated to establish a consistent policy framework across IHA member organizations for the management of complaints. The principles outlined are:

- accessibility
- impartiality
- simplicity
- speed of redress
- confidentiality
- improvement in patient care (learning lessons).

The hospital manager has responsibility for managing the complaints process and their role is pivotal in local resolution, ensuring prompt completion of a thorough investigation, providing someone to act impartially and objectively, and being an 'advocate' for the aggrieved.

It is imperative that learning from complaints is an integral part of the process. The independent sector's report of complaints in 2001 concluded that all complaints reaching the final stage did so because of poor management handling at the first and second stages. Accountability for handling the complaint was the key message. Poor adherence to timescales for getting back to the patient was also an issue. Therefore, the messages are: take ownership of the issue and try to work within the required timescales. If this is not possible, then communicate the reasons why to the patient.

RELEVANT COMPETENCY

'Engage in, develop and disengage from therapeutic relationships through the use of appropriate communication and interpersonal skills.'

(UKCC 2001a)

The sub-component 'utilize a range of effective and appropriate communication and engagement skills' is particularly relevant to handling complaints, where effective communication is essential.

SUMMARY

Handling complaints well is important for all members of the health care profession and, in particular, they provide an opportunity to improve the service.

HEALTH AND SAFETY

The Health and Safety at Work Act (1974) requires NHS and independent organizations to ensure the health and safety of their employees. Incidents involving staff can result in time off due to minor injuries, stress, temporary or permanent disability and even death. They can also incur costs, e.g. staff replacement costs, compensation payments, fines and higher insurance premiums. Poor attention to health and safety issues can have detrimental effects on the quality of services, staff morale and public opinion about health care organizations.

In 1999 the government launched the Improving Working Lives Campaign (DoH 1999b) in which NHS trusts are required to invest in staff training and development, apply zero tolerance on violence, reduce workplace accidents and sickness absence, and provide better occupational health and counselling services.

EXERCISE
Try to find out what your own trust is doing in respect of Improving Working Lives.

Towards the end of 1999, the Department of Health launched the Controls Assurance initiative in England (see above) – through publication of a set of standards for risk management. The Health and Safety Controls Assurance standard states:

'there is a need for a managed environment which ensures as far as is reasonably practicable the health, safety and welfare of patients, staff, visitors, contractors and all others who are affected by the activities of the organisation'.

In June 2000 the government published a strategy statement (DoH 2000b) setting out how it and the Health and Safety Commission will work together to revitalize health and safety with the use of the following targets:

- to reduce the number of working days lost per 100,000 workers from work-related injury and ill health by 30% by 2010
- to reduce the incidence of fatal and major injury accidents by 10% by 2010
- to reduce the incidence of cases of work-related ill health by 20% by 2010
- achieve half the improvement under each target by 2004.

In addition, the Health Service Circular HSC 1999/229 requires trusts to reduce the incidence of violence to staff by 30% by 2003.

Reporting of incidents in all health care organizations should include:

- violence (physical and verbal)
- slips/trips/falls
- needlestick/sharps injuries
- musculo-skeletal disorders
- sensitization to such substances as latex
- contact with hazardous substance
- health care associated infections.

Health and safety monitoring should include the cost of health and safety incidents to the trust/ independent sector organizations.

High on the agenda for all health care professionals are manual handling incidents. Every year several thousand nurses and other health professionals leave the NHS due to back injury. While back injury is viewed by many as an occupational hazard, the number of cases involving litigation is growing, e.g. a registered nurse was awarded £410,000 compensation in a case which is seen as a landmark victory for those who have suffered injury at work (*Daily Mail* 17th October 2002).

REFLECTION POINT

What precautionary arrangements for manual handling are in place in your workplace?

A comprehensive strategy for addressing health and safety must be in place which is owned by the trust/independent sector CEO, together with the health and safety adviser, the human resources director, the head of occupational health, the head of facilities and estates, and a representative from each relevant department, e.g. A&E and critical care. However, it is ultimately about individual responsibility – strategies are useless unless enacted by individuals. Nurses must take individual responsibility within a corporate strategy and must be professionally confident enough to challenge bad practices, i.e. be active not passive.

Comprehensive occupational health services should be provided to employees, both in the NHS and the independent sector, and should include:

- pre-employment medicals
- routine employment screening

- immunization programmes
- investigations of incidents
- rehabilitation/managed return to work advice
- confidential counselling service
- general lifestyle advice, e.g. smoking, fitness.

The Improving Working Lives standard was to be met by NHS organizations in England by April 2003 (DoH 1999b). It requires employers to demonstrate a commitment to flexible working practices, such as flexi-time, annual hours agreements, flexible retirement, career breaks and reduced hours options – a challenge for both the NHS and the independent sector.

In ensuring that the appropriate health and safety measures are in place, the hospital, clinic or care home needs to ensure compliance with the legislation listed in Box 15.6.

Box 15.6 Legislation relevant to health and safety

- Health and Safety at Work Act (1974)
- Management of Health and Safety at Work Regulations (1999)
- Workplace (Health, Safety and Welfare) Regulations (1992)
- Provision and Use of Work Equipment Regulations (1999)
- Electricity at Work Regulations (1989)
- Health and Safety (First Aid) Regulations (1981)
- Control of Substances Hazardous to Health Regulations (COSHH) (1999)
- Manual Handling Operation Regulations (1992)
- Reporting of Injuries, Diseases and Dangerous Occurrences Regulations (RIDDOR) (1985)

DECONTAMINATION

Decontamination is a combination of processes, including cleaning, disinfection and/or sterilization, used to render re-usable surgical instruments safe for further use. Failure to decontaminate surgical instruments properly can lead to post-operative infection and other problems, such as spread of disease. Recent concerns have concentrated on the spread of variant Creutzfeldt Jakob disease (vCJD). Failure to maintain decontamination equipment and sustain proper working practices can raise health and safety issues for staff. The government's decontamination initiative was described in Health Service Circulars 178 and 179 in August 1999 (Kerr 2002).

The level of decontamination required varies according to the equipment itself, the procedure being carried out and the environment in which it is performed. For example, some equipment simply needs to be washed and disinfected, while invasive equipment needs to be washed, sterilized and then protected from further contamination. In the UK, surgical instruments are generally sterilized using a standard high-temperature steam cycle. Some instruments that cannot withstand high temperatures, particularly flexible endoscopes, are disinfected using chemical solutions.

Recent first-hand decontamination audit experiences, both within trusts and in the independent sector, have highlighted many fundamental operational difficulties that professionals working in front-line patient care face, as the ever increasing demands for quality are balanced against clinical governance and professional competency. A root and branch shift in practices will be needed at all levels in the 'decontamination chain' if hospital-acquired infection is to be kept under control. This will require holistic commitment from all members of the team involved in the management of medical devices, from procurement through to end-user.

Leadership and accountability, through recent controls assurance decontamination standards, is crucial, as is education and training, and monitoring of performance and progress. The Departments of Health for all four countries in the UK have launched an array of standards and initiatives to address theoretical iatrogenic (caused by treatment) infection risks, but responsibility without authority and resources will not meet patient's expectations.

The modernization of decontamination processes within the NHS and the independent sector is a long-term process, not a one-off event. There must be a commitment to ensure that the momentum to raise standards continues and that there are appropriate precautions, based on evidence and scientific advice, to ensure patient safety.

RELEVANT COMPETENCIES

'Based on the best available evidence, apply knowledge and an appropriate repertoire of skills indicative of safe nursing practice.'

(UKCC 2001a)

The sub-component 'engage with, and evaluate, the evidence base which underpins safe nursing practice' is particularly relevant to health and safety. Reflect again on the government's targets to reduce the number of working days lost through work-related injuries and, in particular, take into consideration safer manual handling policies that are evidence based and ensure that your practice is appropriate.

'Contribute to public protection by creating and maintaining a safe environment of care through the use of quality assurance and risk management strategies.'

(UKCC 2002)

The sub-component 'identify environmental hazards and eliminate and/or prevent them where possible' is particularly relevant. Adequate cleaning and sterilizing of instrumentation is essential to ensure that the environmental hazards that relate to the decontamination agenda are either eliminated and/or prevented.

SUMMARY

Health and safety issues should always be at the forefront, particularly when the environment is frequently pressurized. Thinking about safety needs to be a reflex action prior to any task being taken. Decontamination has been raised from the bottom to the top of most NHS trust's/independent sector organization's agendas. The importance of maintaining this momentum cannot be overemphasized for the safety of all patients and yourselves.

MEDICINES MANAGEMENT

Any risk management strategy would not be complete without a medicine management policy to ensure that measures are in place for the safe management and secure handling of medicines. All health care organizations should have a written medicines policy and procedure, accessible to staff, and covering all aspects of medicines systems and medical gases:

- ordering, procurement, receipt, storage, administration and disposal of medicines
- action to be taken in case of adverse reactions
- error reporting to encourage an open reporting system and a non-blame culture.

The recent agenda of the extension of nurse prescribing (DoH 2002c) and the use of patient group directives must, equally, have their own policies and procedures. When nurse prescribing and patient group directives are used, they must comply with Department of Health/Medicines Control Agency guidance. It is important that medicines prescribed and labelled, and received against a prescription for a named patient, are not used for any other patient. A procedure should also be in place for the self-administration of medicines by the patient, in particular concerning safe storage. Information must be given to patients about the use, benefits and potential harm of prescribed medication.

THE EXPERT PATIENT

All health care organizations/professionals need to be patient-centred, e.g.:

- focus on the things that matter to patients
- get patient and carer perspectives on what happens
- see if patients, carers and the public have a say in things
- provide people with information on how good services are.

The modernization agenda requires an increasingly patient-centred approach to health care delivery. An open culture that challenges historical practice by re-designing processes and procedures ensures that lessons are learnt and shared and a patient focus is achieved.

A central theme of *The Expert Patient* report (Kirkness 2000) is that we need to extend the government's concept of the expert patient – everyone should be better informed or more expert. In 1979, Bennett wrote:

'The greatest benefit could come in the future if patients could take on more responsibility for their bodies and minds.... Doctors then may come to acknowledge .... that doctoring is something of a joint venture between patient and healer, in which the doctor serves as a guide.'

If Bennett were writing today, he would be sure to acknowledge the role of all health professionals in view of the number of nurse and therapist-led services. However, health care professionals alone cannot provide the level of understanding and support many people need. The self-help movement, the fastest growing component of the human service industry, is filling the vacuum.

The visiting card of 20th century medical culture, 'Doctor knows best', created an unhealthy dependency. But now it is to be torn up in favour of patient partnership and sharing: shared information, shared evaluation and shared responsibility. At least, this is the theory. An increasingly patient-centred approach to health care delivery implies organizing services around the patient pathway, rather than on functional lines. As a consequence, new ways of working emphasize flexibility in professional and other roles. Specialist knowledge and roles will remain important, but increasingly so in advising and training other staff, patients and carers, as well as in hands-on patient care.

Health care staff, particularly doctors and nurses, are ceasing to be possessors of unique knowledge and have to adopt new ways of working. Patients will expect more continuity and convenience of care. In the case of chronic conditions, they are partners in the management of their condition, not passive consumers. Ensuring that service issues are patient-centred is essential, particularly when taking into consideration the management of risk (see above).

RELEVANT COMPETENCIES

'Create and utilize opportunities to promote the health and well-being of patients, clients and groups.'

(UKCC 2001a)

The sub-component 'provide relevant and current health information to patients, clients and groups in a form which facilitates their understanding and acknowledges choice/individual patients', is particularly relevant. Patients need information on how good services are.

'Formulate and document a plan of nursing care, where possible in partnership with patients, clients, their carers and family and friends, within a framework of informed consent.'

(UKCC 2001a)

The need for health professional/patient partnerships cannot be overemphasized.

MANAGEMENT OF ABUSE AND VIOLENCE

The management of abuse and violence is an essential component of a risk management programme. In *Practioner–Client Relationships and the Prevention of Abuse*, the Nursing and Midwifery Council (NMC) (2002h) spells out precisely what is expected from practitioners in their relationship with clients, and defines six categories of abuse (see Box 5.1). It describes how professional boundaries allow a client and practitioner to interact safely in a therapeutic relationship, which is based on meeting the client's needs, and how a breach of professional boundaries is an abuse of power which acts against the best interests of the client. It also describes how the growing consumer movement in health care has led to demands for better standards of care and for clients to have the right to take decisions about their own treatment.

The publication describes how zero tolerance of abuse should be reflected throughout the organization and reiterates what has already been described above about how good communication channels that maximize feedback from clients, practitioners and managers, as well as risk management processes and regular audits of practice, including critical incidents and near misses, will all help in the prevention and detection of abuse.

It is particularly important that training is provided at the induction stage in the handling of abuse, which includes the recognition of the types of abuse, the possible sources of the abuse and the handling of suspected and/or alleged abuse.

REFLECTION POINT

Stop and think for a moment about how zero tolerance is applied where you work. Is the policy effective?

MANAGING VIOLENT PATIENTS

All health care organizations should have a local policy for managing violent patients. Characteristics of the human and physical environment have a powerful effect in mitigating and preventing or exacerbating and precipitating the manifestations of violence.

The following factors are important in ensuring violence is reduced:

- experience, training and supervision, motivation and numbers of staff
- facilities provided for staff, patients and visitors such as space, security, comfort and activities
- organization and management of the environment according to principles and policies that are shared with patients.

Training in aggression control techniques is essential in particular environments and especially where patients are cared for in secure mental health settings. In these settings, the importance of good leadership, structured staff roles and predictable routines cannot be over-emphasized. When properly used and explained, restraint can be acceptable both to users of services and to staff. Restraint, when skilfully applied by trained and supervised staff according to monitored protocols and in the context of other methods of care, is an effective and safe means of coping with overtly violent behaviour. Seclusion is unnecessary if restraint is properly applied in association with other methods of good clinical practice. Compliance with training in managing abusive behaviour and injuries from patient violence is essential for all health care professionals.

The Department of Health recently commissioned an overview to assess the overall needs of NHS staff (working in non-mental health settings) in relation to the provision of training in the recognition, prevention and management of violence and aggression and conflict resolution. The government has also launched a zero tolerance campaign, which includes patient warnings against harassment and bullying and details of the possible consequences of such actions.

The Employment National Training Organization is working with the Health and Safety Executive and key stakeholders to develop standards in conflict management. It is hoped that these standards will be useful to people in a range of jobs where there is the potential for verbal or physical violence.

SUMMARY

Zero tolerance of abuse and the management of violent patients have been taken on board at national level, and it is important that they stay there.

CONTINUING PROFESSIONAL DEVELOPMENT

Continuing professional development (CPD) is essential to the risk management agenda. Health care is increasingly delivered through non-hierarchical teamworking, which requires a different set of skills and attitudes from those traditionally deployed. People have a right to expect that those caring for them are still competent to practise, however long ago they qualified/gained their licence to practise.

A characteristic of much education and training in health care is the need for a substantial amount of teaching and supervised practice in the workplace. It is simply not possible to train as a hands-on deliverer of care in the classroom, although the recent return of clinical skills laboratories is welcome. That is not to say that there is not a continuing debate about the balance between theory and practice and the best way to integrate the two. One of the key features of the health sector is the high proportion of professionally qualified staff.

Although the NHS may dominate in many parts of the health care sector, it must be remembered that the independent and voluntary sectors in conventional health care and the whole complementary therapy sector are significant in their own right, with their own distinctive education and training needs in managing risk.

GOVERNMENT DEPARTMENTS

The Department of Health in England and the health departments in the other countries are responsible for the overall education and training strategy for the NHS. They directly fund much non-medical professional education (in England through a devolved system using NHS organizations for commissioning known as Workforce Development Confederations) and much non-professional training (again, either directly or through a devolved system). The Department for Education and Skills (DfEE) in England (and its equivalents elsewhere) is the other department with a major interest in the health field, by virtue of the significant role of the health sector within higher education and vocational training.

REGULATORY BODIES

The regulatory bodies such as the NMC, Health Professions Council and the General Medical Council (GMC) all have functions relating to determining the professional competencies and academic awards required for admission to their particular register; most also have, or will shortly have, functions relating to post-qualifying training, CPD and the development requirements for re-validation or re-registration. Their role in specifying competencies and educational requirements is justified by their overall purpose of protecting the public by ensuring fitness to practise. The NMC and the Health Professions Council will ensure that this happens.

In conventional health care, most are statutory bodies dealing with those who offer direct patient care. Operating department assistants/practitioners have a voluntary register but discussions are taking place with regards to their admission to the Health Professions Council. In the complementary therapy sector most are non-statutory (the exceptions being osteopathy and chiropractice), with consequent varying degrees of effectiveness.

HIGHER EDUCATION

Most higher education institutions (HEIs) in the UK have an interest in teaching and research in the health field. The Quality Assurance Agency for Higher Education (QAA) is a significant player, as efforts are made to align the quality assurance processes of the agency, regulatory bodies and, for those professions where it is the funding agent, the NHS/health departments.

OTHER TRAINING PROVIDERS

Further education is an important provider in the technical field, and to some extent in the training of health care assistants, although some of the latter training is provided within the NHS or independent sector – or by university nursing departments.

Sector skills councils (previously National training organizations)

Healthwork UK (New Skills for Health) was the national training organization (NTO) for the sector covering all four countries. There have been significant links to the work of other NTOs, particularly the Training Organization for Social Care (TOPSS – which also has a bid in to become a sector skills council) and the Voluntary Sector National Training Organization (VSNTO). Links with training in social work and social care may become closer with the development of NHS care trusts, providing both health and social care. Sector skills councils have a responsibility to address the education and training needs of managing risk in conjunction with workforce development confederations in England and the associated bodies in the other four countries.

Employers

Employers in the conventional health care sector in England have, from April 2001, been organized into workforce development confederations (DoH 2000e), which succeeded education and training consortia. These commission and manage education and training for all clinical staff covered by the NHS education levy; work with key professional groups to ensure the delivery of adequate numbers of properly trained staff; work with employers in developing and commissioning training programmes for all staff reflecting the needs of the sector; and work with postgraduate deans on the management and delivery of postgraduate medical and dental education. In addition to NHS trusts, health authorities and primary care groups/trusts, they will involve social services departments, the voluntary and independent sectors, the armed forces and the prison service. Confederations will be the key link between the health sector and regional development agencies and local learning and skills councils.

A workforce planning review has also been carried out in Wales and Scotland. Both are mirroring changes underway in England.

Budget

Levies have been combined from April 2002 into a single multi-professional education and training levy (MPET). This will enable resources to be used more flexibly to support multi-professional learning and workforce development in its widest sense.

Vocational training

Vocational training is provided through a mix (largely) of higher and further education, and in-house and commercial provision, and is essential to ensure that staff are trained to manage risk in both health and social care. A survey published in 2000 shows that by September 1998, a cumulative total of 246,407 registrations for Scottish/National Vocational Qualifications (S/NVQs) in care had been recorded by the awarding bodies, together with 213 for physiological measurement and 4802 for operating department practice/support. By the same date, 80,091 certificates had been recorded for care S/NVQs, together with 89 for physiological measurement and 2674 for operating department practice/support. The care S/NVQs cover both health and social care and it is not known how many people working in the health sector hold, or are working towards, S/NVQs. It is, however, known that, of all the care sector certificates awarded in 1997/8, 33.9% went to staff employed by the NHS, 21.6% by the independent sector, 11% by voluntary organizations and 9.3% by social services (Employment Surveys and Research Unit 2000).

In the independent sector, there are, in many cases, well-developed workforce development systems. Commercial disciplines demand well-founded short-term workforce planning. The sector is a major provider of vocational training and also provides clinical placements for students. In a survey conducted in 1999 by the Independent Healthcare Association (1999) 69% of the acute providers who responded reported providing clinical placement in the previous year, 85% of the mental health providers and 71% of the community care providers. However, in about half of the organizations responding there was no formal education post for staff development, although a good range of post-registration training opportunities for nurses and the allied health professions were recorded or accredited.

e-Learning

An e-learning (electronic, on-line learning) strategy is being developed for the NHS in England that will embrace all forms of education and training for all groups in the workforce. This will be incorporated into the role of the NHS university, which will provide widespread and effective access to web-based learning, and will develop relevant learning materials and packages, in addition to NHS-based or accredited e-learning resources.

ACCREDITATION AND QUALITY ASSURANCE

For NHS-funded professional education, the Department of Health has contracted the QAA to develop (UK wide) subject benchmarking statements for courses which lead to an academic and professional qualification coterminously, and a quality assurance review process that integrates the interests of QAA, the regulatory bodies and the NHS as funders.

S/NVQs are subject to the well-established accreditation and quality assurance mechanisms of the 1996/7 Education Act Regulatory Authorities, NTOs, awarding bodies and work-based verifiers and assessors. An interesting move is the development of national occupational standards (NOSs) for some professions, e.g. public health or, in a closely analogous field, the proposed new 3-year programme for social workers. It is the policy of the UK health departments that regulatory bodies should be encouraged increasingly to express their requirements for professional competencies in NOS terms. Occupational standards will be further described.

Many NHS, independent and voluntary sector organizations have achieved Investors in People accreditation. In England the NHS's Improving Working Lives Standard (DoH 1999b) has important components relating to the provision of learning and development opportunities for all staff. The Welsh Plan for the NHS seeks to encourage lifelong learning through ensuring that all staff have personal development plans, and that all health organizations prepare career development planning programmes. In July 2002 it became compulsory in England for all staff within the NHS to have a personal development plan.

BREAKING DOWN PROFESSIONAL BOUNDARIES

The boundaries between primary and secondary care are continually shifting, with a greater range of conditions, such as a number of the long-term medical conditions, capable of being managed in primary care. The same applies to professional boundaries. Similarly, the links between health and social care are becoming closer, with the government's proposals for joint 'care trusts' in England currently the subject of legislation. The changing workforce programme is now looking at a patient-centred reason for multi-professional learning and the need to reduce the number of different professionals delivering different 'fragments' of health care for patients.

The demands for better regulation of non-professionally qualified 'support workers' will increase the need for these staff to possess NVQs or other relevant qualifications.

Increasing the breadth of a job is being addressed, e.g. the health care practitioner pioneered by Kingston Hospital in the medical assessment unit, which extends nurse and therapist roles to become almost interchangeable with junior doctors, as is increasing the depth of a job, e.g. the roles of nurse and therapy consultants, and reallocating tasks within traditional hierarchies, e.g. changes in the respective roles of radiologists, radiographers and assistants.

Greater emphasis on teamworking, flexibility of qualifications and new roles all suggest the need for more multi-professional education. Post-qualifying, the trend to a multi-professional approach has been apparent for some years. Increasingly, there is a trend towards the same approach in pre-qualifying education, with significant integration taking place in places such as St George's Hospital Medical School/Kingston University and Southampton University. In England, there are moves towards a common learning experience for all pre-registration students, with a particular emphasis on communications skills, and common clinical placements as well as classroom activity. Although multi-professional education at pre-registration level is in its infancy, it is likely to grow significantly over the next decade.

A significant driver in maintaining and upgrading the skills of existing staff is the trend towards periodic registration or re-validation required by the statutory regulatory bodies. You will be aware that nurses, midwives and health visitors have a form of periodic registration that requires practitioners to demonstrate CPD through a portfolio, and the GMC is implementing a re-validation scheme for doctors. It is likely that the new Health Professions Council will explore similar requirements. The Department of Health is providing earmarked funding for CPD in the NHS in England and is actively considering a lifelong learning strategy for all members of the workforce, which will be linked to the NHS University. A CPD website is being launched in Wales to provide all staff with direct access to learning and other materials that will help them with their CPD.

Among the key skills gaps and shortages are:

- IT skills
- communication skills
- management skills
- work-based assessment/verification/clinical supervision skills
- in some health care professions, there is difficulty in recruiting academic/teaching staff and a need to upgrade the skills of those in the field
- there is a significant demand for counselling skills (and some complementary therapies) among conventional health care practitioners.

REFLECTION POINT

Do you feel that you need further development in any of the above areas? If you do, investigate whether further training and development is available within your trust.

OCCUPATIONAL STANDARDS AND S/NVQS

As stated above, it is the policy of the Department of Health to promote the use of occupational standards within the health sector. The National Assembly for Wales has similar objectives. This is not to say that S/NVQs will, or should, replace professional qualifications.

Historically, work on occupational standards in the health sector has concentrated on the non-professional workforce. By 1991, an integrated suite of standards and awards became available to health and care support workers. By 1997, a total of 31 S/NVQs had been developed from these standards. A complete revision of the standards and the awards structure was finalized in 1998. This reduced the number of S/NVQs to nine and introduced a number of improvements to language, clarity of definition and integration of units.

NOSs are competency frameworks encapsulating skills, knowledge and application of competent performance within an occupational setting, e.g. mental health. They are consensus statements of good practice produced in a modular format. They describe what an individual must be able to do across a defined range of activity, to what standard (performance criteria) and what underpinning knowledge is required. In future, their overall objectives are likely to be:

- to identify sections of the workforce where occupational mapping and functional analyses have not yet been commissioned
- to map further potential uses of occupational standards
- to promote to employers the wider use of occupational standards in their sector.

The current position with the NTO Healthwork UK (to become Skills for Health) is summarized in Table 15.1.

Table 15.1 Healthwork UK (to become Skills for Health) progress on occupational standards

Service areas and domains	Current status
Public health	2-year Department of Health contract in place with negotiations with other departments
	Faculty of Public Health and other key stakeholders support project
	1996/7 Education Act Regulatory Authorities funding for mapping
Mental health	Leading joint NTO work
	Link to Department of Health Mental Health National Service Framework Workforce Action Team in England
	1996/7 Education Act Regulatory Authorities funding for mapping
Drugs and alcohol	Leading joint NTO work
	Cabinet Office request
	1996/7 Education Act Regulatory Authorities funding for mapping
Complementary medicine	Homeopathy standards developed with Faculty support
	Shared strategy developed with Department of Health
	Application for funding to complete standards in reflexology and aromatherapy submitted to 1996/7 Education Act Regulatory Authorities funding for mapping
	Proposal for gaining future funding being considered by Healthwork UK Executive Board
Cancer	Department of Health contract to project manage development of standards for breast cancer screening services
	1996/7 Education Act Regulatory Authorities funding for mapping standards
	Support from College of Radiography
Support staff	1996/7 Education Act Regulatory Authorities funding for mapping
	Department of Health involvement in UK-wide steering group
Oral health	Qualifications being developed for dental nurses with contract from Department of Health
	Standards development for dental technicians with contract from Department of Health
	1996/7 Education Act Regulatory Authorities funding for mapping
	Support from professional bodies and General Dental Council
Elderly people	Working with TOPSS leading on standards development
Learning disabilities	Working with TOPSS leading on standards development

NTO = national training organization; TOPSS = Training Organization for the Personal Social Services.

RELEVANT COMPETENCIES

A number of the competencies ensure that the pre-registration student upholds the position that professional development and knowledge acquired through education and training are at the top of the agenda.

'Demonstrate a commitment to the need for CPD and personal supervision activities in order to enhance knowledge, skills, values and attitudes needed for safe and effective practice.'
'Demonstrate key skills.'

(UKCC 2001a).

The sub-component to the second competence listed, 'detail literacy, numeracy, information knowledge and management and problem solving', is particularly relevant.

SUMMARY

Education and training must be at the top of the agenda to ensure that risk management and how it is handled are the subject of regular training sessions.

CONCLUSION

This chapter ended with information about aspects of various educational developments in order to emphasize that CPD is integral to taking forward the harmonization of risk management into everyday work. You should now understand the role of effective clinical governance in managing risk positively, the importance of managing complaints and having in place a revitalized health and safety strategy. The 'decontamination chain' has been explained – which requires commitment from purchaser through to end-user, including having training and effective management processes in place. The safe management and secure handling of medicines are a key part of any risk management strategy.

The description of the role of the patient and patient partnership has also been explored, along with the management of abuse and violence. Consumer representation is now an essential part of regulatory bodies, such as the NMC, and other agencies, such as the National Patient Safety Agency.

It is appropriate to finish with the following statement:

'To fail to learn is unforgivable – Either we manage human error or human error will manage us.'

CHAPTER 16

WORKING WITHIN A HEALTH CARE TEAM

Nigel Northcott

INTRODUCTION

This chapter examines teamworking as a Nursing and Midwifery Council (NMC) requirement for nurse registration (NMC 2002a). It establishes the fundamental nature of health care to be a 'team sport', where individual excellence can and should occur, but in a setting that acknowledges and celebrates the contribution of the team. Teams, like leaders, are not born; they arise as a result of certain characteristics of the members and activities designed to bring their efforts together. The characteristics of effective teams are considered in this chapter along with issues that arise with teamwork. The extent of teamworking within health care is explored using a number of examples. Pointers are given to ways to help teams function and become established. An invitation is given to you to consider that indeed 'no man [sic] is an island unto himself', especially where health care is concerned. Health care occurs in a context that requires collaboration and co-operation – teamwork.

WHAT IS A TEAM?

The noted preacher John Donne stated, 'No man is an island, entire of itself' to illustrate our need for unity in spiritual and secular matters. We are inter-dependent individuals who have evolved to live and function in families, groups and teams. It may be that team game playing is an attempt to allow us to get back in touch with our primeval need to work and function collectively as 'hunter gatherers' who evolved 'in part' because they learnt to collaborate, or perhaps it is an obvious example of team-working which emphasizes the importance of co-operation and collaboration.

Reinertsen (1998) identifies that for some health care professionals training appears to hone their individual skills and leaves them feeling like a solo performer. But like for a Wimbledon tennis champion or prima ballerina, individual success is based upon the input and actions of others. Clemmer *et al.* (1998) assert that a single doctor may have difficulty preventing exacerbations in patients with chronic asthma; good results are much more likely if they work as part of an effective team or well managed organization. The white paper *Caring for People* emphasizes, '... no single professional discipline can encompass the whole picture' (DoH 1989c).

REFLECTION POINT

Clemmer *et al.* (1998) suggest, 'More often than not, a balanced team that passes well will beat an equally talented team full of players who hog the ball'. Are you in a team of ball huggers? Are there some individuals in the teams you work in that hog the ball? Are you in a team that passes well and is balanced?

It is recognized that some health care staff will need, and will have, refined personal skills that will enable them to rise to the top of their profession. Professional staff, such as nurse consultants, clinical nurse specialists and even 'modern matrons', will, however, need the co-operation of many other staff to enable them to do their work. Reinertsen (1998), in comparing doctors to all-star athletes, emphasizes that they do not all make the transition to becoming a 'player-coach' from their training as a solo performer. We are never an island entire of itself; we live and work in social groups that are more or less formed into teams.

Large numbers of staff are employed in the NHS and many of these staff identify that they work in a team, or as is often the case, in a number of teams. They recognize the other people that they work alongside and have established some form of relationship with those other staff. Whether these associations can be called teams and what are the key dimensions of teams is the subject of this chapter.

REFLECTION POINT

Can you recall playing hockey or football at school? Can you remember the frantic scene of all 20 youngsters chasing the ball with no sense of position or relationship? Only the goalkeepers stand in their allocated position and even they might wander up the field if they have too little action. You might also recall the sound of these games as each player tries to be heard; the shouting of advice and often criticism dominating the playing field. Did such games illustrate teamwork?

Alternatively you might have played netball. In netball, each player has a set position, you have to pass the ball from player to player, you cannot wander around the court as the players depend on each other for success.

Are you in teams that rush around chaotically with no sense of personal place or group direction? Do you understand your place in the scheme of care delivery? Do you work in a functioning team – or are you in what is more like an under 11s sports team?

Teams are different people with different skills working towards the same goal(s) or as Katzenbatch and Smith (1993) put it:

'A team is a small number of people with complementary skills who are committed to a common purpose.'

If we take the netball analogy further, we can identify that the effective team will not only have tall people that are good at scoring goals. These players will need defenders and attackers to feed them the ball if they are to score. Goal scorers would be no good as goalkeepers or defenders, where stopping others from scoring is most important. Attackers need to be able to run, catch and throw accurately, but have no need to be able to score goals; they are not allowed to! In netball, as in all teams, some skills overlap and are duplicated, others are unique to certain players or team members.

In a health care setting, e.g. an operating theatre, it is easy to see how many people make up the team and how important each person is. However, it is evident what their similarities and differences are. Their individual skills are of equal valuable to the team. Such a team needs:

- domestic/housekeeping staff – to ensure an hygienic environment
- engineers and maintenance staff – to ensure lighting, heating and ventilation
- sterile supply staff – to sterilize and prepare the equipment
- porters – to bring patients to and fro
- nurse – to care for patients throughout the operative experience
- surgeons – to perform the operations
- anaesthetists – to put patients to sleep and more importantly, wake them up!
- laundry staff – to provide clothing for staff in the theatre.

The list would probably stop at around 50 people for one operation. While some staff are multi-skilled and can do a number of tasks, each one has their own part to play in ensuring the success of the team.

FORMING A TEAM

Problems in teams

The fact that a number of professional and ancillary staff are required to work together within health care is no guarantee that a 'team' will emerge. Problematic areas for staff working within teams include:

- understanding the purpose of inter-professional working
- understanding the role of others
- professional rivalry and tribalism
- exclusion of the significance of others

- ownership of resources
- effective assessment (Mathias *et al.* 1997).

REFLECTION POINT

Think of teams that you work within and or belong to, past or present, and consider the bullet points listed above. Which of the factors inhibited teamwork in your experience? Which of the factors were identified and managed to ensure an effective teamwork result?

The points identified by Mathias *et al.* (1997) offer insight into the workings of teams, and when explored carefully they reveal a number of issues.

Understanding the purpose of inter-professional working. The need to understand the purpose of inter-professional working reminds us that working in the same building or department as other staff, in itself, does not provide for teamworking. The need and purpose for the staff in any one team to work together needs to be explicit and understood by the members.

Understanding the role of others within a team. Implicit in the importance of appreciating what others do, is the need to understand your own role in the team. As in a netball team, all the 'players' need to know their role and how it interacts with the roles of others. Without this appreciation, confusion and poor performance will arise.

Professional rivalry and tribalism. The conflict and rivalry that exists among the different members of a team are often the cause of poor performance. In the netball team the attackers are quick to blame the defenders if the result goes against them and vice versa. The different professional staff in a team may feel their role is paramount, failing to realize it is the collective efforts of all the players that brings about results. Instead of emphasizing the differences between staff as a means to separate them, it will be more fruitful to celebrate the differences and unite on the common ground.

Exclusion of the significance of others. How often do some members of the team forget the input of others, who may be less qualified or of lesser status, yet are just as important to the team's performance?

Ownership of resources. Given our cash-limited health service, resources will be scarce and will need to be used wisely. Unfortunately, history has favoured some professional groups over others, and resource allocation is not always equitable. This has been the source of much health care inter-professional and inter-team rivalry. In his book on sociological aspects of decision-making in hospitals, Chabliss (1996) identifies the higher status and economic authority of doctors compared to nurses and indeed patients. For many years medicine has been the 'gatekeeper' to resources and services within the health care and many services can still only be accessed by medical authorization.

Effective assessment. Having the evidence about the effectiveness – or not – of the organization and its activities is essential to good teamwork. Unless all the evidence and information about a problem is collated and analysed together, the chances of prescribing an effective plan of action to resolve it diminish. Single pieces of information, or a single profession's perspectives on health issues, rarely provide an appropriate or accurate basis for diagnosis and treatment.

Collaboration and co-operation

Returning to Mathias *et al.*'s (1997) point about tribalism, we recognize the importance of Berwick's (1996) modernization message for the NHS; working collaboratively and co-operatively against a common enemy, disease – not each other. For years an intriguing academic game, prisoners' dilemma, has been played to illustrate collaboration and co-operation (Box 16.1). In the game, as in life and work, collaboration and co-operation lead to the best all round results.

Box 16.1 Prisoners' dilemma

Each player or team of players is invited either to co-operate or defect over a series of games with the object being to achieve the highest possible score over the series. Each player or team is invited secretly to choose the letter A (to co-operate) or B (to defect). The choices are made public simultaneously and are scored as follows:

- if both players choose to co-operate they both score 3
- if one player defects and their opponent does not, they score 4 and 1, respectively
- if both players defect they both score 2.

Over a series of games it is usual for co-operation to be chosen at the outset and for a number of turns thereafter, until one team or individual risks defection. If their opponent stays with co-operation they gain a 4/1 advantage. Subsequent rounds become less predictable as opponents try and outwit each other to score 4/1 but avoid 1/4 or 2/2.

Eventually opponents 'learn' that co-operation, which gains a 3/3 score, is the better option for both parties.

Phases in team development

Are the staff who work together a team? The answer to this question will depend upon their ability to establish a number of key characteristics, and even if they do, Tuckman (1965) suggests they will need to pass through a number of stages before they become fully functional. The forming, storming, norming and performing stages that he describes are widely promoted as keys phases in team development.

- *Forming* is the first stage and is characterized by uncertainty about purpose, structure and leadership. Members feel their way and only when they start to think of themselves as part of a team/group do they move on into the next phase.
- *Storming* involves inter-group conflict; having accepted themselves as part of a group, issues like control become paramount.
- *Norming* allows cohesion to arise out of conflict and group identity and values to replace individual thinking.
- *Performing* occurs when each member knows their place, and achieving group tasks becomes more important than the dynamics of the team.

SUMMARY

- Teams are more than a number of people gathered together.
- Teams need 'players' with different skills.
- People working together are not intrinsically a team, nor are they necessarily successful.

TEAMS IN HEALTH CARE

The illustration of an operating theatre, mentioned above, indicates the size and complexity of teams that work in health care. Such a team is a large number of people pulling together towards a common goal.

Consider your current work situation. How many teams do you work within? How many different professions and individuals are involved?

If your current work situation is within a hospital ward, you might recognize a number of staff as part of the multi-professional team. In an acute psychiatric ward these might include:

- relatives
- psychiatrists
- medical students
- psychologists
- nurses
- physiotherapists
- occupational therapists
- volunteers
- clinical nurse specialists
- nursing students
- health care assistants
- music therapists
- pharmacists
- chaplains.

In a community setting these might include:

- relatives
- neighbours
- health visitors
- community nurses
- community pharmacist
- voluntary groups
- social services
- social care staffing agencies
- religious organizations
- GP.

Not all the staff will be actively involved in the care of patients all the time, but they are members of the multi-professional team who together care for the patients. Each profession makes an individual contribution to a common goal.

REFLECTION POINT

Identify the multi–professional team that you work within. Do you work in any other teams at the same time?

You have probably identified a number of additional teams, e.g.:

- the team of nurses in your ward/department/faculty
- the whole hospital/trust nursing team
- the team of nurses you work with.

In many health care settings 'team nursing' is practised (Waters 1985). You may have experience of being a member of a nursing team while on a placement. These are often named after colours, such as the red team, and are responsible for the care of a group of patients. Team nursing arose in the 1980s as a way of ensuring more holistic care. Before this much nursing care was based on 'task allocation'; each nurse would be given tasks to perform depending upon their experience and ability. Junior nurses might spend a whole shift washing patients and making beds. Their more senior colleagues would do dressings and administer medications. Arranging discharges was left to the most senior nurses.

Team nursing includes patient allocation and promotes 'total patient care'; the same nurses doing all the care for a number of patients. This gives more continuity to patient care and increases job satisfaction for nurses. It also became popular because, to ensure work is allocated to nurses according to their ability, it places together a group of nurses with different levels of ability. Between them, they care for their group of patients, with the more senior nurses supervising their less experienced colleagues.

Beyond this is the team of nurses who work on a single ward or department. These nurses will be a team under the leadership of the ward manager, ward sister/charge nurse or similarly titled nurse. This team will provide the care for patients across the whole managerial area. There is also the team of nurses that exists within a hospital or trust. It might be argued that at this level the nurses are no longer actually a team. Indeed it would certainly be stretching the point of teamwork to suggest that all nurses in the country are in a team. The key dimensions of a team are explained later in this chapter.

CODE OF PROFESSIONAL CONDUCT

Section 4 of the *Code of professional conduct* (NMC 2002a) sets out the responsibilities for a registered nurse, midwife or health visitor with regards to teamwork.

'As a registered nurse or midwife, you must co-operate with others in the team.'

(NMC 2002a, p6)

- Section 4.1 confirms the extent of the team and in particular that the patient/client and their family should be included together with members from across the health, voluntary and social care sectors
- Section 4.2 emphasizes respectful co-operation within teams
- Sections 4.3 and 4.4 indicate the vital importance of communications within teams
- Sections 4.5 and 4.6 confirm that individual roles within the team carry individual accountability and this includes accountability to develop skills in others and avoid inappropriate delegation
- Section 4.7, requiring co-operation in investigations, reminds us of the larger organizational teams that we may also be part of.

SUMMARY

We all operate in a number of teams at the same time. Teams have a specific focus and can be made up of very different individuals.

EFFECTIVE TEAMS

Over the past 20 years the author has helped a number of groups of health care staff work effectively as a team. During this time a number of theoretical perspectives have proven useful to help their understanding. However, most striking have been the views of many of these teams on the key characteristics of a team. To examine the views that teams have on their underlying foundations, the author invites them to undertake the following exercise.

EXERCISE

Your team/group has been marooned on a desert island. It is hospitable; plenty of fruit and nuts to eat, fresh water and a climate that rarely exceeds 22°C or drops below 15°C. A ship may pass the island in 2 months time, but escape by other means is impractical, given the currents in the sea. Agree six rules/principles/structures that you will live by, to ensure a harmonious and productive existence on the island. What six would you suggest?

The six that have emerged most often from groups of staff are:

- agreeing on the need for *leadership*
- establishing *group goals* – direction/vision
- identifying effective *communications* strategies
- agreeing to show *respect* – for each other, themselves and resources
- having *clear roles* for each member – according to skills and allowing for learning
- sustaining group and individual *morale* – optimism and humour.

Each of these six points is fundamental to a successful team. Indeed, it is the establishment of these characteristics that makes a group of people who work together, move on to become the more effective unit of work, a team.

REFLECTION POINT

Think of a team that you work within, or have worked within, and decide to what extent these six points exist or existed within that team.

LEADERSHIP

REFLECTION POINT

Note the term leadership has been used in preference to a leader. Why do you think this is so? What ideally do you want from a leader/leadership?

Groups of staff usually realize the importance of having someone to co-ordinate the efforts of the team, but often shy away from suggesting 'a leader'. Groups who do not suggest leadership or a leader often state it is because their experience of leadership is less than satisfactory. Many groups suggest a co-ordinator, facilitator or even rotating leadership among them, rather than a leader. The suggestion of rotation is closer to the best choice than groups often realize. Rotation, however, to them often means taking turns. The type of rotation that offers a highly effective method of leadership is to place the best person in charge for the task in hand.

White and Lippitt's (1960) ideas have shaped thinking about leadership for many years. Their three leadership styles, which are often immediately recognized, are cited by groups as a reason not to offer leadership/a leader as one of their structures or principles:

- autocratic – bossy, highly productive only when present
- democratic – tries to please all, may please none, time lost in the process
- laissez faire – gets little done and does not care!

The autocratic or authoritarian leader is effective when present, but rules by fear. Performance drops off when they are off-duty. This approach is recognized as valuable in emergencies when no one objects to strong command, e.g. during a cardiac arrest. The democratic leader is less effective than the autocratic one, but the work rate is sustained in their absence. This approach makes all the staff feel valued, but often is so concerned with making sure everyone is represented, that indecision and lack of direction can occur. The laissez faire leader has little impact on performance or direction and will frequently be usurped by strong team members. The lack of direction and support leave staff confused and undervalued and little is achieved.

The notion of a benevolent dictator, with processes that are democratic but a clear sense of the desired product, was raised by Vaughan and Pilmoor (1989); it is like the 'transformative leader' described by MacGregor Burns (1978). Transformational leadership offers a number of features:

- develop a shared vision
- inspiration and communication
- valuing others
- challenge and stimulation
- development of trust
- enabling others.

Manthey (1994), the vision behind the Leading in Empowering Organization's (LEO) programme of leadership training, established in 2000, for nurses in the UK, offers a view of all four styles of leadership (Figure 16.1). This indicates the optimum style of leadership or leader as one that is focused on the goals and supporting the team, a style advocated by many, but practised by few! Senge (1990) suggests that an effective leader offers vision with nurturing. While keeping sight of the goals and direction, Senge (1990) advocates bringing the team with you and selling your ideas to them. By being mindful of the team members, ensuring they help shape the direction, they are groomed to become leaders themselves.

REFLECTION POINT

Have you experienced leadership or a leader that is inspirational and visionary, and supportive and nurturing of the 'followers'?

Overall a team needs a leader to co-ordinate the effort, and one who is prepared to stand back and allow leadership from another member who is better equipped to focus the team on a particular issue

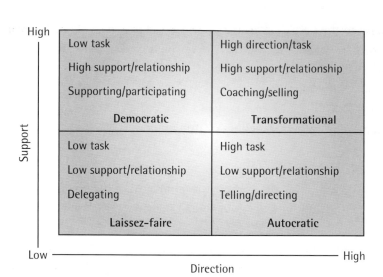

Figure 16.1 Leadership grid (Manthey 1994; Hersey *et al.* 1996)

or need. Preferably, the leader will combine the needs of the team members with achieving the collective goals.

GOALS

The Duke of Plazatoro, in Gilbert and Sullivan's Gondoliers, had a clear sense of where he was going:

> 'In enterprise of marshal kind when there was any fighting, he led his regiment from behind. He found it less exciting! But when away his regiment ran his place was at the fore oh!'

Where a team is going – or at least aiming for – is essential if the members are to pull together. On the desert island (see above), groups often suggest building a shelter, storing food and allocating activities, which all help the group identify its purpose. Some groups suggest that they should explore collective goals and, occasionally, phrases, such as 'What are we aiming to achieve?' or 'What would be a successful outcome of the experience?', are raised. Without a clear sense of purpose, goals or outcomes, any team will flounder, and as identified earlier, one of the key purposes of leadership is to establish direction for the team.

EXERCISE

On the desert island, what happens if one member decides they would rather stay, another feels so claustrophobic they have to try and escape, and the others wait for the ship?

You can imagine the difficulties that arise among six or seven people if one refuses to build the shelter and concentrates on building a raft. Another sees no point in building a fire to attract attention; indeed, they might even sabotage this for fear any rescue party insists they leave. Another member sees no point in any discipline; in the 2 months before the ship arrives, they want to do as they wish and have a good time. Without agreed goals and direction, the group on the island remains one made up of individuals and not a team. In teamwork the needs of the team must take preference over the needs of the individuals. While individual goals are valued and may help shape the team goals, they must remain less important.

Many groups doing the 'desert island' activity discuss goals and some suggest these should be SMART goals (Armstrong 1994):

- stretching (or as others have suggested, specific)
- measurable
- agreed
- realistic
- time related.

These five dimensions create goals that all team members can focus upon and from which they recognize that the whole is greater than the sum of the parts. Their being measurable allows the team to monitor progress, and being agreed recognizes and accommodates the input of all the team members. Realistic offers the team challenges that are stretching but will not lead to disappointment if they are out of reach. Time-related suggests the goals are those that need addressing at this time and that a timeframe for achievement should be agreed.

The seven players in a netball team may all be good players in their own right, but by coming together as a team and working collectively towards specified goals, they achieve better results than the sum of their parts. It is worth considering again that a team is a small number of people with complementary skills who are committed to a common purpose (Katzenbatch and Smith 1993).

COMMUNICATIONS

How common purpose is reached and sustained is the third dimension of effective teams – communication. Most groups suggest that on the desert island (see above), regular meetings to co-ordinate the activities will be essential. These meetings will be used to allocate work, monitor group members' well-being, keep track of resources and help maintain morale. It is interesting, as a facilitator, to ask groups doing the 'desert island' activity whether they have regular meetings at work, and if so whether they are effective.

REFLECTION POINT

Think of a work situation that you have been in recently, or are in, and describe how effective communications were/are. Do you know the team goals? How frequently were/are meetings held? How well do you know what is going on?

If leadership is truly product- and process-orientated, communications will be paramount as a means of establishing the direction for the team, and for monitoring success in reaching the vision/goals. Communications will also allow for the well-being of the team to be monitored. Figure 16.2 (Adler 1996) offers a model for communications; this indicates the complexity of the activity and emphasizes that communications is a two-way process. Indeed, communications should be measured by response and not by output. Whether it takes the form of a written message or instruction, a verbal request or a facial expression, the sender must check the response of the receiver(s), and not assume that it has been received.

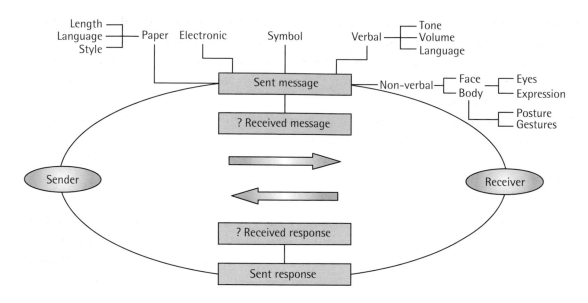

Figure 16.2 Model for communications (Adler 1996)

Within teams the efforts of the members are co-ordinated and combined to achieve agreed goals; this requires sensitive and accurate communication, especially if each members is to know what is expected of them.

ROLES

Identification of the role that each person should undertake on the 'desert island' is often accompanied by suggestions of rotation of some roles and tasks, to ensure no one person always does unpleasant tasks. This approach is highly commendable but may be unrealistic.

REFLECTION POINT
How should the roles within a team be allocated?

If you introduce a rota system, it will ensure fair allocation of work, but will result in less than satisfactory performance if individuals are allocated to work that they are unable to undertake. Imagine an operating theatre where all the roles are allocated on a daily basis; an anaesthetist on one day, technician the next, porter the next! In the definition of teamwork used at the start of this chapter, Katzenbatch and Smith (1993) identified 'complementary skills', which suggests that team members may not all possess the same skills. Belbin (1997) has, over a number of years, developed ideas about the roles that are required in effective teams. His research strongly supports the idea that teams are made up of different people with common goals:

- *co-ordinator* – a confident and trusting individual who seeks to ensure all members can contribute, while remaining in overall control. The co-ordinator (leader) encourages decision-making, monitors effectiveness and holds the team together. This cohesion is achieved by recognizing the abilities of others
- *shaper* – an energetic individual who seeks solutions, if necessary by pressurizing others. Shapers focus on goals, but tend to be rather volatile and easily frustrated

- *plant* – creative and imaginative and with unorthodox ways of working and solution finding. Plants are not always good with people, but are excellent with brainstorming ideas
- *resource-investigator* – who communicates extremely well; networking and developing contacts to help solve problems. They need new challenges to keep them interested, but with these, will be enthusiastic and resourceful
- *monitor-evaluator* – who is more interested in rationality than feelings, but will carefully analyse options and offer well thought through solutions
- *teamworker* – who is sociable and helps the team members to gel and work together. Teamworkers are not in themselves particularly effective at creating solutions, but work tirelessly to encourage the team to succeed
- *implementers* – who are highly practical and like moving ideas into actions. A reliable member, who may seem somewhat inflexible, but brings a disciplined approach to getting to the answer
- *completer* – who is a stickler for detail and will ensure the finished product is the best the team can offer. May be rather anxious about getting solutions, but will thoroughly review work to ensue quality
- *specialist* – who has little breadth but makes up for this by offering specific knowledge and skills with single minded determination.

REFLECTION POINT
What role do you contribute to teams? Does the role vary according to which team it is?

Belbin recognizes this list provides a tall order if you are working with an established team. It is not easy or appropriate to 'remove' people to bring in the right 'Belbin' character. However, this should not stop a team leader and the members from examining the list to ensure new staff complement existing staff and to develop the range of skills Belbin's research identifies. If nothing else, Belbin reminds us that members of teams are not all skilled at the same thing and we should therefore not rotate roles without careful thought. Many staff can multi-skill and undertake a variety of activities, but this does not suggest all staff and all activities are fully exchangeable. In the netball team, the 'shooter' would do badly if rotated to the wing or to defence. Their catching and shooting skills having little use in areas where running and stopping others from attacking are required.

However, roles should not be seen as static and staff should be offered regular opportunities to review their performance through appraisal schemes and their personal development plan (see Chapter 18). The leadership role that nurtures the team members places great importance on helping them to develop new skills. However, the goals of such schemes should be carefully negotiated to ensure they meet individual and team goals, and provide the support required to help achieve the goals provided by the leader.

RESPECT

Most groups on the 'desert island' recognize the need for respecting privacy and land use; and many allocate toilet areas. Not all extend this respect to areas such as:

- respect for resources – using resources carefully to avoid waste
- respect for each other – having regard for the rights of all other members
- respect for the leadership – and being loyal to the agreed goals of the team

- respect for differences in opinion
- respect for themselves.

REFLECTION POINT
Have you ever felt you were not respected in the workplace? Do you feel resources are respected where you work?

It is while discussing respect that many groups on the 'desert island' appreciate the inter-locking nature of the six structures. Respect for team goals, leadership and each other's roles will allow the 'small number of people with complementary skills to achieve a common purpose' (Katzenbatch and Smith 1993), that is teamwork. Without this respect the satisfaction and achievements of the team will be diminished.

MORALE

For about 15 years the teams I have worked with have offered and accepted five structures and processes essential to effective teams. In the past year, however, the author has introduced/accepted the importance of morale. The author senses this is in part a result of the increasing demands within the NHS to be more efficient and effective, but also reflects changes in society. The author senses the 'get on with it' attitude that arose post-war influenced health care considerably and staff had little awareness of individual rights.

The past few years have seen growing awareness of rights and a more collaborative and open society in which reasoning has replaced orders. Changes in the status of women, recognition of individual rights and consumerism have led to a need to ensure the morale and well-being of all staff are respected. Teams in the 21st century are increasingly driven by collective purpose, mutual regard and respect, and less by authority. Many teams identify the importance of humour and enjoyment in the workplace.

REFLECTION POINT
What is it like where you work? What is the morale like? Is there a sense of enjoyment as well as achievement?

HABITS OF EFFECTIVE TEAMS

Covey (1989) describes three levels of maturity that can equally apply to teams as to individuals:

- dependency: you – you care for me, I can blame you
- independence: I – I can do it, I am to blame, I can choose
- Interdependence: we – we can do it, we can combine and create.

To achieve the third level of maturity, individuals must function collaboratively and collectively within 'teams'. Covey (1989) offers seven habits as tools to move along the personal maturity scale. The first three are of character and the remaining four of personality and behaviour:

- habit 1 – between stimulus and response there is choice – responsibility! Seek to create, choose and initiate. Learn to be proactive

- habit 2 – create a vision, have personal and organizational mission statements; have leadership of self and the organization
- habit 3 – prioritize, manage time and delegate. Identify importance and urgency, allocate time accordingly
- habit 4 – seek solutions that are win-win, or 'no-deal' – agree to disagree agreeably
- habit 5 – listen and understand, before seeking or expecting a hearing
- habit 6 – seek solutions by combining resources and collaborating and co-operating
- habit 7 – gain personal renewal by physical, mental, social/emotional and spiritual means.

These seven habits offer a very similar picture to the one that has emerged in groups completing the 'desert island' exercise.

WORKING IN TEAMS: CONFLICT RESOLUTION

REFLECTION POINT
How do you resolve conflict? In your experience what is the most common means of resolving conflict?

Combining the resources and characters of a number of individuals into a team is not without its difficulties and at times conflict and tensions may arise. Tradition has it that conflict is bad and something to be avoided, and that good mangers resolve conflict. Current thinking is that conflict is natural and if managed skilfully can have a positive impact on work and performance. Thomas (1976) suggested that conflict is held in balance by two opposing factors:

- satisfying self (assertiveness)
- satisfying others (co-operation).

These two dimensions will be brought close together when individuals function within a team. They are displayed graphically in Figure 16.3 and there are five possible outcomes for conflict.

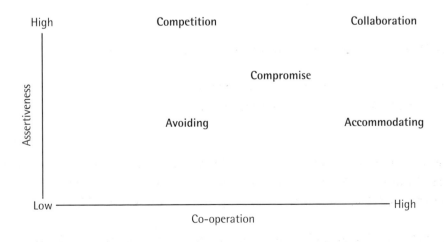

Figure 16.3 Conflict outcomes: assertiveness and co-operation (Thomas 1976)

Avoidance

Avoidance is the most frequent response to conflict. Both parties withdraw from the conflict by suppressing their position, allowing the conflict to simmer just below the surface. Short-term this option causes the least demand for both parties, but long-term the most difficulties.

Competition

Competition is the 'win–lose' option and, like the choice in prisoner's dilemma to defect (Box 16.1), results in success for one party at the expense of the other. This action gives rise to resentment because the losing party will feel they have been imposed upon and violated by the other. It may solve the immediate conflict but not without longer-term impact.

Accommodation

Like competition, accommodation is a 'win–lose' option, where one party gives way to the other. The 'self sacrifice' of the less assertive member will be at a cost. Indeed, giving way may even be manipulative, 'they gave way then, so later it will be my turn'; or the less assertive member may adopt a victim mode and foster resentment for the 'winning' member.

Compromise

Compromise is often offered as the best option for conflict resolution. It is often the quickest, but is very much half win/half lose. Each side, by giving way, has helped resolve the conflict, but has not been able to assert its preferred solution, so no side fully wins.

Collaboration

This is the 'win–win' option that is achieved by offering alternative solutions until one that suits both parties is identified. In this way no resentment is created and the parties may learn the possibility of mutual conflict resolution.

While collaboration is the best option, the option to agree to disagree agreeably is also a collaborative means to resolve conflict. Given that teams are made up of different people, a degree of conflict is inevitable – the means to resolve it, however, are not. Johns (1992) offered insight into the façade of the team with no conflict. The 'harmonious team' that denies conflict and presents a picture of complete togetherness, fails to appreciate the reality of conflict and the need to resolve it constructively.

CULTURE

Conflict resolution does not occur in a vacuum; the social context and culture will be highly influential. Hawkins and Shohet (1989) identify five distinct cultures that may operate and play a major role in the success of a team and its effectiveness in the workplace. These five cultures offer very different ways of working:

- personal pathology
- bureaucratic culture

- watch your back culture
- reactive/crisis culture
- learning/development culture.

REFLECTION POINT

From the titles offered for the five types of culture, can you identify the culture where you work?

The five cultures do not exist in pure form; many organizations and teams have a combination of several of them.

Personal pathology

In this culture assumptions are made about the need to coerce staff to perform, and sanctions are used to help coerce, control and motivate staff. Scapegoats are identified if things go wrong and blame is attributed to individuals. This culture uses external rewards, such as money, and fails to recognize that the success of the team will reward the members.

Bureaucratic culture

The clearly laid down rules, regulations and lists of procedures of a bureaucracy inhibit the performance of team members by prescribing how and when work should be undertaken. This can strip them of their individuality and diminish the benefits, clearly recognized by Belbin (1997), of bringing different people together. This culture is dominated by rules, which in more constructive organizations will be replaced by reasons and guidelines.

Watch your back culture

This functions by 'showing up' other teams or individuals who are failing in an arena of competition. It is a culture where sharpening the competitive edge exists, rather than genuinely and broadly ensuring development, and is one where elitism arises.

Reactive/crisis culture

This is a problem-solving culture where attention focuses on immediate problems with no concern for development or visionary activities. This culture operates in many busy teams, especially if the leadership is autocratic.

Learning/development culture

This culture best illustrates the effective team and is one where growth, development and learning are all central. The notion of the 'learning company' (Pedlar *et al.* 1991) is a clear example of this culture, which has the following features:

- learning is seen as a lifelong activity for all staff
- all work situations may potentially create learning opportunities

- problems are learning opportunities
- good practices arise from exploring learning cycles
- feedback exists at all levels and is ongoing
- time is an expected dimension of change
- regular review and evaluation are part of the individual and organizational activity.

TEAMBUILDING

'The shared aims of a team are obviously important but do not occur by spontaneous generation. They need to be hammered out, discussed and debated and by joint agreement put into practice.'

(Calman 1994)

REFLECTION POINT

At this point you may wish to summarize your learning by listing the main features of a well functioning, effective team.

To foster teambuilding, McGregor (1960) offered the following features:

- an informal relaxed atmosphere
- a lot of focused discussion in which all members participate
- a well understood task or objective that members are committed to
- every idea is listened to
- there is disagreement, but with resolution not domination – consensus decision-making
- criticism is frequent, frank and relatively comfortable; personal attacks are rare
- free expression exists
- action is promoted by clear assignment of tasks
- a leader does not dominate; the issue is not control but getting the job done.

The existence of teams within health care is not in doubt, their effectiveness, however, may be. Many staff fail to realize they are part of a team, and teams may not fully understand the issues and factors that influence teamworking.

Teambuilding recognizes that a state of perfection never exists and all staff and teams can enhance their performance and benefit from educational activities to enhance their interdependence. On occasions teambuilding is undertaken to rescue teams that have become dysfunctional or to assist new teams to establish effective working practices. It focuses on three dimensions:

- task review
- process review
- context review.

The task review allows the team to re-establish or create the direction, vision or goals that will enable the different members of the team to pull together and function inter-dependently. Within this review, the roles team members need to fulfil can be explored. Task review allows teams to focus on tasks that they are required, collectively, to achieve and as such the work is intellectual rather than emotional. The process review examines the ways of working – the communication strategies, the conflict resolution techniques and the respect shown. In this area the emotional dynamics of the team are explored and addressed and it is here that Tuckman's (1965) four stages of team development are most likely to be identified. The contextual review examines the culture, morale and relationship between group members.

Teambuilding often uses active learning with activities designed to allow staff to explore their performance in simulations that offer insight into their world of work. Given careful debriefing and analysis, activities such as the 'desert island' exercise can and have assisted teams to examine their ways of working, evaluate them and 'build' better strategies. Health care needs staff who can fly the plane solo in an emergency, but more often is best delivered by a team of individuals who complement each other and focus on the common goal of resolving the disease of the patient or client.

SUMMARY

Teams bring small numbers of individuals with complementary skills together to achieve a common purpose. Working in teams requires a number of supportive environmental factors, including culture and conflict resolution.

CONCLUSION

Teamworking is something that we have all done in social, educational, recreational and work settings, and have observed in many aspects of human endeavour. Effective teams win the world cup, win sporting success, succeed in business and provide effective health care. Teams do not happen; they require a number of key features and characteristics to build and sustain them. This chapter used a number of illustrations and your reflections to help you appreciate teamwork against the backdrop of the NMC requirements for registered nurses, midwives and health visitors.

CHAPTER 17

SUPPORTING PRACTITIONERS IN GIVING HIGH QUALITY CARE

John Fowler

INTRODUCTION

Supporting practitioners in giving high quality care is an important issue for all nurses ranging from the new student nurse to the experienced practitioner. The subject of support relates to all the Nursing and Midwifery Council (NMC) requirements for pre-registration nursing programmes (UKCC 2001a), but six of the competencies specifically identify the importance of supporting practitioners and the way that this influences the quality of patient care.

This chapter presents you with three approaches to providing support: mentorship, preceptorship and clinical supervision. At times it asks you to reflect upon your previous experience of giving or receiving support and to identify areas of good practice or issues of concern. At other times you will be introduced to new ideas based upon theories or current research. You will be encouraged to explore how these new ideas relate to your clinical practice. Finally, there are a number of scenarios that present you with real life situations to explore; you will be asked to identify the issues within the scenarios and suggest possible ways forward.

The six competencies (UKCC 2001a), as listed below under the following headings, that specifically identify the importance of supporting practitioners and the way that this influences the quality of patient care are:

- *professional and ethical practice*:
    - manage oneself, one's practice and that of others, in accordance with the NMC *Code of professional conduct (NMC 2002a)*, recognizing one's own abilities and limitations
- *care delivery*:
    - engage in, develop and disengage from therapeutic relationships through the use of appropriate communication and interpersonal skills
- *care management*:
    - contribute to public protection by creating and maintaining a safe environment of care through the use of quality assurance and risk management strategies
    - delegate duties to others, as appropriate, ensuring that they are supervised and monitored
- *Personal and professional development*:
    - demonstrate a commitment to the need for continuing professional development and personal supervision activities in order to enhance knowledge, skills, values and attitudes needed for safe and effective nursing practice
    - enhance the professional development and safe practice of others through peer support, leadership, supervision and teaching.

REFLECTING ON YOUR OWN EXPERIENCE OF GIVING AND BEING SUPPORTED

It is very easy for the experienced nurse to forget the feelings and emotions that they had as a new student nurse entering the clinical area for the first time; or as the new staff nurse being left in charge and given 'the keys'. For most nurses these situations contain a mixture of emotions: excitement, fear, embarrassment and pride. Having survived the experience the nurse can then look back with a sense of achievement and accomplishment. Success in one situation gives confidence for the next and, no matter how experienced we become, there will always be new and challenging experiences.

REFLECTION POINT

Take some time to think about the first time that you had any direct contact with a patient.

- When was it?
- How did you feel prior to the event?
- How did you feel during the contact?
- How did you feel afterwards?
- How did the more senior nurse who was looking after you support you?

Now ask the same questions to someone with a similar amount of experience as yourself and compare your experiences. Finally, ask the same questions of an experienced nurse – see if you can find someone who registered over 10 years ago, and compare their experiences with yours and those of your peers. Having done this, reflect on what has been said to you. What is common to peoples' experiences? What is valuable in terms of the support that was offered? What can you do in terms of supporting others as you become more experienced?

At this 'one-to-one' interactional level the support of staff focuses upon our interpersonal skills of empathy, communication, genuineness and often a sense of humour. These are crucially important and will form the underlying theme of much of this chapter. The support of staff, however, cannot be seen in isolation from the wider strategic issues that are involved in the delivery of health care. How could the senior nurse give time to the new student if the staffing levels are not adequate? Who is responsible for the student's nursing care? Being part of a team is, in itself, very supportive, but is teamwork something that just happens (see Chapter 16)? To help you answer these questions and examine the wider strategic issues, the English National Board for Nursing, Midwifery and Health Visiting (ENB) 10 key characteristics of professional development are used as a framework to explore these organizational issues.

10 KEY CHARACTERISTICS OF PROFESSIONAL DEVELOPMENT

The ENB (1990, 1991) identified 10 key characteristics for the development of professional practice. These were developed from a research study that identified a framework of professional development for registered practitioners. At that time they formed the central structure of the ENB Higher Award and, although the ENB and Higher Award no longer exist, the 10 key characteristics still form a core framework for practice development. The characteristics are:

- accountability
- clinical skills
- use of research
- teamwork
- innovation
- health promotion
- staff development
- resource management
- quality of care
- management of change.

REFLECTION POINT
What do these characteristics mean to you? How do you think that each of the 10 key characteristics relates to supporting registered practitioners in giving high quality care? Jot down a few ideas about each of the characteristics, then compare your ideas with those below.

Accountability

There needs to be clarity about who is responsible for what. This is particularly important for the registered nurse mentoring the student nurse. It is also relevant when registered staff are undergoing extended skill training or changing specialities. Who holds the authority for the action that is being undertaken? What degree of autonomy is there within the role? Who is responsible and accountable for the nursing care of the patient/client? These are legitimate questions when undertaking a new post or even within a span of duty.

Clinical skills

Clinical skills are usually a combination of psychomotor, cognitive and affective skills – what we do, why we do it and how we do it. It is important not to overwhelm the student with the volume or complexity of skills that they will ultimately be expected to master. However, it is also important to allow the student to participate and develop appropriate skills, under supervision. In terms of support, students will find it useful to know what they are expected to do, over what time frame and to what degree of expertise. This is where learning objectives, opportunities and outcomes can form a supportive framework, giving guidance and promoting understanding for the clinical team.

Use of research

Supporting staff is not a precise science, in which action 'A' plus action 'B' will inevitably result in 'C'. There is no simple formula for giving support that will work for all people in all situations. You will need to develop strategies that work for 'you', using evidence from a wide variety of sources. Several research-based principles are described later and the ENB 10 key characteristics are in themselves based on research undertaken with practitioners, managers, patients and a range of other stakeholders (ENB 1990). Use the principles discussed in this chapter, review some of the papers referenced and reflect upon your own experience to develop your own way of supporting staff. Ask for, and be accepting of, feedback from your students and be willing to change and adapt your ways of working based on new and evolving ideas.

Teamwork

Working with a group of people has the potential for being a supportive, enriching experience or conversely a negative and draining one. Teamwork is the essential difference. Any new member of staff entering into an established group will very soon experience and try to make sense of the dynamics within that group. Take a few minutes to reflect on a group of staff you work with. Is it a positive, supportive experience? One that welcomes newcomers for the skills, experience or questions that they bring? Or is it one that has different factions? Where one group does not talk to another? Where the social rules change depending on whom you are working with? Teamwork inevitably involves the multi-professional team and part of the responsibility of the senior members of the various disciplines is to develop positive teamwork within their own discipline and then between others (see also chapter 16).

Innovation

The provision of health care has changed, is changing and will continue to change. Certain illnesses that 10 years ago required a patient to undergo major surgery and remain hospitalized for 2 weeks are now treated by day surgery. Although the principles of care that remain at the heart of nursing remain unchanged, the ways of delivering nursing and health care are changing almost daily. Dealing positively with innovation as it affects you and your team will help others who work with you to respond in a similar way. Avoidance, negativity or denigration of new ideas will help create a spiral of decline for both you and those who work with you. A positive and enthusiastic approach, whatever your place within the team, will support and help others as they come to terms with new ideas. Enthusiasm is not the same as unquestioning acceptance of any new idea. Enthusiasm is about openness, energy and a willingness to explore. It is infectious and supportive.

Health promotion

The physical and psychological health of nursing staff can be viewed from both short- and long-term perspectives. In the short term, the senior officers have a responsibility to maintain a safe environment, provide support and training in areas such as moving and handling, safe handling of blood and waste products, and organizing debriefing following traumatic events. Longer-term support strategies may include the provision of coffee areas away from the immediate environment, a sports and social club, and a staff support and counselling service. At a more operational level, a number of teams could organize an occasional social event in which staff have a chance to meet and relate to one another in a fun way. Encouraging and supporting staff who have chosen to stop smoking, lose weight or take some exercise can often be done by personal encouragement and peer group support. A positive approach to the health care of staff will increase their health and well-being and should indirectly influence the health and well-being of patients.

Staff development

At a formal level, staff development is about identifying a person's learning needs, helping them to form a plan of action to meet those development needs, supporting them as they develop, and then ensuring that these skills and abilities are utilized accordingly. Support will involve motivating and encouraging but may also require the support of money and time, to gain appropriate clinical experience or attend suitable courses. At a more informal level, staff development is about taking an interest in what our colleagues are doing, drawing upon their experience and not resenting their development. When you are asked to give a talk or attend a meeting, then consider taking a more inexperienced nurse with you, or suggest to the person inviting you, that this other nurse would be a very suitable person and that you would support them in their preparation for the talk/meeting. So often we only send a replacement when we ourselves are either too busy or just do not want to go.

Resource management

Supporting staff takes time and money. In an outcome-driven health service with limited resources, both time and money need to be used efficiently and effectively. This means planning and management. Staff who are working longer hours and taking on extra shifts to cover for shortages will soon become demoralized and possibly ill if they feel that no one in authority knows, cares or is trying to do anything to counteract the staff shortage. Staff who feel that they will never get on a course, or gain promotion because their 'face does not fit', will also become demoralized and, if opportunity allows, will probably leave the job and possibly nursing. Resource management is not about having unlimited resources. It is about fighting for resources as well as the efficient, effective and fair management of what is available. Some managers use such resources as a means of controlling staff, when actually the correct use of such resources is in enabling staff to do the job for which they are employed.

Quality of care

If all grades of staff work in a positive, supportive atmosphere where reflection on clinical practice is encouraged, and issues of concern are voiced and discussed, then the result can only be an increase in the quality of patient care. Support that is superficial and tokenistic, either at a strategic or operational level, will suggest to staff that this is an appropriate standard to set, not only for support of others, but for other issues such as quality of care, health and safety, patient education and infection control.

Management of change

There can be few workplaces that have not undergone significant change in the past 5 years. People vary in their reactions to change, some welcoming it, others resisting or accepting the inevitable. Whatever people's reaction to change is, everyone will experience a drain on their physical and psychological energy. Supporting people prior, during and after the process of change is an important element in the management of change. Involvement, communication and ownership are important principles highlighting the way that individuals should be valued within the change process. If individuals feel valued, they will also feel supported.

SUMMARY

Supporting staff to give high quality care needs to be addressed at two levels. First, at the one-to-one interactional level focusing on communication, empathy and genuineness; and second, at a strategic level. The ENB 10 key characteristics are a useful way of exploring the strategic level.

HELPING PEOPLE LEARN FROM EXPERIENCE: EXPERIENTIAL LEARNING

Learning how to nurse has a number of parallels with learning how to swim. Unless you actually get in the water, you are not going to learn. However, if you jump in at the deep end on your first attempt you will probably swallow considerable amounts of water before, hopefully, scrabbling to the side and vowing never to go swimming again. Likewise, if your first experience in nursing was a placement on an intensive care unit, caring for a patient with gangrenous wounds or caring for an unpredictable aggressive patient, then the experience, if not putting you off nursing altogether, would be highly traumatic.

Having established that the student nurse is in the equivalent of their 'safe depth', there are two important principles in helping someone learn and develop nursing skills. First, they have to feel confident and safe in the clinical area, sure that even if they did get out of their depth, there would be a 'lifeguard' on the side to pull them to safety. Second, once they have mastered some of the elements of nursing, the doggy paddle equivalent, they then need to learn from people who are more experienced than themselves. Steinaker and Bell (1979) identified this form of learning – learning from experience – as experiential learning and developed a taxonomy of five levels (Box 17.1).

Box 17.1 Experiential learning taxonomy (Steinaker and Bell 1979)

- Exposure – observation, inactive participation
- Participation – actively engages in activities with supervision
- Identification – student performs skills competently with minimal supervision

- Internalization – student feels ownership of skill and is comfortable in its performance
- Dissemination – student can transfer the skill to other areas and wishes to convey the skill to others

Imagine yourself as a student nurse allocated to a new placement. Initially you will feel very new. You will be exposed to a number of new staff, patients, medical conditions and the layout of the ward or community placement. There will be new or different social etiquette, rules, policies and procedures. At this initial level the student takes on a largely inactive participation role, one of observer. As the student begins to feel more comfortable in this new environment then they will begin to participate and actively engage in the activities. At this level the student requires close supervision and support as they develop new skills, attitudes and behaviours. With time, practice and feedback the student moves to the third level in which they perform these new skills competently with minimal supervision. At the fourth level, the student takes ownership of the new skills, attitudes and behaviours. They will appear at ease and comfortable with this developing role. Finally, at the fifth level the student begins to apply and transfer these skills to new areas and begins to teach them to others. Thus, the swimmer goes from standing on the side observing others, to jumping in, getting to grips with the basics under close supervision, swimming within their own depth, swimming several lengths, and finally helping others and becoming an instructor and lifeguard.

REFLECTION POINT

Think about the above example and your own level of expertise; are you just learning to paddle or are you a strong swimmer?

Now put yourself in the position of the nurse's mentor. Is your role static as the student progresses or do you need to take on different roles as the student works through these different taxonomy levels?

RELATIONSHIP OF THE MENTOR/SUPERVISOR TO THE STUDENT

At the first level (Box 17.2), that of 'exposure', the mentor has to take on a motivating role: to encourage the student to take an interest in the clinical area, to see the rewards and pleasures of working with this client group and to make them feel safe. They need to encourage the student to jump in the water. At the second level of 'participation', the mentor acts as a catalyst, helping the student to take an active part, putting them in the right place at the right time, encouraging progress and praising the achievement of small targets. As the student develops competence in certain skills, the level of 'identification', the mentor needs to stand back, but at the same time maintain an adequate distance to safeguard the student and the client – they act as a moderator. As the student moves to the fourth level, 'internalization', the mentor takes on the role of sustainer, helping the student to maintain their interest. Finally, as the student enters the level of 'dissemination', the role of the mentor is to give feedback and advice – to act as an honest critic.

Box 17.2 Experiential learning taxonomy: mentor role and function (Steinaker and Bell 1979)

- Exposure – motivator: to encourage the student to gain an interest
- Participation – catalyst: to assist and encourage the student to take an active part
- Identification – moderator: to safeguard the student and client

- Internalization – sustainer: to help the student transfer the skill to other areas and re-motivate if necessary
- Dissemination – critic: to give feedback and advice

By analogy, those of you who are parents will have realized that the role and skills required to parent a baby are different from those required to parent a toddler and are totally different from those required for teenagers and young adults.

IMPLICATIONS

REFLECTION POINT

What are the implications of the theory of experiential learning to professional development, clinical practice, supporting staff and teaching and assessing?

The implications of the experiential learning taxonomy can be summarized as:

- the role of the mentor/teacher encompasses different function and these change over time
- some people may feel more competent with one function than another
- learning occurs over a time – it is a process
- the role of the student changes over time
- some students may be better at one stage of the process than others
- both student and teacher are equal, but with different roles.

REFLECTION POINT

Take some time to reflect on how the ideas contained within experiential learning relate to you.
- How do they relate to your experience of entering new clinical areas?
- How do they relate to you learning about a new clinical procedure?
- How do they relate to you as an existing or future mentor?
- How do they relate to your future professional development?
- How do they relate to the way you support staff?

EXERCISE

Think through the following scenarios – discuss them with a colleague. If you were the mentor, how would you deal with the following students?

Scenario Jane is an 18-year-old student nurse. She is on her first clinical placement, a busy medical ward, and you are her mentor. During an initial brief assessment of her learning needs you form an opinion of her as being very nervous, even frightened, and not really saying much. You have a busy morning in front of you, five quite dependent patients and two empty beds are likely to be filled by emergency admissions. Jane's placement is scheduled for 3 days a week for the next 6 weeks. She will be working with you for most, but not necessarily all, of this time.

You are busy and Jane is very nervous. How are you going to handle this first morning? How are you going to structure her 6-week placement? At this stage, what will you tell her you will be expecting from her, and what will you tell her she can expect from you?

Scenario Sally is 19 years old. She has previous experience as a health care assistant and this is her second clinical placement. Her first placement was in the community and now she is on a 6-week placement on a surgical ward. She works three shifts a week and you are her mentor. Following your initial meeting with Sally you have formed an opinion that she is a very confident person, keen to undertake as many dressings and drug administration rounds as she can. You are a little concerned that she appears over-confident for her length of experience and, while not wishing to dampen her enthusiasm, feel concerned that she does not appear to appreciate her limitations.

How are you going to handle this first morning – you are busy and Sally is very keen to take an active role? How are you going to structure her 6-week placement? At this stage, what will you tell her you will be expecting from her, and what will you tell her she can expect from you?

SUMMARY

People learn from practical experiences in a different way from how they learn from a textbook. Steinaker and Bell's (1979) experiential learning taxonomy is a helpful way of understanding how people learn from practical experiences.

TEACHING

In a small scale research study the author asked a number of staff what they found most valuable and most supportive from trained staff in terms of their teaching, mentoring and support (Fowler 1995). A considerable number of different examples were given which could be categorized into five main areas: assessment, negotiation, listening, explaining and feedback.

- *Assessment of the person's previous knowledge and experience.* This was seen as important because it not only acknowledged and valued the student's previous background, but it also allowed the mentor to build upon the previous knowledge.
- *Being willing to negotiate regarding the process and focus of supervision/teaching.* It was not 'the teacher knows best' attitude but the recognition that both the mentor and the student had a valuable perspective on what was required. The mentor could draw upon their experience of the learning opportunities relating to their clinical area, and the experiences of past students; the student could draw upon the knowledge of their own abilities and their strengths, needs and weaknesses.
- *Listening to what the student has to say about what they learn from a specific experience.* At its simplest, this can take the form of a question and answer session, being genuinely interested in what the student has done and learned, resisting the temptation to jump in and take over the conversation. The more advanced skills of listening will also enable the mentor to assist the student in reflecting upon clinical practice, and patient interactions, encouraging a deeper understanding of events.
- *Being able to explain ideas and knowledge in an easily understandable way.* Students valued both informal and formal teaching sessions but not if the session confused them or went over their heads. They valued someone who could explain ideas and facts to them in an easy to understand way.

● *Commenting on good practice, not just criticizing the weak areas.* Feedback is an important aspect of a nurse's professional development, particularly in relation to any specific learning outcomes. All the specialist practitioner qualifications require students to have a mentor/supervisor who is responsible for giving them feedback on their developing specialist skills. If done in a positive and supportive way, then feedback can be a powerful means of identifying strengths and weaknesses, and shaping and developing advanced nursing skills. The students in this study commented that it was the combination of commenting on their good practice as well as criticizing their weak areas that was important.

REFLECTION POINT

How do these above areas relate to your own experience?

A MODEL OF CLINICAL TEACHING

For the outsider, nursing structures which encompass management, leadership and support can appear complex and confusing.

EXERCISE

How do you answer the following relatively simple questions:

● Who is your manager?
● Who provides professional leadership?
● Who provides advice on clinical issues?
● Who do you turn to for career guidance?
● Who supervises your clinical practice?
● Who do you turn to for support following a difficult shift?

Ask these questions to four or five other nurses, ranging from a junior staff nurse to a senior nurse or clinical nurse specialist.

You will probably find that for the more junior nurse the 'ward sister', or the equivalent, combines most of those roles. However, as nurses become more experienced and specialized, no single person has the knowledge, skills, experience or authority to fulfil such roles. Here lies the somewhat confusing complexity of the management, leadership and support structures within nursing. There are a number of different ways that nurses are given support, guidance and teaching on a fairly routine basis:

● working with more experienced staff
● in-service training sessions
● staff handovers
● at coffee breaks
● debriefing following traumatic events
● clinical supervision
● preceptorship
● individual performance review
● mentoring

- reflection
- study days
- courses
- talking with friends.

This is not an exhaustive list. What other forms of support, guidance and teaching have you experienced?

What structure is there to all these differing support processes? How do they all relate to one another? The model in Figure 17.1 attempts to give some meaning to these various structures by identifying two continuums, 'task-centred' versus 'patient-centred' and 'planned' versus 'ad hoc'. Task-centred events are those that focus on a particular nursing procedure, a series of skills, an aspect of physiology or psychology or any fairly discrete body of knowledge. Patient-centred events are those that are generated by a particular patient or group of patients, e.g. a patient's medical condition, nursing problems, social environment or general management. Planned activities are those which are planned in advance and put in the diary. Ad hoc activities are those things that happen on the spur of the moment. They may be a response to a traumatic event or occur simply because the ward is quiet and there is time to do some teaching or sit down and discuss a particular patient. Using these two continuums we can begin to give some structure to the support and teaching processes that exist within the structure and management of nursing.

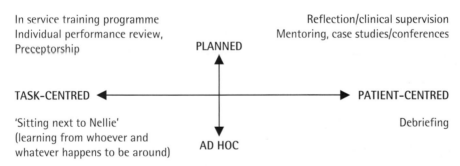

Figure 17.1 A model of clinical teaching

Thus, processes that are planned and task-centred are those such as in-service training programmes, individual performance reviews, preceptorship, moving and handling study days, asthma care study days and some post-registration courses. Activities that are planned but patient-centred are those such as clinical supervision, patient hand-overs and case studies, reflection and possibly mentoring, although this can be task-centred depending on the style adopted. Situations that are patient-centred but ad hoc usually focus on some form of emergency or traumatic event, following which staff take time to discuss what has happened and how it was handled, and the effects that it has had on staff – debriefing. Finally, there is the intersection of ad hoc and task-centred events. This is typified by the phrase 'sitting next to Nellie' – the belief that by working alongside a more experienced person we will pick up some useful tips and ways of working.

EXERCISE

Think through each of the four approaches above and identify the strengths and weaknesses of each one. Then compare your ideas with those in Table 17.1.

Table 17.1 A model to analyse clinical teaching

	Strength	Weakness
Planned and task-centred	Structured, allows important aspects to be highlighted, rules and guidelines can be clearly set, people generally feel comfortable with structure	The paperwork and completion of a list of learning outcomes can override the principle of what the structure was set up for
Planned and patient-centred	Patient care and associated nursing actions form the focus of development	Requires considerable skills from the supervisor/mentor to use patient-centred situations in a positive way
Ad hoc and task-centred	Tends to occur because all parties want it to; therefore, it is usually relevant and positive	Important aspects may not get covered and there maybe a lack of structure and depth to support or learning
Patient-centred and ad hoc	Relevant and immediate to the needs of the clinical area and of the staff	Requires considerable skill of the senior staff. Events that are not stressful in themselves, but may become so over time, are often overlooked

SUMMARY

Teaching in the clinical area can be planned and task-centred, planned and patient-centred, ad hoc and task-centred, or patient-centred and ad hoc.

MENTORSHIP

Although the idea of experienced nurses directing less experienced nurses in their clinical work has been in existence since the days of Florence Nightingale, the idea of a mentoring relationship is a far more recent concept, appearing in the nursing literature from about 1980 onwards (Darling 1984). Woodrow (1994) suggests that the nursing profession's sympathetic acceptance of a humanistic philosophy, in both its clinical practice and nurse education, has led to an embracing of partnership between learners and teachers, staff and patients.

The terms mentorship, preceptorship and clinical supervision have found their way into the everyday language of the clinical nurse (Burnard 1990; Maggs 1994). Some people appear to use them interchangeably, recognizing little or no difference between them. This is understandable, as they have a common theme regarding a nurturing relationship, usually between an experienced person and someone new to the situation. Mentorship is probably the most ambiguous term:

'Finding a definition of mentorship is not difficult. The problem lies in selecting one from the many available and widely contrasting definitions.'

(Earnshaw 1995, p274)

Nevertheless, mentoring is a frequently used term, both within and outside nursing. It is often used in everyday nursing conversation but appears to mean different things to different people. Many of the more substantive reviews of mentoring within the nursing profession make reference to the historical derivation of the term 'mentor' from Homer's Odyssey, in which Odysseus entrusts the upbringing of his son Telemachus to Mentor, a trusted advisor and friend (Donovan 1990; Earnshaw 1995). Mentoring within the business and professional world often utilizes a close relationship between an experienced and less experienced person to help them through a transitional period in their life, or more usually, their career. The relationship seems to vary from intense interpersonal experiences to formalized organizational programmes (May 1982; Hagerty 1986).

There are two distinctive ways in which the term mentoring is used within nursing in the UK: one concerned with student nurses and the other with registered nurses. The ENB (1989; 1993) gave the role of mentor prominence within nurse education by stipulating that each student nurse should have a mentor throughout the clinical placements of their training. It defined this as someone who would, by example, facilitate, guide and support the learner in the development of new skills, new behaviours and new attitudes (ENB 1993). Later, the ENB altered the focus regarding the supervision of students. The 'mentor' was to take on the full responsibility for the teaching, assessing and support of the student.

'The term mentor is used to denote the role of the nurse, midwife or health visitor who facilitates learning and supervises and assesses students in the practice setting. Different professional groups use differing terminology. The term assessor is often used to denote a role similar to that of the mentor as defined in this publication.'

(ENB/DoH 2001)

In 2002 the ENB ceased to exist; however, the role and function of the mentor as defined above continues to be the standard for student supervision.

For most nurse training curricula, the mentor is a clinically-based nurse, who mentors the student for the time that they are learning in their clinical area, normally 4–12 weeks. This means that the student will have a number of different mentors throughout their pre-registration period – one for each clinical placement and 10–15 throughout their 3 years of preparation. There are only rare examples where the same mentor is attached to a pre-registration student for all or most of their training (Morris *et al.* 1988).

As well as the specific use of mentoring for student nurses, the term is also used for a more general relationship between registered nurses in the UK (Burnard 1990; Maggs 1994; Butterworth 1998). Here, the term is not well defined and tends to have a wide usage. It ranges from a committed and intense relationship, focusing on personal and professional development of the mentee, to a general pairing of a new staff member with a more experienced one, for induction and orientation to a new area. Thus, the term 'mentor' may be used to describe any of the following:

- the supporting and facilitating relationship between a student nurse and a registered nurse
- a long-term, nurturing and professional development relationship between senior and less experienced registered staff
- someone who shows you where to hang up your coat and takes you to coffee on your first day.

REFLECTION POINT

Think back through your experience, both before and during your nursing career, and identify people who have acted as a mentor to you. Was this a formal system as occurs in some schools and colleges – sometimes called a buddy or pairing system, or was there someone 'older and wiser' who seemed to have time for you, someone who you respected? What was that relationship like? What did you get out of that relationship? What do you think the other person got out of it?

Mentoring relationships occur in all walks of life, sometimes spontaneously but at other times they are planned and organized. The nursing profession, like many other professional and business organizations, recognizes the potential benefits that such a relationship offers, both to the members and the organization. However, trying to capture and replicate the richness of that relationship to make it available for all staff has proved difficult.

Scenario Joan, aged 32, has been a staff nurse for 5 years on the same ward. One year ago you were appointed as the nurse in charge of that ward. You are a similar age to Joan but have greater clinical experience. Having worked with Joan for the last year you have developed respect for her experience in this speciality but feel she is not really achieving her potential. She does her clinical work well but never seems to volunteer for anything new and seems to avoid teaching students and new staff. She appears to be someone who would benefit from a positive, nurturing relationship with someone more experienced – a mentoring relationship.

You make a list of the various staff who you consider may be appropriate mentors (see below). Think through each of the people listed and identify the strengths and weakness of using each one, based upon the information given. Having done that, decide who to approach to act as Joan's mentor. Finally, think through how you are going to set up this mentoring relationship and identify some key steps that you will need to make.

- You – You are the ward manager and have wider clinical experience; you know Joan's strengths and where she needs to develop, and feel that you have a good working relationship
- Staff nurse Jenny Smith, aged 39. She has been on the ward for 10 years and is a very capable staff nurse. She works part-time, has two young children and a very mature outlook on life. She is a supportive person and a good friend of Joan's
- July Brown, a clinical nurse specialist, aged 42. She frequently comes to the ward to give advice on patient care and holds a number of informal teaching sessions with staff. She is well respected by staff and will always give advice when asked
- Susan Peters, a professional development officer for the trust. She is 45 years old and has a previous clinical background in your specialty. She runs a 2-day counselling course for the trust and has a reputation for being a caring Personal study
- Sally Walters, a ward manager within the same directorate. She is the same age as you and has been a personal friend of yours for a number of years. You know that she would be very happy to take on this role as a mentor for Joan.

SUMMARY

The term mentorship is used and defined in different ways: in the business world, as a one-to-one relationship during a transitional period; for student nurses, as the person who is responsible for the teaching, supervision and assessment of the student while on a clinical placement; and as a general supportive relationship for any member of staff.

PRECEPTORSHIP

Preceptorship is similar to mentoring. In the US, the term is used to describe the support, teaching and direction that student nurses receive while on clinical placement. This includes developing a learning contract (Andrusyszyn and Maltby 1993), teaching (Williams *et al.* 1993), clinical socialization (Ouellet 1993; Dibert and Goldenberg 1995), developing clinical competence and confidence (Myrick and Barrett 1994). In addition, it is used to describe a general orientation and teaching programme for new or junior staff (Dibert and Goldenberg 1995; Dushmohamed and Guscott 1998). Peutz (1985) differentiates preceptorship from mentoring in that it has a more active teaching and supervision role.

The term preceptorship is a relatively recent introduction to the UK nursing language. It has a specific use that arises from the United Kingdom Central Council for Nursing, Midwifery and Health Visiting (UKCC) post-registration education and practice project (PREP) (UKCC 1990, 1994b). Recommendations 1 and 2 state that:

'There should be a period of support for all newly registered practitioners to consolidate the competencies or learning outcomes achieved at registration (4.4). A preceptor should provide the support for each newly registered practitioner (4.10).'

This was later expanded (UKCC 1993) to include not only newly registered nurses, but also those moving to an unfamiliar area, and the UKCC expressed that this support should extend for a minimum of 4 months. Although not introduced as a statutory requirement, the UKCC (1993) stated that this should be introduced as good practice. Preceptorship has been introduced within nursing in a fairly consistent way across the UK (Ashton and Richardson 1992; Gately 1992; Brennan 1993; Burke 1994; Skyte 1997). It is seen as a short-lived programme (Burke 1994), with the focus on the acquisition of knowledge and skills designed specifically to enable the newly registered nurse to work safely and effectively in a new environment. Although there is an emphasis on assessing this nurse's individual needs (Ashton and Richardson 1992), the focus is on the programme of development and support, rather than the one-to-one relationship common to the mentor literature (Brennan 1993).

Thus, the practice of preceptorship, as it is used within the UK, has a fairly precise and well-defined role. It is defined by the UKCC (1994b) and distinguishes certain groups of staff with specific needs and then identifies a particular way of meeting those needs for an identified period of time. Guidelines on issues, such as accountability of the practitioner, are also fairly well explained. Once the period of preceptorship has finished the registered nurse is subject to whatever staff development processes are available in their place of employment. This may be a poorly structured system or it may be a formal clinical supervision process incorporating a formalized staff development programme.

EXERCISE

Talk to some of the more experienced staff you are working with and ask them about their experiences of preceptorship.

Scenario Sarah is a newly registered nurse. She is due to start work on your ward in 2 weeks time. The ward manager has asked you to be her preceptor. You have been qualified for just over a year and this is the first time you will have been a preceptor. There is a well structured preceptorship pack, which contains learning outcomes and a weekly schedule.

- Identify the concerns and questions that you would have at this stage in this situation. Discuss these concerns with a more experienced staff nurse in your clinical area.
- Now try and predict what Sarah's concerns and questions. How would you deal with these?
- When would you try and set up your first meeting with Sarah? Before she starts or on her first day?
- How would you try and personalize the well structured, but somewhat formal, preceptorship pack?
- What sort of support would you want in taking on this new role. Who would you look to for this support?

The above scenario is an example of the most common type of a preceptorship relationship: a newly qualified nurse being preceptored by someone with more experience, but not so experienced that they have forgotten what it was like to be in that situation. There are other occasions when preceptorship is required but the situation is more complicated. It is important to make sure that the person asked to be the preceptor has the experience, skills and support to take on the more complex roles.

Scenario Peter trained as a nurse in 1982. After working as a staff nurse for 8 years he left the profession and worked as a tour guide for an international coach holiday company. A year ago he left the coach company and worked as a care assistant in a nursing home. He then decided to return to nursing and undertook a return-to-practice course. This course updated him on recent developments and provided a placement for him on the ward in which he would work as a staff nurse. Following successful completion of this course and re-registration, he was offered a permanent post on your ward. The ward manager has asked if you would be Peter's preceptor for the next 4 months.

- How are you going to assess Peter's learning needs?
- In what way is this preceptorship relationship different from that of a mentoring relationship (see above)?
- You are 15 years younger than Peter and have much less life experience than him. How will this affect the preceptorship relationship?
- For Peter's first 2 weeks on the ward he can work in a supernumerary capacity. How would you want to structure this time?
- Reflecting on the ward that you are currently working on, identify, in order or priority, 10 learning outcomes that you would want Peter to achieve in the first 8 weeks of his work.
- How would you organize the support and feedback you give Peter throughout this period of preceptorship?

If you feel this scenario is beyond your current experience and abilities, then discuss it with a more experienced registered nurse on your ward. Have they ever experienced something similar? If so, how did they deal with the situation? How would you deal with this situation?

SUMMARY

The term preceptorship is used in two main ways. In the US, it refers to the relationship, in the clinical area, between the trained nurse and the student. It is predominantly a teaching relationship. In the UK, it refers to a supportive, teaching relationship for the newly qualified nurse.

CONTINUING PROFESSIONAL DEVELOPMENT

Continuing professional development (CPD) is underpinned by a philosophy which seeks to counter the tendency to see an initial qualification as the end of a process, rather than a phase of lifelong learning (Thompson 1995). The UKCC, via the PREP, formally acknowledged the need for ongoing development for all nurses, midwives and health visitors following their initial registration (UKCC 1990, 1994b). This was part of a move towards lifelong learning, changing ways of work and developing emphasis on CPD (Wallace 1999). Thompson (1995, p89) identifies three elements to CPD:

- in-service training – developing and strengthening links between ideas, action and practice
- line management supervision, focusing upon clinical practice and interventions
- appraisal – helping people to maintain a clear focus on what they are trying to achieve (the focus is on the positive and constructive side of appraisal).

Development reviews or appraisals were introduced into the NHS in the form of individual performance reviews (IPRs) in 1986 to apply to the new breed of 'general managers' (Harrison *et al.* 1990). They were intended to complete the 'pyramid of objective setting' from ministerial reviews to individual managers (Harrison *et al.* 1990, p135). IPRs predominated at the more senior levels of health service management and tended to have a large economy and efficiency agenda. With regard to the general manager culture, in which they were introduced, short-term targets for financial savings dominated. When IPRs are used at more clinical levels they usually involve an annual meeting with the line manager, when the interviewee makes a general review of their performance and identifies any needs that they have. They are useful in developing longer-term objectives for the individual and relating them to organizational goals (Harrison *et al.* 1990).

Thompson (1995) sees CPD as contributing to maintaining motivation and increasing job satisfaction; he also feels that if it involves reflective practice then it becomes an important way of integrating theory and practice. In the early 1980s Benner researched the various levels of expertise with which nurses practised. *Novice to Expert* (Benner 1982) became a standard text for any nurse advancing their clinical career. Based upon the work of Dreyfus and Dreyfus (1980), Benner discussed five stages of proficiency, from novice, advanced beginner, competent, proficient, to expert, and described an expert nurse as:

'The expert nurse with her/his enormous background of experience, has an intuitive grasp of the situation and zeros in on the accurate region of the problem without wasteful consideration of a large range of unfruitful problem situations'.

(Benner 1982, p405)

Benner was identifying that some nurses had greater skills, experience and expertise than others, a fact accepted within the nursing profession, but not well documented at that time. Prior to 1990, a nurse in the UK, once registered, was free to practice, even following a break in service of many years, without any further training, support or assessment. PREP (UKCC 1990) brought in a number of changes regarding support, CPD and re-registration. As discussed above, it introduced a period of preceptorship for newly registered nurses. Also, following a break of service of more than 5 years, a nurse has to undergo a period of study and professional updating, and to be eligible for periodic re-registration, a nurse, midwife or health visitor must complete a period of 35 hours of study every 3 years and maintain a portfolio of professional development.

REFLECTIVE PRACTICE

The use of reflective practice is central in much of the discussion regarding CPD. The work of Argyris and Schon (1974) has been influential in a number of professions where the interaction of theory and its application to practice settings is integral. This work prompted interest in the use of reflective practice, initially within nurse education and also in clinical nursing practice. Schon (1987, 1991) identifies two types of reflection: reflection-on-action and reflection-in-action. The concept of reflection-on-action has been used in traditional nurse education settings, either in the clinical area or later in a classroom (McCaugherty 1991). Reflection-in-action occurs while the practice is being undertaken and, according to Schon, has the potential to influence its decisions and outcomes.

REFLECTION POINT
Why do you think reflection plays an important part in helping staff to give high quality care?

The use of reflective practice, particularly reflection-on-practice, was attractive to nursing because it offered a solution to the theory–practice gap that was recognized in the 1970s and 1980s (Birch 1975; Gott 1984). When reflection forms part of a structured learning experience, then theory and practice become more integrated, and theory informs practice and practice informs theory (Clark et al. 2001). This idea fitted with the concept of nursing as a practice-based profession and the theory of learning from experience developed by Kolb (1984) in the 1980s.

On clinical placement the student's 'mentor' became a key figure in helping the student to reflect on practice. The general move to develop a more questioning profession was being articulated to some extent by the emphasis on reflection on what the student saw and did. Most reviews of reflective practice acknowledge various stages of reflection (e.g. Mezirow 1981; Schon 1991; Johns 1993) and the difficulty of undertaking this process in isolation (Johns 1993). Reflective practice was thus welcomed within the nursing profession (Snowball et al. 1994; Marrow et al. 1997; Johns 1997) as a useful tool, particularly to help students integrate theory and practice. However, the use of reflection-in-practice and reflection-on-practice by experienced registered staff was not so evident. Atkins and Murphy (1993), in their review of the literature on reflection, stated that reflection must involve the self and must lead to a changed perspective. This is echoed by Snowball et al. (1994, p1235):

'It is clear in the literature that the involvement of self is a crucial element of the reflective process.'

Atkins and Murphy (1993) state that for reflection to occur the individual needs to be minimally defensive and be willing to work in collaboration with others. While this openness and willingness to 'expose the self' is appropriate for some staff, it is an exercise that many people find difficult to accomplish without support and guidance from a skilled and caring person. The clinical supervision relationship offered an opportunity for reflection on clinical practice by registered nurses under the guidance of a more experienced clinician. It is here that CPD, the practice of reflection and the role of clinical supervision come together for all registered nurses (Dooher et al. 2001). Prior to the early

1990s, implementation of reflective practice had been with student nurses or those staff on a post-registration course. It was seen as a valuable tool, but required a structure that certainly was not present in any systematic way within the nursing profession at that time. Clinical supervision offered an infrastructure for reflection-on-practice for all registered nursing staff.

SUMMARY

CPD and reflective practice are important ways of enhancing the development of high quality care.

CLINICAL SUPERVISION

In 1993, the Department of Health NHS Management Executive (DoH 1993b) published a strategic document, *A Vision for the Future*. This aimed to give overall direction and focus to the contribution that nurses and midwives could make to the NHS. It was the first time that the term clinical supervision had been used in a way that implied the introduction of a systematic structure. The document (paragraph 3.27) described clinical supervision in broad terms that included: development, individual responsibility, consumer protection, self-assessment and reflection.

EXERCISE

Talk to some experienced nurses and ask them about their experiences of clinical supervision.

MODELS

In the early 1990s, a number of accounts appeared describing how clinical supervision could work, or was working, in a variety of clinical settings. Different models of clinical supervision began to emerge. At the more humanistic end of the spectrum, Faugier (1992) described a growth and support model of the supervisory relationship. This focuses on, first and of prime importance, the relationship between the individuals. Then, using the interactions within the relationship, it focuses on the role of the supervisor to facilitate both educational and personal growth for the supervisee. At the same time, the relationship must be one that provides support for the developing clinical autonomy of the supervisee. Faugier describes many of the humanistic qualities associated with such growth and support, e.g. generosity, openness, humanity, sensitivity and trust. Chambers and Long (1995) identify a similar facilitative model of growth and support based on the relationship between the supervisor and supervisee. These approaches have their roots in a humanistic school of counselling (Farrington 1995), with its focus on self-awareness and personal growth.

From a more behaviourist perspective, Nicklin (1995) argues that clinical supervision could become rhetoric, promoting the illusion of innovation without producing change. While supporting the developmental elements, he feels that tangible outcomes are required. He proposes that clinical supervision be used to analyse issues and problems, clarify goals and identify 'strategies for goal attainment and establish an appropriate plan of action'. Nicklin (1997) developed these ideas into a six-stage process of supervision. Focusing on practice, it starts with practice analysis, problem identification, objective-setting, planning, implementation action and evaluation. Nicklin (1995) states that the process of clinical supervision should complement other managerial and professional processes and that clinical supervision should not develop as a vehicle for diluting or fragmenting managerial responsibility. This 'outcome' approach, with its focus on problem identification and problem-solving, has its roots in a behavioural school of psychology (Farrington 1995), with the focus of supervision being on what the supervisee is doing for the client.

PRINCIPLES

People's experiences of clinical supervision vary widely. Three principles, however, appear to be core (Fowler 1996; Figure 17.2):

● at least two people meeting together for the purpose of clinical supervision
● using 'reflection' to focus upon clinical practice
● meetings are structured and organized.

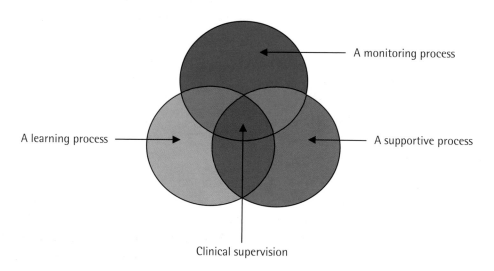

Figure 17.2 Interactive process of clinical supervision

The purpose and function of clinical supervision can encompass one or a combination of the following (Fowler 1995):

● a learning process
● a supportive process
● a monitoring process.

Senior staff who work predominantly on their own may develop clinical supervision in a way that allows them to meet in a small supportive peer group. Junior staff nurses will require a clinical supervision relationship that focuses largely on a learning, challenging process. For others, a combination of all three processes defines the purpose of clinical supervision. The more specialized the nurse, the more specific the relationship they will require. A nurse practitioner may value the opportunity to work with a medical consultant in developing a new area of practice. A ward manager may use clinical supervision to provide an opportunity to reflect on their leadership style with the director of nursing or with a group of peers. The important principle with clinical supervision is that it is your time to reflect upon your practice. The supervisor is there to help you do that, not to tell you what to do.

REFLECTION POINT

Think through your own experiences, if any, of clinical supervision. Write down what you consider the purpose to be. How do your experiences relate to:

- a learning process, which could range from a junior member of staff learning specific skills to the experienced ward sister who wants to develop research skills of finance management
- a support process which might include the discussion of difficult clinical or working conditions
- a monitoring process, which could range from informal, formative feedback to formal summative assessments, with quality assurance of defined standards falling somewhere in the middle.

Once you have identified the purpose of clinical supervision for your own practice, you need to consider who should be your supervisor? This may be someone who is appointed by the ward manager, but most areas will try to match the two people together and allow the supervisee some say in who their supervisor is going to be. The general rule for the choice of appointment as supervisor is someone who is enthusiastic to take on the role and who has the appropriate experience. The more experienced and specialized you become, the harder it will be to find a more experienced supervisor.

Once you have identified your ideas as to the purpose of clinical supervision and have an identified supervisor, you then need to be clear regarding certain ground rules. These may have been well thought out within your area of work, or they may be areas that you and your supervisor need to explore in the early stages of your supervision. Consider the following:

- What is the relationship between the supervisor and supervisee, the structure of the supervisory sessions, issues of confidentiality, record keeping. It is likely that there will be some hospital guidelines for some of these issues. The important principle is to relate the ground rules to the purpose of clinical supervision and to your needs. The 'contract' and 'record keeping' for a junior staff nurse is likely to be quite different from that of an experienced ward manager or clinical specialist. However, the principles may be quite similar.
- It is important to identify the time involvement as this will help you set realistic targets. The manager, supervisor and supervisee should all agree the amount of time to be invested in the process. You need to identify how long and how often you are going to meet. Again, this may vary for different staff. As a general guide, more inexperienced staff will need shorter periods of supervision fairly often, maybe an hour a week; experienced staff may require a longer session, but not as often, maybe an afternoon every month.
- The supervisor, supervisee and manager all need to develop a simple agreement on what is expected of all parties involved. A danger with the implementation of clinical supervision is that there are good intentions at the planning stage but it never gets beyond two or three sessions, because the practical issues have not been thought through and planned for. If you know that your ward gets very busy at certain times of the year, then how will you safeguard clinical supervision time? What happens when someone moves wards? Do they keep their supervisor? You cannot predict all the eventualities, but try to identify common probabilities. The agreement or contract should be used to strengthen the process of clinical supervision, not to inhibit it.

> **Scenario** You have just taken up a new post on an acute admissions ward. You have been qualified 6 months and this is your second ward. There is a strong culture of clinical supervision on the ward and the ward manager has suggested that Peter Young could be your supervisor. You have worked with Peter for a few shifts and respect his professional skills, knowledge and attitudes to work. You feel that this would be a good match and he and you agree to meet up the following week. Peter asks you to come to that meeting with some ideas as to what you want from the clinical supervision relationship.
>
> - Identify the areas that you would like the first 3 months of clinical supervision to focus on.
> - What questions will you ask Peter regarding the structure and ground rules?

> **Scenario** David has been registered for 3 years. You are the 'F' grade on the ward and have just been asked to be his clinical supervisor. You have arranged your first meeting for the following week – a 1-hour meeting at the end of the early shift.
>
> - How will you plan this first session? Consider the venue, content and focus of the session. Are you going to ask David to do any preparatory work prior to coming to the meeting?
> - What are your long-term goals for clinical supervision with David? How often are you going to meet? How are you going to structure the sessions?

If clinical supervision is going to result in a warm, challenging, reflective relationship, then both the supervisor and supervisee have to commit themselves to the relationship. A good way of demonstrating commitment is for both parties to prepare for the session and regard the meeting as a high priority. The supervisee needs to feel an equal partner with the supervisor. The experience and knowledge of the supervisor should lead the direction of the supervision, but not dominate it. Both people should feel equally in control of the situation and the 'agenda'; if there is something important to discuss, then you should feel free to discuss it.

The more specialist and independent the practitioner becomes, the greater is the need for a formalized system of clinical supervision. Whereas staff working in a ward team may have a number of informal opportunities for support, discussion and development, the same cannot always be said for staff working in isolated specialized posts.

SUMMARY

Clinical supervision offers a way of safeguarding and monitoring standards, development of practice and support of practitioners. It requires commitment of time, openness to reflect on practice and maturity to admit weakness and be willing to learn new ideas and skills.

CONCLUSION

The support required by staff to enable them to give high quality patient care must be developed at a strategic level, e.g. UKCC policy on preceptorship and clinical supervision; at an organization level, e.g. establishing adequate staffing levels and coffee areas; and at a personal interactional level, e.g. developing listening and mentoring skills. Skills that are common to all supportive relationships are:

- assessment of the person's previous knowledge, experience and concerns
- being willing to negotiate about the process and focus of the relationship

- listening to what the person has to say about what they are experiencing
- explaining ideas and knowledge in an easily understood way
- commenting on good practice as well as exploring areas where development is needed.

At an individual level, each of us has a responsibility to support and care for colleagues who we have daily contact with. This may take the form of formal preceptorship, mentoring or clinical supervision relationships, but it also involves informal means, such as having coffee together or organizing the occasional night out to celebrate a birthday or engagement. Remember people's names and treat them as individuals, greet the pharmacist by name as they enter the ward, thank the domestic by name as they finish for the day, leave a note for the night staff thanking them for the way that they sorted out the problem the night before. These are little things that everyone can do at no extra cost but they make our working environment a much more positive place to work in. The way that we treat each other will reflect upon the way we treat our patients.

CHAPTER 18

MAINTAINING A LICENCE TO PRACTISE: YOUR CAREER AS A PROFESSIONAL NURSE

Jane E Schober

INTRODUCTION

This chapter provides a comprehensive overview of the personal and professional requirements nurses require to maintain their licence to practise. Ultimately, the purpose of fulfilling these requirements is to maintain standards which result in the delivery of optimum care standards for those needing nursing and health care. Career opportunities for nurses are also explored, as are the factors influencing career choices and career management.

When we visit, and are cared for by, a doctor, nurse or any member of the multi-professional team, our expectations are that they will be competent to practise. This expectation is central to the relationship between the public and health care professionals. It is considered so important within the nursing profession that all nurses are required to meet certain criteria which are used to monitor their licence to practise and thus their suitability to practise as a registered nurse. When nurses register with the Nursing and Midwifery Council (NMC), they have successfully completed a course of study and been declared fit to practise nursing in the UK through the fulfilment of a range of practice, academic and professional requirements. As with a driving licence, a licence to practise nursing depends on nurses exercising their responsibilities in accordance with statutory, professional and employment requirements. Much of the responsibility to fulfil these requirements lies with each nurse as an accountable practitioner but should be supported, for example, by the existence of policies in the workplace, the NMC *Code of professional conduct* (NMC 2002a) and professional standards (UKCC 2001a).

All branches of nursing have a range of roles and expectations for nurses when they register. The successful acquisition of a role, e.g. as a staff nurse, usually depends on a process of selection which relies on thorough preparation and self-presentation to ensure that any career development opportunity is pursued appropriately. With these demands in mind, this chapter seeks to provide the guidance necessary for nurses to maintain their licence to practise and to support the process of career development.

NMC REQUIREMENTS TO MAINTAIN A LICENCE TO PRACTISE NURSING

Since 2000, the requirements for student nurses to enter a branch programme – and subsequently to be declared fit to practise as a registered nurse – have been clearly described (UKCC 2001a). They take the form of competencies which are assessed theoretically and practically throughout a pre-registration study programme. Chapter 2 discusses the competencies which address the four domains:

- professional and ethical practice
- care delivery
- care management
- personal and professional development (UKCC 2001a).

The publication of the NMC *Code of professional conduct* (NMC 2002a) provided a means of linking the required standards of professional conduct with the legal requirements for nurse education charged to the NMC by The Nursing and Midwifery Order (2001) under the Health Act (2000) (see also Chapters 2 and 16). Hence, these form the foundation for the professional development of all nurses. Because the focus of this chapter is on maintaining a licence to practise and the management of career opportunities, the professional development and expectations of nurses are discussed and explored here.

The *Code of professional conduct* states in clause 6:

'As a registered nurse or midwife, you must maintain your professional knowledge and competence'.

(NMC 2002a, p8)

This does not apply to nurses only; indeed this criterion is also one of the seven values found at the beginning of the *Code of professional conduct* and, as such, is a value shared by all the health care regulatory bodies in the UK. The *Code* goes on to describe ways in which this may be demonstrated and what the duties and responsibilities of a nurse are to achieve them.

REFLECTION POINT

Consider the criteria in section 6 of the *Code of professional conduct*. Make a list of how a registered nurse may work towards the achievement of each of these. Think about the resources needed for their achievement and who could, and should, help in this process.

Before considering the resources in any detail, reflect on any pre-registration experiences relevant to this process. First, there are the competencies and outcomes relating to professional development which should be demonstrated in order to enter the branch programme. These form the basis for the teaching and learning experiences during pre-registration courses as follows:

'Demonstrate responsibility for one's own learning through the development of a portfolio of practice and recognize when further learning is required:

- identify specific learning needs and objectives
- begin to engage with, and interpret, the evidence-base which underpins nursing practice.

Acknowledge the importance of seeking supervision to develop safe nursing practice.'

(UKCC 2001a, p20)

The emphasis here is on personal learning, personal reflection and taking responsibility for this process. The development of a portfolio of practice is evidence of the student nurse's learning experience, but this only occurs with supervision and support. From the period of the common foundation programme, there are professional and personal expectations that focus on the student's learning experiences in practice and their understanding of research and theoretical evidence relating to practice. Thus, the scene is set for personal and professional development. By the end of a branch programme the competencies demand that the responsibility for ongoing learning and continuing professional development (CPD) extends beyond personal responsibility for learning to the skills necessary to support the personal and professional development of others.

The UKCC (2001a) personal and professional development competencies for entry to the register are:

- demonstrate a commitment to the need for CPD and personal supervision activities in order to enhance knowledge, skills, values and attitudes needed for safe and effective nursing practice:
  - identify one's own professional development needs by engaging in activities such as reflection in, and on, practice and lifelong learning
  - develop a personal development plan which takes into account personal, professional and organizational needs
  - share experiences with colleagues and patients and clients in order to identify the additional knowledge and skills needed to manage unfamiliar or professionally challenging situations
  - take action to meet any identified knowledge and skills deficit likely to affect the delivery of care within the current sphere of practice

- enhance the professional development and safe practice of others through peer support, leadership, supervision and teaching
  - contribute to creating a climate conducive to learning
  - contribute to the learning experiences of others by facilitating the mutual sharing of knowledge and experience
  - demonstrate effective leadership in the establishment of safe nursing practice (UKCC 2001a, p21).

It is from this background that registered nurses embark on their professional careers. The personal and professional competencies are far-reaching and demand that nurses have been assessed to demonstrate the necessary skills which meet these criteria prior to registration. This, then, is the foundation for all registered nurses. It is this combination of the adherence to the *Code of professional conduct* and the fulfilment of post-registration requirements for maintaining the licence to practise nursing, which emphasizes the nursing profession's pledge to provide competent practice. However, this process does not occur without support and resources.

REFLECTION POINT

Look again at your resources list from the reflection point above. You may find that they fall into particular categories, such as support from staff and colleagues, learning resources, financial support and study time, information and skill development, e.g. in relation to teaching and supervision. This is a tall order. However, it emphasizes what registered nurses are responsible for within this domain and clarifies that all registered nurses have a duty and responsibility to initiate the necessary activities for these requirements to be met.

The NMC provides clear requirements to maintain a licence to practise, which apply to all nurses registered with it. A set of post-registration and practice standards (PREP) have been designed to support this process of maintaining the best possible care for patients. In essence, they support the process of updating yourself in the relevant practice area, personal reflection and decision-making, supporting practice development and the promotion of optimum care of patients. The PREP standards, which it should be emphasized are legal requirements, are as follows:

- practice standard – you must have worked in some capacity by virtue of your nursing or midwifery qualification during the previous 5 years for a minimum of 100 days (750 hours), or have successfully undertaken an approved return-to-practice course
- CPD standard – you must have undertaken and recorded your CPD over the 3 years prior to the renewal of your registration. All registered nurses have been required to comply with this standard since April 1995. Since April 2000, registrants need to have declared on their Notification of Practice (NOP) form that they have met this requirement when they renew their registration (NMC 2002g, p4).

(The NOP form is sent as part of the re-registration documentation and is returned to the NMC with the renewal fee every 3 years.)

So far, elements of the *Code of professional conduct* and the PREP requirements have been considered. It can be seen that they serve to protect the public by setting clear standards for practice, professional development, behaviour and decision-making. It is through the pursuit of these demands that the competencies necessary for registration may be further developed throughout a nursing career.

RETURNING TO PRACTICE

Many nurses have a break in service of 5 years or more. If this is the case, then nurses are unable to fulfil the practice standard without successfully completing a return-to-practice course. These are available across the UK and are usually 5 days or more in length. The courses are validated by the NMC and provide participants with input relating to health and social policy, practice-related updates and support to enhance professional development. Details of courses in Scotland, Wales and Northern Ireland are available on the NMC website and for England, from NHS Careers (see Appendix 4, Useful addresses).

The NMC requirements for renewal of registration are summarized in Box 18.1. The personal professional profile is a key tool with which each nurse can maintain details of their professional life as well as being a document which may be requested by the NMC for audit purposes.

Box 18.1 NMC requirements for the renewal of registration

- Completion of the notification of practice form giving details of qualifications and area of practice
- Signed declaration that the PREP requirements have been met:
  - PREP practice standard: 100 days (750 hours) of practice in the 5 years prior to renewal
  - PREP CPD standard: completion of 5 days or 35 hours. Learning activity relevant to your practice during 3 years prior to renewal
- Maintenance of a personal professional profile
- Compliance with the NMC audit

MAINTAINING A PERSONAL PROFESSIONAL PROFILE

For nurses who have registered in recent years the profile has become an integral part of pre- and post-registration activities. For student nurses, it now serves as a means of recording learning needs and experiences and a record of the elements of evidence-based learning. In many higher education institutions (HEIs), it forms a component of course assessment; thus students are encouraged to use it as a basis for tutorials and dialogue with experienced nurses. It is a valuable means of professional support. Although the NMC competencies refer to it as a portfolio, there are marked similarities between the terms profile and portfolio and they are often used interchangeably. There is, therefore, a natural extension of the process of profile maintenance between the pre- and post-registration periods, making it a personal record of professional development.

For registered nurses the profile is a record of professional development and career progression. The minimum PREP requirement is the record of evidence of any CPD activity, but it may also include:

- biographical information
- the record of qualifications, academic and professional
- a summary of current and previous posts
- details of relevant responsibilities and activities, e.g. management roles, interest groups, research activities and publications
- the record of education and formal learning experiences, e.g. courses, study days and updates, conference attendance and teaching activities

- a record of working hours during the previous 3 years
- reflection and evaluation of performance; this may also include critical incident analysis as well as examples of feedback from mentors and peers
- personal and professional objectives; this may be in the form of an action plan.

Other tips

The profile is a live document and should be kept up to date. For nurses who work closely with a preceptor or mentor, the profile is a tool which may serve to shape and prioritize dialogue relating to practice, and professional and career development. It is also a useful tool to support job applications and to develop the analytical skills necessary for reflective practice.

Aim to use a clear structure and an index, and record and date all entries. The profile may be completed in the Welsh language. Care should be taken to ensure confidentiality, particularly if incidents or examples from practice are described and analysed. Names should always be omitted.

LIFELONG LEARNING

The links between CPD and PREP represent an important part of lifelong learning. The notion that individuals are responsible for their learning is made clear in developments such as the portfolio and the achievement of practice and CPD standards. Support for this process is essential through preceptorship, mentoring and effective role models (see Chapter 19).

SUMMARY

To maintain a licence to practise nursing all registered nurses must:

- protect the public through adhering to professional standards
- comply with the NMC *Code of professional conduct*
- meet the PREP standards
- maintain a personal professional profile.

MANAGING CAREER OPPORTUNITIES

Understanding the available options for registered nurses, as well as consideration of career opportunities, serves to support the process of professional development. As nurses are personally accountable for their practice (NMC 2002a), it is essential that personal, professional and career decision-making is as effective as possible.

Regardless of the choice of branch, there is a wide range of career options for nurses. Making an informed choice, and one which will result in a positive work role, places demands on any applicant. Over the years, the job market has fluctuated greatly from times of job shortages to the current position where there are many vacancies all over the UK. The government drive to recruit more nurses has resulted in increases in student numbers with the resulting pressure on students when applying for their first-choice staff nurse post. Competition for many posts in acute hospitals or larger units can be great and the way each nurse prepares for and proceeds with career choices will impact significantly on all stages of a career.

FACTORS AFFECTING CAREER CHOICES

Initially, the pursuit of career opportunities depends on a range of factors and resources:

- employment opportunities
- educational and training opportunities
- career guidance opportunities for nurses
- work, personal and social needs
- information relating to career options
- career pathways for nurses
- preparation for selection procedures and interviews.

Employment opportunities

Historically, most newly-registered nurses have opted to apply for a D grade or equivalent staff nurse post local to their higher education institution, or elsewhere in their base country. There are many employment opportunities for nurses depending on qualifications, skills and experience. Box 18.2 illustrates both the range of options as well as the potential further learning demands on registered nurses who have already completed at least a 3-year course of full-time study. Progress through the tiers of grades in the NHS or private health sectors, or diversification into non-clinical roles, usually requires further qualifications, skills and role developments.

Box 18.2 Key employers of nurses in the UK

- Charitable organizations, e.g. Macmillan nurses, King's Fund
- Further education colleges
- HM Forces e.g. army, navy and air force
- Higher education institutions (universities)
- Local authorities
- NHS trusts, including primary care trusts
- Nursing agencies
- Occupational health services
- Overseas development services, e.g. British Red Cross
- Independent health care organizations
- Pharmaceutical companies
- Professional organizations, e.g. Royal College of Nursing
- Publishing houses
- Statutory bodies, e.g. the NMCI
- Trade unions

Sources of employment information

Knowing the employment options is crucial to any career or role development. Seeking information through advertisements is only a part of the process. If you aspire to a particular role, have ambitions and have your sights set on a particular path, then information gathering is the essential first step. Key sources of employment information are summarized in Box 18.3. These will be complemented by knowledge of:

- qualifications and other professional requirements necessary to apply
- required previous experience
- terms and conditions of employment, e.g. contract and salary details
- employment policies, e.g. family-friendly policies, health and safety policies
- role specification for the post-holder
- employment opportunities for the post-holder
- details of the induction programme and staff training
- details of staff appraisal and support networks
- evidence of quality assurance mechanisms.

Box 18.3 Sources of employment information

- Parent organization websites, e.g. NHS, NMC, RCN, local trusts
- Human resources departments for local employment information
- Prospectuses for university details
- Specialist journals for specialist posts
- Libraries for local information
- National and local press for job advertisements
- Internal communications, newsletters
- Staff notice boards

Some of this information will feature on an advertisement, but usually only key elements of the role are outlined. Later in the chapter, guidance is offered on the process of applying for a post.

Educational and training opportunities for nurses

Following registration, most nurses recognize that they have reached a stage when, despite the achievements of registering as a nurse, learning is just beginning in relation to many facets of their chosen role. The generation of a personal development plan (see above) may be supported by attention to education and training opportunities. Recognition of the demands of professional nursing practice and the support needed to maintain standards of practice is manifest in the provision of:

- work-based learning: this is characterized by opportunities to learn relevant skills and competencies in the workplace which are assessed. Successful outcomes may result in the award of academic credits if the course or module has been approved using academic approval criteria. This is a relatively new scheme that is supported by the Department of Health, Working Together, Learning Together recommendations (DoH 2001q) for lifelong learning
- Royal College of Nursing Study Hours: this scheme, which is approved by the RCN Accreditation Unit and promoted through the Nursing Standard CPD articles, is a means for nurses to

quantify the number of hours of learning undertaken (see Appendix 4, Useful addresses). These can be used as evidence for the NMC PREP requirements as 2 points are awarded for every hour of study

- CPD: this is characterized by opportunities for learning following registration (and may include work-based learning). Higher education institutions (HEIs) work in partnership with NHS trusts to identify, prepare and gain approval and necessary contracts for the provision of courses. These are subject to academic and professional approval by the NMC and HEI provider. Courses are offered through modular schemes using the credit accumulation and transfer scheme (CATS), where academic credits are awarded following successful outcome at the academic level approved for the stage of the course.

> **Scenario** Jasmine Robertson is a registered mental health nurse, who has worked full time in a community psychiatric day centre for 18 months. She has a Diploma in Higher Education (Mental Health Nursing). Following a performance review, she has the support of her line manager to apply for a BSc (Hons) nursing course. The purpose of this would be to facilitate her development in relation to the academic study of nursing and to undertake modules in the theory and practice of research methodology and counselling.

The achievement of a Diploma level course results in the award of: 120 CATS points – Level 1, 120 CATS points – Level 2. The requirement of a first degree course [either a BA (Hons) or BSc (Hons)] is the achievement of a further 120 credits at Level 3 – usually the third year of a full-time 3-year degree course. The CATS scheme allows applicants to transfer previously acquired points to a course of further study which would be subject to approval under the approval of prior learning scheme (APL). In addition, approval of prior experiential learning (APEL) may also be assessed by the course admissions team, as this may also be counted. Jasmine's academic achievement and professional experience may result in her only needing to complete the Level 3 modules which would usually be undertaken over 2 years part-time or 1 year full-time.

There is a wide range of modules and courses for registered nurses. They are based in HEIs and trusts. Your ability to undertake a course of study will usually depend on:

- relevance to the applicant and their workplace needs
- available funding – applicants may be asked to self-fund
- the nature, content, level and availability of the course
- the study leave approval processes.

Making the most appropriate choices relating to ongoing education may be supported by career guidance advice and information.

Career guidance opportunities for nurses

Making career choices is a complex process. Avoiding mistakes in the choice of new posts, courses of study and career changes depends on each of us being aware of the range of possibilities and options available, as well as being conversant with the necessary information and skills to succeed with, for example, an application. Historically, career guidance for nurses has been limited to national and local sources of career information and experienced nursing staff providing opportunities for nurses to explore, discuss and review their career options. Job availability remains a key factor in the process of career management. While this cannot be underestimated, it is important that nurses aspire to their optimum potential through making effective career choices.

Work, personal and social needs

All career decisions may be influenced by personal and social factors. In recent years, changes in working patterns have become evident, in particular, in relation to the increase in numbers of those working part-time, returning to nursing and pursuing more flexible working practices.

REFLECTION POINT

Consider the factors important to you in a choice of job or career change. What is particularly helpful here is what motivates you. You may find the following categories helpful: work needs, personal needs and family and social needs.

Now examine Box 18.4, which lists the factors found to be important to nurses making career choices (Schober 1990). They influence motivation and, in particular, job satisfaction, which is central to the sense of well–being at work.

Box 18.4 Factors affecting career choices (Schober 1990)

Work needs:
- Need to work
- Promotion
- Motivation and opportunities to learn and develop professionally
- Interest/commitment to the work and role
- Range of responsibility
- Dynamics of the team and management structure

Personal needs:
- Job satisfaction
- Job security
- Status of the role
- Salary
- Reluctance to change roles
- Terms of the contract

Family/social needs:
- Family need for income
- Child care availability
- Availability of accommodation
- Travelling distance from home
- House prices
- Support of partner/family members

There is much discussion in the nursing and national press about the concerns over the terms and conditions of nurses in work and their pay levels. Given high house prices and cost of living expenses, the influence of these factors should not be underestimated. Indeed, many employers have introduced initiatives such as flexible working and family-friendly policies to support nurses. Nurses, however, identify other factors which emphasize the importance of job satisfaction and positive work relationships. Stechmiller and Yarandi (1992) found that the quality of supervision, promotion opportunities and the meaningfulness of work were more influential than pay and job security.

Schober (2000) suggests a range of factors influencing job satisfaction in a clinical post (Box 18.5). They may also serve to help nurses in the process of deciding their preferred clinical placement.

Box 18.5 Factors influencing job satisfaction in a clinical post

- Factors relating to care and the patient/client group
- The clinical speciality
- The pace of work, e.g. patient turnover, day care
- Opportunities to develop the nurse–patient relationship
- Opportunities for and support for learning
- Team membership and support
- Staff support network
- Style of leadership
- Staff morale
- Opportunities for professional development

REFLECTION POINT

Consider your favourite clinical placement(s). To what extent did the factors listed in Box 18.5 influence your choice? To confirm your choice, it may help you to place these in order of importance and compare them with your needs, as listed in Box 18.4.

You may find a pattern emerging, which will help you to feel confident about what is important to you when choosing a role and, just as importantly, what you would not enjoy or would be disadvantageous to your ways of working.

Information relating to career options

Understanding what motivates nurses in work needs to be supported by sound advice and information. It is rare to find career officers or counsellors in the health services but there are often highly motivated lecturers, managers and clinical staff willing to offer advice. The preceptorship and mentor systems are additional ways of finding support (see Chapter 17). Despite this type of networking, it is a challenge for staff to keep abreast of the career information available and necessary for sound decision-making. Information may relate to:

- current career options
- job availability
- career pathways
- in-service education and training
- courses of study
- prerequisites to promotion and development, e.g. a teaching qualification.

Career pathways for nurses

Whether nurses opt to develop a career that includes the pursuit of promotion, working full time and/or working until retirement is a personal decision. More nurses appear to be opting for periodic career breaks, part-time working and flexibility to meet domestic needs. Trends in working patterns also show that more nurses are working in the private sector and up to 47% take a career break – mainly maternity leave (Seccombe *et al.* 1993). With more nurses returning to practice, the expansion of community nursing roles, e.g. practice nurses, and initiatives such as the 'modern matron' and nurse consultants (see Chapter 19), there is a wide range of available posts.

Traditionally, nurses pursued a clinical pathway until professional development and promotion opportunities resulted in the acceptance of a teaching, management or research role. Nowadays, the grading structures for nurses demand the integration of these three activities with clinical responsibilities to a greater or lesser extent throughout the grading scheme (Box 18.6). Ultimately, this structure supports the opportunity for nurses to remain in clinical practice and have an advancing clinical career, rather than finding promotion by opting for educational or managerial posts.

Box 18.6 Role specifications and clinical grades

E grade role specifications usually include:
- Experience (usually 1 year) and satisfactory performance in the speciality
- Previous teaching experience
- Experience of supervising students and/or other staff
- Evidence of effective interpersonal, teamworking and communication skills
- Evidence of the development of leadership skills
- Evidence of research appreciation and evidence-based practice
- Personal and professional updating and development
- The English National Board (ENB), or equivalent, qualification in the speciality
- Teaching qualification (e.g. ENB 998)

F grade role specifications usually include:
- All the E grade specifications
- The potential to lead a team
- Experience in the speciality (usually 2 years)
- Evidence of clinical and managerial skills

G grade role specifications usually include:
- All the F grade specifications
- Experience in the speciality (e.g. 3–5 years)
- Evidence of clinical, managerial, educational and leadership skills
- Evidence of the potential to undertake research
- Qualifications or advanced study relating to the speciality
- The potential for innovative practice

H grade role specifications usually include:
- All the G grade specifications
- Proven leadership ability
- Evidence of relevant managerial, educational and research ability
- Potential to initiate and respond to policies, innovations and quality initiatives

NHS PAY SYSTEM AND IMPLICATIONS FOR NURSES

In 1999, the white paper Agenda for Change (DoH 1999e) promised a fairer pay system for nurses and health professionals. The introduction of revised pay structures has been slower than planned but will impact on a wider agenda than pay. Conditions of service, clearer career progression paths and the number of pay bands will additionally be affected. More consistent schemes for appraising staff and supporting professional development will feature, as well as the NHS job evaluation scheme, which will support the aim to deliver equal pay for work of equal value.

The job evaluation scheme will consider a range of factors including:

● communication and relationship skills
● knowledge, training and experience
● analytical and judgemental skills
● planning and organizational skills
● responsibilities for patient/client care
● responsibilities for policy implementation
● responsibilities for research and development
● physical, mental and emotional effort
● working conditions (Leifer 2002).

Implementation of these proposals has begun and is subject to modifications following feedback from the 12 pilot sites in England which test the scheme. Eight pay bands are likely to replace the A–H nursing pay grades (Box 18.6). This new pay system will apply to all NHS staff in the UK from 2004/5, except doctors, dentists and senior managers. The implementation of the new scheme is based on a full set of job profiles, which will assist in the choice of pay band for existing staff, a job evaluation scheme and a new terms and conditions handbook.

It is worth noting that, despite significant improvements in the clinical career opportunities for nurses across the specialities, the characteristics required for progression and promotion often necessitate the development of managerial, educational and research abilities. This can be seen encapsulated within the roles of 'modern matrons' and nurse consultants.

THE SPECIALIST PRACTITIONER

Opportunities for nurses to undertake courses leading to specialist practitioner roles have facilitated learning relating to clinical practice, care and programme management, practice development and clinical practice leadership (UKCC 2001d). Courses are available and may relate to any speciality, although the UKCC (2001e) specified standards relating to:

● general practice nurses
● community mental health nurses
● community learning disability nurses
● community children's nurses
● public health nurses/health visitors
● occupational health nurses

- home/district nurses
- school nurses.

The availability of courses leading to specialist practitioner qualifications may be found on the websites of the education bodies for nurses in each of the countries in the UK and the NHS website. More detailed explanations of the content of courses are found in HEI prospectuses, HEI websites and from senior nurses, lecturers and lecturer–practitioners in the NHS trusts.

CAREER PATHWAYS IN EDUCATIONAL, MANAGERIAL AND RESEARCH ROLES

So far, consideration has been given to the development of a clinical career pathway. Career pathways may also facilitate emphasis on teaching, management and research roles. Currently, one in four nurses works outside the NHS, so it is vital that nurses are aware of the necessary information to make informed decisions at all stages.

Sources of information for these roles include:

- UK websites for career information (see Appendix 4, Useful addresses); each UK country has a website containing information relating to roles and available courses. Some, e.g. Northern Ireland, include details of the centres offering specific courses
- statutory organizations, e.g. the NMC, provide details of statutory requirements for specific roles, re-registration and educational requirements for key roles, e.g. nurse teachers
- professional organizations, e.g. the RCN (see Appendix 4, Useful addresses), provide details of services to members, professional guidance and support and learning opportunities, e.g. conferences and professional forums. The *RCN Bulletin* also provides information on job opportunities
- educational opportunities fall into different categories. Details of professional/statutory courses and continuing education are available from the NMC, Health Professionals Wales, NHS Education for Scotland and the Northern Ireland Practice and Education Council (see Appendix 4, Useful addresses)
- open learning (see Appendix 4, Useful addresses) and additional educational opportunities are available from HEIs, the RCN and professional journals.

Embarking on a pathway which focuses on research, management or education demands that the applicant has undertaken appropriate academic preparation as well as completing necessary pre-requisites for the role.

Nursing research

The expectation that research is applied in practice settings is specified at the outset of all pre-registration courses. Opportunities for nurses to participate in research processes have increased in recent years, as nurse education was integrated within HEIs and more opportunities developed for nurses to study aspects of nursing beyond diploma level. Research posts exist in a range of sectors, although mainly in university departments, specialist research centres and through specifically funded research projects. When considering a research post, there are a number of issues influencing the role:

- length of contract: it is often fixed-term and for a short period, e.g. 1 year, especially for research assistants
- role specification: may demand unsocial hours for data gathering
- opportunities for education and training: examine what is available and what skills are expected
- consider the available resources, e.g. office accommodation, secretarial support and IT facilities
- teaching requirements and responsibilities for disseminating research outcomes that may be through writing papers, seminar presentation and conferences
- opportunities for promotion to senior roles, e.g. a readership or a professorial position: consider the available research activity and funding, the work of the research active staff, the history of research activity within the department and evidence of quality assessment. The research assessment exercise (RAE) ranking is a valuable measure of the quality of previous research outputs. Currently, this assessment invites academic departments to submit evidence of research activity every 4 years. The score is an indicator of quality and activity and a useful guide for potential applicants, as well as influencing the degree of funding the HEI receives from the relevant funding body

Whatever the research activity, whether it be as part of a clinical role, a course of study or a specific post, the potential is there to contribute to the growing body of nursing knowledge, as well as the evidence-base for practice. The use of research findings is integral to teaching and education roles.

Teaching and education

As with research, teaching and learning may be exercised at all levels of experience. Indeed, there is a professional expectation for nurses to teach others, disseminate information and promote learning within the process of patient care. Support for this begins during pre-registration programmes, although it is following registration that those intent on specific teaching roles have the opportunity to undertake them. One of the key developments in nursing in recent years has been the recognition of the value of learning in practice settings and the necessity to balance the emphasis of teaching between the theoretical perspectives necessary for academic attainment and the practice skills essential to the quality of patient interventions. The competency-based curriculum and the standards required of pre-registration programmes (UKCC 2001e) are central to this process. Subsequently, changes to the preparation of nurse teachers have facilitated educational pathways for the preparation of practice educators and for those wishing to teach in a practice environment, as well as opportunities for preparation as a lecturer to teach in an academic department in an HEI.

Teaching courses are now equivalent to 1 year full-time study and result in a recordable teaching qualification on the NMC register. Most courses are part-time, which enables applicants to maintain their professional role. The courses have a range of entry requirements including:

- a degree or equivalent qualification
- entry on the NMC register
- 3 years full-time practice experience (or equivalent) with student nurses in the past 10 years
- evidence of professional knowledge.

These courses demand study at postgraduate diploma level and may lead to a Master of Arts degree in many institutions. Details of these courses are available from the NMC website.

Nurses embarking on this career pathway will need to consider carefully the implications of these two means (or pathways) of achieving a teaching qualification. The choice may ultimately be influenced by the nature and responsibility of their current role. The employer, therefore, may recommend that the completion of one of the pathways is essential to the professional development of the nurse. It would be necessary, as with many courses, for the candidate to negotiate study leave and support for funding.

Career opportunities for those willing to teach usually demand both a teaching qualification as well as evidence of academic attainment at master's level in a subject relevant to the post. Most practice educators are employed in the NHS and most lecturers in the HEI sector. However, the partnerships which exist to support students at pre- and post-registration levels facilitate opportunities for both parties to work closely together to achieve learning objectives and other educational requirements. Terms and conditions of service, as well as role specifications, differ in a number of ways and candidates should explore these carefully.

Lecturer–practitioner roles (see Chapter 19), although not as numerous, exist to span the academic and practice-based learning environments. Most require a teaching qualification but are often limited to a fixed-term contract, which may deter some applicants. Historically, these posts have been more closely allied to the educational support of registered nurses in specialist clinical areas.

Nurse management

As with teaching, management is integral to the role of any registered nurse but will increase in complexity and emphasis as more senior roles are adopted. Nurse managers exist at all levels in the NHS and independent sector and significant opportunities exist for nurses to manage effectively from the point of registration, as there is immediate responsibility for the management of patient care, self, personal and professional development.

Beyond the initial management responsibilities required of staff nurses, for example, nurse managers who lead teams of staff and manage departments, units and significant caseloads also have responsibilities which include:

- monitoring standards of practice
- clinical governance
- staff recruitment and retention
- audit of nursing and clinical services
- managerial and clinical leadership
- staff support and development
- policy implementation
- financial management.

More and more nurse managers are graduates and, for many posts, this is a pre-requisite with posts having a specific practice base. It is recognized that senior managers benefit from educational opportunities that address skills such as leadership, the management of change and innovation, team building, conflict management, project development and quality assurance systems. The development of IT services relating to patient care management and outcomes requires ongoing updating of staff.

These skills are often featured in degree courses that focus on, for example, health service management and nursing studies. Scrutiny of prospectuses and HEI websites will reveal the key features of such courses.

SUMMARY

Managing a career pathway depends on:

- acquisition of relevant information
- scrutiny of employment opportunities
- self-assessment of family, work and social needs
- maximizing personal and professional development opportunities
- maintaining professional standards.

PREPARATION FOR SELECTION PROCEDURES AND INTERVIEWS

Making career decisions depends on a range of factors, including those summarized above relating to the management of a career pathway. Embarking on the process of applying for a post demands additional skills. Whether a nurse is considering a first post, a new post, promotion opportunities or a complete change in a clinical area, there is a range of issues to consider. The RCN (1995b) suggests the following are important to the quality of a working environment because they support individuals at work:

- value is given to nurses and nursing
- teamwork is evident
- staff are supported
- training and education opportunities are evident
- successes are celebrated
- mistakes are regarded as opportunities for learning
- ability is regarded as an asset rather than a threat.

In addition, employee-friendly policies facilitate a positive working environment and should be explored for their relevance to your needs as a potential employee as part of the process of seeking information about a post.

REFLECTION POINT

Consider the importance to you of the following features:

- any flexible working opportunities: school holiday contracts, flexi-time, self-rostering and special shifts
- a workplace crèche or nursery
- paternity, parental and adoption leave
- emergency carer leave
- career breaks
- counselling and advice services
- sabbatical leave.

These provide nurses with a useful guide to what to expect from a working environment. They combine to make a positive workplace where the leader(s) encourages an approach to work in which individuals are valued, supported and praised. Dissatisfaction usually occurs when one or more of these features is absent. So, they may serve to help you decide whether it is opportune to consider a change of post.

Before applying for any post a range of information is needed to produce an effectively planned application:

- location of the post
- role description
- terms and conditions of service
- length of the contract
- grade of the post
- pre-requisites, e.g. qualifications and required experience
- care management systems
- patient quality outcomes
- management style in the unit
- opportunities for support and preceptorship (as relevant to grade)
- teaching and learning opportunities
- appraisal scheme
- closing date for applications.

THE INFORMAL VISIT

Although not always possible, an informal visit to a new work area is invaluable. It gives you the opportunity to gain insight into the atmosphere, the environment and the attitudes of staff. More pertinently, much may be gleaned from such a visit and may convince you about pursuing the application.

WRITING A CURRICULUM VITAE

One of the most important documents associated with any application is your curriculum vitae (CV). You use this tool to demonstrate to a potential employer that you have the necessary skills and experience for a post. You can submit your CV with your application form as it may include details that an application form does not request. It may also be used for speculative applications and in response to an advertisement that requests you apply in writing.

There is no standard format for a CV but there are key features that should be included:

- personal details
- qualifications and educational background
- work and professional experience
- professional activities
- personal activities, e.g. voluntary work.

A suggested format is offered in Box 18.7 and it may be modified depending on the post applied for and the details requested by the employer.

Box 18.7 Format for your curriculum vitae

<table>
<tr><td colspan="2" align="center">**Curriculum Vitae**</td></tr>
<tr><td>Name:</td><td></td></tr>
<tr><td>Address:</td><td></td></tr>
<tr><td>Contact phone no.:</td><td></td></tr>
<tr><td>E Mail:</td><td></td></tr>
<tr><td>PIN no:</td><td>Expiry date:</td></tr>
<tr><td>Qualifications:</td><td>Professional qualifications, with dates, should be listed.
Educational awards, with dates and the college/university attended</td></tr>
<tr><td>Previous experience:</td><td>List all previous relevant employment, with dates and highlight your current post</td></tr>
<tr><td>Professional activities:</td><td>These may include details of publications, in-service education and training/CPD activities, membership of professional groups, conferences attended and papers given, and research activities</td></tr>
<tr><td>Personal:</td><td>You may wish to include reference to relevant details of other activities, e.g. voluntary work, committee membership but this is not essential</td></tr>
</table>

EXERCISE

This is your opportunity to create or revise your own CV. Consider the format in Box 18.7 and complete the details for yourself. Aim to identify any queries or uncertainties and compare them with the following additional tips:

- note that the request for date of birth is omitted, this is not necessary on a CV
- explain any gaps in your employment history, e.g. to raise a family, to undertake voluntary work
- use action words to explain particular achievements, responsibilities and activities, e.g. organized, produced, implemented, managed and developed
- keep the presentation clear and well laid out, and limit the number of font styles and type faces
- avoid abbreviations which may not be familiar
- use good quality paper
- enclose a covering letter with your CV. This may be used to highlight key points and their relationship to the post applied for.

COMPLETING THE APPLICATION FORM

Application forms are central to the first stage of the selection process and are used for short-listing suitable candidates. They should be completed to the highest possible standard and contain relevant and factual information. Ensure that all requested information is given and, where relevant, include your CV. Application forms are usually photocopied so, to ensure a positive presentation, type the form or use black ink unless requested to do otherwise. One of the most demanding sections on an application form is the question concerning why you are applying for this post. This is usually referred to as supporting information and should be written in a way that links your skills and qualities with the skills and experience required for the post. Prepare this carefully and organize it logically. It may be useful, for example, to use the subheadings on the role description to organize your supporting information.

The health assessment form

Usually, applicants are requested to complete a health assessment form which is sent to the occupational health department and should remain confidential to that department. Any health-related declaration may result in being called for an interview with an occupational health nurse.

Previous convictions

If requested, you must declare any previous convictions, even those that occurred over 10 years ago. If the post requires you to work with vulnerable people, then the employer will check your police record.

Choosing referees

Usually, two referees are requested, one being the previous employer or the educational institution if you are applying for your first post after registration. Referees are asked a range of questions about the applicant and should be prepared for the task. Liaise closely with your referees; they should be fully conversant with your plans, have worked with you in a senior position or have knowledge of your professional capabilities over a period of time. Their support is essential and referees should be honest enough to discuss any reservations they might have about the suitability of an application. Maintain contact with referees and give them feedback about the outcomes of interviews as they may be needed for a number of years in some cases.

THE INTERVIEW

The complexity of the interview procedure will usually depend on the seniority of the post. A range of interview techniques may be used; the most common is the panel interview where there may be between two and four members present.

Preparation

Thorough preparation for the interview is essential, particularly as candidates are usually nervous and aware of the competitive nature of the event. This should include:

- familiarity with and understanding of the role specification
- consideration of how your experience and skills link with the requirements of the role
- being prepared to expand on any detail on the application form and CV
- being familiar with relevant professional and practice-related initiatives
- details of how you keep up-to-date with local and national initiatives and fulfil CPD and PREP requirements

- preparing questions you expect to be asked and practising a mock interview with colleagues, for example
- planning the journey to the interview and the necessary timing
- ensuring you are smartly dressed and well-presented.

The presentation

Many selection procedures request that the candidates prepare a presentation on a given topic which is usually closely related to the job. The time allowed for this is usually included and is often 15–20 minutes. Aim to prepare colour acetates or a power point presentation if you have the skills and the necessary equipment is available. A brief summary of the presentation may be prepared and copied for each panel member. The presentation is usually delivered prior to the interview.

The interview

Panel interviews are commonly used, as they allow a range of interested parties to meet and assess the candidates. Panel members mainly include the line manager, a member of the human resources team, a representative of any associated partner organization and a senior member of the unit of department staff.

Panel members tend to ask the same questions of each candidate and may follow them up with secondary questions to encourage a detailed response. The areas of questioning relate to key areas and will reflect the demands of the post. They may include:

- background details: biographical details are checked and reasons for the application are explored. Reference is made to the application form and CV
- clinical and practice-related details: clinical posts will require exploration of relevant practice-related issues including, for example, reflection of skills, problem-solving-based questioning and understanding of current issues
- professional issues: professional awareness and how up-to-date you are may be explored. Questions which explore your professional values and commitment may also be asked
- teaching and management issues: issues such as team-working, leadership potential, teaching and preceptorship experience may all be explored.

The interview is your opportunity to communicate your qualities and skills. It is also a time for you to demonstrate your enthusiasm, commitment and professionalism. Maintain good eye contact with the questioner and other panel members, avoid rushing into a response, rather pause and reflect on your answers. If necessary, ask the panel to clarify a question if it is not clear to you.

Following an interview

The outcome of an interview may not be communicated for anything from a number of hours to a number of days after the event. If you are offered a post, then you are in a position to discuss the start date, pay scale and any other contractual detail when the contract arrives. If any aspect of the contract is unclear, seek advice from the human resources department initially. Avoid resigning from your current post until you have received the offer of the post in writing. An unsuccessful outcome is disappointing but you should gain from any feedback as to your performance, suitability for the post and advice for the future.

SUMMARY

When considering a career move:

- gather thorough information about the post
- maintain an up-to-date CV
- plan an informal visit
- liaise closely with your referees
- relate your supporting information on the application form to the role specification
- prepare a well-presented application form
- rehearse necessary elements of the interview
- prepare key responses and questions.

CONCLUSION

This chapter examined the relationship between the nurse's responsibilities for maintaining a licence to practise nursing and the associated NMC requirements. The general public expects and deserves to be cared for by competent accountable practitioners and nurses are charged to deliver standards of care to meet this requirement.

Nurses need support to progress and develop their careers. Professional standards relating to re-registration, education, training and conduct exist to facilitate this process and each nurse is responsible for the maintenance and development of professional knowledge and skills. Career opportunities are many and varied and may not always result in promotion. Successful career moves not only reflect professional development but also thorough planning, networking and professional commitment. It is hoped that the guidance offered in this chapter will help to support the process of career development and the realization of your professional potential.

CHAPTER 19

CONSULTANCY: THE FUTURE FOR NURSING ROLES?

Nicky Hayes

INTRODUCTION

This book is aimed at nurses who are just beginning their careers. This chapter offers a glimpse of what may be ahead for some practitioners – consultant level practice, which is a relatively new level of practice within the NHS. The background to the creation of consultant nurse, midwife and health visitor posts is described, and there is a discussion of the political, practical and theoretical facets of the roles. Consultancy in nursing, midwifery and health visiting is new, evolving and its effects are largely unknown. To some it is controversial. This discussion will draw on three case studies to illustrate consultant practitioner roles in practice, and it will explore the structure and functions of the roles. Finally, it asks, 'where do we go from here?'

CONSULTANCY AND THE POLITICAL AGENDA

Consultant nursing, midwifery and health visiting within the NHS is a relatively new concept, with the first appointments in the four countries of the UK being announced in 1999/2000. Until the creation of these posts, there was no widely agreed definition of the concept of consultant practice within the professions. Any practitioner could set up as an independent consultant should they wish, providing their own terms of reference as to what consultancy meant, in either public services or independent practice. The regulatory bodies do not at present register or record consultants and there are currently no data on the number of practitioners who work as independent consultants. It may be suggested that few practitioners appear to have taken up this career option. By contrast, NHS consultant nursing, midwifery and health visiting was announced with much publicity within the national press. It formalized the concept of consultant practice and has remained high profile following the launch of the first posts.

From the announcement of an initial 141 posts in England, the numbers of consultant nurse, midwife and health visitor posts have continued to increase. They now exist in a range of specialities and NHS trusts across the UK. The first of 12 initial posts to be announced by the Chief Nursing Officer in Scotland were in Public Health, Midwifery and Services for Older People (Scottish Executive 2000b); in Wales, the Assembly Secretary for Health and Social Services announced the first 11 posts in August 2000; in Northern Ireland eight posts were initially announced (DHSS, Northern Ireland 1999).

Many practitioners in the UK, when completing their training for registration today, might wonder where their career will lead and whether consultancy will be relevant to them as an option for future practice, either within the NHS, or independently within private practice. This chapter explores the concept of consultancy within nursing, midwifery and health visiting, examines its launch within the NHS, and sets out some discussion around the development of formal consultant posts and what the future may hold for them. The discussion draws mainly on the English documentation and experience. Scottish, Welsh and Northern Ireland health departments have developed their own proposals and documentation, although to date the development in consultant posts is in accordance with the English government proposals. The documents of each of the four countries of the UK are not therefore discussed further in this chapter.

CONSULTANT POSTS

The Department of Health's strategy for nursing, midwifery and health visiting in England (DoH 1999d) sets out the NHS vision of nurse, midwife and health visitor consultant posts. The proposals for these posts reflect the Department's perceived need to provide a stronger focus for clinical leadership and improvement of services, for which the development of senior posts is identified as key. The link between clinical leadership and standards of care is made explicit in the strategy, along with recognition of the need for an:

> 'organizational climate that enables the next generation of leaders to challenge orthodoxy, to take risks and to learn from experience.'
>
> *(DoH 1999d, p53)*

A clear quality agenda for consultant practitioners is therefore set, but the selling point of these posts does not rest on leadership and quality issues alone; there is also a significant emphasis on career development opportunities for nurses, midwives and health visitors. The strategy also explicitly addresses a perceived need to retain senior and experienced staff:

'These posts will provide a new opportunity for experienced and expert nurses, midwives and health visitors who wish to remain in practice to do so. These posts significantly extend the career ladder enabling those nurses, midwives and health visitors who might otherwise have entered management or left the profession to advance their careers and improve their pay'.

(DoH 1999d, p32)

CAREER PROGRESSION

The Department of Health view fits with the received wisdom that, historically, nurses who wish to progress their career beyond the level of senior sister have found their choices restricted to predominantly non-clinical roles in management or, if not in management, then in education or occasionally research. Once started along one of these career paths, it has been increasingly difficult for some nurses to go back to the bedside. The reasons for this might include the lack of financial incentive as identified in *Making a Difference* (DoH 1999d).

REFLECTION POINT
Stop for a moment and think whether you might in future years be tempted to move into a nursing role that is less 'hands-on'; alternatively, what might induce you to stay at the bedside?

It is reasonable to speculate that other likely disincentives to return to the bedside might include: the physically strenuous nature of some of the work, unsocial shift patterns, child care issues and fluctuating levels of morale within the profession. A gradual loss of practice in clinical skills might also add distance from direct caring if nurse managers, educators and researchers channel and increase their skills in other directions. Nurses who are simply taking a career break for family or other reasons face a similar range of constraints and choices when deciding whether to resume a hands-on role. But it is pay which tends to have the highest profile, when concerns about the attrition rate are aired, with salary often gaining headlines in the popular nursing and general press. This, in turn, reflects and informs public perception of the key factors which underlie the problems with retention of qualified nurses. For example, following a recent above-inflation pay award, the popular nursing press continued to take up the issue of pay at all levels of the profession, and to draw on comparisons of pay levels with other public services to support their argument.

POTENTIAL BENEFITS OF CONSULTANCY

The development of consultant roles was embedded within political issues from its inception, and the pay issue is one of the most visible of these, capturing sympathetic public interest and providing a quantifiable demonstration of political interest. It would be wrong, though, to conclude that general interest in consultant nursing, midwifery and health visiting is only about pay.

The public

Popularly, the new consultants were tagged 'supernurses' and there was much publicity about their high level skills and discussion about how they might be effective. The NHS vision of the benefits of consultant posts was as part of a 'package of measures to help improve quality and services' (NHS Executive 1999b), but public expectation may well be caught by more specific potential benefits of the posts. There has been tremendous public support for higher rewards for nurses, as discussed above. These new roles are also likely to be perceived as high profile, leadership figures who inspire confidence that standards are being raised at the bedside – as with the concept of 'matron', the consultant is likely to have popular appeal as a role with a mandate directly to improve care. Accountability, visibility and leadership are all qualities that are meaningful to the public and press when care standards are at issue. Consultant nurses, midwives and health visitors may be popularly envisaged as champions of the patient and the service. Although on a darker note, as one consultant nurse, new to post, recently remarked to the author, '…and when there is some major catastrophe in the hospital, will it be my name on the headlines of the local press?'

Nurses

For aspiring consultant practitioners, the opportunity to expand and apply clinical skills and take responsibility for decision-making might be as much, if not more, of an incentive to apply for the consultant post than the opportunity to earn a higher salary. Career development opportunities mean more than money. Consultant practitioners may in some circumstances take on responsibilities such as the admission and discharge of patients, acceptance and making of referrals, and prescribing, all of which add extra dimensions and challenges to their role. The opportunity to take on a consultant level role also offers recognition of the practitioner's experience, knowledge and skills. The acquisition, through many sources of learning and practice, of academic, practical and personal knowledge may not be fully embodied in a formal qualification. The consultant *title* and *role* offers a meaningful endorsement of practitioners' abilities to make senior, professional decisions and judgements and to apply their accumulated knowledge and skills.

Patients

For patients, benefits include access to nurses, midwives and health visitors whose skills are enhanced and enabled. Consultant posts provide patient access to recognized expert nursing advice and care, including care within the framework of nurse-led services. Consultant posts in speciality areas of traditional nursing expertise, such as stoma care, palliative care and pain control, all offer patients access to specific expert practitioners, with confidence that they are receiving what is recognized by the service as being the highest level care and advice.

NHS EXECUTIVE GUIDANCE ON CONSULTANT POSTS

Much of the above discussion of the potential benefits of consultancy in nursing, midwifery and health visiting is pure speculation. More objectively, the launch of the roles was accompanied by a formal outline of how the roles would be structured and how the consultants would be expected to make a difference to patient services.

Following the publication of *Making a Difference* (DoH 1999d) and the Prime Minister's initial announcement that nurse, midwife and health visitor consultant posts were to be created, some specifics about the consultant roles were set out in a circular issued by the NHS Executive for action by health authorities, NHS trusts, primary care groups and regions (NHS Executive 1999b). This outlined the core components of the posts:

- an expert practice function
- a professional leadership and consultancy function
- an education, training and development function
- a practice and service development, research and evaluation function.

While detailed job descriptions were left to local determination, the guidance clearly set out that at least 50% of each post was to be used in working directly with patients, clients or communities. This specification was a landmark in the development of senior nursing roles, in that it defined a practice function as one in which the practitioner must work clinically, i.e. directly with patients – a parallel with medical consultants who work a number of clinical 'sessions' each week, seeing and treating patients.

Expert practice function

The expert practice function of consultant nurses, midwives and health visitors was described as including a number of possible features:

- making and receiving referrals
- exercising independent or delegated prescribing rights
- drawing on advanced knowledge and exercising clinical skills of the highest order
- exercising a high degree of professional autonomy
- making critical judgements of the highest order
- making decisions where precedents do not exist
- advising and supporting colleagues where standard protocols do not apply.

From this list of features, it is hard to imagine a consultant nurse, midwife or health visitor whose approach to practice was 'hands-off' or indirect. Later in this chapter, three examples are described of a practising consultant's work; these illustrate how the NHS Executive guidelines have been interpreted by employers and implemented within practice by practitioners.

Professional leadership and consultancy function

In addition to working directly with patients, the new consultant posts were described as providing a professional leadership and consultancy function. The issue of leadership has already been identified as central to the NHS vision of developing patient services and quality. It could be argued that without this component, the role of consultant practitioner could be difficult to distinguish from other senior roles, such as nurse practitioner, lecturer–practitioner or specialist nurse. Consultant leadership has a crucial role in setting and improving standards, and helping to deliver better services. The NHS guidance specifies that this is to be achieved by working with colleagues at a number of levels, providing expert advice to individuals or teams, and providing consultancy across the wider organization and across organizational boundaries. This is an interesting development for a profession whose practitioners largely work within a defined caseload or unit, and who, with the exception of senior managers, have had little opportunity for influencing strategic planning or working across organizations. The examples given later also illustrate the extent to which consultants are making this happen within different specialities.

REFLECTION POINT

Take a few minutes to write down what the roles of nurse practitioner, lecturer–practitioner or specialist nurse mean. Have you come across these types of practitioners? What do you think they might do?

Education, training and development function

The education, training and development function emphasizes the role consultants could develop in educating and teaching, with a strong emphasis on forming links with universities, possibly as joint appointments. A joint appointment is a job that is split between two organizations, with the postholder spending a proportion of their time working for each one. A joint appointment is one of the examples described below of a current consultant role. It is compared with the role of lecturer–practitioner, which is another type of joint appointment. It will be suggested that under some circumstances, roles such as lecturer–practitioner could provide a route for some practitioners to develop towards consultant. Currently there is no specific training or formal preparation for the role of consultant nurse, midwife or health visitor. This is why it is not a registerable or recordable qualification with the regulatory bodies. The availability of suitably prepared consultants is an important issue for future development of the role.

Practice and service development, research and evaluation

The fourth role function, practice and service development, research and evaluation is closely tied in with professional leadership and consultancy. Consultants are described as:

'… working at the forefront of practice innovation – drawing on their professional knowledge and expertise to determine how to deal with ambiguous, unique, or novel problems, creating precedents and generating, monitoring and evaluating practice protocols…'

(NHS Executive 1999b, p5)

Involvement in practice development and clinical governance and working at the forefront of quality innovations cannot be achieved without high level leadership skills and the ability to work across organizations. Expectations of consultants' involvement in research and evaluation are correspondingly high:

'Consultant practitioners will have a track record of scholarship and the appraisal and application of research in practice; and in many cases formal research expertise'.

(NHS Executive 1999b, p8)

With nursing research arguably not enjoying as high a profile and reputation as medical research, consultant practitioners are likely to be expected to add credibility to nursing research within their specialities, both by carrying out their own research, and by assimilating research evidence into practice, and disseminating findings to other practitioners.

The author has suggested that nursing research does not enjoy a very high profile in comparison with medical research. This is quite a controversial statement – what do you think of the profile of nursing research? Is it just down to consultant practitioners to raise the profile?

SUMMARY

- The vision for consultant posts is set out in *Making a Difference (DoH 1999d)*.
- Clinical leadership and raising standards of care are fundamental to the posts.
- Consultant posts provide a career opportunity for nurses to remain by – or return to – the bedside.
- There is a strong political agenda around consultancy.
- The NHS Executive has defined four core components of consultant posts: an expert practice function; a professional leadership and consultancy function; an education, training and development function; and a practice and service development, research and evaluation function, with 50% of time to be spent in clinical practice.

WHAT IS CONSULTANCY?

DEFINITION

As discussed above, the NHS Executive (1999b) provides an outline of the components of the consultant nurse, midwife and health visitor role, including a 'professional leadership and consultancy function'. Implicit features of the consultancy function include the provision of expert advice, both within and outside the profession, acting as a resource, setting standards, developing practice and influencing strategic planning. In addition, the consultant nurse, midwife or health visitor role is described as including functions in education, research and clinical practice; altogether this is a very broad role definition which goes beyond narrow or basic definitions of *consultant* or *consultancy*.

The *Collins English Dictionary* defines a consultant as:

'a physician, esp. a specialist, who is asked to confirm a diagnosis … a physician or surgeon holding the highest appointment in a particular branch of medicine or surgery in a hospital … a specialist who gives expert advice or information.… a person who asks advice in a consultation'.

Compared with the dictionary definition, consultancy in nursing, midwifery and health visiting is indeed a much broader concept. The dictionary definition describes an expert advice element and this can be seen to fit part of the consultant practitioner role. Second, there is also an analogy between the doctor's role in diagnosis in medicine and that of the expert nurse, midwife or health visitor who confirms a nursing problem. Third, the notion of the consultant practitioner being at the highest level of practice concurs with the dictionary definition of the consultant holding the highest appointment in a branch of medicine or surgery in a hospital.

SCOPE OF SETTINGS OF THE CONSULTANT ROLE

In other ways, the consultant nurse, midwife and health visitor goes far beyond this definition, in terms of both the components of the role and the scope of settings in which they might work. The consultant nurse, midwife and health visitor has the four role functions outlined above. Consultant practitioners work within critical care, mental health, chronic disease management, child health and many other areas of health care. The distribution of consultant practitioner posts also extends beyond the boundaries of hospitals into primary care – consultant practitioners currently work in primary care services, such as intermediate care and nurse-led walk-in centres, as well as a range of posts within acute and community hospitals.

MANAGEMENT CONSULTANT

A different type of consultant, employed by health services from time to time, is the management consultant, who is contracted to advise on organizational rather than clinical issues. This is a very different model of consultancy, since it relates to advising or solving problems on specific projects or issues; it is time-limited, purchased on an ad-hoc basis and independently provided. The NHS nurse, midwife and health visitor consultants are employed by and accountable to the NHS, mostly on full-time contracts. In this case also, the NHS consultant role functions would appear far to exceed that of most forms of intermittent or short contract consultancy.

CONCEPTS AND MODELS OF CONSULTANCY IN THE GENERAL AND MEDICAL LITERATURE

Consultant as technical adviser

There is quite a large general literature on consultancy but little of it discusses the new type of NHS nursing, midwifery and health visiting consultancy. Within health and social care, Gallessich (1982a) describes the basic role of the consultant as that of technical adviser. Interestingly, she suggests that consultants may or may not assume the role of healer (Gallessich 1982a, p104). This description is partly contradicted by the new roles; the expert practice component of a consultant nurse, midwife or health visitor is described by the NHS Executive (1999b) as spending 50% of the time in direct contact with patients, clients or communities. While this is not defined as a 'healing' role, it could be argued that it is analogous to it because direct client contact is highly likely to include a therapeutic component. Gallessich's implication that consultants do not always have this therapeutic component is therefore now out of date – the definition and expectations of consultancy in nurse, midwife and health visitor practice have developed and changed since the 1980s. Where Gallessich's model of consultancy does have more resonance with the NHS model is in the way in which consultants may effect change in the consultee or in which the consultee effects changes in their work. NHS consultants are expected to '... exercise leadership to support and inspire colleagues' (NHS Executive 1999b, p7) and therefore are likely to influence and effect changes in their colleagues and the way in which they work.

Consultant models

Elsewhere, Gallessich (1982b) makes links with the concept of professionalization and describes six models of the consultant:

- consultant as educator and trainer
- clinical consultant
- mental health consultant
- behavioural consultant
- organizational consultant
- programme consultant.

The consultant nurse, midwife or health visitor role, as outlined earlier in this chapter, probably fits elements of all these models but the overall emergent model in the NHS is different. This is hardly surprising since the NHS model reflects both the needs and expectations of the health service in the 21st century and the perceptions and expectations of politicians, employees and the public. It has drawn on previous literature and models of consultant roles but has been shaped by many factors, expectations and constraints. This is why the literature alone does not provide a full picture of where the new NHS roles have come from, or where they are at. There is, however, a small specific literature on nurse consultancy, and this will now be considered.

CONCEPTS AND MODELS OF NURSE CONSULTANCY IN THE NURSING LITERATURE

Differentiating consultancy from pre-existing roles

Earlier it was suggested that one of the issues in defining consultancy within nursing, midwifery and health visiting is that of differentiating it from pre-existing roles, such as nurse practitioner, nurse specialist and lecturer–practitioner. This is supported by Wright (1992) who suggests that many nurses within the NHS, such as managers, teachers, clinical specialists, sisters and charge nurses, have previously acted in a consultant capacity, without actually adopting the title of consultant. He suggests that this capacity has been manifested in terms of giving advice on nursing practice to others. It can be seen from this that difficulty in defining nursing roles is not a new issue, and that it is partly driven by opinion and subjectivity. Consultancy has probably formed an integral element of many types of nursing, midwifery and health visitor role in the past, but it has been informally defined or unacknowledged, unless the practitioner has set up independently as a consultant service. The new consultant roles have a more formal definition and explicit remit, which consequently makes it difficult to draw direct comparison with aspects of these other roles.

Leadership and breadth of role. It was suggested earlier that it is the leadership aspect of consultant practice which is key to understanding the difference between consultancy and some of these other roles. Another possible differentiating aspect is that of the breadth and level of the consultant role. Abley (2001), for example, emphasizes the significance of the level of strategic involvement that occurs in the role of consultant nurse for vulnerable adults. Strategic working involves the evaluation, planning and development of services, often at high levels within an organization and across organizational or professional boundaries. This type of work may be exhibited by other types of senior clinical roles, but the key difference is that it is not necessarily integral to all other roles or to be expected of them by definition. For example, there are aspects of some nurse specialist roles that are similar to those of some consultant practitioner roles, e.g. the expert advice function. Both the consultant and the specialist nurse might provide, in some cases, a similar level of expert advice on specific clinical issues and problems. It could be argued, however, that consultancy provides this expert advisor function much more broadly and at higher level, such as providing a higher level of advice and strategic input to organizations as a whole, and at a regional and national level.

Multi-dimensionality. The consultant role may also add more dimensions to practice than other types of practitioners. This multi-dimensionality of the consultant nurse role was modelled by Manley (1997) who identified the role as consisting of:

- expert practitioner
- educator, enabler and developer
- researcher
- expert and process consultant
- transformational leader.

She outlines a role which is weighted towards the second and fifth of these points, i.e. the consultant practitioner as a change agent, a role which transforms the organizational culture as a prerequisite towards quality (Manley 2000). Her view, then, is that the consultant practitioner is working at a high level and has an influence beyond their immediate client or patient caseload, across the clinical team, culture and organization within which they work. Manley's description of the dimensions of the consultant can be compared with the aims of a consultant nurse post cited by Wright (1992), which was set out by Johnson *et al.* (1989):

- to retain a senior nurse with a high level of clinical, educational, research and management expertise at clinical level
- to demonstrate and encourage excellence in nursing
- to support the conduct of nursing research at clinical level and application of findings
- to act as a resource person to clinical nurses and senior management as an expert in nursing practice for the elderly patient.

Manley's description of the consultant is far more explicit in its description of the leadership aspect of the role, in which she emphasizes the consultant's role in transforming organizational culture. The earlier model described by Johnson *et al.* (1989) leaves the leadership function more implicit, in that it aims for the consultant to model expert practice and advice, research and excellence in nursing.

Political implications of leadership

The elements identified by Manley and Wright all appear embedded in the vision for consultant practice set out in *Making a Difference* (DoH 1999d). It would seem that the leadership function has assumed a higher priority and profile over the past decade (DoH 1999d). This is partly political: the Labour government has developed a modernization programme and it relies on strong nursing, midwifery and health visiting leadership to achieve it (DoH 1999d, p52). The NHS agenda cannot be separated from politics and consultancy is embroiled within this.

Leadership issues are fundamentally important to consultant practice in the 21st century, but the concept of expert practice is also a strong theme which runs through the literature and manifests in a commitment for NHS consultant practitioners to spend at least 50% of their time engaged in clinical practice, working directly with patients, clients or communities.

EXPERT NURSING AND CONSULTANT PRACTICE

There is a large literature which attempts to identify what constitutes an 'expert' level of practice. The best known work is that of Benner (1984), who identifies attributes such as focusing on patient's problems and providing solutions, managing complex situations, and having vision. Benner's model is famously based upon a psychological model of how pilots learn; she has applied this to nursing, supported by analysis of interviews with nurses and observations of nursing practice. Nearly 20 years later, one of the four role functions of the new NHS consultant practitioner role is still described as 'expert practice' (see above).

REFLECTION POINT

Benner's model of skill acquisition is relevant to pre-registration nursing. She describes the development of skills from novice level, through advanced beginner to competent, proficient then expert level. 'Expert' is the highest level that she describes. Where do learner nurses sit on this hierarchy? Do you think it is possible for a learner to be an expert in some aspects of care, or for a consultant to be a novice?

Expert and consultant practice: an example

To explore in a little more depth what 'expert practice' is currently taken to mean, an extract from a NHS hospital trust's consultant nurse job description is shown in Box 19.1. It provides a few pointers as to how the consultant nurse is looked upon to provide expert professional judgements and opinion, particularly in this case in working in a multi-professional way and as an expert resource at organizational level. Benner's work suggests that it is a capacity to make high level decisions and solve patient-centred problems that distinguishes this level of practice from that of less experienced and skilled practitioners. The consultant nurse job description states that the post-holder will 'act as an adviser … within the Trust' and 'develop and lead nurse-led services…', both of which are activities which require the consultant to exercise high levels of professional judgement while applying their skills to patient-focused problems.

Box 19.1 Extract from a consultant nurse (health of older people) job description (Barnet and Chase Farm Hospitals NHS Trust, 2001)

- Be a clinical expert in the field of nursing, with a particular emphasis on the care of older people
- Determine therapeutic programmes of care, based on evidence, to improve health outcomes or quality of life following and during illness

- Demonstrate expertise in multi-professional working, and in the assessment, treatment, management and evaluation of patients, aimed at maximizing the individual's independence, to reduce hospital length of stay, improve quality of life and, where appropriate, enable patients to live at home/other residential setting
- Be effective in developing a robust network of professionals and organizations, working in partnership to meet the health care needs of older people
- Identify needs and promote the development of evidence-based nursing, integrating pathways and standards of care for nursing older people
- Act as an adviser for the care of older people in nursing within the Trust
- Promote cross-boundary working by co-ordinating all relevant agencies to ensure effective provision of care
- Develop and lead nurse-led services through demonstrating and exercising high degrees of professional autonomy
- Supply and administer a range of medicines under patient group directives
- Make and receive referrals

Higher level practice and consultant practice

Since Benner's work on expert practice, the UKCC (now the NMC) engaged in much debate around the nature of higher level practice, specifically about what may be termed either *advanced* or *higher level* practice. Advanced practice proved to be extremely elusive to define in terms of the tasks that a practitioner might perform. The UKCC's Advanced Practice Project resulted in a decision not to set standards for advanced practice. It made this decision on the grounds that advanced practice was not about tasks, but about a broader concept of nursing, midwifery and health visiting:

'…a checklist of standards would be in direct conflict with the dynamic and autonomous nature of advancing practice…'

(UKCC 1997)

Subsequently, the Higher Level Practice Pilot Project produced standards and competencies for higher level practice and at the time of press these are awaiting further consideration by the NMC as to their role in regulating practice, including that of consultant practitioners. The Report of the Higher Level of Practice (HLP) pilot (UKCC 2002) refers to the contribution that the HLP standard has made to the consultant nurse, midwife and health visitor initiatives across the four countries of the UK. The NHS guidance on the appointment of nurse, midwife and health visitor consultants states that:

'The UKCC's recent work on 'a higher level of practice' holds out the prospect of a system that will provide professional recognition – in the interests of public protection – denoting a threshold level of attainment and practice competence commensurate with minimum expectations for appointment to a consultant practitioner post, and could therefore serve as a helpful eligibility criterion'.

(NHS Executive 1999b, p9)

Although this UKCC project was carried out before the new NHS consultant posts were developed, and does not define the nature of *expert* practice, it is relevant and informative to the appointments that have been made. The HLP standard is not in itself a sufficient condition for appointment because the decision to appoint is based on a judgement about the candidate's experience, qualifications and current professional practice and whether or not these match the expectations of the post (NHS Executive 1999b, p9). Consultant practitioners are not required to demonstrate competency in specific tasks in order to define their practice as lying at a higher or expert level. This is endorsed by the HLP project report which states that:

'A higher level of practice has been clearly articulated in the form of a threshold and *generic* standard which. ... was applicable to all health care settings and described a *level* of practice, rather than a speciality or role'. (author's italics)

(UKCC 2002, p6)

This does not preclude specific role functions being outlined, such as in the job description in Box 19.1; in this case, part of the expert function is described as to 'supply and administer a range of medicines under patient group directives' – superficially a task, although in fact it is a role function, which is underpinned by considerable higher level knowledge and the exercise of a high degree of professional autonomy. This specific role function of the post is derived from directions given in the original Health Service Circular (NHS Executive 1999b).

Nursing practice is by its nature extremely complex and in the literature it has been theorized that nurses use many sources of knowledge (see, for example, Carper 1978) and deal with multiple tasks and demands when providing care. Although it may not be possible to break down expert practice into easily understood tasks, there is still a responsibility for practitioners to exercise professional accountability for their actions, and to demonstrate that their actions are effective.

Local competency frameworks

Consultant practitioners who are employed by the NHS must also account to their organizations for their activity, and participate in appraisal and review of their performance. As explained above, there are currently no nationally set specific standards or competencies for employers to use in appraising their new consultants. The generic higher level of practice standard and competencies, which may be used to develop eligibility criteria, may provide a future form of professional recognition, but these are awaiting consideration or adoption by the new NMC. Some employers may therefore choose to develop their own competency frameworks, which might be specific to the organization or to the speciality in which the consultant is based. An example is given in Table 19.1 of draft competencies for consultant nurses and midwives that were developed at King's College Hospital as part of the trust competency framework for nursing and midwifery staff in July 2000. This is used as a basis for individual competency generation.

Definition of competency

It will be seen that this attempt at specifying competencies at a consultant level is in fact quite general and parallels the job descriptions of the three case studies that follow. It is difficult to measure quantitatively how a practitioner 'takes the lead', or 'acts as the highest source of authority'. The literature on competency has not offered any universal definition of what competency itself means, let alone at an expert level. While *et al.* (1995) identify competence as something that a practitioner:

'... knows and can do under ideal circumstances, that is, potential; while performance is actual situation behaviour, that is, what is done in the real life context.'

Table 19.1 Extract from a local competency framework (King's Healthcare NHS Trust)

Nursing and midwifery professional competency area	Draft competency level for consultant practitioner
Delivery of care	Takes the lead within the trust and demonstrates advanced professional independence in an area of practice
	Acts as the highest source of authority and specialist expertise within the trust, setting and monitoring standards of practice
	Formulates local, and influences the setting of national, policy, guidelines and procedures related to an area of professional nursing/midwifery practice

The UKCC used the term competence to describe: '… the skills and ability to practise safely and effectively without the need for direct supervision…' (UKCC Commission for Nursing and Midwifery Education 1999). This is the level of competence that is expected of all qualified nurses and applies to consultant practitioners as well as to newly qualified staff nurses. In the terms of pre-registration nurse training, the UKCC further stated that 'the outcomes and competencies expressed will be achieved under the direction of a registered nurse'. Competency statements can give access to evaluation and appraisal of a practitioner's performance in clinical practice, but have been criticised on the grounds of whether they accurately assess the range of qualities required of nurses (Ashworth and Morrison 1991). As practitioners become more advanced and work at higher levels and in increasingly complex ways, it is likely to become more difficult to analyse and articulate what they do in the phraseology of competency or performance indicators. As pointed out earlier, there is a subjective element in defining nursing roles – finding ways of evaluating objectively the new roles is a challenge that both employer and practitioner will have to meet.

REFLECTION POINT

Take a few minutes to think about what competency means to you and what you have to achieve in order to qualify as a registered nurse. How do these draft competencies for consultant nurses compare with the UKCC's competencies for care delivery (UKCC 2001a)?

SUMMARY

- Consultant nurse, midwife and health visitor roles are broader than traditional medical or surgical consultant roles.
- The consultant practitioner roles are different from management consultants.
- The new consultant nurses, midwives and health visitors are employed by the NHS.
- The new roles have formalized the concept within nursing, midwifery and health visiting.
- Consultant level practice is distinguishable from that of specialist level partly by the leadership function and strategic level at which consultants work.
- Benner (1984) described 'expert' level as a capacity to make high level decisions and solve patient-centred problems.

- Expert practice is difficult to analyse and express as performance indicators or competencies.
- The UKCC (now NMC) set a higher level practice (HLP) standard, which is recommended by the NHS Executive guidance on consultant appointments as a 'helpful eligibility criterion'.
- Employers may set local, specific competencies.

CONSULTANT NURSING: SOME CASE STUDIES

Consultant nurses and midwives now work within a wide range of health care, both within primary care and hospitals. The guidance that was issued on the consultant posts outlined the four role functions of the consultant practitioner, but in practice these functions will inevitably be manifested and interpreted in different ways. To give an example of this, Table 19.2 provides summary descriptions of three different consultant nurse roles. These are drawn from the individual job description of each post.

- Case 1 is drawn from the job description of the author's post as a full time consultant nurse in health care of older people in a London teaching hospital.
- Case 2 outlines more detail of the consultant role which was described earlier (Table 19.1); this consultant also works within the speciality of health care of older people, but the post is structured as a joint appointment with a university and therefore can be described as a senior lecturer–consultant practitioner role.
- Case 3 is that of a consultant nurse in pain management.

Each role is described within the role functions defined by the NHS Executive, which formed a starting point for all the new consultant roles. The way in which each job description interprets each role is, however, unique.

COMPARISON BETWEEN JOB DESCRIPTIONS

In Table 19.2, the original wording of the consultants' job descriptions has been retained as closely as possible. The terminology varies slightly across the three job descriptions, but it is possible to identify key features and discrepancies within each role function. For example, within the expert practice function, posts 1 and 3 specify that the consultant will hold a caseload of patients, while post 2 does not. This post, by contrast, is quite specific that the expert practice function will include, 'Supply and administer a range of medicines under patient group directions', a specification which is absent from the other two job descriptions. By not holding a named caseload of patients, it could be queried whether a consultant practitioner is fulfilling the requirement to spend 50% of their time working directly with patients, clients or communities. In this case, however, the post-holder fulfils her clinical commitments in a different way. Her clinical work is largely generated through referrals for consultation and expert practice with patients across the hospital in which she is based, including the accident and emergency department and medical wards. These patients may not form part of an ongoing caseload, since consultation may be made on an ad-hoc basis, without clinic or bedside follow-up necessarily

Table 19.2 Summary descriptions of three consultant nurse roles

Functions of the consultant nurse as identified by the NHS Executive	Case 1: Consultant nurse in health care of older people	Case 2: Senior lecturer–consultant practitioner in health care of older people	Case 3: Consultant nurse in pain management
Expert practice function	Hold a caseload of patients where the main need is nursing, in collaboration with the multi-disciplinary team, acting as the highest level of nursing authority Provide high quality advanced health care to patients Contribute to the development of co-operative working between different professions and teams	Clinical expert in the field of nursing, determine therapeutic programmes of care, develop and lead nurse-led services Promote cross-boundary working and demonstrate expertise in multi-professional working Be effective in developing a robust network of professionals and organisations Identify needs and promote development of evidence-based nursing Act as an adviser within the Trust Supply and administer a range of medicines under patient group directions Make and receive referrals	Hold a caseload of patients referred from hospital doctors, GPs and community/primary care nursing teams, for whom she/he is responsible Accountability for care will be shared between the nurse consultant and the referrer and close communication links will need to be established

Professional leadership and consultancy function	Anticipate and identify key team strategic issues facing the speciality	Lead practice and professional development	To take the lead in identifying gaps in service provision arising from unmet need and to ensure that these are raised and solutions sought
	Subsequently to act as a facilitator in managing change, ensuring full involvement of multi-disciplinary team members	Lead changes in the area of systems and processes for the effective referral and assessment of patients for rehabilitation	Act as a role model and work with health care teams in their settings, assessing and managing clients who present with pain
	Make creative decisions, demonstrating ability to analyse the local and strategic implications of decision-making	Inspire, facilitate and support colleagues	To lead, in collaboration with the multi-disciplinary team, a regular audit programme of practices and procedures, assessment tools and treatment strategies for pain relief
	Develop the skills and expertise of senior team members	Work collaboratively with other health care professionals	To develop communication networks to support practitioners and practice development and lead workshops, seminars and conferences to share and promote excellence in practice
		Be an innovative, creative leader	
		Contribute to the corporate clinical governance agenda	
		Develop and promote partnership working in inter-professional health care	
		Contribute to formulating strategy for service development	
		Value the contributions of all colleagues	
		Compare and share best clinical practice	
Education, training and development function	Link with relevant education establishments	Work in partnership with the university network and collaborate with other centres of excellence and departments	To have close links with the university and to teach formally on courses where pain assessment and management are an integral component, developing curricula jointly with the university
	Identify educational and development opportunities with external agencies with the aim of improving cross-boundary working	Contribute to the education training and development of others	

(Continued)

Table 19.2 (*Continued*)

Functions of the consultant nurse as identified by the NHS Executive	Case 1: Consultant nurse in health care of older people	Case 2: Senior lecturer–consultant practitioner in health care of older people	Case 3: Consultant nurse in pain management
	Develop education and training to enable nurses and colleagues to achieve the required competencies Utilize research knowledge as a basis for improving standards of practice within the speciality	Liaise with clinical managers in relation to educational initiatives Lead a culture of continuous improvement and practice development in nursing Act as a mentor and clinical supervisor Lead environments for lifelong learning	To hold regular sessions for both hospital and community/primary care teams to develop pain assessment and management skills to benefit patient care
Practice and service development, research and evaluation function	Set a clear direction on service planning, and lead in discussions on the requirements of the nursing service Formulate local policy within the department and disseminate best practice through the trust Influence the setting of national policy, guidelines and procedures in relation to the care of older people Develop links with external agencies To commission independently research studies within own area of personal expertise	Review current systems and processes for referral and assessment Work with patients, carers and community groups in delivering patient/user-responsive services Initiate research into key functions of the nurse's role Create a culture of research Ensure that the fundamental and essential benchmarks are applied Actively disseminate through publishing, regional, national and international networks	To ensure that good quality data is available on patient outcomes and demographics which will be available for audit or research requirements Ensure that information and advice is available to clients, carers and colleagues on the range and accessibility of services for the assessment, management and strategies for pain relief on both a formal and informal basis To participate actively in research and to identify areas requiring further investigation

being made, but they form the core of her clinical work. The original guidance on the composition of the consultant roles, while stating that the posts should be constructed so that at least half the time is available to patients, clients or communities, does not actually specify that this should be organized within an ongoing caseload.

In the professional leadership and consultancy function, multi-disciplinary and partnership working is a shared theme, within an expression of various examples of leadership and change management.

A further difference between the posts is in the education, training and development function; the pain management post specifies that the consultant nurse will '... teach formally on courses where pain assessment and management are an integral component ...'. This post is not set up as a lecturer–consultant post in the way that post 2 is, yet it has a strong formalized education component. The post-holder contributes to formal university teaching on a regular basis. Post 1, by contrast, specifies a link with relevant education establishments but does not indicate a formal university teaching component to the post.

FROM JOB DESCRIPTION TO OBJECTIVES: INTERPRETING GUIDELINES AND DESCRIPTIONS IN PRACTICE

Specific cases

While job descriptions give an outline of what functions an organization wishes the postholder to fulfil, the interpretation of the job description into practice depends upon the individual and their work environment. The author's experience of developing a consultant role is one of evolution and challenge, with many choices to be made about actions to be undertaken: time management is a major issue, especially in terms of deciding where clinical time is best directed. Expert practice, in her case, has evolved to include running nurse-led clinics based in a day hospital, as well as providing nursing advice to the acute and rehabilitation inpatient services for older people. This advice is accessed and offered at a range of levels within the trust:

- provision of advice on the care of individual inpatients who have complex care needs
- assessment, planning and implementation of specialist care of individual clinic patients
- advice at a trust-wide level on service development and identification of the local nursing agenda in caring for older people.

By comparison, the consultant nurse in case 2 has developed a broader role, as discussed above, which offers advice on the care of older patients on medical wards and in the A&E department, but does not include a clinic or formal patient caseload. The pain consultant nurse cited in case 3 runs a clinic and holds a caseload of patients, but works more closely with primary care colleagues than either of the other consultants. All three consultant nurses describe their work as being highly involved proportionally across all four areas of the role functions, although this does not seem to be the case nationally (see below).

The national picture

A broader picture of the work of consultant practitioners is provided by a recent preliminary evaluation of the establishment of nurse, midwife and health visitor consultants, in which Guest *et al.* (2001)

surveyed all consultants in post in February 2001. This study provides an initial evaluation of the progress in setting up and working in the role, and offers an objective insight into the diversity of experiences of the new consultants and how they have assimilated the functions of the role into practice.

Guest *et al.* found that most consultants were involved across all four role functions: expert practice; professional leadership and consultancy; education, training and development; research and evaluation. Consultants rated the most important roles to be within the category of *leadership* followed by *expert practice*, and these were the categories in which they had the highest level of involvement. The average time spent with patients was 44%, which is close to the 50% practice commitment specified by the NHS Executive.

Role engagement. Of particular interest was Guest *et al.*'s analysis of role engagement of consultants, i.e. the variety of patterns of activity that consultants undertake. Initially they identified what they called 'super-specialist' and 'designer–developer roles'. The 'super-specialist' role has been described as a focused specialist consultant who undertakes advanced and technical clinical practice, manages a caseload of patients, accepts referrals, discharges patients and works closely with doctors. The 'designer–developer', while still a clinical expert, might have a broader role which includes a stronger emphasis on practice development and organizational change; a visionary who engages in inter-agency and cross-boundary collaboration (S. Redfern, personal communication, 2001). This dual model is not, however, fully representative of how the consultant roles have emerged over their first year: Guest *et al.*'s further analysis has identified five role profiles which can be summarized as:

- *high involvement profile* (18% of posts): high involvement across most of the four areas of activity
- *dual focus profile* (19%): high involvement in two of the main areas, but medium or low in the other two
- *single focus profile* (29%): concentrating high involvement in one area while the rest are medium or low
- *medium involvement profile* (14%): medium activity in two areas and low engagement in the other two
- *low involvement profile* (22%): low level of engagement in at least three of the areas and no more than moderate engagement in the other.

Guest *et al.* suggest that there is considerable variation in practice among consultants. The three individual consultant roles discussed above probably fit within the high involvement profile, but it would seem from Guest *et al.*'s survey that this is not the norm for all consultant posts.

Level of involvement in previous job. Guest *et al.* further suggest that any differences between consultants' practice are associated with levels of involvement in the post-holder's previous job, i.e. those who were already doing these activities in a previous job were more likely to be doing them in their present job. The survey report does not provide examples of this, but the idea can be explored by relating one of the specific cases presented above to the role this consultant held previously.

The senior lecturer–consultant practitioner working in health care of older people previously held the post of lecturer–practitioner. She describes her consultant role as being similar to her role as a lecturer–practitioner, but more extended and higher powered, with a larger range of clinical problems to solve. She describes her lecturer–practitioner role as a 'wonderful training ground' for the post that she currently holds. A comparison between the two roles is presented in Table 19.3. This contrasts the practice, leadership and consultancy aspects of the two roles.

Table 19.3 Comparison of aspects of the role of lecturer–practitioner and senior lecturer–consultant practitioner

Role function	Lecturer–practitioner role	Senior lecturer–consultant practitioner role
Expert practice, professional leadership and consultancy	Advisor, implementation of evidence-based practice	Advisor, implementation of evidence-based practice
	Implementation of evidence-based practice is influenced by research awareness, clinical knowledge and experience, high level professional judgement, involvement with patients and carers, and by local level involvement in policy issues	Implementation of evidence-based practice is influenced by research awareness, clinical knowledge and experience, high level professional judgement, involvement with patients and carers, and by local, regional and national level of involvement in policy issues
	Local leadership function with limited involvement in strategic planning and work beyond unit level	Strong local leadership function which also extends into involvement at high level within the organization, and contribution to regional and national level practice and policy development

This consultant has raised the level of her practice and involvement from that of a lecturer–practitioner, so that she is engaged within more levels of her organization, providing higher level leadership and influence than before, and contributing more significantly to strategic planning and policy issues.

The role of lecturer–practitioner has been modelled by Newman *et al.* (2001), in terms of the implementation of the four components of evidence-based practice: research evidence, patient preferences, utilization of professional expertise and utilization of available resources. The senior lecturer–consultant practitioner described above, has continued to engage in implementation of evidence-based practice, but has significantly raised the level at which she engages, crossing over into regional and national involvement, and increasing her influence and leadership at all levels. Her consultancy function has built upon her experiences as a local advisor and clinical expert, and her education, development and research activities have also developed from a basis that was laid down in the previous role. This example would seem to support Guest *et al.*'s (2001) suggestion that level of involvement as a consultant depends upon level of involvement in the consultant's previous job.

SUMMARY

- Consultant posts are structured around the four role functions but each is interpreted uniquely.
- Consultants may hold a caseload of patients but the way in which they organize their clinical work varies according to the trust, speciality and post-holder.

- Three role profiles describe how practising consultants allocate their time across the role functions.
- The senior lecturer–consultant practitioner practices at a higher level than lecturer–practitioner, although there are some similarities in how evidence-based practice is promoted by both roles.

FUTURE DEVELOPMENT OF CONSULTANT ROLES: WHERE NEXT?

The question that the author is often asked about her job, and hears asked of others is, 'Where next?' Now that the structure of nursing has been extended to include this new, highest level, will there be any further level to achieve, or different direction for professional practice to take in the future? Within medicine and surgery, the consultant post is, as the dictionary definition quoted earlier states: '… the highest appointment in a particular branch of medicine or surgery in a hospital'. As a clinician, the consultant physician or surgeon does not usually move on to a higher level. They remain the expert clinician and leader, heading up their team or firm, responsible for the treatment of their caseload of patients. In adopting the same terminology for the highest level of practice, it could be suggested that nursing practice may finally have reached its highest level. By its own definition, consultancy in nursing involves demonstration of an expert level of practice – and there is currently no higher definition of clinical practice than that of expert to achieve.

EXPECTATIONS AND PERCEPTIONS

The survey by Guest *et al.* (2001) asked consultant nurses for their perceptions, experiences and evaluations of the consultant role. When the rewards of the role were identified, 80% of those surveyed reported that the role provided high personal growth and development opportunities. Furthermore, 52% believed that the job had good career opportunities, although the type of opportunities were not specified. One way of exploring consultants' current expectations of their career development is to examine their support networks and learning sets, and form an unscientific feel for this from their reflections and discussions. A facilitator of a consultant nurse action learning set in the London region recently provided an opinion on her group's expectations (E. Hedgecock, personal communication, 2002). She suggests that many consultant nurses and midwives express relief at 'being out of the managerial chain' and has some interesting speculations to offer on future possible role developments – perhaps into an equivalent role to medical director, or new strategic, regional level roles.

FUTURE HEALTH POLICY AND ITS INFLUENCE

As leaders within their clinical specialisms, it is probably partly up to the consultants themselves to shape their future roles and careers, should consultancy in itself not be seen as the end of the line. However, the political agenda that was identified earlier should not be forgotten; although nurses have been able to develop consultant-type roles for some time, it was not until the publication of *Making a Difference* (DoH 1999d) and the announcement by the Prime Minister, that NHS consultant practitioner roles were formalized and able to proliferate. Future role developments may well be constrained by political imperatives and either expedited or inhibited according to the way that the political wind might blow. Health policy is fickle; terms of government in the UK last a maximum 5 years, and within this time, the government must implement its policies, please the electorate and hope to be re-elected to govern for a further term. Nurses have to believe that they are part of the vehicle by which each government delivers its agenda, because their future roles partly depend upon the will of ministers and the political importance of nursing itself.

A related issue, which may either constrain or enable the appointment of further consultant practitioners, is that of resources. Funding within the NHS is dependent upon health policy, and the future of roles such as nurse, midwife and health visitor consultants is crucially dependent upon resources – with the average salary of a consultant nurse in 2001 being £34,000, NHS trusts have to be convinced that the value of a consultant post is effective in financial terms compared to that of other, cheaper, front-line staff.

The future for consultancy in nursing is not all in the lap of the politicians. Professional nurses may chose to practice independently as consultants, as they have always been able to do. Also, consultant nurses have already made their mark on nursing and potentially have a significant role to play in shaping the future of nursing developments. To be more concrete about the contribution that consultants are making to patient care, however, there is a need to carry out further evaluation and research into the roles and to be clear about what consultancy and expert practice really mean, and what impact the new roles are having on practice development, education and research.

PREPARATION AND DEVELOPMENT OF FUTURE CONSULTANTS

A final issue which will shape the supply and demand for future consultants is that of preparation and development into the role. Experience of roles such as specialist nurse or lecturer–practitioner may provide some useful preparation, but currently there are no pre-requisite posts or courses which qualify a nurse, midwife or health visitor to be a consultant practitioner. The NHS guidance is clear that there is no intention to develop or specify any particular programme of study as preparation for a consultant nurse, midwife or health visitor post. The expectation is, nonetheless, that these practitioners will be qualified and experienced to a high level:

'The nature of consultant practitioner posts will demand a portfolio of career-long learning, experience and formal education, usually up to or beyond master's degree level; research experience and a record of scholarship and publication will become the norm for appointments of this sort.'

(NHS Executive 1999b, p8)

With the initial registered nurse qualification in England set at diploma level, it can be seen that there is significant academic progression required for nurses who ultimately aspire to consultant level. The availability of future consultants crucially hinges on the provision of access for qualified nurses to higher education, research and publication. This partly requires motivation and aspiration on the part of individual practitioners, but also needs the support of employers – both non-NHS and NHS trusts – higher education and the political process to ensure that the resources are in place at every level to facilitate the progression of aspiring consultant practitioners.

SUMMARY

- Most consultant practitioners report that the role has high personal growth and development opportunities, despite there being no current career structure beyond consultant.
- Future development of nursing roles is constrained by the fickle nature of political agendas; resource issues are an important factor.
- Preparation for consultant posts is not formalized.

CONCLUSION

This chapter has provided an overview of the literature and policy background on consultant nurses, and a summary of the current establishment of consultant posts. Consultancy in nursing would appear to be emerging with a broader model than medical and other types of consultancy, and with a strong emphasis on expert level practice, leadership, strategic working, practice development, education and research. It is a multi-dimensional role and one which demands a highly skilled and experienced practitioner to fulfil it. It has been suggested that there are two basic models of the consultant practitioner, with potentially several different variants emerging from that.

By exploring the cases of three different real-life NHS consultant posts, it has been shown that while they share four basic role functions, there is variation in the ways in which individual consultants interpret their roles, and in the way that different organizations define the roles in the first place.

There is currently little formal evaluation of consultant nurse, midwife and health visitor roles, and for this reason this exploration and discussion has probably been somewhat subjective in places, certainly reflecting the views of the author, who is herself a practising consultant nurse. This lack of scientific evidence of role evaluation is inevitable while the roles of consultant practitioners are in their infancy. It is important for the future development of nursing, midwifery and health visiting roles that further research and evaluation of these is carried out.

It is hoped that this chapter has given a feel for what might be possible, rather than what has to be, and that practitioners of the future will see themselves, too, as potential pioneers of new nursing roles. As a final personal view, Box 19.2 offers the author's account of a day in her working life. This is intended to give just a glimpse into the reality of a consultant nurse's role, seen through the activity of a typical working day.

Box 19.2 A day in the working life of a consultant nurse for older people

07.30	I arrive at my office, have a cup of tea and prepare my day. I finish preparing a presentation ready for a conference I have been invited to speak at in a few weeks' time. The presentation is about nursing and health policy for older people.
08.30	Research meeting. I am leading a research project into the use of hip protectors with older inpatients. (Hip protectors are a type of customized underwear which prevents hip fracture if the person falls.) I meet regularly with the project nurse and other members of the research team.

09.30   Clinical work. This is one of my fixed clinical sessions on our acute assessment unit for older peo-ple. I spend two sessions per week here (two mornings). My role on the unit is to provide consul-tancy, in the form of expert nursing practice and advice. I work closely with the consultant geriatrician and all other members of the multi-professional team. Any member of the team can refer patients to me for advice.

         Part of my role on the unit is to lead a multi-disciplinary review meeting once a week. Patient goals and discharge plans are set and reviewed at this meeting. The senior house officer, physio-therapist, occupational therapist and staff nurse attend today's meeting.

         After the review meeting, I work with patients. For example, one patient I see was admitted last night, and has complex care needs. This patient has severe pain from an ischaemic right leg, mul-tiple necrotic ulcers, and high risk of complications due to reduced mobility, poor nutritional state, urinary incontinence and depression. I work with the patient and staff nurse to prioritize prob-lems, review nursing management and to provide care. I refer to the pain team and tissue viabil-ity nurse specialist. I also talk to the patient's relatives. I have a 'hands-on' approach, but it is the ward-based nursing team who provide ongoing care, therefore I work with them, advising, role modelling and developing practice. Good working relationships and communication are vital.

13.00   Lunch-time departmental academic meeting. This is a weekly multi-professional meeting within our Department of Health Care for Older People. There is a visiting academic speaker and lunch is sponsored by a drug company.

14.15   Day hospital. I meet with the team to discuss a new nurse-led clinic that I am setting up for older people with Parkinson's disease. As the consultant for this clinic, I take named responsibility for the care of patients, accept direct referrals from all professional groups, and take responsibility for discharge from the service. Patients will not routinely have a medical review at this clinic, but I will refer for medical advice if necessary, either from a neurologist or a geriatrician. All patients will be offered assessment, care and advice, including access to the expertise of our Parkinson's disease specialist nurse. This afternoon we discuss how the clinic will run and our methods for evaluation. It is an opportunity for teaching and practice development. I use part of the time for formal teaching about the use of patient assessment tools.

16.00   I go to one of the surgical wards to see a patient who requires assessment of continuing care needs. Part of my role as consultant nurse for older people is to act as a point of referral for older patients on the acute wards, who are likely to need a complex care package on discharge, or a move to a nursing home. When a patient is referred to me, I advise the team whether they are suitable for transfer to our continuing care assessment ward. In this case, I accept the patient and place him on the waiting list for a bed. I provide two consultant sessions per week to the contin-uing care assessment ward itself.

16.30   Back to the office. Deal with phone calls, emails and general correspondence. I then continue with some work, which I am doing with the health authority, on review of the nursing assessment of older people who require continuing care. Today I continue some associated paperwork and emails, and prepare for a meeting at the health authority tomorrow.

18.45   Go home.

APPENDIX 1

CODE OF PROFESSIONAL CONDUCT

This Code of professional conduct *was published by the Nursing and Midwifery Council (NMC) in April 2002 and it came into effect on 1 June 2002.*

As a registered nurse or midwife, you are personally accountable for your practice. In caring for patients and clients, you must:

- respect the patient or client as an individual
- obtain consent before you give any treatment or care
- protect confidential information
- co-operate with others in the team
- maintain your professional knowledge and competence
- be trustworthy
- act to identify and minimize risk to patients and clients.

These are the shared values of all UK health care regulatory bodies.

Introduction

1.1 The purpose of the *Code of professional conduct* is to:
- inform the professions of the standard of professional conduct required of them in the exercise of their professional accountability and practice
- inform the public, other professions and employers of the standard of professional conduct that they can expect of a registered practitioner.

1.2 As a registered nurse or midwife, you must:
- protect and support the health of individual patients and clients
- protect and support the health of the wider community
- act in such a way that justifies the trust and confidence the public have in you
- uphold and enhance the good reputation of the professions.

1.3 You are personally accountable for your practice. This means that you are answerable for your actions and omissions, regardless of advice or directions from another professional.

1.4 You have a duty of care to your patients and clients, who are entitled to receive safe and competent care.

1.5 You must adhere to the laws of the country in which you are practising.

2 As a registered nurse or midwife, you must respect the patient or client as an individual

2.1 You must recognize and respect the role of patients and clients as partners in their care and the contribution they can make to it. This involves identifying their preferences regarding care and respecting these within the limits of professional practice, existing legislation, resources and the goals of the therapeutic relationship.

2.2 You are personally accountable for ensuring that you promote and protect the interests and dignity of patients and clients, irrespective of gender, age, race, ability, sexuality, economic status, lifestyle, culture and religious or political beliefs.

2.3 You must, at all times, maintain appropriate professional boundaries in the relationships you have with patients and clients. You must ensure that all aspects of the relationship focus exclusively upon the needs of the patient or client.

2.4 You must promote the interests of patients and clients. This includes helping individuals and groups gain access to health and social care, information and support relevant to their needs.

2.5 You must report to a relevant person or authority, at the earliest possible time, any conscientious objection that may be relevant to your professional practice. You must continue to provide care to the best of your ability until alternative arrangements are implemented.

3 As a registered nurse or midwife, you must obtain consent before you give any treatment or care

3.1 All patients and clients have a right to receive information about their condition. You must be sensitive to their needs and respect the wishes of those who refuse or are unable to receive information about their condition. Information should be accurate, truthful and presented in such a way as to make it easily understood. You may need to seek legal or professional advice, or guidance from your employer, in relation to the giving or withholding of consent.

3.2 You must respect patients' and clients' autonomy – their right to decide whether or not to undergo any health care intervention – even where a refusal may result in harm or death to themselves or a fetus, unless a court of law orders to the contrary. This right is protected in law, although in circumstances where the health of the fetus would be severely compromised by any refusal to give consent, it would be appropriate to discuss this matter fully within the team, and possibly to seek external advice and guidance (see clause 4).

3.3 When obtaining valid consent, you must be sure that it is:
- given by a legally competent person
- given voluntarily
- informed.

3.4 You should presume that every patient and client is legally competent unless otherwise assessed by a suitably qualified practitioner. A patient or client who is legally competent can understand and retain treatment information and can use it to make an informed choice.

3.5 Those who are legally competent may give consent in writing, orally or by co-operation. They may also refuse consent. You must ensure that all your discussions and associated decisions relating to obtaining consent are documented in the patient's or client's health care records.

3.6 When patients or clients are no longer legally competent and thus have lost the capacity to consent to or refuse treatment and care, you should try to find out whether they have previously indicated preferences in an advance statement. You must respect any refusal of treatment or care given when they were legally competent, provided that the decision is clearly applicable to the present circumstances and that there is no reason to believe that they have changed their minds. When such a statement is not available, the patients' or clients' wishes, if known, should be taken into account. If these wishes are not known, the criteria for treatment must be that it is in their best interests.

3.7 The principles of obtaining consent apply equally to those people who have a mental illness. While you should be involved in their assessment, it will also be necessary to involve relevant people close to them; this may include a psychiatrist. When patients and clients are detained under statutory powers (mental health acts), you must ensure that you know the circumstances and safeguards needed for providing treatment and care without consent.

3.8 In emergencies where treatment is necessary to preserve life, you may provide care without patients' or clients' consent, if they are unable to give it, provided you can demonstrate that you are acting in their best interests.

3.9 No one has the right to give consent on behalf of another competent adult. In relation to obtaining consent for a child, the involvement of those with parental responsibility in the consent procedure is usually necessary, but will depend on the age and understanding of the child. If the child is under the age of 16 in England and Wales, 12 in Scotland and 17 in Northern Ireland, you must be aware of legislation and local protocols relating to consent.

3.10 Usually the individual performing a procedure should be the person to obtain the patient's or client's consent. In certain circumstances, you may seek consent on behalf of colleagues if you have been specially trained for that specific area of practice.

3.11 You must ensure that the use of complementary or alternative therapies is safe and in the interests of patients and clients. This must be discussed with the team as part of the therapeutic process and the patient or client must consent to their use.

4 As a registered nurse or midwife, you must co-operate with others in the team

4.1 The team includes the patient or client, the patient's or client's family, informal carers and health and social care professionals in the NHS, independent and voluntary sectors.

4.2 You are expected to work co-operatively within teams and to respect the skills, expertise and contributions of your colleagues. You must treat them fairly and without discrimination.

4.3 You must communicate effectively and share your knowledge, skill and expertise with other members of the team as required for the benefit of patients and clients.

4.4 Health care records are a tool of communication within the team. You must ensure that the health care record for the patient or client is an accurate account of treatment, care planning and delivery. It should be consecutive, written with the involvement of the patient or client wherever practicable and completed as soon as possible after an event has occurred. It should provide clear evidence of the care planned, the decisions made, the care delivered and the information shared.

4.5 When working as a member of a team, you remain accountable for your professional conduct, any care you provide and any omission on your part.

4.6 You may be expected to delegate care delivery to others who are not registered nurses or midwives. Such delegation must not compromise existing care but must be directed to meeting the needs and serving the interests of patients and clients. You remain accountable for the appropriateness of the delegation, for ensuring that the person who does the work is able to do it and that adequate supervision or support is provided.

4.7 You have a duty to co-operate with internal and external investigations.

5 As a registered nurse or midwife, you must protect confidential information

5.1 You must treat information about patients and clients as confidential and use it only for the purposes for which it was given. As it is impractical to obtain consent every time you need to share information with others, you should ensure that patients and clients understand that some information may be made available to other members of the team involved in the delivery of care. You must guard against breaches of confidentiality by protecting information from improper disclosure at all times.

5.2 You should seek patients' and clients' wishes regarding the sharing of information with their family and others. When a patient or client is considered incapable of giving permission, you should consult relevant colleagues.

5.3 If you are required to disclose information outside the team that will have personal consequences for patients or clients, you must obtain their consent. If the patient or client withholds consent, or if consent cannot be obtained for whatever reason, disclosures may be made only where:
- they can be justified in the public interest (usually where disclosure is essential to protect the patient or client or someone else from the risk of significant harm)
- they are required by law or by order of a court.

5.4 Where there is an issue of child protection, you must act at all times in accordance with national and local policies.

6 As a registered nurse or midwife, you must maintain your professional knowledge and competence

6.1 You must keep your knowledge and skills up-to-date throughout your working life. In particular, you should take part regularly in learning activities that develop your competence and performance.

6.2 To practise competently, you must possess the knowledge, skills and abilities required for lawful, safe and effective practice without direct supervision. You must acknowledge the limits of your professional competence and only undertake practice and accept responsibilities for those activities in which you are competent.

6.3 If an aspect of practice is beyond your level of competence or outside your area of registration, you must obtain help and supervision from a competent practitioner until you and your employer consider that you have acquired the requisite knowledge and skill.

6.4 You have a duty to facilitate students of nursing and midwifery and others to develop their competence.

6.5 You have a responsibility to deliver care based on current evidence, best practice and, where applicable, validated research when it is available.

7 As a registered nurse or midwife, you must be trustworthy

7.1 You must behave in a way that upholds the reputation of the professions. Behaviour that compromises this reputation may call your registration into question even if is not directly connected to your professional practice.

7.2 You must ensure that your registration status is not used in the promotion of commercial products or services, declare any financial or other interests in relevant organizations providing such goods or services and ensure that your professional judgement is not influenced by any commercial considerations.

7.3 When providing advice regarding any product or service relating to your professional role or area of practice, you must be aware of the risk that, on account of your professional title or qualification, you could be perceived by the patient or client as endorsing the product. You should fully explain the advantages and disadvantages of alternative products so that the patient or client can make an informed choice. Where you recommend a specific product, you must ensure that your advice is based on evidence and is not for your own commercial gain.

7.4 You must refuse any gift, favour or hospitality that might be interpreted, now or in the future, as an attempt to obtain preferential consideration.

7.5 You must neither ask for nor accept loans from patients, clients or their relatives and friends.

8 As a registered nurse or midwife, you must act to identify and minimize the risk to patients and clients

8.1 You must work with other members of the team to promote health care environments that are conducive to safe, therapeutic and ethical practice.

8.2 You must act quickly to protect patients and clients from risk if you have good reason to believe that you or a colleague, from your own or another profession, may not be fit to practise for reasons of conduct, health or competence. You should be aware of the terms of legislation that offer protection for people who raise concerns about health and safety issues.

8.3 Where you cannot remedy circumstances in the environment of care that could jeopardize standards of practice, you must report them to a senior person with sufficient authority to manage them and also, in the case of midwifery, to the supervisor of midwives. This must be supported by a written record.

8.4 When working as a manager, you have a duty toward patients and clients, colleagues, the wider community and the organization in which you and your colleagues work. When facing professional dilemmas, your first consideration in all activities must be the interests and safety of patients and clients.

8.5 In an emergency, in or outside the work setting, you have a professional duty to provide care. The care provided would be judged against what could reasonably be expected from someone with your knowledge, skills and abilities when placed in those particular circumstances.

Further information

This *Code of professional conduct* is available on the NMC website at www.nmc-uk.org. Printed copies can be obtained by writing to the Publications Department, Nursing and Midwifery Council, 23 Portland Place, London W1B 1PZ, by fax on 020 7436 2924 or by e-mail at publications@nmc-uk.org. A wide range of NMC standards and guidance publications expand upon and develop many of the professional issues and themes identified in the *Code of professional conduct*. All are available on the NMC website. A list of current NMC publications is available either on the website or on request from the Publications Department as above.

Inquiries about the issues addressed in the *Code of professional conduct* should be directed in the first instance to the NMC's professional advice service at the address above, by e-mail at advice@nmc-uk.org, by telephone on 020 7333 6541/6550/6553 or by fax on 020 7333 6538.

The NMC will keep this *Code of professional conduct* under review and any comments, suggestions or requests for further clarification are welcome, both from practitioners and members of the public. These should be addressed to the Director of Policy and Standards, Nursing and Midwifery Council, 23 Portland Place, London W1B 1PZ.

APPENDIX 2

REQUIREMENTS FOR PRE-REGISTRATION NURSING PROGRAMMES

Introduction

1 This document provides an update on the UKCC's requirements for pre-registration nursing programmes, following the publication of the report of the Council's Commission for Education, *Fitness for practice* (1999). The legislative background is set out below, followed by the UKCC's requirements for pre-registration nursing programmes. These requirements should be read in conjunction with the rules to implement the new pre-registration nursing programmes and Statutory Instrument 2000 No. 2554, *The Nurses, Midwives and Health Visitors (Training) Amendment Rules Approval Order 2000*.

Legislative background

2 The *Nurses, Midwives and Health Visitors Act 1997*, section 2 (3), requires the Council, by means of rules, to determine the standard, kind and content of training to be undertaken with a view to registration. Section 6 (1) (b) of the act requires the National Boards for Nursing, Midwifery and Health Visiting to ensure that the programmes meet the UKCC's requirements.

3 In circular PS&D/89/04(B), the UKCC made clear that, as a result of consultation with the profession and others, its requirements for content should not be included in the legislation, thus enabling flexibility and development. This policy remains unchanged.

Kind and standard of programmes

4 The kind and standard of pre-registration nursing programmes leading to registration on parts 12, 13, 14 or 15 of the UKCC's register are currently set out in statutory instrument 1989 no. 1456, *The Nurses, Midwives and Health Visitors (Registered Fever Nurse Amendment Rules and Training Amendment Rules) Approval Order 1989*.

5 Statutory Instrument 2000 No. 2554 enables the implementation of 'new' pre-registration nursing programmes to meet the recommendations of the Commission for Education, as accepted by the Council.

6 The new programmes will comprise a one year common foundation programme (CFP) and a two year branch programme. The amended rules will give details as to how these lengths of time may be varied in particular circumstances. The requirement for the overall length of the course to be of three years duration containing 4,600 hours must continue to be met. Programmes leading to admission to part 12 of the register must meet the requirements of European Directive 77/453/EEC. Further details are published in Registrar's letter 15/2000.

7 The balance between practice and theory in the new programmes should normally be 50 per cent practice and 50 per cent theory in both CFP and branch programmes. A period of clinical practice of at least three months, towards the end of the pre-registration programme, is required to enable students to consolidate their education and their competence in practice.

8 The minimum academic standard of pre-registration nursing programmes remains that of a diploma of higher education.

Requirements for the content of programmes of preparation leading to registration on parts 12, 13, 14 or 15 of the register

9 The content of the curriculum for pre-registration nursing programmes should be that which will enable the achievement of the outcomes for entry to the branch programme and of the competencies for entry to the register.

10 The outcomes and competencies are set out in section 3 of this document and should be read in conjunction with the accompanying guiding principles.

11 In general terms, the CFP should be the foundation on which all further nursing preparation is based. To ensure transferability to any branch programme, students should have experience of each designated area of practice (branch) during the CFP. The branch programme should be an integral development of the theory and practice of nursing from the CFP and the core content commenced in the CFP should be extended into the branch programmes. This will also provide opportunities for appropriate shared learning between the branches.

12 Each branch programme is directed towards a specific area of nursing practice; children, adults, people with mental health problems or people with learning disabilities.

13 In order to provide a knowledge base, the following should be explored, using contemporary theoretical perspectives:
- professional, ethical and legal issues
- the theory and practice of nursing
- the context in which health and social care is delivered
- organisational structures and processes
- communication
- social and life sciences relevant to nursing practice
- frameworks for social care provision and care systems.

Nursing competencies – guiding principles

14 These guiding principles establish the philosophy and values underpinning the UKCC's requirements for programmes leading to entry to the register as a registered nurse. These principles provide the foundation for the outcomes/competencies for entry to the branch programmes and to the register and should be reflected in the pre-registration nursing programmes. The guiding principles relate to professional competence and fitness for practice. As practice takes place in the real world of health care delivery, it is inextricably linked to other aspects of fitness, that is fitness for purpose, professional academic awards and professional standing.

Preparation: fitness for practice

15 The primacy of practice underpins the competencies and must be reflected in all programmes of preparation for entry to the register.

Practice-centred learning

16 The primary aim in pre-registration nursing programmes is to ensure that students are prepared to practise safely and effectively to such an extent that the protection of the public is assured. On this basis, it is a fundamental principle that programmes of preparation are practice-centred and directed towards the achievement of professional competence.

Theory and practice integration

17 Safe and effective practice requires a sound underpinning of the theoretical knowledge which informs practice and is in turn informed by that practice. Such knowledge must therefore be directly related to, and integrated with, practice in all programmes leading to registration as a nurse. The competencies, and preparation for such competencies, must therefore reflect a breadth of practice and of learning.

Evidence-based practice and learning

18 Within the complex and rapidly changing health care environment, it is essential that practice is informed by the best available evidence. This commitment is reflected in the competencies. It includes searching the evidence base, analysing, critiquing and using research and other forms of evidence in practice, disseminating research findings and adapting practice where necessary. This must be reflected throughout all programmes of preparation.

Service: fitness for purpose

19 Nursing must relate to the changing needs of the health services and the communities which they serve, responding to current and future need.

Provision of care

20 Orientation must be towards practice which is responsive to the needs of various client groups across different care settings. This will be reflected in the capacity to assess needs, diagnose and plan, implement and evaluate care in such circumstances. Care practice must not only reflect collaborative working with other members of the care team but must also empower patients and clients, and their carers, actively to participate in the planning, delivery and evaluation of care. These principles must be reflected in all programmes of preparation leading to entry to the register.

Management of care

21 The nursing role involves a capacity not only to participate actively in care provision but also to accept responsibility for the effective and efficient management of that care, practised within a safe environment. This involves the capacity to accept accountability, to take responsibility for the delegation of aspects of care to others, and effectively to supervise and facilitate the work of such carers. It also involves the capacity to work effectively within the nursing and wider multi-disciplinary team, to accept leadership roles within such teams, and to demonstrate overall competence in care and case management.

A health for all orientation

22 In keeping with the orientation towards holistic care, the emphasis must be one which avoids a narrow disease-oriented perspective and instead encompasses a health promotion and health education perspective. This extends beyond a disease orientation to a commitment to health for all, irrespective of class, creed, age, gender, sexual orientation, culture or ethnic background. Principles of equity and fairness are fundamental professional values which must be reflected in the competencies and addressed directly in all programmes of preparation.

Lifelong learning

23 The rapidly changing nature of health care reflects a need for career-wide continuing professional development and the capacity not only to adapt to change but to identify the need for change and to initiate change. The provision of safe and effective health care and appropriate responsiveness to the changing needs of services and patients or clients cannot be achieved by adhering to rigid professional boundaries. The competencies must therefore include the capacity to extend the scope of practice and to address lifelong learning skills within all programmes of preparation.

Quality and excellence

24 The practice-centred competencies essential in nursing are not separate and insular professional aspirations. They are directly linked to the wider goals of achieving clinical effectiveness within health care teams and agencies, with the ultimate aim of achieving high quality health care. In this respect, assuring the quality of nursing care is one of the fundamental underpinnings of clinical governance. It is therefore necessary that nursing competencies encompass the capacity to contribute to this wider health care agenda and quality must be addressed within all programmes of preparation.

Recognition: fitness for award

25 Education for practice must be established at the level and pace of learning commensurate with the demands of complex and professional practice. Education for practice must be designed to meet the needs of the health services and communities and be structured to meet the specific needs of the profession.

Level of learning

26 The level of learning must be such as to facilitate the achievement of knowledge, understanding and skill acquisition, and the development of critical thinking, problem-solving and reflective capacities essential to complex professional practice. The UKCC has set the level of learning essential for underpinning the achievement of the identified competencies to be at a minimum of diploma of higher education standard.

Nature of learning

27 Given the primacy of practice as the required focus of programmes of preparation, learning must involve the integration of relevant and sound theoretical knowledge, with knowledge and

experience derived from practice. The UKCC values such learning as being the essence of professional education. Therefore, the UKCC expects that the philosophy explicit in programmes of preparation reflects the value of practice-centred education.

Access and credit

28 All programmes of preparation should value prior learning and, by so doing, provide wide access to programmes and advanced standing in year one through appropriate accreditation of relevant prior learning.

Flexibility, integrity and progression

29 Programmes of preparation should provide flexibility without compromising overall integrity and progression. This is achieved through modular design and the structuring of the programme into a common foundation and branch element. The three conditions (flexibility, integrity and progression) serve to ensure that modularisation does not compromise cumulative learning, leading to progression to the branch at the end of year one and entry to the register at the end of year three. This allows for maximum flexibility and provides a part-way point of exit and re-entry.

Educational quality

30 Programmes of preparation must be established upon sound academic and professional quality assurance processes which address professional learning and, in particular, the professional competencies to be achieved. In this respect, the UKCC recognises that professional nurse education must be academically rigorous. Educational quality will be achieved through partnership and collaboration involving all stakeholders, including service users, education purchasers, service providers, educational institutions, higher education quality assurance agencies and the statutory regulatory system.

Responsibility: fitness for professional standing

31 The UKCC values the rights implicit in the social contract between the profession and society to participate in the health care of individuals, families and communities. Such rights also carry obligations. These include not only the responsibility to provide competent, safe and effective care but also responsibility for the highest standards of professional conduct and ethical practice.

Adherence to the *Code of professional conduct*

32 An essential condition of entry to the profession is the acceptance and internalisation of the *Code of professional conduct*, which all registered nurses, midwives and health visitors must uphold. The *Code of professional conduct* provides the foundation for the competencies and must be reflected at all stages of programmes of preparation.

Responsibility and accountability

33 As members of a profession, registered nurses must take personal responsibility for their actions and omissions, and fully recognise their personal accountability. Each individual practitioner must be

able to make sound decisions in respect of their: personal professional development; practising within the scope of their personal professional competence and extending this scope as appropriate; delegating aspects of care to others and accepting responsibility and accountability for such delegation; and working harmoniously and effectively with colleagues, patients and clients and their carers, families and friends.

Ethical and legal obligations

34 The *Code of professional conduct* requires all practitioners to conduct themselves and practise within an ethical framework based fundamentally upon respect for the well-being of patients and clients. While various rule-oriented and principle-based ethical models may assist in informing ethical decisions, within modern health care settings ethical dilemmas are by definition complex. Practitioners must recognise their moral obligations and the need to accept personal responsibility for their own ethical choices within specific situations based on their own professional judgement. In making such choices, practitioners must be aware of, and adhere to, legal as well as professional requirements.

Respect for individuals and communities

35 All members of the profession must demonstrate an inviolable respect for persons and communities, without prejudice, and irrespective of orientation and personal, group, political, cultural, ethnic or religious characteristics. Care must be provided without prejudice and in an anti-discriminatory fashion. No member of the profession should convey any allegiance to any individual or group which opposes or threatens the human rights, safety or dignity of individuals or communities, irrespective of whether such individuals or groups are recipients of care.

Nursing competencies

36 The UKCC uses the term competence to describe '...the skills and ability to practise safely and effectively without the need for direct supervision...' (*Fitness for practice*, 1999)

37 The pre-registration nursing programme should be designed to prepare the student to be able, on registration, to apply knowledge, understanding and skills when performing to the standards required in employment and to provide the nursing care which patients and clients require, safely and competently, and so assume the responsibilities and accountabilities necessary for public protection.

38 The development of nursing programmes arises from the premise that nursing is a practicebased profession, recognising the primacy of patient and client well-being and respect for individuals and is founded on the principles that:
- evidence should inform practice through the integration of relevant knowledge
- students are actively involved in nursing care delivery under supervision
- the *Code of professional conduct* applies to all practice interventions
- skills and knowledge are transferable
- research underpins practice
- the importance of lifelong learning and continuing professional development is recognised.

39 The outcomes and competencies expressed will be achieved under the direction of a registered nurse.

Domain	Outcomes to be achieved for entry to the branch programme
Professional and ethical practice	**Discuss in an informed manner the implications of professional regulation for nursing practice** • demonstrate a basic knowledge of professional regulation and self-regulation • recognise and acknowledge the limitations of one's own abilities • recognise situations which require referral to a registered practitioner. **Demonstrate an awareness of the UKCC's** *Code of professional conduct* • commit to the principle that the primary purpose of the registered nurse is to protect and serve society • accept responsibility for one's own actions and decisions.
Professional and ethical practice	**Demonstrate an awareness of, and apply ethical principles to, nursing practice** • demonstrate respect for patient and client confidentiality • identify ethical issues in day to day practice. **Demonstrate an awareness of legislation relevant to nursing practice** • identify key issues in relevant legislation relating to mental health, children, data protection, manual handling, and health and safety, etc.
Professional and ethical practice	**Demonstrate the importance of promoting equity in patient and client care by contributing to nursing care in a fair and anti-discriminatory way** • demonstrate fairness and sensitivity when responding to patients, clients and groups from diverse circumstances • recognise the needs of patients and clients whose lives are affected by disability, however manifest.

Competencies for entry to the register – Professional and ethical practice

Manage oneself, one's practice, and that of others, in accordance with the UKCC's
Code of professional conduct, recognising one's own abilities and limitations

- practise in accordance with the UKCC's *Code of professional conduct*
- use professional standards of practice to self-assess performance
- consult with a registered nurse when nursing care requires expertise beyond one's own current scope of competence
- consult other health care professionals when individual or group needs fall outside the scope of nursing practice
- identify unsafe practice and respond appropriately to ensure a safe outcome
- manage the delivery of care services within the sphere of one's own accountability.

Practise in accordance with an ethical and legal framework which ensures the primacy of patient and client interest and well-being and respects confidentiality

- demonstrate knowledge of legislation and health and social policy relevant to nursing practice
- ensure the confidentiality and security of written and verbal information acquired in a professional capacity
- demonstrate knowledge of contemporary ethical issues and their impact on nursing and health care
- manage the complexities arising from ethical and legal dilemmas
- act appropriately when seeking access to caring for patients and clients in their own homes.

Practise in a fair and anti-discriminatory way, acknowledging the differences in beliefs and cultural practices of individuals or groups

- maintain, support and acknowledge the rights of individuals or groups in the health care setting
- act to ensure that the rights of individuals and groups are not compromised
- respect the values, customs and beliefs of individuals and groups
- provide care which demonstrates sensitivity to the diversity of patients and clients.

Domain	Outcomes to be achieved for entry to the branch programme
Care delivery	**Discuss methods of, barriers to and the boundaries of effective communication and interpersonal relationships** • recognise the effect of one's own values on interactions with patients and clients and their carers, families and friends • utilise appropriate communication skills with patients and clients • acknowledge the boundaries of a professional caring relationship. **Demonstrate sensitivity when interacting with and providing information to patients and clients**
Care delivery	**Contribute to enhancing the health and social well being of patients and clients by understanding how, under the supervision of a registered practitioner, to:** • contribute to the assessment of health needs • identify opportunities for health promotion • identify networks of health and social care services.
Care delivery	**Contribute to the development and documentation of nursing assessments by participating in comprehensive and systematic nursing assessment of the physical, psychological, social and spiritual needs of patients and clients** • be aware of assessment strategies to guide the collection of data for assessing patients and clients and use assessment tools under guidance • discuss the prioritisation of care needs • be aware of the need to reassess patients and clients as to their needs for nursing care.

Competencies for entry to the register – Care delivery

Engage in, develop and disengage from therapeutic relationships through the use of appropriate communication and interpersonal skills

- utilise a range of effective and appropriate communication and engagement skills
- maintain and, where appropriate, disengage from, professional caring relationships which focus on meeting the patient's or client's needs within professional therapeutic boundaries.

Create and utilise opportunities to promote the health and well-being of patients, clients and groups

- consult with patients, clients and groups to identify their need and desire for health promotion advice
- provide relevant and current health information to patients, clients and groups in a form which facilitates their understanding and acknowledges choice/individual preference
- provide support and education in the development and/or maintenance of independent living skills
- seek specialist/expert advice as appropriate.

Undertake and document a comprehensive, systematic and accurate nursing assessment of the physical, psychological, social and spiritual needs of patients, clients and communities

- select valid and reliable assessment tools for the required purpose
- systematically collect data regarding the health and functional status of individuals, clients and communities through appropriate interaction, observation and measurement
- analyse and interpret data accurately to inform nursing care and take appropriate action.

Care delivery | **Contribute to the planning of nursing care, involving patients and clients and, where possible, their carers, demonstrating an understanding of helping patients and clients to make informed decisions**

- identify care needs based on the assessment of a patient or client
- participate in the negotiation and agreement of the care plan with the patient or client and with their carer, family or friends, as appropriate, under the supervision of a registered nurse
- inform patients and clients about intended nursing actions, respecting their right to participate in decisions about their care.

Care delivery | **Contribute to the implementation of a programme of nursing care, designed and supervised by registered practitioners**

- undertake activities which are consistent with the care plan and within the limits of one's own abilities.

Demonstrate evidence of a developing knowledge base which underpins safe nursing practice

- access and discuss research and other evidence in nursing and related disciplines
- identify examples of the use of evidence in planned nursing interventions.

Demonstrate a range of essential nursing skills, under the supervision of a registered nurse, to meet individuals' needs, which include: maintaining dignity, privacy and confidentiality; effective communication and observational skills, including listening and taking physiological measurements; safety and health, including moving and handling and infection control; essential first aid and emergency procedures; administration of medicines; emotional, physical and personal care, including meeting the need for comfort, nutrition and personal hygiene.

Competencies for entry to the register – Care delivery

Formulate and document a plan of nursing care, where possible in partnership with patients, clients, their carers and family and friends, within a framework of informed consent

- establish priorities for care based on individual or group needs
- develop and document a care plan to achieve optimal health, habilitation and rehabilitation based on assessment and current nursing knowledge
- identify expected outcomes, including a time frame for achievement and/or review in consultation with patients, clients, their carers and family and friends and with members of the health and social care team.

Based on the best available evidence, apply knowledge and an appropriate repertoire of skills indicative of safe nursing practice

- ensure that current research findings and other evidence are incorporated in practice
- identify relevant changes in practice or new information and disseminate it to colleagues
- contribute to the application of a range of interventions to support patients and clients and which optimise their health and well-being
- demonstrate the safe application of the skills required to meet the needs of patients and clients within the current sphere of practice
- identify and respond to patients and clients' continuing learning and care needs
- engage with, and evaluate, the evidence base which underpins safe nursing practice.

Care delivery	**Contribute to the evaluation of the appropriateness of nursing care delivered**
	• demonstrate an awareness of the need to assess regularly a patient's or client's response to nursing interventions
	• provide for a supervising registered practitioner, evaluative commentary and information on nursing care based on personal observations and actions
	• contribute to the documentation of the outcomes of nursing interventions.
Care delivery	**Recognise situations in which agreed plans of nursing care no longer appear appropriate and refer these to an appropriate accountable practitioner**
	• demonstrate the ability to discuss and accept care decisions
	• accurately record observations made and communicate these to the relevant members of the health and social care team.

Provide a rationale for the nursing care delivered which takes account of social, cultural, spiritual, legal, political and economic influences

- identify, collect and evaluate information to justify the effective utilisation of resources to achieve planned outcomes of nursing care.

Evaluate and document the outcomes of nursing and other interventions

- collaborate with patients and clients and, when appropriate, additional carers to review and monitor the progress of individuals or groups towards planned outcomes
- analyse and revise expected outcomes, nursing interventions and priorities in accordance with changes in the individual's condition, needs or circumstances.

Demonstrate sound clinical judgement across a range of differing professional and care delivery contexts

- use evidence-based knowledge from nursing and related disciplines to select and individualise nursing interventions
- demonstrate the ability to transfer skills and knowledge to a variety of circumstances and settings
- recognise the need for adaptation and adapt nursing practice to meet varying and unpredictable circumstances
- ensure that practice does not compromise the nurse's duty of care to individuals or the safety of the public.

Domain	Outcomes to be achieved for entry to the branch programme
Care management	Contribute to the identification of actual and potential risks to patients, clients and their carers, to oneself and to others and participate in measures to promote and ensure health and safety • understand and implement health and safety principles and policies • recognise and report situations which are potentially unsafe for patients, clients, oneself and others.
Care management	Demonstrate an understanding of the role of others by participating in inter-professional working practice • identify the roles of the members of the health and social care team • work within the health and social care team to maintain and enhance integrated care.
Care management	Demonstrate literacy, numeracy and computer skills needed to record, enter, store, retrieve and organise data essential for care delivery

Competencies for entry to the register – Care management

Contribute to public protection by creating and maintaining a safe environment of care through the use of quality assurance and risk management strategies

- apply relevant principles to ensure the safe administration of therapeutic substances
- use appropriate risk assessment tools to identify actual and potential risks
- identify environmental hazards and eliminate and/or prevent them where possible
- communicate safety concerns to a relevant authority
- manage risk to provide care which best meets the needs and interests of patients, clients and the public.

Demonstrate knowledge of effective inter-professional working practices which respect and utilise the contributions of members of the health and social care team

- establish and maintain collaborative working relationships with members of the health and social care team and others
- participate with members of the health and social care team in decision-making concerning patients and clients
- review and evaluate care with members of the health and social care team and others.

Delegate duties to others, as appropriate, ensuring that they are supervised and monitored

- take into account the role and competence of staff when delegating work
- maintain one's own accountability and responsibility when delegating aspects of care to others
- demonstrate the ability to co-ordinate the delivery of nursing and health care.

Demonstrate key skills

- literacy – interpret and present information in a comprehensible manner
- numeracy – accurately interpret numerical data and their significance for the safe delivery of care
- information technology and management – interpret and utilise data and technology, taking account of legal, ethical and safety considerations, in the delivery and enhancement of care
- problem solving – demonstrate sound clinical decision-making which can be justified even when made on the basis of limited information.

Domain	Outcomes to be achieved for entry to the branch programme
Personal and professional development	Demonstrate responsibility for one's own learning through the development of a portfolio of practice and recognise when further learning is required - identify specific learning needs and objectives - begin to engage with, and interpret, the evidence base which underpins nursing practice. Acknowledge the importance of seeking supervision to develop safe nursing practice

Competencies for entry to the register – Personal and professional development

Demonstrate a commitment to the need for continuing professional development and personal supervision activities in order to enhance knowledge, skills, values and attitudes needed for safe and effective nursing practice

- identify one's own professional development needs by engaging in activities such as reflection in, and on, practice and lifelong learning
- develop a personal development plan which takes into account personal, professional and organisational needs
- share experiences with colleagues and patients and clients in order to identify the additional knowledge and skills needed to manage unfamiliar or professionally challenging situations
- take action to meet any identified knowledge and skills deficit likely to affect the delivery of care within the current sphere of practice.

Enhance the professional development and safe practice of others through peer support, leadership, supervision and teaching

- contribute to creating a climate conducive to learning
- contribute to the learning experiences and development of others by facilitating the mutual sharing of knowledge and experience
- demonstrate effective leadership in the establishment and maintenance of safe nursing practice.

Further copies of this document are available by writing to the UKCC's Distribution Department, 23 Portland Place, London W1B 1PZ, by e-mail at publications@ukcc.org.uk or by fax on 020 7436 2924. It can also be accessed on the UKCC's website at www.ukcc.org.uk. Enquiries should be referred to Pam Walter or Janice Gosby at the address above, by e-mail at pamwalter@ukcc.org.uk or janicegosby@ukcc.org.uk or by fax on 020 7333 6696.

APPENDIX 3
USEFUL ADDRESSES

Organizations offering advice for applicants to pre-registration nursing courses

Diploma programmes

Nursing & Midwifery Admissions Service (NMAS)
Rosehill
New Barn Lane
Cheltenham
Gloucestershire
GL52 3LZ
Tel: 01242 223707 (Applications)
Tel: 01242 544949 (General Enquiries)
Fax: 01242 544962
Website: www.nmas.ac.uk

Degree programmes

Universities & Colleges Admissions Service (UCAS)
New Barn Lane
Cheltenham
Gloucestershire
GL52 3LZ
Tel: 01242 227788 (Applications)
Tel: 01242 222444 (General Enquiries)
Fax: 01242 221622
Website: www.ucas.ac.uk

VISA queries for applicants from non-EEA countries

Immigration & Nationality Directorate
The Home Office
Lunar House
40 Wellesley Road
Croydon
CR9 2BY
Tel: 020 8686 0988

Bursaries and financial support

England:

The NHS Student Grants Unit

Room 212C Government Buildings

Norcross

Blackpool

FY5 3TA

Tel: 01253 655655

Fax: 01253 655660

Scotland:

The Students Awards Agency for Scotland

3 Redheughs Rigg

South Gyle

Edinburgh

EH12 9HH

Tel: 0131 4768212

Wales:

The NHS (Wales) Student Awards Unit

Human Resources Division

The National Assembly for Wales

Cathays Park

Cardiff

CF10 3NQ

Tel: 029 2082 6886

Northern Ireland:

The Department of Higher and Further Education

Training and Employment

Student Support Branch

4th Floor Adelaide House

39–49 Adelaide Street

Belfast

BT2 8FD

Tel: 028 9025 7777

Careers information for nurses, midwives and health visitors and information regarding continuing education

NHS Careers

PO Box 376

Bristol

BS99 3EY

Tel: 0845 6060655

Website: advice@nhscareers.nhs.uk

NHS Education for Scotland

22 Queen Street

Edinburgh

EH2 1NT

Tel: 0131 2267331

Website: careers@nhs.org.uk

Northern Ireland Practice & Education Council

Carter House

79 Chichester Street

Belfast

BT1 4JE

Tel: 028 9023 8152

Health Professionals Wales

Floor 2

Golate House

101 St. Mary's Street

Cardiff

CF10 1DX

Tel: 029 2026 1400

Fax: 029 2026 1499

Email: info@wnb.org.uk

Applications for diploma courses in Scotland

NBC Catch
PO Box 21
Edinburgh
EH2 1NT
Tel: 0131 2476622
Fax: 0131 2262492

Open and distance learning providers for nurses, midwives and health visitors

Distance Learning Centre
South Bank University
Southwark Campus, 103 Borough Road
London
SE1 0AA
Tel: 020 7815 8254

The Open University
Walton Hall
Milton Keynes
MK7 6AA
Tel: 01908 274066

Royal College of Nursing
Distance Learning
20 Cavendish Square
London
W1G 0RN
Tel: 020 7409 3333

Emap Healthcare Open Learning
Greater London House
Hampstead Road
London
NW1 7EJ
Tel: 020 7874 0600

Open University in Wales
24 Cathedral Road
Cardiff
CF11 9SA
Tel: 029 2039 7911

Professional and regulatory bodies related to nursing, midwifery and health visiting

Nursing and Midwifery Council
23 Portland Place
London
W1B 1PZ
Tel: 020 7637 7181
Fax: 020 7436 2924
Email: nmc-uk.org

NMC Registration Department
United Kingdom registration – Tel: 020 7333 9333
Outside EU enquiries – Tel: 020 7333 6600
Professional advice – Tel: 020 7333 6541 Email: advice@nmc-uk.org
Professional conduct – Tel: 020 7333 6564 Email: conduct@nmc-uk.org
Finance – Tel: 020 7333 6652 Email: finance@nmc-uk.org

The King's Fund
11–13 Cavendish Square
London
W1G 0AN
Tel: 020 7307 2400
Fax: 020 7307 2801
www.kingsfund.org.uk

Royal College of Midwives
15 Mansfield Street
London
W1G 9NH
Tel: 020 7312 3535
Website: www.rcm.org.uk
RCN Direct
Tel: 08457 726100 (24 hour information and advice for RCN members)

Royal College of Nursing
20 Cavendish Road
London
W1M 0AB
Tel: 020 7409 3333
Website: www.rcn.org.uk

Community Practitioners and Health Visitors Association
40 Bermondsey Street
London
SE1 3UD
Tel: 020 7939 7000
Website: www.msfcphva.org

British Association of Counselling (BAC)
1 Regent Place
Rugby
Warwickshire
CV21 2PJ
Tel: 01788 550 899
Fax: 01788 562 189
Email: bac@bac.co.uk
Website: www.counselling.co.uk

Other useful contacts

NHS Pensions Agency
200–220 Broadway
Fleetwood
Lancashire
FY7 8LG

UNISON
1 Mabledon Place
London
WC1H 9AJ
Tel: 020 7388 2366

Institute of Psychiatry
16 De Crespigny Park
London
SE5 8AF
Tel: 020 7703 5411

RCN Nurseline

The Nurseline service offers career information and guidance, help with problems at work or personal issues and help and support to all nurses and midwives even after they have retired from the profession. They are also able to search databases for information on courses and professional development.

Tel: 020 7647 3463 (10am–4pm Monday to Friday)
Fax: 020 7647 3589
Email: nurseline@rcn.org.uk

20 Cavendish Square
London
W1G 0RN
Website: www.rcn.org.uk

RCN Counselling Service

Tel: 0845 769 7064 (9am–4pm Monday to Friday)
The RCN counselling service offers free professional counselling for members and student members.

WING – Working Injured Nurses Group

Provide help to nurses who are suffering or have suffered illness or injury in the course of their work.
Tel: 020 7647 3465
Email: WING@rcn.org.uk

REFERENCES

Abley, C. (2001). The nurse consultant. *Nursing Older People* 13(8), 34–5

Acheson, D. (1998). *Independent Inquiry into Inequalities in Health.* HMSO, London

Adler, N. (1996). Communicating across cultural barriers. In: Billsberry, J. (ed.) *The Effective Manager.* Sage, London

Agenet/RCN (1999). *Gerontological Nursing Research – The Case for Developing a User Focused Agenda.* Report of a workshop to discuss the future of gerontological nursing research, organized by AgeNet and the Royal College of Nursing, London, December 1998

Aggleton, P., Chalmers, H. (2000). *Nursing Models and Nursing Practice.* Macmillan, Basingstoke

Ahern, K., McDonald, S. (2002). The beliefs of nurses who were involved in a whistleblowing event. *Journal of Advanced Nursing* 38(3), 303–9

Akinsanya, J., Cox, G., Crouch, C., Fletcher, L. (1994). *The Roy Adaptation Model in Action.* Macmillan, Houndmills

Alderson, P. (1996). Sociological aspects of adolescent health and illness. In: Macfarlane, A. (ed.) *Adolescent Medicine.* Royal College of Physicians, London

Alderson, P. (2000). *Young Children's Rights: Exploring Beliefs, Principles and Practice.* Jessica Kingsley Publications, Philadelphia, p22–48

Alford, D.M., Futrell, M. (1992). Wellness and health promotion of the elderly. *Nursing Outlook* 40(5), 221–6

Allen, D. (2000). Negotiating the role of expert carers on an adult hospital ward. *Sociology of Health and Illness* 22(2), 149–71

Anderson, C., Rubenach, S., Mhurchu, C. (2000). Early discharge plus home based rehabilitation reduced length of initial hospital stay but did not improve health related quality of life in patients with acute stroke. *Evidence-Based Nursing* 3(4), 127

Andrusyszyn, M., Maltby, H. (1993). Building on strengths through preceptorship. *Nurse Education Today* 13, 277–81

Anonymous (2000). *Hospice and Palliative Care Services in the United Kingdom and the Republic of Ireland. Hospice Information Services.* St Christopher's Hospice, London

Anonymous (2001). News: Bristol report finally published. *Bulletin of Medical Ethics* 169, 3–8

Anonymous (2002). The Shipman Inquiry: The First Report. www.the-shipman-inquiry.org.uk/reports.asp

Antrobus, S., Kitson, A. (1999). Nursing leadership: influencing and shaping health policy and nursing practice. *Journal of Advanced Nursing* 29(3), 746–53

Apfel, R.J., Simon, B. (1985). Patient therapist sexual contact – psychodynamic perspectives in the causes and the results. *Psychotherapuetic Psychosomatics* 43, 57–62

Appleby, J., Walshe, K., Ham, C. (1995). *Acting on the Evidence.* Health Services Management Centre, University of Birmingham

Argyris, C., Schon, D. (1974). *Theory in Practice.* Jossey Bass, San Francisco

Armstrong, M. (1994). *How to be an Even Better Manager*. Kogan Page, London

Arnold, E., Boggs, K.U. (1999). *Interpersonal Relationships, Professional Communication Skills for Nurses*, 3rd edn. WB Saunders, London

Ashton, P., Richardson, G. (1992). Preceptorship and PREP. *British Journal of Nursing* 1(3), 143–6

Ashworth, P., Morrison, P. (1991). Problems of competence-based education. *Nurse Education Today* 11, 256–60

Askham, J., Henshaw, L., Tarpey, M. (1995). *Social and Health Authority Services for Elderly People from Black and Minority Ethnic Communities*. London, HMSO

Atkins, S., Murphy, K. (1993). Reflection: a review of the literature. *Journal of Advanced Nursing* 18, 1188–92

Audit Commission (1993). *Children First: A Study of Hospital Services*. HSMO, London

Audit Commission (1999). *First Assessment: A Review of District Nursing Services in England and Wales*. HMSO, London

Baggs, J., Ryan, S.A., Phelps, C.E., Richeson, J.F., Johnson, J.E. (1992). The association between interdisciplinary collaboration and patient outcomes in medical intensive care. *Heart Lung* 21, 18

Baillie, L. (ed.) (2001). *Developing Practical Nursing Skills*. Arnold, London

Baker, C. (1996). Young peoples unit. In: Macfarlane, A. (ed.) *Adolescent Medicine*. Royal College of Physicians, London

Baker, R. (2001). *Harold Shipman's Clinical Practice 1974–1998*. A review commissioned by the DoH. Stationery Office, London

Barber, P. (1998). Developing the 'person' of the professional carer. In: Hinchliff, S., Norman, S., Schober, J. (eds) *Nursing Practice and Health Care: A Foundation Text*, 3rd edn. Arnold, London, p309–36

Bartlett, H., Hind, P., Taylor, H., Wescott, E.J. (1998). *An Evaluation of Pre-registration Nursing Programmes: A Literature Review and Comparative Study of Graduate Outcomes*. Oxford Centre for Health Care Research and Development, Oxford

BBSF (2000). *Motor Neurone Disease. A Guide for Patients and Carers*. British Brain and Spinal Foundation

Beauchamp, T.L., Childress, J.F. (1994). *Principles of Biomedical Ethics*, 4th edn. Oxford University Press, Oxford

Bekeart, S. (2002). Sexual health workshops. *Paediatric Nursing* 14(4), 22–6

Belbin, M. (1997). *Changing the Way We Work*. Butterworth Heinemann, Oxford

Benner, P. (1982). From novice to expert. *American Journal of Nursing* March, 402–7

Benner, P. (1984). *From Novice to Expert: Excellence and Power in Clinical Nursing Practice*. Addison-Wesley, Menlo Park, California

Benner, P., Wrubel, J. (1989). *The Primacy of Caring: Stress and Coping in Health and Illness*. Addison-Wesley, California

Bernard, M., Phillips, J. (2000). The challenge of ageing in tomorrow's Britain. *Ageing and Society* 20(1), 33–54

Bero, L., Grilli, R., Grimshaw, J., Harvey, E., Oxman, A., Thompson, M. (1998). Closing the gap between research and practice: an overview of systematic reviews of interventions to promote the implementation of research findings. *British Medical Journal* 317(17), 465–8

Berwick, D. (1996). Quality comes home. *Annals of Internal Medicine* 125, 839–43

Betts, A. (2002). The nurse as communicator. In: Kenworthy, N., Snowley, G., Gilling, C. (eds) *Common Foundation Studies in Nursing*. Churchill Livingstone, Edinburgh, p259–61

Birch, J. (1975). *To Nurse or Not to Nurse.* Royal College of Nursing, London

Bishop, V. (1998). Clinical supervision: what is it? In: Bishop, V. (ed.) *Clinical Supervision in Practice.* Macmillan Press, London, p1–20

Blane, D. (1988). Health professions. In: Patrick, D.L., Scambler, G. (eds) *Sociology as Applied to Medicine.* Baillière Tindall, London

Blue, L., Lang, E., McMurray, J. *et al.* (2001). Randomized controlled trial of specialist nurse intervention in heart failure. *British Medical Journal* 323, 715–18

Blum, R.W.M., Garrel, D., Hodgman, C.H. *et al.* (1993). Transition from child-centered to adult health-care systems for adolescents with chronic conditions. A position paper of the Society for Adolescent Medicine. *Journal of Adolescent Health* 14, 570–6

Bosanquet, N., Salisbury, C. (1999). *Providing a Palliative Care Service: Towards an Evidence Base.* Oxford University Press, Oxford

Bostrom, J., Suter, W.N. (1993). Research utilisation: making the links to practice. *Journal of Nursing and Staff Development* 9, 28–34

Bowling, A. (1995). The most important things in life: comparisons between older and younger population age groups by gender: results from a national survey of the public's judgements. *International Journal of Health Sciences* 6(4), 169–75

Brace O'Neill, J. (1998). Professional boundaries in pediatric nursing practice. *Journal of Pediatric Health Care* 12(4), 225–7

Bradbury, M. (2000). The good death? In: Dickenson, D., Johnson, M., Katz, J. (eds) *Death, Dying and Bereavement.* Sage, London, p59–63

Bradley, S. (1999). Catherine Wood: Children's nursing pioneer. *Paediatric Nursing* 11(8), 15–18

Brändstädter, J., Greve, W. (1994). The aging self: stabilising and protective processes. *Developmental Review* 14, 52–80

Brandt, P., Weiner, C. (1998). Children's mental health in families experiencing multiple sclerosis. *Journal of Family Nursing* 4(1), 41–64

Brechin, A. (1998). What makes for good care? In: Brechin, A., Walmsley, J., Katz, J., Peace, S. (eds) *Care Matters: Concepts, Practice and Research in Health and Social Care.* Sage, London, p170–87

Brennan, A. (1993). Preceptorship: is it a workable concept? *Nursing Standard* 7(52), 34–6

Briant, S., Freshwater, D. (1998). Exploring mutuality within the nurse–patient relationship. *British Journal of Nursing* 7(4), 204–11

Briggs, A. (1972). *Report of the Committee on Nursing.* HMSO, London

British Medical Association (2001). *The Medical Profession and Human Rights: Handbook for Changing Agenda.* Zed Books, London

British Standards Institute (1999). *Complaints Management Systems: A Guide to Design and Implementation. BS 8600.* British Standards Institute, London

Brykczynska, G. (2000). Not quite the judgement of Solomon. *Paediatric Nursing* 12(9), 6–8

Buckenham, M. (1992). Academic and organisational change. In: Slein, O., Buckenham, M. (eds) *Project 2000: The Teachers Speak.* Campion Press, Edinburgh

Burke, L. (1994). Preceptorship and post registration nurse education. *Nurse Education Today* 14, 60–6

Burke, C., Lugon, M. (1999). Clinical audit and clinical governance. In: Lugon, M., Secker-Walker, J. (eds) *Clinical Governance: Making it Happen.* Royal Society of Medicine Press, London, p61–76

Burnard, P. (1990). The student experience: adult learning and mentorship revisited. *Nurse Education Today* 10(4), 349–54

Burr, S. (2001). Learning from Bristol: acting to improve a cinderella service. *Paediatric Nursing* 13(7), 19–22

Burton Jones, J. (2001). *Involving Relatives and Friends: A Good Practice Guide for Homes for Older People*. Residents and Relatives Association, London

Butler, R. (1969). Ageism: another form of bigotry. *The Gerontologist* 9, 243–6

Butterworth, A. (1998). Clinical supervision as an emerging idea in nursing. In: Butterworth, A., Faugier, J., Burnard, P. (eds) *Clinical Supervision and Mentorship in Nursing*. Stanley Thornes, Cheltenham

Butterworth, A., Carson, J., White, E., Jeacock, J., Clements, A., Bishop, V. (1997). *It is Good to Talk: An Evaluation Study in England and Scotland*. The University of Manchester, Manchester

Calman, K. (1994). Working together: teamwork. *Journal of Inter-Professional Care* 8(1), 95–9

Campbell, A.J. (2001). Purity, pragmatism and hip protector pads. *Age and Ageing* 30, 431–2

Campbell, S., Glasper, E.A. (1995). *Whaley and Wong's Children's Nursing*. Mosby, St Louis

Carpentio, L.J. (1997). *Nursing Diagnosis: Application to Clinical Practice*, 7th edn. Lippincott, Philadelphia

Carper, B. (1978). Fundamental patterns of knowing in nursing. *Advances in Nursing Science* 1, 13–23

Carroll, D., Seers, K. (1998). Relaxation for the relief of chronic pain: a systematic review. *Journal of Advanced Nursing* 27(3), 476–87

Carson, R.A. (1995). Beyond respect to recognition and due regard. In: Toombs, S.K., Barnard, D., Carson, R.A. (eds) *Chronic Illness: From Experience to Policy*. Indiana University Press, Bloomington

Carter, H., McKenna, C., MacLeod, R., Green, R. (1998). Health professionals responses to multiple sclerosis and motor neurone disease. *Palliative Medicine* 12(5), 383–94

Casey, A. (1988). A partnership with child and family. *Senior Nurse* 8(4), 8–9

Casey, A. (1995). Partnership nursing: influences on informal carers. *Journal of Advanced Nursing* 22(6), 1058–62

Caulfield, H. (2002). Legal issues. In: Kenworthy, N., Snowley, G., Gilling, C. (eds) *Common Foundation Studies in Nursing*. Churchill Livingstone, Edinburgh, p123–4

Cavanagh, S.J. (1991). *Orem's Model in Action*. Macmillan, Houndmills

Chabliss, D. (1996). *Beyond Caring*. University of Chicago Press, Chicago

Chadda, D. (2001). Ethnic minority communities still face discrimination in accessing health services. *Physiotherapy Frontline* 7(23), 3

Chambers, M., Long, A. (1995). Supportive clinical supervision: A crucible for personal and professional change. *Journal of Psychiatric and Mental Health Nursing* 2, 311–17

Chandler, T. (2001). Applying teaching skills in practice. In: Hinchliff, S. (ed.) *The Practitioner as Teacher*, 2nd edn. Ballière Tindall, London, p169–93

Charles-Edwards, I. (2001). Children's nursing and advocacy: are we in a muddle? *Paediatric Nursing* 13(2), 12–16

Chesson, R., Macleod, M., Massie, S. (1996). Outcome measures used in therapy departments in Scotland. *Physiotherapy* 82(12), 673–9

CHI (2002a). Nothing about us without us: a patient and public strategy for the Commission for Health Improvement. www.chi.gov.uk/patients/index.shtml

CHI (2002b). Investigations: introduction. www.chi.gov.uk/eng/inv/index.shtml

Christensen, P.J. (1995). *Nursing Process: Application of Conceptual Models*. Mosby, St Louis

Ciliska, D., Cullum, N., Marks, S. (2001). Evaluation of systematic reviews of treatment or prevention interventions. *Evidence-Based Nursing* 4, 100–4

Clark, P.G. (1995). Quality of life, values and teamwork in geriatric care: do we communicate what we mean? *Gerontologist* 35(3), 402–11

Clark, A., Dooher, J., Fowler, J. (2001). *The Handbook of Practice Development.* Quay Books, Mark Allen Publishing, Wiltshire

Clemmer, T., Spuhler, R., Berwick, D., Nolan, T. (1998). Cooperation: The foundation of improvement. *Annals of Internal Medicine* 128, 1004–9

Clinical Guidelines Education Team (2001). *Implementing Clinical Guidelines: A Resource for the Health Care Team.* Ballière Tindall, London

Clinical Resource and Audit Group (1993). *Clinical Guidelines: A Report by a Working Party set up by the Clinical Resource and Audit Group.* National Health Service in Scotland, London

Cochrane, A.L. (1976). *Effectiveness and Efficiency.* Oxford University Press, Oxford and Nuffield Provincial Hospitals Trust, Oxford

Coleman, P., Bond, J., Peace, S. (1993). Ageing in the twentieth century. In: Bond, J., Coleman, P., Peace, S. (eds) *Ageing in Society: An Introduction to Social Gerontology,* 2nd edn. Sage, London, p1–18

Coleman, J.C., Hendry, L.B. (1999). *The Nature of Adolescence.* Adolescence and Society Series. Routledge, London

Coleman, J.C., Scofield, J. (2003). *Key Data on Adolescence.* Trust for the Study of Adolescence, Brighton

Commission of the European Communities (1996). *The Demographic Situation in the European Union.* Commission of the European Communities, Brussels

Congor, J.J., Galmbos, N.L. (1997). *Adolescence and Youth: Psychological Development in a Changing World.* Addison-Wesley Longman, California

Cook, D.G., Strachen, D.P. (1997). Review: parental tobacco smoke increases the risk of asthma and respiratory symptoms in school age children. *Evidence-Based Nursing* 3, 86

Copp, G. (1999). *Facing Impending Death. Experiences of Nurses and Their Patients.* Nursing Times Books, London

Corner, J., Plant, H., A'Hern, R., Bailey, C. (1996). Non pharmacological intervention in lung cancer. *Palliative Medicine* 10(4), 299–305

Costello, J. (2001). Nursing older dying patients: Findings from an ethnographic study of death and dying in elderly care wards. *Journal of Advanced Nursing* 35(1), 5–58

Covey, S. (1989). *Seven Habits of Effective People.* Simon and Schuster, London

Crookes, P.A., Davies, S. (eds) (1998). *Research into Practice.* Baillière Tindall, London, Ch 1, 2 and 4

Cullum, N. (2000). Evaluation of studies of treatment or prevention interventions. *Evidence-Based Nursing* 3, 100–2

Cullum, N. (2001). Evaluation of studies of treatment or prevention interventions. Part 2: applying the results of studies to your patients. *Evidence-Based Nursing* 4, 7–8

Cullum, N., DiCenso, A., Ciliska, D. (1997). Evidence-based nursing: an introduction. *Nursing Standard* 11(28), 32–3

Cullum, N., Deeks, J., Sheldon, T.A. (2000). Review: specially designed products to prevent or heal pressure sores are more effective than standard mattresses. *Evidence-Based Nursing* 3(2), 54

Dalley, G. (1998). Health and social welfare policy. In: Bernard, M., Phillips, J. (eds) *The Social Policy of Old Age: Moving into the 21st Century.* Centre for Policy on Ageing, London

Darbyshire, P. (1994). *Living with a Sick Child in Hospital: The Experiences of Parents and Nurses.* Chapman & Hall, London

Darling, L. (1984). What do nurses want in a mentor? *The Journal of Nursing Administration* 14(10), 42–4

Davies, C. (1995). *Gender and the Professional Predicament in Nursing.* OU Press, Oxford

Davies, C. (1996). A new vision of professionalism. *Nursing Times* 92(46), 54–6

Davies, S. (1999). Empowerment and health: a community development approach to health promotion. In: Purdey, M., Banks, D. (eds) *Health and Exclusion: Victims and Collaborators in Health Care.* Routledge, London, p136–57

Davies, S. (2001). Relatives' experiences of nursing home entry: a constructivist inquiry. Unpublished PhD thesis. University of Sheffield, Sheffield

Davies, S., Nolan, M., Brown, J., Wilson, F. (1999). *Dignity on the Ward: Promoting Excellence in Care.* Help the Aged, London

Dearden, C., Becker, S. (1998). *Young Carers in the UK.* Carers National Association, London

Department of Education and the National Health Executive (1994). *The Education of Sick Children.* Circular no 12/94. Department of Education, London, p1

Department of Health and Social Security and Public Safety (2002). *Investing for Health.* Department of Health and Social Security and Public Safety, Belfast

de Sousa, M. (1998). Making the transition from paediatric to adult care. *Cascade* 26, 4–5

de Sousa, M. (1999). Setting up an adolescent unit: an emergent strategy. In: *The Nurse as a Strategist.* RCN Institute, London

de Sousa, M., Needham, J. (2002). Generation gap. *Nursing Standard* 16(38), 96

DHSS, Northern Ireland (1999). News Release October 4. http://www2.nio.gov.uk/dhsspr.htm

Dibert, C., Goldenberg, D. (1995). Preceptors perception of benefits, rewards, supports and commitment to the preceptor role. *Journal of Advanced Nursing* 21, 1144–51

DiCenso, A. (2001). Clinically useful measures of the effects of treatment. *Evidence-Based Nursing* 4, 36–9

Dimond, B. (1994). Legal aspects of role expansion. In: Hunt, G., Wainwright, P. (eds) *Expanding the Role of the Nurse: The Scope of Professional Practice.* Blackwell Science, Oxford, 54–73

Dimond, B. (1996). *The Legal Aspects of Child Health Care.* Mosby, London

Dingwall, R., Rafferty, A.M., Webster, C. (1988). *An Introduction to the Social History of Nursing.* Routledge, London

DoH (1976). *Fit for the Future* (chairman Court). HSMO, London

DoH (1989a). *The Children Act.* HMSO, London

DoH (1989b). *Working for Patients.* HMSO, London

DoH (1989c). *Caring for People: Community Care in the Next Decade and Beyond.* HMSO, London

DoH (1991a). *Research for Health: A Research and Development Strategy for the NHS.* HMSO, London

DoH (1991b). *The Patient's Charter.* HMSO, London

DoH (1993a). *Report of the Taskforce on the Strategy for Research in Nursing, Midwifery and Health Visiting.* HMSO, London

DoH (1993b). *A Vision for the Future. The Nursing, Midwifery and Health/Visiting Contribution to Health and Health Care.* HSMO, London

DoH (1994a). *The Challenges for Nursing and Midwifery in the 21st Century. The Heathrow Debate, May 1993.* Department of Health, London

DoH (1994b). *The Allitt Inquiry: Independent Inquiry Relating to Deaths and Injuries on the Children's Ward at Grantham and Kesteven Hospital During the Period February–April 1991 (Clothier Report).* HMSO, London

DoH (1995a). *Health of the Nation.* Department of Health, London

DoH (1996). *The Children's Charter.* HMSO, London

DoH (1997). *The New NHS, Modern and Dependable.* NHS, London

DoH (1999a). *Mental Health Act 1983 Code of Practice.* The Stationery Office, London

DoH (1999b). *Working Lives Campaign.* Department of Health, London

DoH (1999c). *National Service Framework for Mental Health.* The Stationery Office, London

DoH (1999d). *Making a Difference: Strengthening the Nursing, Midwifery and Health Visiting Contribution to Health and Healthcare.* Department of Health, London

DoH (1999e). *Agenda for Change – Modernising the NHS Pay System.* The Stationery Office, London

DoH (2000a). *The NHS Plan: A Plan for Investment, A Plan for Reform.* HMSO, London

DoH (2000b). *Revitalising Health and Safety in Great Britain.* Department of Health, London

DoH (2000c). *Extending Independent Nurse Prescribing within the NHS in England: a Guide for Implementation.* Department of Health, London

DoH (2000d). *National Service Framework for Coronary Heart Disease.* The Stationery Office, London

DoH (2000e). *A Health Service of All the Talents: Developing the NHS Workforce.* Department of Health, London

DoH (2001a). *The NHS Plan – An Action Guide for Nurses, Midwives and Health Visitors.* Department of Health, London

DoH (2001b). *Shifting the Balance of Power.* Department of Health, London

DoH (2001c). *Reference Guide to Consent for Examination or Treatment.* Department of Health, London

DoH (2001d). *Learning from Bristol: The Report of the Public Enquiry into Children's Heart Surgery at the Bristol Royal Infirmary 1984–1995*, the Kennedy Report. The Stationery Office, London www.bristol-inquiry.org.uk

DoH (2001e). *Involving Patients and the Public in Healthcare: Response to Listening Exercise.* Department of Health, London www.doh.gov.uk/involvingpatients/listening.htm

DoH (2001f). *The Essence of Care – Patient-Focused Benchmarking for Health Care Practitioners.* Department of Health, London www.doh.gov.uk/essenceofcare.htm

DoH (2001g). *Working Together, Learning Together. A Framework for Lifelong Learning in the NHS.* Department of Health, London

DoH (2001h). *Building a Safer NHS for Patients: Implementing an Organisation with a Memory.* Department of Health, London www.doh.gov.uk/buildsafenhs

DoH (2001i). *The National Service Framework for Older People.* The Stationery Office, London

DoH (2001j). *The Care Standards Act.* The Stationery Office, London

DoH (2001k). *The Expert Patient: A New Approach to Chronic Disease Management for the 21st Century.* Department of Health, London

DoH (2001l). *National Clinical Assessment Authority.* Department of Health, London

DoH (2001m). *National Patient Safety Agency.* Department of Health, London

DoH (2001n). *Good Practice in Consent Implementation Guide: Consent to Examination or Treatment.* The Stationery Office, London

DoH (2001o). *National Service Framework for Diabetes.* The Stationery Office, London

DoH (2001p). *Towards a Strategy of Nursing Research and Development.* Department of Health, London

DoH (2001q). *Working Together – Learning Together. A Framework for Lifelong Learning for the NHS.* Department of Health, London

DoH (2002a). *NHS Trust-based Patient Surveys: Inpatients – Acute Hospitals.* Department of Health, London

DoH (2002b). *Delivering the NHS Plan – Next Steps on Investment, Next Steps on Reform.* Department of Health, London

REFERENCES

Dolan, B., Holt, L. (2000). *Accident and Emergency Theory into Practice.* Ballière Tindall, London, p189–98

Donabedian, A. (1966). Evaluating the quality of medical care. *Milbank Memorial Fund Quarterly* 44(2), 166–206

Donabedian, A. (1980). *The Definition of Quality and Approaches to its Assessment.* Health Administration Press, Ann Arbor, MD

Donovan, J. (1990). The concept and role of mentor. *Nurse Education Today* 10, 294–8

Dooher, J., Clark, A., Fowler, J. (2001). *Case Studies on Practice Development.* Quay Books, Mark Allen Publishing, Wiltshire

Downer, P. (2002). Nursing theory and nursing care. In: Kenworthy, N., Snowley, G., Gilling, C. (eds) *Common Foundation Studies in Nursing.* Churchill Livingstone, Edinburgh, Ch 13

Doyle, K.A., Maslin-Prothero, S. (1999). Promoting children's rights: the role of the children's nurse. *Paediatric Nursing* 11(8), 23–5

Dreyfus, S., Dreyfus, H. (1980). A 5 Stage Model of Mental Activities Involved in Directed Skill Acquisition. [Unpublished study cited in Benner, P. (1982). Novice to expert. *American Journal of Nursing* March, 407]

Driscoll, J. (2000). *Practising Clinical Supervision: A Reflective approach.* Baillière Tindall, London

Driscoll, J., Teh, B. (2001). The contribution of portfolios and profiles to continuing professional development. *Journal of Orthopaedic Nursing* 5, 151–6

Duff, L.A., Kitson, A.L., Seers, K., Humphries, D. (1996). Clinical guidelines: an introduction to their development and implementation. *Journal of Advanced Nursing* 23, 887–95

Duff, L., Loftus-Hills, A., Morrell, C. (2000). *Implementation Guide: Clinical Guidelines for the Management of Venous Leg Ulcers.* Royal College of Nursing Institute, London

Dunn, C., Beegan, A., Morris, S., Powell, T. (1998). *The Kings Fund PACE Project in West Berkshire: Improving the Care of Patients with Leg Ulcers.* Royal Berkshire and Battle Hospitals NHS Trust in conjunction with West Berkshire Priority Care Services

Dushmohamed, H., Guscott, A. (1998). Preceptorship: A model to empower nurses in rural health settings. *Journal of Continuing Education in Nursing* 29(4), 154–60

Dyer, C. (2002). Woman sues for not being warned about the psychological effects of abortion. *British Medical Journal* 324, 1477

Earnshaw, G. (1995). Mentorship: The student's view. *Nurse Education Today* 15, 274–9

Eccles, M., Freemantle, N., Mason, J. (2001). Using systematic reviews in clinical guideline development. In: Egger, M., Davey Smith, G., Altman, D.G. (eds) *Systematic Reviews in Health Care. Meta-analysis in Context*, 2nd edn. BMJ Books, London

Edwards, S. (1997). Measuring temperature. *Professional Nurse* 13(2), S5–7

Edwards, S. (1998). Malnutrition in hospital patients: where does it come from? *British Journal of Nursing* 7, 954, 956–8, 971–4

Eiser, C. (1993). *Growing Up with a Chronic Disease: The Impact on Children and their Families*, 2nd edn. Jessica Kingsley Publishers, London

Elkind (1968)

Ellefsen, B. (2001). Changes in health visitors' work. *Journal of Advanced Nursing* 34(3), 346–55

Ellwood, P. (1988). Shattuck lecture – outcomes management: a technology of patient care. *New England Journal of Medicine* 318, 1549–56

Employment Surveys and Research Unit (2000). *Care Sector NVQ Take-up Survey 1999.* Employers Organisation for Local Government, London

ENB (1989). *Preparation of Teachers, Practitioners/Teachers, Mentors and Supervisors in the Context of Project 2000.* English National Board for Nursing, Midwifery and Health Visiting, London

ENB (1990). *A New Structure for Professional Development. The Framework for Continuing Professional Education and the Higher Award.* English National Board for Nursing, Midwifery and Health Visiting, London

ENB (1991). *Framework for Continuing Professional Education for Nurses, Midwives and Health Visitors.* English National Board for Nursing, Midwifery and Health Visiting, London

ENB (1993). *Regulations and Guidelines for the Approval of Institutions and Courses.* English National Board for Nursing, Midwifery and Health Visiting, London.

ENB/DoH (2001). *Preparation of Mentors and Teachers. A New Framework of Guidance.* English National Board for Nursing, Midwifery and Health Visiting/Department of Health, London

Epstein, A. (1990). The outcomes movement – will it get us where we want to go? *New England Journal of Medicine* 323, 266–70

Eraut, M. (1994). *Developing Professional Knowledge and Competence.* The Falmer Press, London

Erikson, E.H. (1968). *Youth and Crisis.* Faber and Faber, London

Erikson, E.H. (1987). The human life cycle. In: Schlein, S., Erikson, E.H. (eds) *A Way of Looking at Things. Selected Papers from 1930 to 1980.* W.W. Norton, New York, p595–610

Esmond, G. (2000). Cystic fibrosis: adolescent care. *Nursing Standard* 13(14), 47–52

European Association for Palliative Care (1989). *Newsletter No 1.* European Association for Palliative Care, Milan

Evandrou, M. (1998). Great expectations: social policy and the new millennium elders. In: Bernard, M., Phillips, J. (eds) *The Social Policy of Old Age: Moving into the 21st Century.* Centre for Policy on Ageing, London

Evans, G. (2001). A rationale for oral care. *Nursing Standard* 15(43), 33–6

Evans, M. (1999). *Ethics: Reconciling Conflicting Values in Health Policy*, Policy Futures for UK Health No. 9. Nuffield Trust, London

Evans, R. (1998). Be glad the patients are complaining. *Nursing Standard* 12(19), 18–20

Evans, S. (1998). Beyond the mirror: a group analytic exploration of late life depression. *Aging and Mental Health* 2(2), 94–9

Evers, H.K. (1981). Multidisciplinary teams in geriatric wards: myth or reality? *Journal of Advanced Nursing* 6, 205–14

Ewins, D., Bryant, J. (1992). Relative comfort. *Nursing Times* 88(52), 61–3

Exall, K., Johnston, H. (1999). Caring for carers coping with stroke. *Nursing Times* 95(11), 50–1

Fairweather, M., Border, R. (2001). *Living Wills and Enduring Powers of Attorney.* The Stationery Office, London

Farrington, A. (1995). Models of clinical supervision. *British Journal of Nursing* 4(15), 876–8

Faugier, J. (1992). The supervisory relationship. In: Butterworth, T., Faugier, J. (eds) *Clinical Supervision and Mentorship in Nursing.* Chapman & Hall, London

Faulder, C. (1985). *Whose Body Is It? The Troubling Issue of Informed Consent.* Virago Press, London

Fay, B. (1987). *Critical Social Science.* Polity Press, Cambridge

Feder, G., Eccles, M., Grol, R., Griffiths, C., Grimshaw, J. (1999). Using clinical guidelines. *British Medical Journal* 318, 728–30

Feigenbaum, A.V. (1963). *Total Quality Control.* McGraw-Hill, New York

Feldman, S. (1999). Please don't call me 'dear': older women's narratives of health. *Nursing Inquiry* 6, 269–76

Field, D., Copp, G. (1999). Communication and awareness about dying in the 1990s. *Palliative Medicine* 13, 459–68

Field, M.J., Lohr, K.N. (eds) (1992). *Guidelines for Clinical Practice. From Development to Use.* National Academy Press, Washington, DC

Fiorentino, L., Phillips, D., Walker, D., Hall, D. (1998). *Health and Social Care in the Community* 6(4), 260–70

Fisher, B., Neve, H., Heritage, Z. (1999). Community development, user involvement, and primary health care: community development has much to offer to primary care groups. *British Medical Journal* 318(7186), 749–50

Fisk, M. (1999). *Our Future Home: Housing and Inclusion of Older People in 2025.* Help the Aged, London

Fletcher, L., Buker, P. (1999). *A Legal Framework for Caring: An Introduction to Law and Ethics in Health Care.* Macmillan Press, London

Flynn, R. (1992). *Structures of Control in Health Management.* Routledge, London

Ford, P., McCormack, B. (1999). The key attributes of a gerontological nurse specialist. *Nursing Standard* 13(33), 31

Fowkes, F.G.R. (1982). Medical audit cycle. *Medical Education* 16, 228–38

Fowkes, F.G.R., McPake, B.I. (1986). Regional variations in outpatient activity in England and Wales. *Community Medicine* 8, 286–91

Fowler, J. (1995). Nurses perceptions of the elements of good supervision. *Nursing Times* 91(22), 33–7

Fowler, J. (1996). The organisation of clinical supervision within the nursing profession. *Journal of Advanced Nursing* 23, 471–8

Fraser, S., Atkins, J. (1990). Survivor's recollections of helpful and unhelpful emergency nurse activities surrounding the sudden death of a loved one. *Journal of Emergency Nursing* 16(1), 13–16

Frasier (1986). Gillick v W Norfolk and Wisbeach Area Health Authority. 1AC 112

Freidson, E. (1970). *Profession of Medicine.* Mead, New York

Fulton, F., Gottesman, D. (1996). In: Wright, B. (ed.) *Sudden Death. A Research Base for Practice,* 2nd edn. Churchill Livingstone, p11

Gabbay, J., McNicol, M.C. Spilby, J. *et al.* (1990). What did audit achieve? Lessons from the preliminary evaluation of a year's medical audit. *British Medical Journal* 301, 526–9

Gallessich, J. (1982a). Diverse approaches to consultation. In: *The Profession and Practice of Consultation.* Jossey-Bass, p87–108

Gallessich, J. (1982b). Evolution: the social context. In: *The Profession and Practice of Consultation.* Jossey-Bass, p17–48

Garner, J., Ardern, M. (1998). Reflection on old age. *Aging and Mental Health* 2(2), 92–3

Gately, E. (1992). PREPP: From novice to expert. *British Journal of Nursing* 1(2), 88–91

Gatford, J.D., Anderson, R.E. (1998). *Nursing Calculations,* 5th edn. Churchill Livingstone, Edinburgh

Gerrish, K., Husband, C., Mackenzie, J. (1996). *Nursing for a Multiethnic Society.* Open University Press, Milton Keynes

Gibbs, G. (1988). *Learning by Doing. A Guide to Teaching and Learning Methods.* Further Education Unit, Oxford Polytechnic, Oxford

Gibson, F., Nelson, W. (2000). Oral hygiene. In: Huband, S., Trigg, E. (eds) *Practices in Children's Nursing: Guidelines for Hospital and Community.* Churchill Livingstone, Edinburgh, p179–88

Gibson, P.G., Coughlan, J., Wilson, A.J. *et al.* (1998). Review: self management education for adults with asthma improves health outcomes. *Evidence-Based Nursing* 1(4), 117

Gillam, S. (ed.) (2001). *What has New Labour Done for Primary Care?* King's Fund, London

Girvin, J. (1998). *Leadership and Nursing.* Macmillan Press, London

Glasper, E.A., Ireland, I. (eds) (2000). *Evidence-Based Child Health Care: Challenges for Practice.* Macmillan Press, Basingstoke, Ch 5 and 15

GOLD – Global Obstructive Lung Disease Initiative (2001). *The Phase 111 Gold Initiative* http://www.goldcopd.com

Gott, M. (1984). *Learning Nursing.* Royal College of Nursing, London

Gould, D. (2001). Pressure ulcer risk assessment. *Nursing Standard* 11(5), 43–9

Greener, M. (2002). Hit the spot. *Nursing Standard* 16(4), 18

Greengross, S., Murphy, E., Quam, L., Rochon, P., Smith, R. (1997). Aging: a subject that must be at the top of the world agendas. *British Medical Journal* 315, 1029–30

Greenhalgh and Co. (1994). *The Interface Between Junior Doctors and Nurses: A Research Study for the Department of Health.* Executive Summary. Greenhalgh and Co. Management Consultants, Cheshire

Greenhalgh, T, (1997). How to read a paper: Assessing the methodological quality of published papers. *British Medical Journal* 315, 305–8

Grey, W. (2000). Right to die or duty to live? The problem of euthanasia. In: Dickenson, D., Johnson, M., Katz, J.S. (eds) *Death, Dying and Bereavement.* Sage, London, p270–83

Griffiths, P. (2000). Commentary. *Evidence-Based Nursing* 3(4), 126–7

Grimby, A. (1993). The influence of urinary incontinence on the quality of life of elderly women. *Age and Ageing* 22, 82–9

Grimley Evans, J. (1994). Can we live to be a healthy hundred? In: *A Healthy Old Age.* Medical Research Council, London

Grimshaw, J., Russell, I.T. (1993). Effect of clinical guidelines on medical practice: a systematic review of rigorous evaluations. *Lancet* 342, 1317–22

Grundy, E., Bowling, A. (1999). Enriching the quality of extended life years: identification of the oldest old with a very good and very poor quality of life. *Aging and Mental Health* 3(3), 199–212

Guest, D., Redfern, S., Wilson-Barnett, J. *et al.* (2001). *A Preliminary Evaluation of the Establishment of Nurse, Midwife and Health Visitor Consultants.* King's College, London

Guyatt, G.H., Meade, M.O., Jaeschke, R.Z. *et al.* (2000). Practitioners of evidence-based care. *British Medical Journal* 320, 954–5

Haas, B.K. (1999). Clarification and integration of similar quality of life concepts. *Image: Journal of Nursing Scholarship* 31(3), 215–20

Hagerty, B. (1986). A second look at mentors. *Nursing Outlook* 34(1), 16–24

Haines, A., Jones, R. (1994). Implementing findings of research. *British Medical Journal* 308, 1488–92

Hall, J. (2000). The nature of pain. *Nursing Times* 96(24), 37–40

Hall, J. (2002). Assessing the health promotion needs of informal carers. *Nursing Older People* 14(2), 14–18

Ham, C. (1998). Retracing the Oregon trail: the appearance of rationing and the Oregon Health Plan. *British Medical Journal* 316, 1965–68

Hamer, S., Collinson, G. (1999). *Achieving Evidence-Based Practice: A Handbook for Practitioners.* Ballière Tindall, London

Hanford, L., Easterbrook, L., Stevenson, J. (1999). *Rehabilitation for Older People: The Emerging Policy Agenda.* King's Fund, London

Harris, A. (1999). Impact of urinary incontinence on the quality of life of women. *British Journal of Nursing* 8(6), 375–80

Harrison, S., Hunter, D., Marnoch, D., Pollitt, C. (1990). *The Dynamics of British Health Policy.* Unwin Hyman, London

HAS (1998). *'Not Because They are Old': An Independent Inquiry into the Care of Older People on Acute Wards in General Hospitals.* Health Advisory Service, London

Hawkins, P., Shohet, R. (1989). *Supervision in the Helping Professions.* Open University Press, Milton Keynes

HEA (1998). *The UK Smoking Epidemic – Deaths in 1995.* Health Education Authority, London

Heath, H. (2000). The nurse's role in assessing an older person. *Elderly Care* 12(1), 23–4

Hector, W. (1968). *Modern Nursing.* Heinmann, Oxford

Help the Aged (1999). *Dignity on the Ward: The Future of Hospital Care for Older People.* Conference Report. Help the Aged, London

Henderson, V. (1966). *The Nature of Nursing: a Definition and its Implications for Practice.* Macmillan, New York

Henderson, V. (1969). *Basic Principles of Nursing Care: The Nature of Nursing. A Definition and its Implications for Practice Research and Education.* ICN, Basel

Henderson, J., Goldacre, M., Yeates, D. (1993). Use of hospital in-patient care in adolescence. *Archives of Disease in Childhood* 69, 559–60

Herbert, R.A., Alison, J.A. (1996). Cardiovascular function. In: Hinchliff, S.M., Watson, R. (eds) *Physiology for Nursing Practice,* 2nd edn. Ballière Tindall, London

Hersey, P., Blanchard, K., Johnson, D. (1996). *Management and Organisational Behaviour: Utilizing Human Resources,* 7th edn. Prentice-Hall, Englewood Cliffs, New Jersey

Hibbs, P. (1988). *Pressure Area Care for the City and Hackney Health Authority.* City and Hackney Health Authority, London

Hickey, J.V. (1992). *The Clinical Practice of Neurosurgical Nursing,* 3rd edn. JB Lippincott, Philadelphia

Hill, J.E. (1993). Caring for the dying patient. In: Hinchliff, S.M., Norman, S.E., Schober, J.E. (eds) *Nursing Practice and Health Care,* 2nd edn. Arnold, London, p812–38

Hinchliff, S. (1998). Lifelong learning in context. In: Quinn, F. (ed.) *Continuing Professional Development in Nursing: A Guide for Practitioners and Educators.* Stanley Thornes (Publishers) Ltd, Cheltenham, p34–58

Hopayian, K. (2001). The need for caution in interpreting high quality systematic reviews. *British Medical Journal* 323, 681–4

Hospital Standards. (2003). *The National Service Framework for Children, Young People and Maternity Services.* Department of Health, London

Huband, S., Trigg, E. (2000). *Practices in Children's Nursing.* Churchill Livingstone, Edinburgh

Humphris, D., Littlejohns, P. (1996). Implementing clinical guidelines: preparation and opportunism. *Journal of Clinical Effectiveness* 1(1), 5–7

Hunt, J. (1981). Indicators for nursing practice: the use of research findings. *Journal of Advanced Nursing* 6(3), 189–94

Hunt, G. (1992). Project 2000 – Ethics, ambivalence and ideology. In: Slein, O., Buckenham, M. (eds) *Project 2000: The Teachers Speak.* Campion Press, Edinburgh

Husband, L., Henry, C. (2002). Palliative care and care of the dying. In: Kenworthy, N., Snowley, G., Gilling, C. (eds) *Common Foundation Studies in Nursing,* 3rd edn. Churchill Livingstone, Edinburgh, p483–507

Hutchfield, K. (1999). Family-centred care: a concept analysis. *Journal of Advanced Nursing* 29(5), 1178–87

Iliffe, S., Lenihan, P. (2001). Primary care for older people: putting research into practice. *Community Practitioner* 73(12), 867–9

Independent Healthcare Association (1999). *Report to the Department of Health on the Provision of Clinical Placements in Independent Sector Acute, Mental Health Hospitals and Nursing Homes.* Independent Healthcare Association, London

Independent Healthcare Association (2002). *Handling Patients' Complaints – A Code of Practice for Members of the Independent Healthcare Association.* Independent Healthcare Association, London

International Association for the Study of Pain (1992). *Management of Acute Pain: A Practical Guide.* IASP Publications, Seattle

International Council of Nurses (2000). *Participation of Nurses in Health Services Decision Making and Policy Development.* ICN, Geneva

Jackson, J.A. (1970). *Professions and Professionalization.* Cambridge University Press, Cambridge

Jasper, M. (1996). *Evaluating Care and Effecting Change.* Unit study guide. Distance Learning Centre, South Bank University, London

Jevon, P., Ewens, B. (2001). Assessment of a breathless patient. *Nursing Standard* 15(16), 48–53

JM Consulting Ltd. (1998). *The Regulation of Nurses, Midwives and Health Visitors.* JM Consulting Ltd., Bristol

Johns, C. (1992). Ownership and the harmonious team. *Journal of Clinical Nursing* 1(2), 89–94

Johns, C. (1993). Professional supervision. *Journal of Nursing Management* 1, 9–18

Johns, C. (1997). Reflective practice and clinical supervision – Part 1 The reflective turn. *European Nurse* 2(2), 87–97

Johns, C. (2000a). *Becoming a Reflective Practitioner: A Reflective and Holistic Approach to Clinical Nursing, Practice Development and Clinical Supervision.* Blackwell Science, Oxford

Johns, C. (2000b). Becoming a reflective practitioner. In: Johns, C. (ed.) *Becoming a Reflective Practitioner: A Reflective and Holistic Approach to Clinical Nursing, Practice Development and Clinical Supervision.* Blackwell Science, Oxford, Ch 3

Johnson, G., Crombie, I., Davies, H.T.O. *et al.* (2000). Reviewing audit: barriers and facilitating factors for effective clinical audit. *Quality in Health Care* 9, 23–36

Johnson, C.L., Barer, B.M. (1997). *Life beyond 85 Years: the Aura of Survivorship.* Springer, New York

Johnson, M.L., Purdy, E., Wright, S.G. (1989). The nurse as consultant. *Nursing Standard* 5(20), 31–6

Johnston, T. (1972). *Professions and Power.* Macmillan Press, London

Jones, W., Buttery, M. (1981). Sudden death: survivor's perceptions of the Emergency Department experience. *Journal of Emergency Nursing* 7(1), 14–17

Jones, H., Elton, J., Deeth, M., Wheatley, C. (1999). *Leicestershire Grade IV Pressure Ulcer Audit.* c/o J. Elton, University Hospitals of Leicester NHS Trust

Joseph Rowntree Foundation (1999). *Developing a Preventive Approach with Older People.* Joseph Rowntree Foundation, York

Juni, P., Altman, D., Egger, M. (2001). Assessing the quality of controlled clinical trials. *British Medical Journal* 323, 42–6

Katz, J., Sidel, M. (1994). *Easeful Death: Caring for Dying and Bereaved People.* Hodder and Stoughton, London, p16–17

Katzenbatch, J., Smith, D. (1993). *The Wisdom of Teams.* Harvard Business School Press, Boston, MA

Kearns, D., Nadler, D. (1992). *Prophets in the Dark: How Xerox Reinvented Itself and Beat the Japanese.* Harper Business, New York

Keen, J. (2000). In sickness and in wealth. *The Guardian*, November 6

Kemp, C. (1999). Spiritual care: Faiths. In: *Terminal Illness: A Guide to Nursing Care*, 2nd edn. Lippincott, Philadelphia, 56–77

Kerr, D. (2002). Decontamination of surgical instruments. *Healthcare Solutions Infection Control & Sterilisation* 88 –91. Business Briefing. Global Healthcare

King, I. (1981). *A Theory for Nursing: Systems, Concepts, Processes.* John Wiley, Chichester

Kirby, C., Slein, O. (1992). A new curriculum for care. In: Slein, O., Buckenham, M. (eds) *Project 2000: The Teachers Speak.* Campion Press, Edinburgh

Kirk, S., Glendinning, C. (1998). Trends in community care and patient participation: implications for the roles of informal carers and community nurses in the United Kingdom. *Journal of Advanced Nursing* 28(2), 370–81

Kirkness, B. (ed.) (2000). *The Expert Patient.* The Association of the British Pharmaceutical Industry, London

Kitson, A. (1991). *Therapeutic Nursing and the Hospitalised Elderly.* Scutari Press, Harrow

Kitson, A. (1994). Post operative pain management: A literature review. *Journal of Clinical Nursing* 3(1), 7–18

Kitson, A. (1997). Using evidence to demonstrate the value of nursing. *Nursing Standard* 11(28), 34–9

Kitwood, T. (1997) *Dementia Reconsidered: The Person Comes First.* Open University Press, Buckingham

Kivnick, H.Q., Murray, S.U. (1997). Vital involvement: an overlooked source of identity in frail elders. *Journal of Aging and Identity* 2(3), 205–25

Klein, R. (1998). Can policy drive quality? *Quality in Health Care* 7(Suppl), S51–3

Kohner, N. (1994). *The Moral Maze of Practice.* King's Fund, London

Kolb, D. (1984). *Experiential Learning: Experience as the Source of Learning and Development.* Prentice Hall, New Jersey

Korgaonkar, G., Tribe, D. (1992). *Living Wills Their Legal Status.* Hertfordshire and District Medico-Legal Society, Hertfordshire

Kübler-Ross, E. (1969). *On Death and Dying.* Macmillan, New York

Kurtz , Z., Hopkins, A. (eds) (1996). *Services for Young People with Chronic Disorders in their Transition from Childhood to Adult Life.* Royal College of Physicians, London

Kyngas, H. (2000a). Compliance of adolescents with diabetes. *Journal of Pediatric Nursing* 15(4), 260–7

Kyngas, H. (2000b). Compliance of adolescents with rheumatiod arthritis. *International Journal of Nursing Practice* 6(5), 261–7

Kyngas, H. (2000c). Compliance of adolescents with chronic disease. *Journal of Clinical Nursing* 9(4), 549–56

Laing and Buisson (2000). *Care of Elderly People: Market Survey 2000*, 13th edn. Laing and Buisson, London

Laming, Lord. (2003). *The Victoria Climbie Inquiry.* Department of Health, HMSO

La Monica, E.L. (1990). *Management in Health Care: A Theoretical and Experiential Approach.* Macmillan, Basingstoke, p242–61

Lancaster, T., Stead, L., Silagy, C., Sowden, A. (2000). Review: advice from doctors, counselling by nurses, behavioural interventions, nicotine replacement therapy and several pharmacological treatments increase smoking cessation rates. *Evidence-Based Nursing* 4(1), 13

Lansdown, R. (1996). *Children in Hospital: A Guide for Family and Carers.* Oxford University Press, Oxford, p43–83

Lansdowne, R. (1998). Listening to children: have we gone too far (or not enough)? *Journal of the Royal Society of Medicine* 91, 457–61

Law, C. (2000). A guide to assessing sputum. *Nursing Times* 96(24), S7–10

Lawton, M.P., Moss, M., Hoffman, C., Grant, R., Hove, T.T., Kleban, M.H. (1999). Health, valuation of life and the wish to live. *Gerontologist* 39(4), 406–16

Layton, A., Moss, F., Morgan, G. (1998). Mapping out the patient's journey: experiences of developing pathways of care. *Quality in Health Care* 7(Suppl), S30–6

Lefrancois, G. (1992). *An Introduction to Child Development.* Wadsworth Publishing, California

Leicestershire Nutrition and Dietetic Services (1998). *Nutritional Screening Tool.* Leicester Royal Infirmary, Leicester

Leidy, N.K., Haase, J.E. (1999). Patients with chronic obstructive pulmonary disease experienced ongoing challenges of preserving their personal integrity. *Evidence-Based Nursing* 2(4)

Leifer, D. (2002). Does it all add up? *Nursing Standard* 16(29), 14–15

Le May, A. (1999). *Evidence-Based Practice.* Nursing Times Clinical Monographs No 1. EMAP Healthcare, London

Lewin, R. (1997). Psychological guidelines for cardiac rehabilitation. In: Thompson, D.R., De Bono, D., Hopkins, A. (eds) *Guidelines for Cardiac Rehabilitation.* Monograph of National Institute of Nursing and the Royal College of Physicians, London

Lewin, R.J.P., Ingelton, I., Newens, A.J., Thompson, D.R. (1998). Adherence to cardiac rehabilitation guidelines: a survey of rehabilitation programmes in the United Kingdom. *British Medical Journal* 316, 1354–5

Liaschenko, J. (1997). Knowing the patient. In: Thorne, S.E., Hays, V.E. (eds) *Nursing Praxis: Knowledge and Action.* Sage, Thousand Oaks

Lightbody, E., Watkins, C., Leathley, M., Sharma, A., Lye, M. (2002). Evaluation of a nurse led falls prevention programme versus usual care: a randomised controlled trial. *Age and Ageing* 31(3), 203–10

Lomas, J. (1993). Diffusion, dissemination and implementation: Who should do what? *Annals of the New York Academy of Science* 703, 226–37

Luft, P., Koch, L.C. (1998). Transition of adolescents with chronic illness: overlooked needs and rehabilitation considerations. *Journal of Vocational Rehabilitation* 10(3), 205–17

Luker, K., Kenrick, M. (1995). Towards knowledge-based practice; an evaluation of a method of dissemination. *International Journal of Nursing Studies* 32, 1, 59–67

Macfarlane, A. (ed.) (1996). *Adolescent Medicine.* Royal College of Physicians, London

MacGregor Burns, J. (1978). *Leadership.* Harper & Row, New York

Maggs, C. (1994). Mentorship in nursing and midwifery education: Issues for research. *Nurse Education Today* 14, 22–9

Mallinson, P., Connell, H., Bennett, M.S., Eccleston, C. (2001). Chronic musculoskeletal and other idiopathic pain syndromes. *Archives of Disease in Childhood* 84, 189–92

Manley, K. (1997). Operationalising an advanced practice/consultant nurse role; an action research study. *Journal of Clinical Nursing* 6, 179–90

Manley, K. (2000). Organisational culture and consultant nurse outcomes part 1 – organisational culture. *Nursing Standard* 14(36), 34–8

Manthey, M. (1994). *Creative nursing management/creative health care management.* In: Miller, D.A. (ed.) Leading an Empowered Organisation. Minneapolis

Marieb, E. (1999). *Human Anatomy and Physiology*, 4th edn. Addison Wesley, California

Marrow, C., Macauley, D., Crumbie, A. (1997). Promoting reflective practice through structured clinical supervision. *Journal of Nursing Management* 5, 77–82

Martin, J.P. (1984). *Hospitals in Trouble*. Oxford, Blackwell

Mathias, P., Prime, R., Thompson, T. (1997). Preparation for interprofessional work: Holism, integration and the purpose of training and education. In: Ovretveit, J., Mathias, P., Thompson, T. (eds) *Interprofesional Working for Health and Social Care*. Macmillan Press, Basingstoke

Maxwell, R.J. (1984). Quality assessment in health. *British Medical Journal* 12(5), 84–6

Maxwell, R.J. (1992). Dimensions of quality revisited: from thought to action. *Quality in Health Care* 1, 17–7

May, K. (1982). Mentorship for scholarliness. *Nursing Outlook* 30, 22–6

Mayo, N.E., Wood-Dauphinee, S., Cote, R. (2000). Prompt hospital discharge with home care improved physical health and community reintegration and reduced initial length of hospital stay after acute stroke. *Evidence-Based Nursing* 3(4), 126

McAlister, F. (2001). Applying the results of systematic reviews at the bedside. In: Egger, M., Davey Smith, G., Altman, D.G. (eds) *Systematic Reviews in Health Care*, 2nd edn. BMJ Books, London

McCaugherty, D. (1991). The use of a teaching model to promote reflection and the experiential integration of theory and practice in 1st year student nurses: An action research study. *Journal of Advanced Nursing* 16, 534–43

McGann, S. (1992). *The Battle of the Nurses*. Scutari Press, London

McGinty, J., Fish, J. (1996). Educational aspects of transition. In: Kurtz, Z., Hopkins, A. (eds) *Services for Young People with Chronic Disorders*. Royal College of Physicians, London, p99–108

McGregor, D. (1960). *The Human Side of Enterprise*. McGraw-Hill, New York

McKinney, J.P., Fitzgerald, H.E., Stommen, E.A. (1977). *Developmental Psychology: The Adolescent and Young Adult*. The Dorsey Press, Homewood, Illinois

McPherson, K., Strong, P., Epstein, A., Jones, L. (1981). Regional variation in the use of common surgical procedures. *Social Science and Medicine* 15, 273–88

McSherry, R. (1997). What do registered nurses and midwives feel and know about research? *Journal of Advanced Nursing* 25(5), 985–98

Meyer, J., Bridges, J., Spilsbury, K. (1999). Caring for older people in acute settings: lessons learned from an action research study in accident and emergency. *NT Research* 4(5), 327–39

Mezirow, J. (1981). A critical theory of adult learning and education. *Adult Education* 32(1), 3–24

Mills, M., Davies, H.T.O., Macrae, W.A. (1994). Care of dying patients in hospital. *British Medical Journal* 309, 583–6

Mills, C. (1997). In: Fulbrooke, P., Buckley, P., Mills, C. *et al.* (1977). On the receiving end: Experience of being a relative in Critical Care. Part 2. *Nursing in Critical Care* 4(4) p179–85

Ministry of Health (1959). *Welfare of Children in Hospital* (Chairman H. Platt). HSMO, London

Minkler, M. (1996). Critical perspectives on ageing: new challenges for gerontology. *Ageing and Society* 16(4), 467–87

Mitchell, J. (2002). The slow road back. *Health Service Journal* 112(5816), 25

Mitchell, P., Koch, T. (1997). An attempt to give nursing home residents a voice in the quality improvement process: the challenge of frailty. *Journal of Clinical Nursing* 6(6), 453–61

Mittman, B.S., Tonesk, X., Jacobson, P.D. (1992). Implementing clinical practice guidelines: social influence strategies and practitioner behaviour change. *Quality Review Bulletin* December, 413–22

Morrell, C., Harvey, G. (2000). *The Clinical Audit Handbook: Improving the quality of care*. Baillière Tindall and Royal College of Nursing, London

Morrell, C., Harvey, G., Kitson, A. (1997). Practitioner based quality improvement: a review of the Royal College of Nursing's dynamic standard setting system. *Quality in Health Care* 6, 29–34

Morris, N., John, G., Keen, T. (1988). Mentors: learning the ropes. *Nursing Times* 84(46), 24–7

Morton-Cooper, A., Palmer, A. (2000). *Mentoring, Preceptorship and Clinical Supervision: A Guide to Professional Roles in Clinical Practice*, 2nd edn. Blackwell Science, Oxford

Moss, F. (1998). Quality in health care: getting to the heart of the matter. In: *The Quest for Excellence: Essays in Honour of Robert J Maxwell*. King's Fund, London

Moss, B. (2002). Palliative care in acute hospitals. *Nursing Times* 98(6), 35–6

Moules, T., Ramsay, J. (1998). *The Textbook of Children's Nursing*. Stanley Thornes Publishers, Cheltenham

Mulhall, A.B., Chapman, R.G., Crow, R.A. (1988). The acquisition of bacterivria. *Nursing Times* 84(4), 61–2

Mulhall, A., Alexander, C., le May, A. (1998). Appraising the evidence for practice: what do nurses need? *Journal of Clinical Effectiveness* 3(2), 54–8

Munro, R. (1999). Together we can do it. *Nursing Times* 9(7), 27

Munshi, S.K., Lakhani, D., Ageed, A., Evans, S.N., Mackness, F., Fancourt, G. (2002). Readmissions of older people to acute medical units. *Nursing Older People* 14(1), 14–16

Murphy, W. (2001). Leadership and community children's nurses. *Paediatric Nursing* 13(10), 36–40

Myrick, F., Barrett, C. (1994). Selecting clinical preceptors for basic Baccalaureate nursing students. *Journal of Advanced Nursing* 19, 194–8

Naidoo, J., Wills, J. (1994). *Health Promotion: Foundations for Practice*. Baillière Tindall, London, p240–7

National Assembly for Wales (2001). *Signposts: A Practical Guide to Public and Patient Involvement in Wales* www.wales.gov.uk/subihealth/content/nhs/signposts/index.htm

National Co-ordinating Centre for NHS Service Delivery and Organization (2001). *Organizational Change: A Review for Health Care Managers, Professionals and Researchers*. NCCSDO, London

National Council for Hospice and Specialist Palliative Care Services (1999). *Palliative Care 2000: Commissioning Through Partnership*. National Council for Hospice and Specialist Palliative Care Services, London

NAWCH (1990). *Setting Standards for Adolescents in Hospital*. Quality Review Series. National Association for the Welfare of Children in Hospital, London

Nazarko, L. (1997). Continence: the whole story. *Nursing Times* 93(43), 63–4, 66, 68

NBS (2000). *Children's Nursing – Core Skills and Competencies*. NBS

Newman, M., Hayes, N., Sugden, M. (2001). Evidence-based practice: a framework for the role of lecturer-practitioner. *Clinical Effectiveness in Nursing* 5, 26–9

Newton, C. (1991). The *Roper–Logan–Tierney Model in Action*. Macmillan, Houndmills

NHS Centre for Reviews and Dissemination (1997). *Effective Health Care 1997: Compression Therapy for Venous Leg Ulcers*. NHS Centre for Reviews and Dissemination, University of York, York

NHS Executive (1993). *A Vision for the Future*. NHS Executive, Leeds

NHS Executive (1996). *Hospital Services for Children and Young People*, 5th report. Minutes of Evidence. House of Commons Health Committee, London

NHS Executive (1999a). *Clinical Governance: Quality in the new NHS*. Health Service Circular, London

NHS Executive (1999b). *Nurse, Midwife and Health Visitor Consultants: Establishing Posts and Making Appointments*, Health Service Circular 1999/217. NHS Executive, Leeds

NHS Executive South East (2000). *The Report of the Inquiry into Quality and Practice within the National Health Service arising from the Actions of Rodney Ledward.* NHS Executive, London

NICE (2001a). *The Guideline Development Process – Information for the Public and the NHS.* National Institute for Clinical Excellence, London

NICE (2001b). *The Guideline Development Process – Information for National Collaborating Centres and Guideline Development Groups.* National Institute for Clinical Excellence, London

NICE (2002). *Compilation: Summary of Guidance Issued to the NHS in England and Wales,* Issue 4, April 2002. NICE, London www.nice.org.uk

Nicklin, P. (1995). Super supervision. *Nursing Management* 2(5), 24–5

Nicklin, P. (1997). A practice centred model of clinical supervision. *Nursing Times* 12(93), 52–4

Nilsson, M., Ekman, S., Sarvimäki, A. (1998). Ageing with joy or resigning to old age: older people's experiences of the quality of life in old age. *Health Care in Later Life* 3(2), 94–110

NMC (2002a). *Code of Professional Conduct.* Nursing and Midwifery Council, London

NMC (2002b). *Council Report Issue 23,* March. Nursing and Midwifery Council, London

NMC (2002c). *Requirements for Pre-registration Midwifery Programmes.* Nursing and Midwifery Council, London

NMC (2002d). *Registering as a Nurse or Midwife in the United Kingdom.* Nursing and Midwifery Council, London

NMC (2002e). *Supporting Nurses and Midwives Through Lifelong Learning.* Nursing and Midwifery Council, London

NMC (2002f). *The PREP Handbook.* Nursing and Midwifery Council, London

NMC (2002g). *Practitioner–Client Relationships and the Prevention of Abuse.* Nursing and Midwifery Council, London

Nolan, M.R. (1997). Health and social care: what the future holds for nursing. Keynote address at Third Royal College of Nursing Older Person European Conference and Exhibition, Harrogate

Nolan, J. (2001). Community care. In: Nolan, M., Davies, S., Grant, G. (eds) *Working with Older People and their Families.* Open University Press, Buckingham, p53–74

Nolan, M.R., Grant, G., Caldock, K., Keady, J. (1994). *A Framework for Assessing the Needs of Family Carers: A Multi-disciplinary Guide.* BASE Publications, Stoke-on-Trent

Nolan, M., Grant, G., Nolan, J. (1995). Busy doing nothing: activity and interaction levels amongst differing populations of elderly patients. *Journal of Advanced Nursing* 22(3), 528–38

Nolan, M.R., Grant, G., Keady, J. (1996). *Understanding Family Care.* Open University Press, Buckingham

Nolan, M., Davies, S., Grant, G. (2001). *Working with Older People and their Families.* Open University Press, Buckingham

Nolan, M., Brown, J., Davies, S., Keady, J., Nolan, J. (2002). *Advancing Gerontological Education in Nursing: Final Report of the AGEIN Project.* Report to the English National Board for Nursing, Midwifery and Health Visiting. University of Sheffield, Sheffield

Norton, C. (1986). *Nursing for Continence.* Beaconsfield Publishers, Beaconsfield

Norton, D., Exton-Smith, A., McLaren, R. (1962). *An Investigation of Geriatric Nursing Problems in Hospital.* National Corporation for the Care of Older People, London

Norwich Union (2002). *The Views of Adolescents and Nurses on the Provision of Healthcare in Hospitals.* Norwich Union Healthcare, Hampshire

Oakley, A. (1989). Who's afraid of the randomised controlled trial? Some dilemmas of the scientific method and 'good' research practice. *Women and Health* 15(4), 25–59

O'Boyle, C.A. (1997). Measuring the quality of later life. *Philosophical Transactions of the Royal Society of London Series B – Biological Sciences* 352(136), 1871–9

Office for National Statistics (1999). *Social Trends 29*. HMSO, London

OPCS (1980). *Classification of Occupations 1980*. HMSO, London

OPCS (1990). *General Household Survey*. HMSO, London

OPCS (1991a). *General Household Survey England and Wales*. OPCS, London

OPCS (1991b). *Population Censuses and Surveys*. OPCS, London

Orem, D. (1995). *Nursing: Concepts of Practice*, 5th edn. Mosby, St Louis

Ouellet, L. (1993). Relationship of a preceptorship experience to the views about nursing as a profession. *Nurse Education Today* 13, 16–23

Oxman, A. (1994). *No Magic Bullets: A Systematic Review of 102 Trials of Interventions to Help Health Care Professionals Deliver Services More Effectively and Efficiently*. North East Thames Regional Health Authority, London

Packer, T. (2000). Does person-centred care exist? *Journal of Dementia Care* 8(3), 19–21

Parasuraman, A., Zeithaml, V.A., Berry, L.L. (1985). A conceptual model of service quality and its implications for future research. *Journal of Marketing* 49, 41 50

Parasuraman, A., Zeithaml, V.A., Berry, L.L. (1988). SERVQUAL: A multiple item scale for measuring consumer perceptions of service quality. *Journal of Retailing* 64, 12–40

Parker, M.J, Gillespie, L.D., Gillespie, W.J. (2001). Review: hip protectors reduce hip fracture after falls in elderly people living in institutions or supported home environments. *Evidence-Based Nursing* 3(4), 23

Parkes, C.M. (1972). *Bereavement Studies of Grief in Adult Life*. Penguin, Harmondsworth

Parkes, C.M. (1986). *Bereavement*. Penguin, London

Parkes, C.M. (2000). Bereavement as a psychosocial transition, processes of adaptation to change. In: Dickenson, D., Johnson, M., Katz, J. *Death, Dying and Bereavement*. Sage, London, p325–31

Pearson, A. (1996). *Nursing Models for Practice*. Butterworth Heinmann, Oxford

Peate, I. (1993). Nurse administered oral hygiene in the hospitalised patient. *British Journal of Nursing* 2(9), 459–62

Pedlar, M., Burgoyne, J., Boydell, T. (1991). *The Learning Company*. McGraw Hill, New York

Pellatt, G. (2001). Caring for the person with impaired mobility. In: Baillie, L. (ed.) *Developing Practical Nursing Skills*. Arnold, London

Pencheon, D. (1998). *Evolution of an Evidence-based Approach to Health Care Decision Making: Changing the Culture*. Evidence-based Health Advice Workshop 4–5 November 1998

Peplau, H. (1988). *Interpersonal Relationships in Nursing*. Putnam, New York

Peplau, H.E. (1992). *Interpersonal Relations in Nursing: A Conceptual Frame of Reference for Psychodynamic Nursing*, 2nd edn. Macmillan, Basingstoke

Peutz, B. (1985). Learning the ropes from a mentor. *Nursing Success Today* 2(6), 11–13

Phillipson, C., Biggs, S. (1998). Modernity and identity: theories and perspectives in the study of older adults. *Journal of Aging and Identity* 3(1), 11–23

Place, B. (2000). Pulse oximetry: benefits and limitations. *Nursing Times* 96(26), 34

Place, B., Graham, S. (2000). Non-invasive vital organ assessment. *Nursing Times* 96(20), S6–9

Porter, E. (1995). A phenomenological alternative to the 'ADL Research Tradition'. *Journal of Aging and Health* 7(1), 24–45

Pound, P., Ebrahim, S. (2001). Patients in stroke units have better outcomes, but receive less personal nursing care. *Evidence-Based Nursing* 4(4), 128

Pownceby, J. (1996). *The Coming of Age Project.* The Cystic Fibrosis Trust, Kent

Poxton, R. (1998). Community care for older people: taking the broad view for radical change. *Managing Community Care* 6(1), 13–19

Prophet, H. (ed.) (1998). *Fit for the Future: the Prevention of Dependency in Later Life.* Continuing Care Conference, London

Pyne, R. (1998). *Professional Discipline in Nursing, Midwifery and Health Visiting,* 3rd edn. Blackwell Science, Oxford

Qureshi, H., Bamford, C., Nicholas, E., Patmore, C., Harris, J.C. (2000). *Outcomes in Social Care Practice: Developing an Outcome Focus in Care Management and Use Surveys.* Social Policy Research Unit, University of York

Raphael, B. (1984). *The Anatomy of Bereavement – A Handbook for the Caring Professions.* Hutchinson, London

Raynes, N.V. (1998). Involving residents in quality specification. *Ageing and Society* 18(1), 65–77

RCN (1995a). *The Nursing Care of Older Patients from Black and Minority Ethnic Communities.* Royal College of Nursing, London

RCN (1995b). *A Guide to Planning Your Career.* Royal College of Nursing, London, p5

RCN (1997). *What a Difference a Nurse Makes. An RCN Report on the Benefits of Expert Nursing to Clinical Outcomes in the Continuing Care of Older People.* Royal College of Nursing, London

RCN (1998a). *Guidance for Nurses on Clinical Governance.* Royal College of Nursing, London

RCN (1998b). *The Management of Patients with Venous Leg Ulcers: Recommendations for Assessment, Compression Therapy, Cleansing, Debridement, Dressing, Contact Sensitivity, Training, Education and Quality assurance.* Royal College of Nursing, London

RCN (1999a). *Clinical Practice Guidelines on the Recognition and Assessment of Acute Pain in Children.* Royal College of Nursing, London

RCN (1999b). *Doing the Right Thing, Clinical Effectiveness for Nurses.* Royal College of Nursing, London

RCN (1999c). *Working Well Initiative, Changing Practice, Improving Health: An Integrated Back Injury Prevention Programme for Nursing and Care Homes.* Royal College of Nursing, London

RCN (2000a). *Clinical Governance: How Nurses can get Involved.* Royal College of Nursing, London

RCN (2000b). *The Management of the Patient with Venous Leg Ulcers.* Report of the National Sentinel Audit Pilot Project. Royal College of Nursing, London

RCN (2001). *Blowing the Whistle.* Royal College of Nursing, London

RCN (2002). *Behind the Headlines: A Review of the UK Nursing Labour Market in 2001.* Royal College of Nursing, London

RCP (2000). *The National Clinical Guidelines for Stroke.* Royal College of Physicians, London

Reed, J. (1989). *All Dressed Up and Nowhere to Go: Nursing Assessment in Geriatric Care.* PhD thesis. Newcastle upon Tyne Polytechnic, Newcastle upon Tyne

Reed, J., Bond, S. (1991). Nurses' assessment of elderly patients in hospital. *International Journal of Nursing Studies* 28(1), 55–64

Reed, J., Cook, G., Stanley, D. (1999). Promoting partnership with older people through quality assurance systems: issues arising in care homes. *NT Research* 4(5), 353–63

Reinertsen, J. (1998). Physicians as leaders in the improvement of health care systems. *Annals of Internal Medicine* 128, 833–8

Richardson, J. (1993). Transcultural aspect of paediatric nursing. In: Glasper, E., Tucker, A. (eds) *Advances in Child Health Nursing.* Scutari, London, Ch 7

Ring, L., Davidson, E. (1997). Patients' experiences of longterm home oxygen therapy. *Journal of Advanced Nursing* 26, 337–44

Roberts, J., DiCenso, A. (1999). Identifying the best research design to fit the question. Part 1: quantitative designs. *Evidence-Based Nursing* 2, 4–6

Robertson, M.C., Devlin, N., Gardner, M.M. (2001). A home based, nurse delivered exercise programme reduced falls and serious injuries in people >80 years of age. *Evidence-Based Nursing* 5(1), 22

Robinson, S. (1990). Maintaining the independence of the midwifery profession: A continuing struggle. In: Garcia, J., Kilpatrick, R., Richards, M. (eds) *The Politics of Maternity Care: Services for Childbearing Women in Twentieth Century Britain.* Clarendon Press, London

Robinson, J., Elkan, R. (1997). Nursing up to and beyond the year 2000. In: Salvage, J., Heijnen, S. (eds) *Nursing in Europe.* World Health Organization Regional Publications, European Series No. 74, Copenhagen

Rolfe, G., Freshwater, D., Jasper, M. (2001). *Critical Reflection for Nursing and the Helping Professions: A Users Guide.* Models of critical reflection. Palgrave, Hampshire

Roper, N. (2000). *Models for Nursing: Based on Activities for Living.* Churchill Livingstone, Edinburgh

Roper, N., Logan, W., Tierney, A. (1996). *The Elements of Nursing: Based on a Model of Living*, 4th edn. Churchill Livingstone, Edinburgh

Royal Commission on Long Term Care (1999). *With Respect to Old Age: Longterm Care – Rights and Responsibilities.* The Stationery Office, London

Rudd, A.G., Millard, P.H. (1988). What is ageing? *Baillières Clinical Obstetrics and Gynaecology* 2(2), 241–59

Rycroft-Malone, J. (2001). Formal consensus: the development of a national clinical guideline. *Quality in Health Care* 10(4), 238–44

Sackett, D., Richardson, W.S., Rosenberg, W., Haynes, R.B. (1997). *Evidence-Based Medicine: How to Practice and Teach EBM.* Churchill Livingstone, London

Sale, D. (1996). Quality sssurance: for nurses and other members of the health care team. In: *Essentials of Nursing Management*, 2nd edn. Macmillan Press, London

Salvage, J. (ed.) (1993). *Nursing in Action: Strengthening Nursing and Midwifery to Support Health for All.* World Health Organization Regional Publications, European Series No. 48, Copenhagen

Salvage, J. (1998). Nursing today and tomorrow. In: Hinchliff, S., Norman, S., Schober, J. (eds) *Nursing Practice and Health Care*, 3rd edn. Arnold, London

Salvage, J. (2002). *Rethinking Professionalism: The First Step for Patient-Focused Care?* Institute for Public Policy Research, London

Salvage, J., Heijnen, S. (eds) (1997). *Nursing in Europe.* World Health Organization Regional Publications, European Series, Copenhagen

Sandberg, J., Lundh, U., Nolan, M.R. (2001). Spouses who placed partners in care homes experienced emotional reactions to separation and made efforts to maintain their relationship. *Evidence-Based Nursing* 5(1), 32

Schave, D., Schave, B. (1989). *Early Adolescence and the Search for Self: A Developmental Perspective.* Praeger Publishers, New York

Scheidt, R.J., Humphreys, D.R., Yorgason, J.B. (1999). Successful ageing: what's not to like? *Journal of Applied Gerontology* 18(8), 277–82

Schidlow, D.V., Fiel, S.B. (1990). Life beyond pediatrics. Transition of chronically ill adolescents from pediatrics to adult health care systems. *Medical Clinics of North America* 74(11), 13–20

Schober, J.E. (1990). Your career – making the choices. In: Tschudin, V., Schober, J.E. (eds) *Managing Yourself.* Macmillan, London

Schober, J.E. (1998). Nursing: Issues for effective practice. In: Hinchcliff, S., Norman, S., Schober, J. (eds) *Nursing Practice and Health Care,* 3rd edn. Arnold, London

Schober, J.E. (2000). Career opportunities for nurses working with surgical patients. In: Manley, K., Bellman, L. (eds) *Surgical Nursing Advancing Practice.* Churchill Livingstone, Edinburgh

Schon, D. (1987). *Educating the Reflective Practitioner.* Jossey Bass, San Francisco

Schon, D. (1991). *The Reflective Practitioner.* The Academic Publishing Group, Aldershot

Scott, P. (1998). Professional ethics: are we on the wrong track? *Nursing Ethics* 5(6), 477–85

Scottish Executive (2000a). *Our Health: A Plan for Action, A Plan for Change: Commissioning Through Partnership.* National Council for Hospice and Specialist Palliative Care Services, London

Scottish Executive (2000b). *Health Bulletin* 58(4) http://www.scotland.gov.uk/health/cmobulletin/ hb58-02.asp

Seecombe, I., Ball, J., Patch, A. (1993). *The Price of Commitment: Nurses' Pay, Careers & Prospects.* Institute of Manpower Studies, Brighton

Seedhouse, D. (2000). *Practical Nursing Philosophy: The Universal Ethical Code.* John Wiley, Chichester

Seedhouse, D. (2001). *Ethics: The Heart of Health Care.* John Wiley, Chichester

Senge, P. (1990). *The Fifth Discipline.* Doubleday, London

Shaw, P.J. (1999). Science medicine and the future: motor neurone disease. *British Journal of Medicine* 318, 1118–21

Sheehan, J., Crotty, F. (2001). Treatment for depression is an important confounding variable. (Letter). *British Medical Journal* 323, 1376

Sheppard, S. (2000). Pulse oximetry: a case study. *Nursing Times* 96(27), 35

Shipton, H. (2000). Play. In: Huband, S., Trigg, E. (eds) *Practices in Children's Nursing: Guidelines for Hospital and Community.* Churchill Livingstone, Edinburgh, p329–34

Simnett, A. (1986). The pursuit of respectability: women in the nursing profession 1860–1900. In: White, R. (ed.) *Political Issues in Nursing Past, Present and Future.* John Wiley, Chichester

Simpson, H. (1991). *Peplau's Model in Action.* Macmillan, Basingstoke

Singleton, J., McClaren, S. (1995). *Ethical Foundations of Health Care.* Mosby, St Louis

Skyte, S. (1997). PREP The key to safe practice and upholding standards. Learning Curve. *Nursing Times* 1(10), 2–3

Slevin, O. (1992). Knowledgeable doing: the theoretical basis for practice. In: Slevin, O., Buckenham, M. (eds) *Project 2000: The Teachers Speak.* Campion Press, Edinburgh

Smale, G., Tilson, G., Biehal, N., Mars, P. (1993). *Empowerment, Assessment, Care Management and the Skilled Worker.* National Institute for Social Work Practice and Development Exchange. HMSO, London

Smith, P. (1998). Caring for the dying patient: principles of palliative care. In: Hinchliff, S.M., Norman, S.E., Schober, J.E. (eds). *Nursing Practice and Health Care.* Arnold, London, p693–711

Smith, F., Valentine, F. (1999). Value added decisions. *Paediatric Nursing* 11(7), 9–10

Smith, E.A., Young, A.P. (2002). The practitioner as manager. In: Young, A.P., Cooke, M. (eds) *Managing and Implementing Decisions in Health Care.* Ballière Tindall, London, Ch 5

SNMAC (2001). *Caring for Older People: A Nursing Priority.* Standing Nursing and Midwifery Advisory Committee, Department of Health, London

Snowball, J., Ross, K., Murphy, K. (1994). Illuminating dissertation supervision through reflection. *Journal of Advanced Nursing* 19, 1234–40

Soanes, L. (1997). Effect of conflict on the successful formation of nurse–parent relationships. *Journal of Cancer Nursing* 1(4), 191–6

Soothill, K., Mackay, L., Webb, L. (eds) (1999). *Interprofessional Relations in Health Care*. Edward Arnold, London

Spires, A. (2002). Managing cultural diversity in care. In: Kenworthy, N., Snowley, G., Gilling, C. (eds) *Common Foundation Studies in Nursing*, 3rd edn. Churchill Livingstone, Edinburgh, p129–46

Sriven, A., Orme, J. (eds) (1996). *Health Promotion – Professional Perspectives*. Macmillan Press, Basingstoke

Stansfield, G. (2001). Drop in services for schools: health promotion. *Journal of Community Nursing* 15(4), 13

Stechmiller, J., Yarandi, H. (1992). Job satisfaction among critical care nurses. *American Journal of Critical Care* 1(3), 37–44

Steinaker, N., Bell, M. (1979). *The Experiential Taxonomy: A New Approach to Teaching and Learning*. Academic Press, New York

Stevenson, C.J., Pharoah, P.O.D., Stevenson, R. (1997). Cerebral palsy – the transition from youth to adulthood. *Developmental Medicine & Child Neurology* 39(5), 336–42

Steverink, N., Lindeiberg, S., Ornel, J. (1998). Towards understanding successful ageing: patterned changes in resources and goals. *Ageing and Society* 18(4), 441–68

Stocks, J. (1996). Respiration. In: Hinchliff, S.M., Watson, R. (eds) *Physiology for Nursing Practice*, 2nd edn. Ballière Tindall, London

Strauss, A.L., Corbin, J.M. (1988). *Shaping a New Health Care System: the Experience of Chronic Illness as a Catalyst for Change*. Jossey Bass, San Francisco

Strauss, A.L., Corbin, J.M., Fagerhaugh, S. *et al.* (1984). *Chronic Illness and the Quality of Life*. Mosby, St Louis

Stroke Unit Trialists' Collaboration (1998). Organised inpatient (stroke unit) care for stroke (Cochrane Review). In: *The Cochrane Library*, issue 2, 2003. Oxford: Update Software

Sundstrom, G. (1994). Care by families: an overview of trends. In: *Caring For Frail Elderly People: New Directions in Care*. Social Policy Studies No.14, OECD

Sutherland, D. (2000). Ethical issues. In: Bassett, C., Mankin, L. (eds) *Caring for the Seriously Ill Patient*. Arnold, London, p237–52

Taylor, B. (2000). *Reflective Practice: A Guide for Nurses and Midwives*. Open University Press, Buckingham

Teasdale, K. (1998). *Advocacy in Health Care*. Blackwell Science, Oxford

Thayre, K. (1985). *Dynamics of Sudden Death in Accident and Emergency. Lifeline*. National Association of Bereavement Services

Thayre, K., Hadfield-Law, L. (1995). Never going to be easy: giving bad news. RCN. Nursing Update 3. Learning Unit 04. *Nursing Standard* 6(9), No. 50

Thomas, K. (1976). Conflict and conflict management. In: Dunnette, M. (ed.) *Handbook of Industrial and Organizational Psychology*. Rand-McNally, Chicago

Thomas, V., Dines, A. (1994). The health care needs of ethnic minority groups: are nurses and individuals playing their part? *Journal of Advanced Nursing* 20(5), 802–8

Thompson, N. (1995). *Theory and Practice in Health and Social Welfare*. Open University Press, Buckingham

Thompson, D.R., Bowman, G.S., Kitson, A.L., de Bono, D.P., Hopkins, A. (1997). Cardiac rehabilitation services in England and Wales: a national survey. *International Journal of Cardiology* 59(3), 299–304

Tod, A.M., Wadsworth, E., Asif, S., Gerrish, K. (2001). Cardiac rehabilitation: the needs of south Asian cardiac patients. *British Journal of Nursing* 10(16), 1028–33

Torrance, C., Elley, K. (1997). Respiration, technique and observation 1. *Nursing Times* 93(43), S1–2

Townsend, P., Davidson, N., Whitehead, M. (1988). *Inequalities in Health: The Black Report and The Health Divide.* Penguin, Harmondsworth

Tresolni, C.P. and the Pew-Fetzer Task Force (1994). *Health Professions Education and Relationships-Centered Care: A Report of the Pew-Fetzer Task Force on Advancing Psychosocial Education.* Pew Health Professions Commission, San Francisco

Trieschmann, R.B. (1988). *Spinal Cord Injury: Psychological, Social and Vocational Rehabilitation,* 2nd edn. Demas, New York

Trnobranski, P. (1994). Nurse patient negotiation: assumption or reality? *Journal of Advanced Nursing* 19(4), 733–7

Tuckman, B. (1965). Development sequence in small groups. *Psychological Bulletin* 63, 384–99

Tudor Hart, H.J. (1971). The inverse care law. *Lancet* i, 405–12

UKCC (1986). *Project 2000: A New Preparation for Practice.* United Kingdom Central Council for Nursing, Midwifery and Health Visiting, London

UKCC (1990). *The Report of the Post-Registration Education and Practice Project (PREP).* United Kingdom Central Council for Nursing, Midwifery and Health Visiting, London

UKCC (1992a). *The Scope of Professional Practice.* United Kingdom Central Council for Nursing, Midwifery and Health Visiting, London

UKCC (1992b). *The Code of Professional Conduct for Nurses, Midwives and Health Visitors.* United Kingdom Central Council for Nursing, Midwifery and Health Visiting, London

UKCC (1993). *The Councils Position Concerning a Period of Support and Preceptorship.* Registrar's letter 1/1993 Annexe one. United Kingdom Central Council for Nursing, Midwifery and Health Visiting, London

UKCC (1994a). *Post Registration Education and Practice.* United Kingdom Central Council for Nursing, Midwifery and Health Visiting, London

UKCC (1994b). *The Future of Professional Practice – The Councils Standards for Education and Practice Following Registration.* United Kingdom Central Council for Nursing, Midwifery and Health Visiting, London

UKCC (1995). Registrar's Letter 3/1995: *The Council's Position Concerning a Period of Support and Preceptorship.* United Kingdom Central Council for Nursing, Midwifery and Health Visiting, London

UKCC (1996a). *Guidelines for Professional Practice.* United Kingdom Central Council for Nursing, Midwifery and Health Visiting, London

UKCC (1996b). *Clinical Supervision – A Position Statement.* United Kingdom Central Council for Nursing, Midwifery and Health Visiting, London

UKCC (1997). *PREP – The Nature of Advanced Practice.* United Kingdom Central Council for Nursing, Midwifery and Health Visiting, London

UKCC (1998a). *Midwives Rules and Code of Professional Practice.* United Kingdom Central Council for Nursing, Midwifery and Health Visiting, London

UKCC (1998b). *A UKCC Guide for Students of Nursing and Midwifery.* United Kingdom Central Council for Nursing, Midwifery and Health Visiting, London

UKCC (1998c). *Guidelines for Records and Record Keeping.* United Kingdom Central Council for Nursing, Midwifery and Health Visiting, London

UKCC (1999a). *A Higher Level of Practice – Pilot Standard.* United Kingdom Central Council for Nursing, Midwifery and Health Visiting, London

UKCC (1999b). *Code of Professional Conduct.* United Kingdom Central Council for Nursing, Midwifery and Health Visiting, London

UKCC (1999c). *Nursing Competencies Second Stage.* Annexe 1 to JEC/00/0. United Kingdom Central Council for Nursing, Midwifery and Health Visiting, London

UKCC (1999d). *Professional Self Regulation and Clinical Governance.* United Kingdom Central Council for Nursing, Midwifery and Health Visiting, London

UKCC (2000a). *Strategy for Public Involvement.* United Kingdom Central Council for Nursing, Midwifery and Health Visiting, London

UKCC (2000b). *Guidelines for the Administration of Medicines.* United Kingdom Central Council for Nursing, Midwifery and Health Visiting, London

UKCC (2001a). *Requirements for Pre-Registration Nursing Programmes.* United Kingdom Central Council for Nursing, Midwifery and Health Visiting, London

UKCC (2001b). *Professional Conduct Annual Report 2000–2001.* United Kingdom Central Council for Nursing, Midwifery and Health Visiting, London

UKCC (2001c). *Supporting Nurses, Midwives and Health Visitors Through Lifelong Learning.* United Kingdom Central Council for Nurses, Midwives and Health Visitors, London

UKCC (2001d). *Fitness for Practice and Purpose.* The report of the UKCC's post-commission development group. United Kingdom Central Council for Nursing, Midwifery and Health Visiting, London

UKCC (2001e). *Standards for Education and Practice.* United Kingdom Central Council for Nursing, Midwifery and Health Visiting, London

UKCC (2002). *Report of the Higher Level of Practice Pilot and Project.* Executive Summary. United Kingdom Central Council for Nursing, Midwifery and Health Visiting, London (full report is available only on the NMC website at www.nmc-uk.org)

UKCC Commission for Nursing and Midwifery Education (1999). *Fitness for Practice.* United Kingdom Central Council for Nursing, Midwifery and Health Visiting, London

United Nations (1989). *Convention on the Rights of the Child.* United Nations, Geneva

University Hospitals of Leicester (2000). *Oral Risk Indicator Tool.* UHL, Leicester

Valentine, F., Smith, F. (2000). Clinical Governance in acute children's services. *Paediatric Nursing* 12(8), 6–8

Van de Plaats, A. (1997). The homeostatics model and dementia: a new perspective in caregiving. In: Miesen, B.M.L., Jones, G.M.M. (eds) *Caregiving in Dementia: Research and Applications,* 2nd vol. Routledge, London

Vaughan, B., Pilmoor, M. (eds) (1989). *Managing Nursing Work.* Scutari, London

Veeramah, V. (1995). A study to identify the attitudes and needs of qualified staff concerning the use of research findings in clinical practice within mental health care settings. *Journal of Advanced Nursing* 22(5), 855–61

Vickerman, J. (2002). Thorough assessment of functional incontinence. *Nursing Times* 98(28), 58–9

Victor, C.R. (1991). *Health and Health Care in Later Life.* Open University Press, Milton Keynes

Victor, C., Higginson, I. (1994). Effectiveness of care for older people: a review. *Quality in Health Care* 3, 210–16

Vincent, C., Taylor-Adams, S., Chapman, E.J. *et al.* (2000). How to investigate and analyse clinical incidents: Clinical Risk Unit and Association of Litigation and Risk Management Protocol. *British Medical Journal* 320, 777–81

Viner, R.V. (1999). Transition from paediatric to adult care. Bridging the gap or passing the buck? *Archives of Disease in Childhood* 81(3), 271–5

Viner, R.V., Keane, M. (1998). *Youth Matters.* Action for Sick Children, London

Wade, L. (1996). The social world of older people. In: Wade, L., Waters, K. (eds) *Textbook of Gerontological Nursing.* Baillière Tindall, London, p27–48

Walford, S. (1996). The approach of the consultant physician. In: Kurtz, Z., Hopkins, A. (eds) *Services for Young People with Chronic Disorders.* Royal College of Physicians, London, p51–7

Walker, A. (1995). Integrating the family in the mixed economy of care. In: Allen, I., Perkins, E. (eds) *The Future of Family Care for Older People.* HMSO, London

Walker, A., Warren, L. (1996). *Changing Services for Older People: the Neighbourhood Support Units Innovation.* Open University Press, Buckingham

Wallace, M. (1999). *Lifelong Learning – PREP In Action.* Churchill Livingstone, Edinburgh

Walsh, M. (2000). *Nursing Frontiers: Accountability and Boundaries of Care.* Butterworth-Heinemann, Oxford

Walshe, K. (1999). Improvement through inspection? The development of the new Commission for Health Improvement in England and Wales. *Quality in Healthcare* 8, 191–6

Ward, V., Wilson, J., Taylor, L., Cookson, B., Glynn, A. (1997). *Preventing Hospital Acquired Infection: Clinical Guidelines Public Health Service Laboratory.* HMSO, London

Wardman, C. (1991). Norton vs Waterlow. *Nursing Times* 81(13), 74–8

Waterlow, J. (1985). A risk assessment card. *Nursing Times* 81(49), 51–5

Waterlow, J. (1994). *Pressure Sore Prevention Manual.* J. Waterlow, Newtons, Curland, Taunton

Waters, K. (1985). Team nursing. *Nursing Practice* 1(1), 7–15

Waters, K. (1994). Getting dressed in the early morning: styles of staff/patient interaction on rehabilitation wards for elderly people. *Journal of Advanced Nursing* 19(2), 239–48

Watson, A.R. (2002). Rejection, recurrence, or non-adherence. *Lancet* 359, 197

Watts, R., Robertson, J., Thomas, G. (2001). *The Nursing Management of Fever in Children.* A systematic review No. 14. The Joanna Briggs Institute, Adelaide

Weber, W. (2001). France's highest court recognises the right not to be born. *Lancet* 358, 1972

Wells, T. (1980). *Problems in Geriatric Nursing Care. A Study of Nurses Problems in Care of Old People in Hospitals.* Churchill Livingstone, Edinburgh

Wennberg, J. (1987a). The paradox of appropriate care. *Journal of the American Medical Association* 258, 2568–9

Wennberg, J., Freeman, J., Culp, W. (1987b). Are hospital services rationed in New Haven or over utilised in Boston? *Lancet* 1, 1185–9

Wensing, M., Grol, R. (1994). Single and combined strategies for implementing changes in primary care. *International Journal for Quality in Health Care* 6, 115–32

Wensing, M., Grol, R., Van Montfors, P., Smits, A. (1996). Indicators of the quality of general practice cure of patients with chronic illness: a step towards the real involvement of patients in the assessment of the quality of care. *Quality in Health Care* 5, 73–80

Wetle, T. (1998). Challenges and directions for gerontological research beyond 2000. *Australian Journal on Ageing* 17(1), 107–10

Wheeler, K., Leiper, A., Jannoun, L., Chessells, J. (1998). Medical cost of curing childhood acute lymphoblastic leukaemia. *British Medical Journal* 296

While, A. (ed.) (1991). *Caring for Children.* Edward Arnold, London

While, A., Roberts, J., Firzpatrick, J. (1995). *A Comparative Study of Outcomes of Pre-Registration Nurse Education Programme*. King's College London, Department of Nursing Studies. English National Board for Nursing, Midwifery and Health Visiting, London, p9

White, R. (1976). Some political influences surrounding. The Nurses Registration Act 1919. *Journal of Advanced Nursing* 1, 209–17

White, P.H. (1997). Success on the road to adulthood. Issues and hurdles for adolescents with disabilities. *Pediatric Rheumatology* 223(3), 697–707

White, R., Lippitt, R. (1960). *Autocracy and Democracy: an Experimental Enquiry*. Harper & Row, New York

WHO (1993). *Cardiac Rehabilitation and Secondary Prevention: Long Term Care for Patients with Ischaemic Heart Disease*. Briefing letter. World Health Organization Regional Office for Europe, Copenhagen

WHO (1995). *Report of the Global Expert Committee on Nursing*. World Health Organization, Geneva

WHO (1999). *Health 21: The Health for All Policy Framework for the WHO European Region*. World Health Organization, European Health for All series No 6, Copenhagen

WHO (2000a). *The World Health Report 2000 – Health Systems: Improving Performance*. World Health Organization, Geneva

WHO (2000b). *Munich Declaration. Nurses and Midwives – A Force for Health*. Document EUR/00/5019309/6. World Health Organization, Copenhagen

WHO (2000c). European ministerial health summit to focus on nurses and midwives as a force for health. Press release EURO 09/00. World Health Organization, Copenhagen

WHO (2000d). *Nursing and HEALTH21*. World Health Organization, Copenhagen

WHO (2001). *The European Health Report: Summary of Preliminary Findings*. World Health Organization, Copenhagen

Wilkinson, R., Caulfield, H. (2000). *The Human Rights Act: A Practical Guide for Nurses*. Whurr Publications, London

Williams, L. (1995). Is money well spent? *Child Health* 3(2), 68–72

Williams, J., Baker, G., Clark, B. *et al.* (1993). Collaborative preceptor training: a creative approach in tough times. *Journal of Continuing Education in Nursing* 24(4), 153–7

Williamson, C. (2000). Consumer and professional standards: working towards consensus. *Quality Health Care* 9, 190–4

Willis, R. (1979). Bereavement management in the emergency department. *Journal of Emergency Nursing* March/April 5, 35–9

Wills, T., Ford, P. (2001). Assessing older people – contemporary issues for nursing. *Nursing Older People* 12(9), 16–20

Wilson, J. (1998). Clinical governance. *British Journal of Nursing* 7(16), 987–8

Wilson, J.H. (2002). Taking positive action to manage risk in the healthcare organisation. *Clinical, Nursing & Patient Care* C7–9. Campden Publishing

Wise, J. (1997). Patients go hungry in British hospitals. *British Medical Journal* 314, 399

Wistow, G., Lewis, H. (1997). *Preventative Services for Older People: Current Approaches and Future Opportunities*. Nuffield Institute for Health, Anchor Trust, Kidlington

Wong, D., Baker, C. (1988). Pain in children: comparison of assessment scales. *Pediatric Nursing* 14(1), 9–17

Wong, D., Hockenberry-Eaton, M., Winklestein, M., Wilson, D., Ahmann, E. (1999). *Nursing Care of Infants and Children*, 6th edn. Mosby, St Louis

Wood, D. (1998). *How Children Think and Learn*. Blackwell Publishers, Oxford

Woodham Smith, C. (1952). *Florence Nightingale*. Reprint Society Ltd, London

Woodrow, P. (1994). Mentorship: perceptions and pitfalls for nursing practice. *Journal of Advanced Nursing* 19, 812–18

Worden, W. (1991). *Grief Counselling and Grief Therapy. A Handbook for the Mental Health Practitioner*, 2nd edn. Routledge, London

World Medical Association (1999). *The Helsinki Declaration of Medical Research*. World Medical Association, Geneva

Wright, S. (1992). Modelling excellence: the role of the consultant nurse. In: Butterworth, T., Faugier, J. (eds) *Clinical Supervision and Mentorship in Nursing*. Chapman and Hall, London, p203–13

Wright, B. (1996). *Sudden Death. A Research Base for Practice*, 2nd edn. Churchill Livingstone, Edinburgh

Wynsberghe, D.V., Noback, C.R., Carola, R. (1995). *Human Anatomy and Physiology*, 3rd edn. McGraw Hill

Xavier, G. (2000). The importance of mouth care in preventing infection. *Nursing Standard* 14(18), 47–51

Young, K. (1996). Health, health promotion and the elderly. *Journal of Clinical Nursing* 5(4), 241–8

Zahlis, E.H. (2001). The child's worries about the mother's breast cancer, sources of distress in school age children. *Oncology Nursing Forum* 28(6), 1019–25

Zisook, S., Shuchter, S., Dunn, L. (2001). Grief and depression: diagnostic and treatment challenges. *Primary Psychiatry* 8(5), 37–53

FURTHER READING

Chapter 2

Dingwall, R., Rafferty, A.M., Webster, C. (1988). *An Introduction to the Social History of Nursing.* Routledge, London

This text provides a fascinating insight into the development of the history of the nursing profession within a social context. Such an examination allows the reader to reflect on the professionalization of nursing and the impact of the social and political influences on what has become the largest health care workforce.

Garcia, J., Kilpatrick, R., Richards, M. (1990). *The Politics of Maternity Care: Services for Childbearing Women in Twentieth Century Britain.* Clarendon Press, London

An important collection of essays that brings both social and historical perspectives on the developments of midwifery as a profession, with a particular emphasis on the shift in control of childbirth within the professions of midwifery and medicine, and from the women themselves.

Chapter 3

DoH (2001). *The Essence of Care.* Department of Health, London **www.doh.gov.uk/essenceofcare**

A tool to undertake benchmarking activity in the clinical setting. It focuses on eight key aspects of care, including dignity and privacy, confidentiality and record keeping. The benchmark standards have been developed through a process of consensus agreement involving over 2000 patients, professionals and user group representatives. The aspects of care are fundamental to nursing practice and relate closely to the professional standards discussed in Chapter 3.

DoH (2001). *The Report of the Public Inquiry into Children's Heart Surgery at the Bristol Royal Infirmary 1984–1995. Learning from Bristol* (the Kennedy Report). The Stationery Office, London

This report provides a comprehensive examination of standards of care, exploring issues of professional conduct, competence and education, and highlights responsibilities relating to the individual practitioner, managers, regulatory bodies, education providers, NHS organizations and its systems. While lengthy, it is divided into readable sections. It shows how the system of health care lost its focus on the patient and, importantly, how to regain it.

Driscoll, J. (2000). *Practising Clinical Supervision: A Reflective Approach.* Baillière Tindall, London

A practical and easy to read guide about clinical supervision. It demystifies some of the theory surrounding reflection and clinical supervision, and explains the different things needed to get started.

Lewis, D.B. (ed.) (2001). *Whistleblowing at Work.* The Athlone Press, London

A book to expand on the subject of whistleblowing. It explains the legislation around whistleblowing, gives examples across a range of work settings, including health care, and concludes with practical advice about how to whistleblow.

Morton-Cooper, A., Palmer, A. (2000). *Mentoring, Preceptorship and Clinical Supervision: A Guide to Professional Roles in Clinical Practice,* 2nd edn. Blackwell Science, Oxford

This book explains mentorship, preceptorship and clinical supervision, and describes the differences and similarities between them.

National Assembly for Wales (2001). *Signposts: A Practical Guide to Public and Patient Involvement in Wales.* www.wales.gov.uk/subinhealth/content/nhs/signposts.htm

Guidance produced for NHS organizations in Wales to assess current patient and public involvement locally and to develop strategies for involvement for the organization and the population it serves. This is a requirement of Welsh NHS organizations, but the document provides a straightforward introduction into the principles of involvement.

Seedhouse, D. (2000). *Practical Nursing Philosophy: The Universal Ethical Code.* John Wiley & Sons, Chichester

A challenging but refreshing look at professional codes and their shortcomings. It describes an alternative way to approach ethical decision-making in practice.

Chapter 4

Beauchamp, T.L., Childress, J.F. (1994). *Principles of Biomedical Ethics,* 4th edn. Oxford University Press, Oxford

This is a standard work for those seeking an in-depth grounding in the ethical basis of professional practice. Good for describing the nature of ethical theories and professional–patient relationships, and also the concepts of autonomy, non-maleficence and beneficence.

Hursthouse, R. (1987). *Beginning Lives.* Blackwell, Oxford

Written by a philosopher, this book explores the moral status of the fetus and relates it to abortion and women's rights. Also contains a brief but useful overview of the Warnock Report.

Mason, J.K., McCall Smith, A. (1999). *Law & Medical Ethics,* 5th edn. Butterworths, London

An important text which brings together the law and ethics. This book contains strong chapters on issues around the beginning and end of life, as well as confidentiality, consent and negligence. Also helpful in understanding some population issues, including research. Appendices reproduce a number of codes and declarations.

Rumbold, G. (1999). *Ethics in Nursing Practice,* 3rd edn. Ballière Tindall, London

This book is helpful in taking ethical principles and ideas and, through case studies, developing them as they apply to situations which nurses will encounter in day-to-day practice.

Chapter 5

UKCC (2001). *Practitioner–Client Relationships and the Prevention of Abuse* (Learning Resource). United Kingdom Central Council for Nursing, Midwifery and Health Visiting

This pack is based around the policy first published by the UKCC in 1999 and reprinted by the NMC in 2002. It contains distance learning materials for use by individuals or groups and includes written material, a video of scenarios highlighting potential abuses of power in the practitioner–client relationship and a CD-ROM. The pack, a limited edition, was distributed to all establishments responsible for the education of nurses, midwives and health visitors.

Arnold, E., Boggs, K.U. (1999). *Interpersonal Relationships, Professional Communication Skills for Nurses*, 3rd edn. WB Saunders, Philadelphia

This is a useful text for those requiring the theory around communication and relationships. It identifies some practical aspects of interpersonal relationships from a professional perspective and considers regulatory issues from an American viewpoint.

McCullock, C. (1981). *An Indecent Obsession*. Warner Books

This is a novel set in a military hospital in the Pacific. It is a fascinating representation of a nurse–patient relationship stretching the professional boundaries. A good read!

Chapter 6

Baillie, L. (ed.) (2001). *Developing Practical Nursing Skills.* Arnold, London

This is a really good book to dip into! The focus is on developing skills for practice; one of these being assessment. The book uses case studies and scenarios with patients and clients across the age span. Many of the tools for assessment are used in the case studies and the book is well illustrated and referenced.

Nursing with Dignity articles (2002). *Nursing Times* 98(9), 34–5; 98(10), 36–8; 98(11), 37–9; 98(12), 36–7; 98(13), 42–3; 98(14), 39–41; 98(15), 38 40; 98(16), 40–2; 98(17), 36–7

A series of articles reviewing the needs of patient and clients in a multicultural society. The series gives a useful overview of the main religions, faiths and cultures now living within the UK.

Chapter 7

Bero, L., Grilli, R., Grimshaw, J., Harvey, E., Oxman, A., Thompson, M. (1998). Closing the gap between research and practice: an overview of systematic reviews of interventions to promote the implementation of research findings. *British Medical Journal* 317(17), 465–8

A good overview of different approaches to changing health care practice and how effective they are in achieving this.

Cochrane Collaboration (2001). *Cochrane Reviewers Manual.* Cochrane Collaboration, Oxford

The gold standard guide to systematic review methodology.

Crookes, P.A., Davies, S. (eds) (1998). *Research into Practice.* Baillière Tindall, London

Overviews the origins, methodologies of research-based practice and approaches for improving the uptake of research in clinical practice. Useful to those less familiar with the concepts and methods of evidence-based practice.

Cullum, N. (2001). Evaluation of studies of treatment or prevention interventions. Part 2: applying the results of studies to your patients. *Evidence-Based Nursing* 4, 7–8

A useful guide for practitioners on how to interpret and use evidence in making decisions about the care of individual patients.

Dopson, S., Gabbay, J., Locock, L., Chambers, D. (1999). *Evaluation of the PACE Programme: Final Report.* Oxford Healthcare Management Institute, Templeton College, University of Oxford and Wessex Institute for Health Research and Development, University of Southampton

This is a comprehensive evaluation and analysis of the PACE project which involved 16 local implementation projects in different clinical areas. Useful as an overview of the key contextual issues which influence the use of research and the commonalities and differences across different clinical settings and professional groups.

Duff, L., Loftus-Hills, A., Morrell, C. (2000). *Implementation Guide: Clinical Guidelines for the Management of Venous Leg Ulcers.* Royal College of Nursing Institute, London

This guide gives a six-step process for implementing a guideline within a team. Similar guides have been developed by the RCN in other clinical areas, including pain management in children.

Greenhalgh, T. (1997). How to read a paper: Assessing the methodological quality of published papers. *British Medical Journal* 315, 305–8

This paper is part of a BMJ series which explains aspects of critical appraisal in an easy to understand way.

Kitson, A., Harvey, G., McCormack, B. (1998). Enabling the implementation of evidence-based practice: a conceptual framework. *Quality in Healthcare* 7, 149–58

This paper proposes a conceptual framework of key components which influence the utilization of research in clinical practice. While subsequent papers have been written developing these ideas, this initial paper gives a clear overview of the framework.

Lomas, J. (1993). Diffusion, dissemination and implementation: Who should do what? *Annals of the New York Academy of Science* 703, 226–37

A key paper on developments in thinking about the utilization of research in health care practice and in the move away from passive approaches to dissemination and utilization.

Morrell, C., Harvey, G. (2000). *The Clinical Audit Handbook: Improving the Quality of Care.* Baillière Tindall and Royal College of Nursing, London

This book outlines how to use the clinical audit cycle to improve practice and gives useful overviews of how to conduct an audit and of some different approaches to changing practice.

Roberts, J., DiCenso, A. (1999). Identifying the best research design to fit the question. Part 1: quantitative designs. *Evidence-Based Nursing* 2, 4–6

This paper is part of a series which explains critical appraisal and gives a clear explanation of different parts of the process.

Sackett, D., Richardson, W.S., Rosenberg, W., Haynes, R.B. (2000). *Evidence-Based Medicine: How to Practice and Teach EBM*, 2nd edn. Churchill Livingstone, London

This book is sometimes referred to as 'the bible of evidence-based medicine'. It outlines how to ask answerable questions, how to find best current evidence and how to assess the evidence for prognosis, harm and therapy and appraising guidelines.

The Clinical Guidelines Education Team (2001). *Implementing Clinical Guidelines: A Resource for the Health Care Team*. Baillière Tindall, London

This resource pack takes you through five main modules related to implementing clinical guidelines. The pack is designed to be suitable for individual study and also to be worked through with members of a clinical team, enabled by a facilitator.

Chapter 8

Alderson, P. (2000). *Young Children's Rights: Exploring Beliefs, Principles and Practice*. Jessica Kingsley Publications, London and Philadelphia

A useful and concise text that will give the reader an excellent grasp of the rights of children of all ages. An invaluable resource for practitioners as it refers to issues about involving children in decisions and explores the skills required to achieve this. The notion of acting in a child's best interest can only be realized when practitioners have a clear understanding of what that means and how important it is to respect children's rights: this book is useful in guiding practitioners in this area.

Darbyshire, P. (1994). Living with a sick child in hospital: the experiences of parents and nurses. In: *Parents and Nurses Relationships*. Chapman Hall, London, p120–64

A seminal text that is a must for all children's nurses to read. This text explores the complex pressures of a child's hospitalization and the relationship between the parents and nurses. This is gripping and revealing reading, allowing the reader to reflect on their own practice, and the practice of others, when creating partnerships in care.

Dimond, B. (1996). *The Legal Aspects of Child Health Care*. Mosby, London

The Children Act (1989) led to an increased recognition of the legal rights of the child. An understanding of these is crucial in relation to practice, research and teaching. This book explains the law and legal issues, helping practitioners to work within the law and facilitate decision-making in situations where ethical issues are not clear-cut.

DoH (2001). *The Report of the Public Inquiry into Children's Heart Surgery at the Bristol Royal Infirmary 1984–1995 Learning from Bristol – the Recommendations*. The Stationary Office, London **www.bristol-inquiry.org.uk**

This is a large document – the report runs to over 500 pages and has 198 recommendations – but is essential reading to all in health care. The recommendations aim to produce an NHS in which patients' needs are at the centre and in which systems are in place to ensure safe care, and to maintain and improve the quality of care. This is compelling reading and reveals how organizations can fail families. Readers are forced to consider their own practice and reflect on their organization. Recommendations reinforce best practice and therefore practitioners need to be conversant with the report and its findings if they are to play any part in ensuring quality of care continues.

Glasper, E.A., Ireland, L. (eds) (2000). *Evidence-Based Child Health Care: Challenges for Practice*. Macmillan Press, Basingstoke

The contributors in this edited text provide a wide range of impressive topics from clinical practice, management, research and education in the child health arena and in so doing, share a variety of experiences of the everyday challenges of child health care.

Huband, S., Trigg, E. (eds) (2000). *Practices in Children's Nursing.* Churchill Livingstone, Edinburgh

This book is a useful reference for those working with children, both in hospital and the community, in that it discusses a wide variety of child-focused clinical nursing practices, identifying the special needs and problems of infants and children within the context of family-centred care.

Kenworthy, N., Snowley, G., Gilling, C. (eds) (2002). *Common Foundation Studies in Nursing,* 3rd edn. Churchill Livingstone, Edinburgh

Although this text was produced for the Common Foundation Year of all 3-year pre-registration courses, it contains a holistic overview of the theory and principles of practice which can provide a valuable resource for children's nurses well into the branch programme.

Le May, A. (1999). *Evidence-Based Practice.* Nursing Times Clinical Monographs No. 1. EMAP Healthcare, London

This is an authoritative and concise publication that will be an invaluable resource to nurses in practice. It provides an overview as well as directing the reader to other useful reading. It includes some useful tables that summarize the key issues.

Moules, T., Ramsay, J. (1998). *The Textbook of Children's Nursing.* Stanley Thornes (Publishers), Cheltenham

This book is valuable in that it explores many different aspects of children's nursing and increases the learning potential by involving and encouraging the reader to participate in the learning process through undertaking various activities. It clearly highlights the essential roles of the nurse.

Naidoo, J., Wills, J. (2000). *Health Promotion: Foundations for Practice.* Baillière Tindall, London

As health promoters, this book provides nurses with a theoretical framework to enable them to be clear about the intentions and outcomes of interventions designed to promote the health of their patients and clients. Although not child-focused, it provides a wide range of principles and practices which can be readily applied to the care of children and their carers.

NBS (2000). *Children's Nursing – Core Skills and Competencies.* NBS

An excellent, easy to ready document that summarises core skills of children's nurses. A useful tool when considering individual roles and the skills required to become competent. This would be useful for students when thinking about general and specialist practice, and skills within the context of holistic care.

Rolfe, G., Freshwater, D., Jasper, M. (2001). *Critical Reflection for Nursing and the Helping Professions: A Users' Guide. Models of Critical Reflection.* Palgrave, Hampshire

This text offers a guide to all aspects of reflective practice. It offers structured approaches that will guide students through the realities of 'actually doing it'. Supervision, reflective writing and reflective research are also addressed; the interactive writing exercises and points for discussion make this a very useful text for group and individual learning.

Wong, D., Hockenberry-Eaton, M., Winklestein, M., Wilson, D., Ahmann, M. (1999). *Nursing Care of Infants and Children,* 6th edn. Mosby, St Louis

This weighty tome has always been viewed as an excellent teaching text for children's nurses because of the enormous range of information it provides about the health and illness of infants, children and young people. Each new edition offers extensive revision and up-to-date evidence-based practice.

Chapter 9

Alderson, P. (2000). The rise and fall of children's consent to surgery. *Paediatric Nursing* 12(2)

   This article gives a good synopsis of what has happened to the issue of consent in children, written by someone who cares passionately about the rights of children.

Allmark, P. (2000). Pregnant minors: confidentiality issues and nurses duties. *British Journal of Nursing* 11(4)

   Pregnancy in minors is a complex matter where nurses need to know exactly what is needed of them. The author guides the reader clearly through this minefield.

Aynsley-Green, A., Barker, M., Burr, S. *et al.* (2000). Who is speaking for children and young people at the policy level? *British Medical Journal* 321, 229–32

   A joint statement about the need for clear direction at policy level for health care provision.

Bekeart, S. (2002). Sexual health workshops. *Paediatric Nursing* 14(4), 22–6

   Excellent article on how school nurses can deal with the issue of sex education and the prevention of pregnancy.

Dimmond, B. (2001). Legal aspects of consent (when parents are overruled). *British Journal of Nursing* 10(13), 880–1

   A difficult subject explained in easy terms.

Burr, S. (1993). Adolescents and the ward environment. *Paediatric Nursing* 1(1)

   The author shows the unsuitability of paediatric wards for teenagers.

Steven, D. (1992). Lump it or Like it. *Nursing Times* 88(1)

   Read what it is like to be a teenager in hospital.

Chapter 10

Dimond, B. (1999). Patient confidentiality. *British Journal of Nursing* 8, 9–18

   A series of articles that address many of the issues raised by patient confidentiality. The author is a barrister and makes a complex area intelligible.

Mallett, J., Dougherty, L. (2000). *The Royal Marsden Hospital Manual of Clinical Nursing Procedures*, 5th edn. Blackwell Science, Oxford

   This manual gives the latest evidence-based procedures for high quality patient-focused care. A valuable resource for both the student and the experienced nurse.

Hampton, J.R. (1997). *The ECG Made Easy*, 5th edn. Churchill Livingstone, London

   A slim but useful volume, which really does make the ECG easy.

Tortora, G.J., Grabowski, S.R. (1996). *Principles of Anatomy and Physiology*, 8th edn. Harper Collins College, New York

   A thorough grounding in aspects of both anatomy and physiology applied to clinical practice.

Chapter 11

Redfern, S.J., Ross, F.M. (eds) (1999). *Nursing Older People*, 3rd edn. Churchill Livingstone, Edinburgh
This book considers both the practical aspects of caring, and the impact of changing society and health care provision on the older person.

Tortora, G.J., Grabowski, S.R. (1996). *Principles of Anatomy and Physiology*, 8th edn. Harper Collins College, New York
A thorough grounding in aspects of both anatomy and physiology applied to clinical practice.

Chapter 12

Brechhin, A., Walmsley, J., Katz, J., Peace, S. (1998). *Care Matters: Concepts, Practice and Research in Health and Social Care*. Sage, London
Although this book is not explicitly about older people, it considers the nature of 'care' within our society from a range of perspectives and is therefore of relevance to anyone working with older people and family carers. The book aims to address two questions: how can we make sense of the varying concepts of care, and how can good care be defined and evaluated? A number of core principles are identified, including the importance of learning from real experiences of giving and receiving care, and of creating reciprocity within caring relationships.

McCormack, B. (2001). *Negotiating Partnerships with Older People: A Person-Centred Approach*. Ashgate, Aldershot
Based on the findings of a PhD study, this book explores the nature of relationships between older people and nurses in hospital settings. Its focus is the use of language and the way autonomy is presented through the language of health care practice. McCormack explores the many challenges in achieving person-centred care for older people and highlights strategies for creating effective and appropriate partnerships. Extracts from real-life conversations between nurses and older people taken from the research data make riveting reading and help to illustrate many of the shortfalls in current nursing practice.

Nolan, M., Davies, S., Grant, G. (2001). *Working with Older People and their Families: Key Issues in Policy and Practice*. Open University Press, Buckingham
This book reports on the first phase of the AGEIN project (Advancing Gerontological Education in Nursing), a 3½-year project to evaluate programmes of education for working with older people and their families. The book draws upon extensive reviews of the literature in six fields of practice: acute and rehabilitative care, primary care, continuing care, palliative and end of life care, mental health and learning disability. These are complemented with new research data in an attempt to identify how 'person-centred care' can become a reality.

Redfern, S., Ross, F. (eds) (1999). *Nursing Older People*, 3rd edn. Churchill Livingstone, Edinburgh
This book represents a compendium of information on the nursing needs of older people and their families. Now in its third edition, this clear and concise text has provided many students of nursing and other disciplines with a sound grounding in the knowledge-base for practice with older people across a range of care settings.

Warnes, A., Warren, L., Nolan, M. (2000). *Care Services for Later Life: Transformations and Critiques*. Jessica Kingsley Publishers, London

The basic premise of this edited volume is that social and demographic changes have resulted in a need to transform the way that health and social services are delivered. Contributors discuss the implications of current economic, social and political trends for the future development of services, in order that they should become 'fit for purpose'. The book provides numerous illustrations of the ways in which social policy shapes care experiences for older people and their families.

Chapter 13

Dickenson, D., Johnson, M., Katz, J. (eds) (2000). *Death, Dying and Bereavement*, 2nd edn. Open University in association with Sage, London

A comprehensive text produced as a reader. It is a collection of over 60 literary, narrative accounts, poetry, historical and modern perspectives to inform and develop personal and professional insight and understanding. An excellent resource.

Wright, B. (1996). *Sudden Death. A Research Base for Practice*, 2nd edn. Churchill Livingstone, Edinburgh

The source on the issues for relatives and nurses surrounding sudden death. Comprehensive, informative and readable. Empowers you to be able to continue to strive to give the highest quality of care to suddenly bereaved relatives.

Chapter 16

Armstrong, M. (1994). *How to be an Even Better Manager*. Kogan Page, London

A useful handbook of practical ideas about management presented in bullet point form to allow readers easy access to a great deal of material. First published in 1983 and frequently revised to keep it up to date.

Covey, S. (1989). *Seven Habits of Effective People*. Simon and Schuster, London

Stephen Covey based this book on the wisdom gained from a number of other important writers and offers a book that you should buy and use! It offers insight into such important areas as teamwork, individual empowerment and time management.

Hawkins, P., Shohet, R. (1989). *Supervision in the Helping Professions*. Open University Press, Milton Keynes

A book that offers insight into supervision and the broader contexts of organizational working.

Mullins, L. (1996). *Management and Organisational Behaviour*. Pitman, London

First published in 1985 and regularly revised, this weighty tome offers a comprehensive overview of management and organizations. It is an excellent reference source, which is equally accessible as a general reader on management. It has academic depth with a worldly appeal in its style and format. As a nurse manager it is rarely on my bookshelf – it is in constant use!

Chapter 17

Clark, A., Dooher, J., Fowler, J. (eds) (2001). *The Handbook of Practice Development*. Quay Books, Mark Allen Publishing, Wiltshire

This edited book is written by a variety of practitioners, managers and educators and provides a broad overview of the development of practice and quality care. It explores the various ways that practice can develop and looks at a number of influences, such as clinical governance, power, education, multi-professional approaches and the place of audit and research. It is a useful resource for the student nurse as each chapter can be read in isolation.

Dooher, J., Clark, A., Fowler, J. (2001). *Case Studies on Practice Development.* Quay Books, Mark Allen Publishing, Wiltshire

Written as a companion to the more traditional textbook, *The Handbook of Practice Development* (above), this book is a collection of 23 reflective accounts of practitioners' experiences of clinical practice and practice development. It commences with accounts from student nurses through to nurse consultants and nurse practitioners. It provides useful insights into the realities of practice within a complex world of health care. This is an interesting book to read as each person is sharing an important part of their life and work with the reader. Although not a traditional 'text' book, each chapter contains a wealth of truth and theory evolving from clinical experience.

Fowler, J. (ed.) (1998). *The Handbook of Clinical Supervision: Your Questions Answered.* Quay Books, Mark Allen Publications. Salisbury, Wiltshire

For the newly qualified nurse exiting their preceptorship period, clinical supervision should form an integral part of ongoing development and quality assurance. This is a particularly useful book that is designed to give the reader short precise answers to over 50 commonly asked questions on clinical supervision. Students will find it a useful resource in helping them to understand the development of clinical supervision within the nursing profession and the part that supervision has to play in their clinical practice and future professional development.

Lillyman, S., Ward, C. (1999). *Balancing Organisational and Personal Development Needs.* Quay Books, Mark Allen Publishing. Wiltshire

This book provides an operational and strategic approach to understanding how individuals need to be supported to give high quality care. It identifies personal, organizational, professional and governmental needs and wider issues that influence clinical, educational and professional development. It contains a number of appendices which give useful examples of issues such as 'action plans from a training and development strategy' and a 'personal profile proforma'.

Wallace, M. (1999). *Lifelong Learning – PREP in Action.* Churchill Livingstone, Edinburgh

The concept of quality care based upon lifelong learning was at the heart of the UKCC's PREP project in the early 1990s. Maggy Wallace, formally the Director of Standards Promotion for the UKCC, was the architect of the PREP proposals. She explains the context of PREP within lifelong learning, spelling out an individual's responsibilities for developing and maintaining professional expertise.

Chapter 18

NMC (2002). *The PREP Handbook.* Nursing and Midwifery Council, London

This is essential reading for all registered nurses as it contains the statutory requirements for re-registration. Also, it confirms the requirements for any nurse wishing to return to practice after a break of 5 years or more. It is available from the NMC website (see Appendix 4, Useful Addresses) and nursing libraries.

RCN (2001). *Having a Life – An RCN Guide to Employee-Friendly Policies.* Royal College of Nursing, London

This is a useful aid for all nurses considering a job change and what to expect from an employer. RCN members may obtain this from RCN Direct: publication code 001097.

UKCC (2001). *The Professional, Educational and Occupational Needs of Nurses and Midwives Working Outside the NHS.* United Kingdom Central Council for Nursing, Midwifery and Health Visiting, London

This is the report of a UKCC commissioned study of a sample of nurses and midwives who worked outside the NHS. The findings give an interesting insight into their experiences of work, continuing education, support and professional development.

UKCC (2001). *Supporting Nurses, Midwives and Health Visitors through Lifelong Learning.* United Kingdom Central Council for Nursing, Midwifery and Health Visiting, London

The support needed to promote lifelong learning is described and includes reference to preceptorship, continuing professional development and clinical supervision.

Chapter 19

NHS Executive (1999). *Nurse, Midwife and Health Visitor Consultants: Establishing Posts and Making Appointments.* Health Service Circular 1999 /217. NHS Executive, Leeds

This Health Service Circular sets out the full background to the creation of consultant nurse, midwife and health visitor posts. It describes the role functions of the consultant practitioner in detail, and provides guidance for NHS trusts on how the posts could be set up.

Guest, D., Redfern, S., Wilson-Barnett, J. *et al.* (2001). *A Preliminary Evaluation of the Establishment of Nurse, Midwife and Health Visitor Consultants.* Kings College, London

This report is the first published evaluation of the new NHS consultant practitioner posts. While it lacks depth of information about practice and role development, it offers an interesting insight into the range of backgrounds from which the first tranche of consultants came and the challenges encountered. It also offers an analysis of how the role functions are being balanced and broadly interpreted in practice.

INDEX